The Handbook of Zoonotic Diseases of Goats

The Handbook of Zoonotic Diseases of Goats

Edited by Tanmoy Rana

CABI

CABI is a trading name of CAB International

CABI
Nosworthy Way
Wallingford
Oxfordshire OX10 8DE
UK

Tel: +44 (0)1491 832111
E-mail: info@cabi.org
Website: www.cabi.org

CABI
200 Portland Street
Boston
MA 02114
USA

T: +1 (617)682-9015
E-mail: cabi-nao@cabi.org

A catalogue record for this book is available from the British Library, London, UK.

Library of Congress Cataloging-in-Publication Data

Names: Rana, Tanmoy, editor.
Title: The handbook of zoonotic diseases of goats / edited by Tanmoy Rana.
Description: Boston, MA : CAB International, [2024] | Includes bibliographical references and index. | Summary: "Taking a One Health approach, this book provides clear, accurate and comprehensive coverage of the zoonotic diseases of goats. Including information on aetiology, the epidemiology and transmission cycle, clinical symptoms, diagnosis, and prevention and control strategies it covers bacterial, viral, parasitic, rickettsial, and fungal diseases"-- Provided by publisher.
Identifiers: LCCN 2024030822 (print) | LCCN 2024030823 (ebook) | ISBN 9781800622838 (hardback) | ISBN 9781800622845 (ebk) | ISBN 9781800622852 (epub)
Subjects: LCSH: Goats--Diseases. | Zoonoses.
Classification: LCC SF968 .H365 2024 (print) | LCC SF968 (ebook) | DDC 636.3/0896936--dc23/eng/20240916
LC record available at https://lccn.loc.gov/2024030822
LC ebook record available at https://lccn.loc.gov/2024030823

ISBN-13: 9781800622838 (hardback)
9781800622845 (ePDF)
9781800622852 (ePub)

DOI: 10.1079/ 9781800622852.0000

Commissioning Editor: Alexandra Lainsbury
Editorial Assistant: Emma McCann
Production Editor: Rosie Hayden

Typeset by Exeter Premedia Services Pvt Ltd, Chennai, India
Printed and bound in the UK by CPI Group (UK) Ltd, Croydon, CR0 4YY

Contents

Contributors

Gulzhan N. Abuova, South-Kazakhstan State Pharmaceutical Academy, Shymkent, Kazakhstan

Oluwawemimo Adebowale, Department Veterinary Public Health and Preventive Medicine, College of Veterinary Medicine, Federal University of Agriculture Abeokuta, Ogun State, Nigeria

Akansha Agnihotri, Department of Veterinary Medicine, College of Veterinary Science and Animal Husbandry, NDVSU, Jabalpur, Madhya Pradesh, India

Isha Agrawal, Department of Pathobiology, College of Veterinary Medicine, University of Illinois, Urbana-Champaign, USA

Vivek Agrawal, Department of Veterinary Parasitology, College of Veterinary Science and Animal Husbandry, Mhow, NDVSU, Jabalpur, Madhya Pradesh, India

Aliyu Mohammad Bashir, Department of Veterinary Public Health and Preventive Medicine, Ahmadu Bello University, Zaria, Nigeria

Shruti Bhatt, Department of Veterinary Medicine, COVAS, DUVASU, Mathura, India

M. Bhavya Sree, P.V. Narasimharao Telangana Veterinary University, Hyderabad, India

Suman Biswas, Department of Avian Science, West Bengal University of Animal & Fishery Sciences, Kolkata, India

M.N. Brahmbhatt, Department of Veterinary Public Health and Epidemiology, College of Veterinary Science and Animal Husbandry, Kamdhenu University, Anand, Gujarat, India

Gaurav Charaya, Department of Veterinary Medicine, Lala Lajpat Rai University of Veterinary and Animal Sciences, Hisar, Haryana, India

Alok Kumar Chaudhary, Department of Veterinary Medicine, COVAS, DUVASU, Mathura, India

J.H. Chaudhary, Department of Veterinary Public Health and Epidemiology, College of Veterinary Science and Animal Husbandry, Kamdhenu University, Anand, Gujarat, India

Shubhamitra Chaudhuri, Department of Veterinary Clinical Complex, West Bengal University of Animal & Fishery Sciences, Kolkata, India

Nidhi S. Choudhary, Associate Professor, Department of Veterinary Medicine, College of Veterinary Science and Animal Husbandry, Mhow, NDVSU, Jabalpur, Madhya Pradesh, India

Pooja Dawar, Department of Veterinary Medicine, College of Veterinary Science and Animal Husbandry, NDVSU, Jabalpur, Madhya Pradesh, India

Manaswini Dehuri, Department of Veterinary Parasitology, College of Veterinary Science and Animal Husbandry, Odisha University of Agriculture and Technology (OUAT), Bhubaneswar, India

Phelipe Magalhães Duarte, Postgraduate Program in Animal Bioscience, Federal Rural University of Pernambuco (UFRPE), Recife, Pernambuco, Brazil

Z.B. Dubal, Division of Veterinary Public Health, ICAR-Indian Veterinary Research Institute, Izatnagar, Bareilly, Uttar Pradesh, India

Nourhan Eissa, Department of Animal Hygiene and Zoonoses, Faculty of Veterinary Medicine, University of Sadat City, Egypt

Negin Esfandiari, Department of Food Hygiene and Quality Control, Division of Epidemiology, Faculty of Veterinary Medicine, University of Tehran, Tehran, Iran

Meena Goswami, U.P. Pandit Deen Dayal Upadhyay Veterinary University (DUVASU), Mathura, India

Pouneh Hajipour, Department of Pathobiology, Faculty of Veterinary Medicine, Shahid Bahonar University of Kerman, Kerman, Iran

Abbas Rabiu Ishaq, Paws and Claws Specialist Veterinary Clinic, Anas bin Malik Street 3939, Alsahafa District Riyadh, KSA

Md. Saiful Islam, Department of Microbiology and Hygiene, Faculty of Veterinary Science, Bangladesh Agricultural University, Mymensingh, Bangladesh

Supnesh Jain, Department of Veterinary Medicine, Nanaji Deshmukh Veterinary Science University, Jabalpur, Madhya Pradesh, India

Nirmala Jamra, Department of Veterinary Parasitology, College of Veterinary Science and Animal Husbandry, Mhow, NDVSU, Jabalpur, Madhya Pradesh, India

G.P. Jatav, Department of Veterinary Pathology, College of Veterinary Science and Animal Husbandry, Mhow, NDVSU, Jabalpur, Madhya Pradesh, India

Ranbir Singh Jatav, Department of Veterinary Medicine, College of Veterinary Science and Animal Husbandry, NDVSU, Jabalpur, Madhya Pradesh, India; Department of Veterinary Medicine, Nanaji Deshmukh Veterinary Science University, Jabalpur, Madhya Pradesh, India

A.K. Jayraw, Department of Veterinary Parasitology, College of Veterinary Science and Animal Husbandry, Mhow, NDVSU, Jabalpur, Madhya Pradesh, India

J. Jyothi, Department of Veterinary Medicine, P.V. Narasimharao Telangana Veterinary University, Hyderabad, India

J.B. Kathiriya, Department of Veterinary Public Health & Epidemiology, College of Veterinary Science & Animal Husbandry, Kamdhenu University, Junagadh-Gujarat, India

Jasleen Kaur, Department of Veterinary Microbiology, Lala Lajpat Rai University of Veterinary and Animal Sciences, Hisar, Haryana, India

Pradeep Kumar, Department of Veterinary Parasitology COVAS, DUVASU, Mathura, India

Muhammad Mahadi, Paws and Claws Specialist Veterinary Clinic, Anas bin Malik Street 3939, Alsahafa District Riyadh, KSA

Mahmuda Malik, Department of Pathology, Apollo College of Veterinary Medicine, Jaipur, Rajasthan, India

Jinu Manoj, College Central Laboratory, Lala LajPat Rai University of Veterinary and Animal Sciences, Hisar, Haryana, India

Apoorva Mishra, Department of Veterinary Surgery and Radiology, College of Veterinary Science and Animal Husbandry, NDVSU, Jabalpur, Madhya Pradesh, India

Dwarikanath Mohanty, Fisheries and ARD Department, Government of Odisha, India

Naziru Mukhtar, Paws and Claws Specialist Veterinary Clinic, Anas bin Malik Street 3939, Alsahafa District Riyadh, KSA

M. Reza Najafi, Department of Pathobiology, Faculty of Veterinary Medicine, Urmia University, Urmia, Iran

Simant Kumar Nanda, Fisheries and ARD Department, Government of Odisha, India

J.B. Nayak, Department of Veterinary Public Health and Epidemiology, College of Veterinary Science and Animal Husbandry, Kamdhenu University, Anand, Gujarat, India

Sumit Kumar Patel, School of Wildlife Forensic and Health, Nanaji Deshmukh Veterinary Science University, Jabalpur, Madhya Pradesh, India

Nishant Patel, Department of Veterinary Public Health and Epidemiology, College of Veterinary Science and Animal Husbandry, Kamdhenu University, Anand, Gujarat, India

Indu Panchal, College Central Laboratory, Lala LajPat Rai University of Veterinary and Animal Sciences, Hisar, Haryana, India

Salil Pathak, Department of Veterinary Medicine, College of Veterinary Science & Animal Husbandry, NDVSU, Jabalpur, India

Shashi Pradhan, Department of Veterinary Medicine, College of Veterinary Science and Animal Husbandry, NDVSU, Jabalpur, Madhya Pradesh, India

Aditya Pratap, Department of Veterinary Medicine, College of Veterinary Science and Animal Husbandry, NDVSU, Jabalpur, Madhya Pradesh, India

Natalia Pshenichnaya, Clinical Branch of Infectious Diseases Pathology, Central Institute of Epidemiology, Moscow, Russia; Department of Infectious Diseases, Moscow Regional Research Clinical Institute n. a. M.F. Vladimirsky, Moscow, Russia

Md. Tanvir Rahman, Department of Microbiology and Hygiene, Faculty of Veterinary Science, Bangladesh Agricultural University, Mymensingh, Bangladesh

Saindla Rakesh, Department of Veterinary Medicine, College of Veterinary Science & Animal Husbandry, NDVSU, Jabalpur, Madhya Pradesh, India

Tanmoy Rana, Department of Veterinary Clinical Complex, West Bengal University of Animal & Fishery Sciences, Kolkata, India

Yudhbir Rana, Department of Veterinary Medicine, Lala Lajpat Rai University of Veterinary and Animal Sciences, Hisar, Haryana, India

Hafiz Muhammad Rizwan, Section of Parasitology, Department of Pathobiology, KBCMA College of Veterinary and Animal Sciences, Narowal, Sub-campus University of Veterinary and Animal Sciences, Lahore, Pakistan

Kabita Roy, Department of Veterinary Medicine, College of Veterinary Science & Animal Husbandry, NDVSU, Jabalpur, Madhya Pradesh, India

Rajesh Kumar Sahu, Fisheries and ARD Department, Government of Odisha, India

Mukesh Shakya, Department of Veterinary Parasitology, College of Veterinary Science and Animal Husbandry, Mhow, NDVSU, Jabalpur, Madhya Pradesh, India

Barkha Sharma, Department of Veterinary Epidemiology, College of Veterinary and Animal Sciences (COVAS), DUVASU, Mathura, India; U.P. Pandit Deen Dayal Upadhyay Veterinary University (DUVASU), Mathura, India

Binita Kumari Singh, Department of Veterinary Parasitology, College of Veterinary Science and Animal Husbandry, Mhow, NDVSU, Jabalpur, Madhya Pradesh, India

Brejesh Singh, Department of Veterinary Medicine, College of Veterinary Science and Animal Husbandry, NDVSU, Jabalpur, Madhya Pradesh, India

Manoj Kumar Singh, College of Veterinary and Animal Sciences, Sardar Vallabhbhai Patel University of Agriculture and Technology, Meerut, Uttar Pradesh, India

Renu Singh, Department of Veterinary Medicine, COVAS, DUVASU, Mathura, India

Subir Singh, Department of Veterinary Medicine and Public Health, Faculty of Animal Science, Veterinary Science and Fisheries, Agriculture and Forestry University, Rampur, Chitwan, Nepal

Mukesh Kumar Srivastava, Department of Veterinary Medicine, COVAS, DUVASU, Mathura, India

Sina Salajegheh Tazerji, Department of Clinical Science, Faculty of Veterinary Medicine, Science and Research Branch, Islamic Azad University, Tehran, Iran; Young Researchers and Elites Club Science and Research Branch, Islamic Azad University, Tehran, Iran

Sonali Thakur, Department of Veterinary Public Health and Epidemiology, College of Veterinary Science and Animal Husbandry, Kamdhenu University, Anand, Gujarat, India

Amita Tiwari, Department of Veterinary Medicine, College of Veterinary Science and Animal Husbandry, NDVSU, Jabalpur, Madhya Pradesh, India

Shivangi Udainiya, Veterinary Polytechnic College, Bhopal, NDVSU, Jabalpur, Madhya Pradesh, India

Nitin Vaishnav, Department of Veterinary Medicine, College of Veterinary Science and Animal Husbandry, NDVSU, Jabalpur, Madhya Pradesh, India

Aminu Abubakar Zugu, Paws and Claws Specialist Veterinary Clinic, Anas bin Malik Street 3939, Alsahafa District Riyadh, KSA

Preface

Zoonoses are infections that can spread naturally from animals to humans. Zoonotic diseases of goats are generally transmitted due to the occupational exposure of veterinarians, animal breeders and slaughterhouse workers. Airborne zoonotic diseases generally happen among workers of caprine herds. Zoonotic diseases need much more special attention, as most of the emerging infectious diseases of epidemic and pandemic potential of goats belong to that category. In addition, foodborne diseases are generally transmissible from animal to humans through contaminated water or food. Besides, vectors and climate changes are etiological factors for allowing the propagation of infections. Prevention and control measures are to be taken into consideration to reduce/protect the incidence of zoonotic diseases. These preventive measures largely depend on various conditions like economic consequences, the epidemiological status of the zoonoses, local prompt action, the resistance of the microorganism in the environment and the abundance of the infection in wild fauna. The handbook provides a good source of useful information about zoonotic diseases transmitted from animals to humans. The book is helpful for a better understanding of acquiring knowledge about the zoonotic diseases of goats.

The handbook is designed as a single book emphasizing microbial pathogens including bacteria, viruses, fungi and parasites. The book introduces the reader to describe specific diseases that can be transmitted from animals to humans. Various photographs, images and tables are incorporated into the book. The book provides useful information about the etiology, host, transmission route, clinical symptoms and prevention of specific zoonotic diseases.

One Health is a multidisciplinary and holistic approach with a novel perspective applied to animal and public health. The prevention and control of zoonotic diseases can be better realized and ameliorated within the circumstances of the shared environment. Moreover, the effective control of zoonoses requires a 'One Health approach', in which a collaborative understanding and strategy between various professionals can be attributed to producing synergistic effects. The book will be beneficial to all public health professionals including veterinary and medical professionals, to acquire knowledge and information for the deep learning and development of expertise in the particular field of zoonoses. The book may be a reference book for public health professionals and students, including medical and veterinary, and other allied personnel of various disciplines. The book describes the epidemiological and clinical characteristics of various zoonoses, which may help the public health professionals with the incorporation of the 'One Health' taskforce of regional, national and global importance. The contributors read many textbooks, reference books and websites to gather knowledge incorporated in this book. To the best of our knowledge, the book will help readers to gather all of the information about the zoonotic diseases of goats.

Tanmoy Rana
Kolkata, India

Acknowledgements

I express my gratitude to our Hon'ble Vice Chancellor, West Bengal University of Animal & Fishery Sciences, Kolkata, India for proving me the opportunity to edit the book. I also would like to convey sincere thanks to my all contributors who support writing an individual chapter for the book fruitfully. I also convey my gratitude to all zoonoses and public health experts across the world for acquiring knowledge about the zoonotic diseases of goats. I would like to express my sincere regards to Alex Lainsbury, Commissioning Editor, and other members of CABI who actively provide me the opportunity to edit the book. I would also like to thank my family for providing great support and time to finalize the book.

Tanmoy Rana
Kolkata, India

1 Introduction

Shubhamitra Chaudhuri[1]*, Suman Biswas[2] and Tanmoy Rana[1]
[1]Department of Veterinary Clinical Complex, West Bengal University of Animal & Fishery Sciences, Kolkata, India; [2]Department of Avian Science, West Bengal University of Animal & Fishery Sciences, Kolkata, India

Abstract
Zoonotic diseases are highly contagious diseases that spread between animals and humans. It is documented that nearly 75% of recently emerging infectious diseases affecting human beings are of animal origin, whereas about 60% of all human pathogens also have zoonotic potentiality. Most of the zoonotic diseases can be spread through direct contact with infected animals as well as consumption of contaminated food, drinking water or through inhalation. Arthropod vectors, including mosquitoes, flies and ticks, are pests that can spread zoonotic diseases. Generally, zoonoses identified in goats are transmitted by close contact with humans. Breeders, veterinarians and slaughterhouse workers are prone to contamination by zoonotic diseases through occupational activities on the goat farms, where airborne transmission and foodborne diseases also occur. There is a severe risk for transmitting the diseases due to migration of goats, human life styles, improper animal housing and management, which can influence future risks for zoonosis. Monitoring, prevention and control measures are undertaken to prevent further epidemics and to enable the containment of outbreaks. Preventive measures largely depend on the zoonotic potential of pathogens, the epidemiology of the zoonoses, the local scenario and the prevalence of the infective agent in various animals.

Keywords: zoonoses, goat, epidemiology, risk factors, prevention, management

1.1 Introduction

The genesis and spread of various infectious diseases are significantly influenced by the human population, animal population and environmental factors in a particular place or region (Thompson and Kutz, 2019) (Figs. 1.1 and 1.2). Animals are the source of most of the infectious diseases that affect humans. The term zoonosis is a combination of the Greek words *zoon* (animal) and *nosos* (sickness). In 1951 the Expert Committee on Zoonoses of the World Health Organization (WHO) defined zoonoses as 'diseases and infections that are naturally transmitted between vertebrate animals and man'. More recently its definition of a zoonosis was 'any disease or infection that is naturally transmissible from vertebrate animals to humans' (WHO, 2020), but other WHO sources retain the original term 'between'.

According to observations, 61% of all human diseases are zoonotic and, over the past 10 years, pathogens originating from animals or from items containing animal products have been responsible for around 75% of all new human pathogen outbreaks (Rodolakis, 2014). Zoonoses pose a great health hazard to humans as well as animals. The 13 most prevalent zoonoses caused

*Corresponding author: drshubhamitra@gmail.com

 The Handbook of Zoonotic Diseases of Goats (ed. T. Rana)
DOI: 10.1079/ 9781800622852.0001

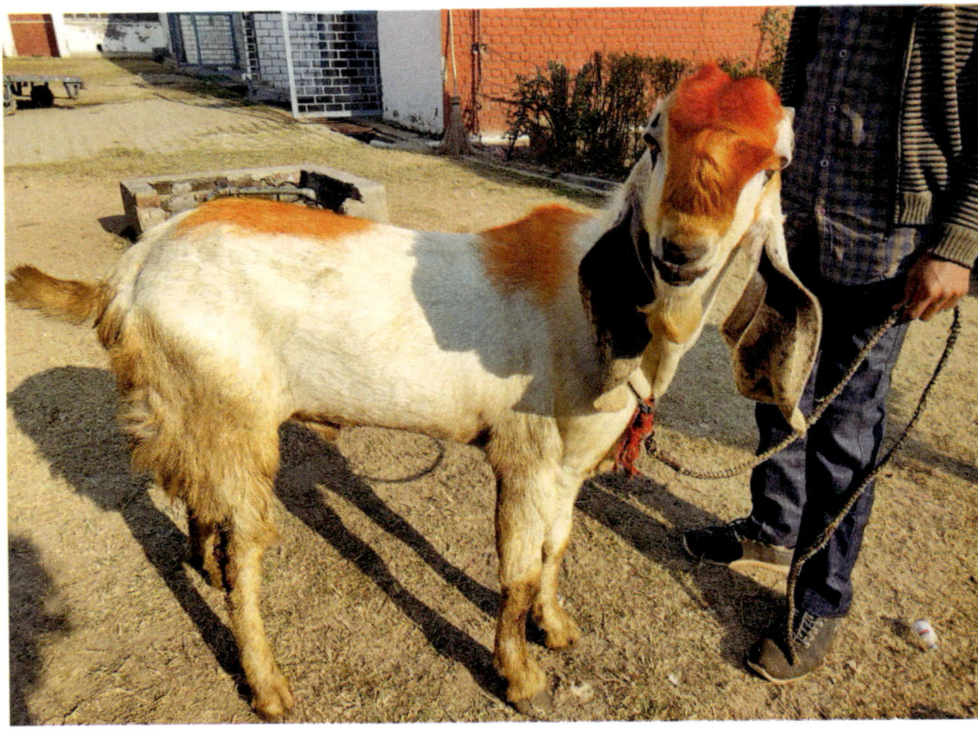

Fig. 1.1. Goat brought into the hospital. (Author's own image.)

2.7 million human fatalities annually in addition to causing 2.4 billion cases of illness, with poor livestock workers in low- and middle-income countries suffering the brunt of this burden (Grace *et al.*, 2012) (Figs. 1.3 and 1.4).

Any kind of infectious agent, including a virus, bacterium, parasite, fungus and many unconventional agents, may act as a zoonotic agent in the case of goats (Fig. 1.5). However, after the incidence of Q fever in the Netherlands from 2007 to 2010 near a large goat farm, we realized that small ruminants like goats could operate as sources of infection to the human population (Ganter, 2015).

1.2 Classification of Zoonotic Diseases

Zoonotic diseases of goats are caused by numerous microorganisms and pathogens. Based on the aetiological agents, goat zoonoses are classified into bacterial zoonoses (e.g. anthrax, brucellosis, leptospirosis, salmonellosis), viral zoonoses (e.g. rabies, Rift Valley fever (RVF)), parasitic zoonoses (e.g. visceral larva migrants, hydatidosis, fasciolosis, cryptosporidiosis), mycotic zoonoses (e.g. ringworm infection, aspergillosis, cryptococcosis), rickettsial zoonoses (e.g. Q fever, epidemic typhus), chlamydial zoonoses (e.g. psittacosis), protozoal zoonoses (e.g. giardiasis, toxoplasmosis, balantidiasis) and diseases due to acellular non-viral pathogenic agents, like transmissible spongiform encephalopathies (Chomel, 2009) (Table 1.1).

Anthroponoses are pathogens transmissible from humans (*anthropos*) to other humans or to animals. Further categories for goat zoonoses include anthropozoonoses, zooanthroponoses, amphixenoses and euzoonoses (Hubálek, 2003). **Anthropozoonoses** are (or were) diseases of animals that can spread to humans. The term **zooanthroponoses** describes (or described) diseases that are spread from humans to animals.

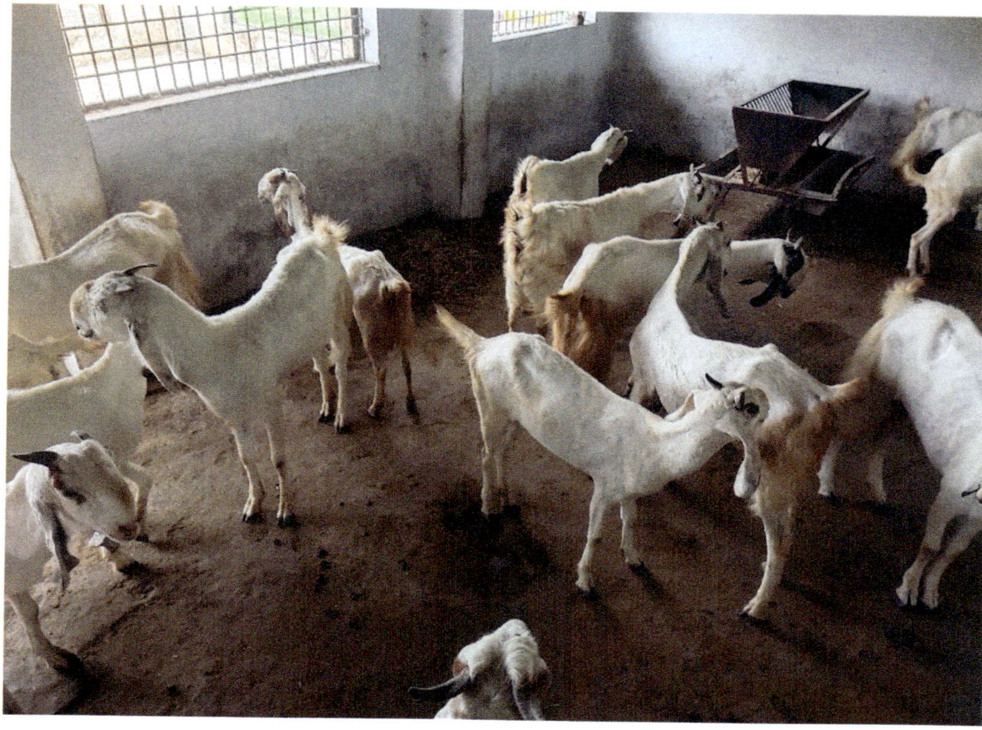

Fig. 1.2. A herd of goats. (Author's own image.)

To avoid confusion between the latter two terms, both are now covered by the term **zoonoses**, which is used to describe diseases that are naturally transmitted between vertebrate animals and humans (Hubálek, 2003). **Amphixenoses** are those diseases that can be transmitted in both directions, from human to animal and vice versa. **Euzoonoses** are those diseases where a human being acts as an obligatory host.

1.3 Factors in Relation to the Prevalence of Zoonoses

Domestic goats sometimes act as amplifying agents for infections that emerge from wild animals, which has a considerable impact on the transmission of many diseases to humans (Morand *et al.*, 2014) (Fig. 1.6). Long ago, it was initially suggested that domestic animals (such as goats) and people have a positive impact on pathogen diversity (McNeill, 1976). Vertebrate animals, including goats, are the source of around 60% of infectious diseases that affect humans (Klous *et al.*, 2016). With the domestication of several vertebrate animals, direct human contact with animals has increased (Pearce-Duvet, 2006). Direct contact, ingestion and inhalation, through the conjunctiva, or biting are the possible modes of transmission for zoonotic bacteria, viruses, parasites, or fungi (Klous *et al.*, 2016). Goats and other domestic animals serve as a reservoir for the viruses that cause domestic zoonoses and can spread the infections to people (Samad, 2011). Pathogens can spread by direct contact or by consuming food made from animals. Anthrax, rabies, brucellosis, campylobacteriosis, leptospirosis, toxoplasmosis, listeriosis, vesicular stomatitis, hydatidosis, Q fever and many others are examples of zoonotic diseases that can be transmitted from goats to humans (Bae and Son, 2011; Samad, 2011).

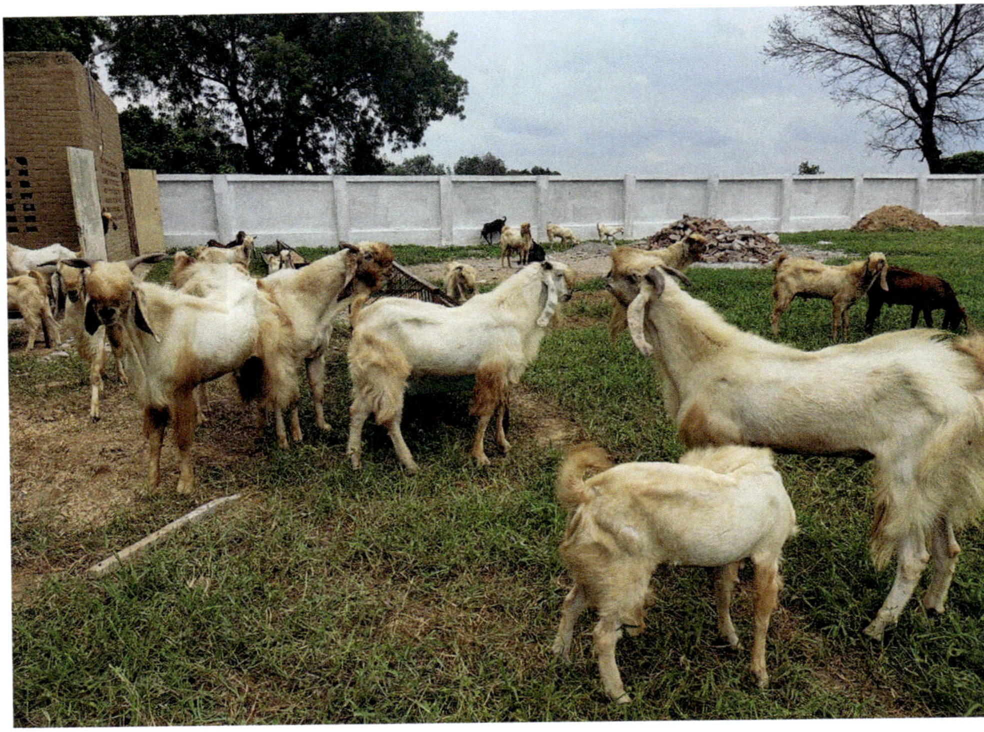

Fig. 1.3. Goats in groups – a source of contamination of diseases. (Author's own image.)

By coming into intimate contact with an infected goat or its products (such as meat, skin, hides, or bones), humans can get infected with anthrax (Goel, 2015). Although it does happen occasionally, human-to-human transmission is extremely uncommon. Globally, between 2000 and 20,000 people are infected by anthrax each year (Goel, 2015). Occasionally, people from India, Bangladesh, Pakistan, the United States, Zimbabwe, Iran, Iraq, South Africa and Turkey are affected with anthrax (Goel, 2015).

Brucellosis is one of the important bacterial zoonoses and it affects about 500,000 humans globally every year (Hull and Schumaker, 2018). The main risk factors for *Brucella melitensis* infection in humans are contact with animals, occupational exposure, food patterns and a lack of hygiene practices. Small ruminants like goats serve as the primary reservoir for human transmission, because human-to-human transmission is uncommon (Ganter, 2015). Contact with infected animals through the conjunctival or oronasal mucosae, particularly during an animal's parturition, can result in the transmission of the disease to humans. Ingesting contaminated animal commodities, primarily dairy products like homemade cheese made from raw goat's milk, can cause infection with brucellosis. Chevon or products made from chevon are less frequently linked to *Brucella* contamination, because they are typically cooked or prepared before consumption. People who by their occupations require frequent contact with goats, such as farmers, butchers, abattoir employees, veterinarians and laboratory personnel, are more likely to get the disease. Additionally, humans can be infected via skin, wool, dung and the upkeep of farm facilities (Blasco and Molina-Flores, 2011; Rodolakis, 2014).

In nations where brucellosis has been controlled, chlamydophilosis is a substantial cause of abortion in goats, and it is the second most significant cause after brucellosis in most other locations, apart from New Zealand. Through inhalation of infectious dust and aerosols during or after abortion or normal parturition,

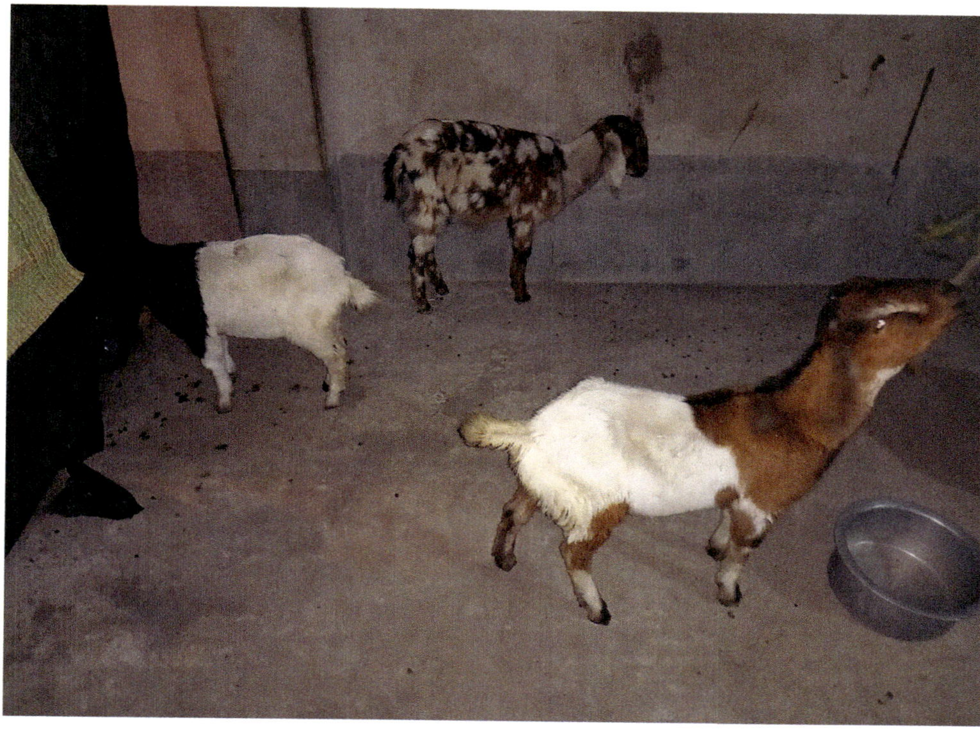

Fig. 1.4. Goats on the farm. (Author's own image.)

Chlamydophila abortus spreads from goats to humans. There is still no vaccine available to prevent human chlamydophilosis. Therefore, prevention focuses on animal disease control, farmer training and general public exposure training. Strict vaccinations, treatment and hygienic practices can help veterinarians and farmers prevent *Chlamydophila* abortions in goats (Rodolakis, 2014).

Mammals, birds, reptiles, amphibians and humans represent the numerous animal species that can be affected with *Coxiella burnetii* infection, causing Q fever. The zoonotic pathogen *C. burnetii* is a big concern because of its low infective dose, especially for people who come into contact with livestock. Affected goat farms pose a particular risk to humans (Eibach *et al*., 2012; Runge *et al*., 2012; Bothe *et al*., 2013). The shedding of *C. burnetii* increases especially during the peri-partum period. The spread of the infection within goat populations depends on prolonged faecal shedding, as well as excretion in milk and urine over weeks. During the period 2007–2009, the Netherlands had faced a severe outbreak of Q fever, with diagnosis of 3523 clinical human cases (Ganter, 2015). The main reason for this outbreak was proximity of aborting goat populations and increased number of susceptible people (Roest *et al*., 2011). By ventilation or goat manure movement, particularly in dry weather conditions, large quantities of the organism may be moved during kidding into the surrounding environment (Berri *et al*., 2003; Tissot-Dupont *et al*., 2004) (Fig. 1.7). These could have an impact on human populations. Worldwide, there is no active sero-surveillance of Q fever in the goat population, but aetiological investigations are frequently carried out in cases of significant peri-parturient losses or following the onset of human disease.

Orf (contagious ecthyma) virus infection affects relatively well-defined 'at risk' populations, such as veterinarians, shepherds and abattoir workers, for whom it is an occupational concern (Nettleton *et al*., 1996). Another risk factor for the disease in humans is unsupervised

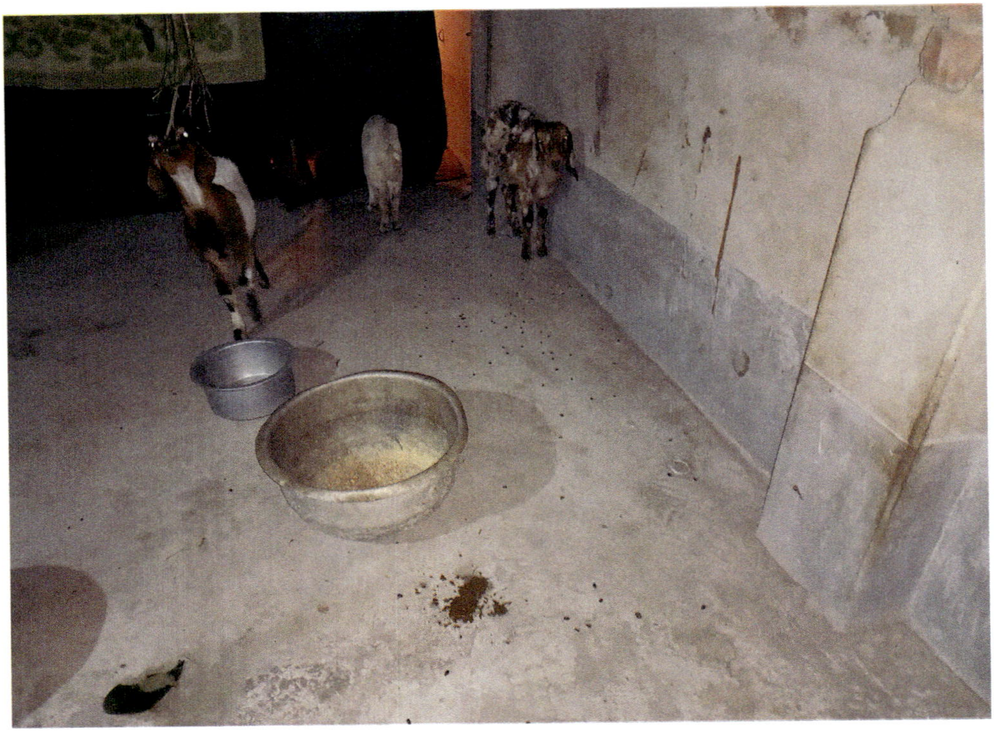

Fig. 1.5. Feeding of goats. (Author's own image.)

goat slaughter or unhygienic household chevon preparation. Non-permeable gloves should be worn while handling goats with orf, open wounds should not be exposed and wounds should be meticulously cleaned with soap and water after handling goats. Additionally, slaughterhouses must ensure that all goats that will be sold or slaughtered are in healthy condition; those that have orf lesions must be properly disposed of. Dermatologists should be made aware of the possibility of orf virus infection and microbiology labs should confirm any suspected infections (Nougairede *et al.*, 2013). The majority of human doctors are not very aware of orf, thus they could mistake orf lesions for cancers or other illnesses that might be fatal, such cutaneous anthrax.

Humans can get RVF through handling infected goats, placentas, blood, flesh, or body fluids, or by being bitten by mosquitoes. The virus can also be spread through drinking raw milk from infected goats (Rodolakis, 2014). Different vector control strategies, like sterilization of male mosquitoes by radiation, or destruction of mosquito bedding by means of larvicides, are a good option in tropical countries. In the face of viral outbreaks, however, actions to control the vectors are largely palliative and ineffective. Restrictions or prohibitions on the movement of animals have little impact on the progression of an outbreak within infected areas, but they can slow the spread of the virus from infected to uninfected areas. The disease can only be effectively controlled through vaccination of susceptible animals (Rodolakis, 2014). For veterinary application, modified attenuated or inactivated vaccines have been developed.w

1.4 Zoonotic Diseases and Public Health Importance

The effects of zoonoses on human and animal health are numerous. The impact of zoonoses can be measured using factors including disease

Table 1.1. Major goat zoonoses with aetiological agents, transmission and brief clinical signs in goat and humans.

Disease	Aetiological agent	Clinical signs in goats	Clinical signs in humans	Major transmission route
BACTERIAL ZOONOSES				
Anthrax	*Bacillus anthracis*	High rise in body temperature; Loss of rumination; Oedema of the pharynx and pulmonary region; Dyspnoea with cerebral anoxia; Sudden death	Cutaneous form: skin sore on hands, arms, face and neck; malignant oedema GI form: nausea; vomiting; diarrhoea; abdominal cramps with inappetence Respiratory form: throat pain; laboured breathing with spontaneous coughing	Ingestion or inhalation of virgin bacterial spore
Brucellosis	*Brucella melitensis, Brucella abortus*	Haemorrhagic discharge from external vagina with concurrent stillbirth or abortion; Orchitis or epididymitis in buck; Arthritis in chronic case with huge weight loss	Undulant fever with flu-like syndrome; Occasional arthritis and liver damage; Miscarriages	Ingestion of contaminated materials like feed, water etc.
Leptospirosis	*Leptospira interrogans*	Acute form: inappetence/anorexia; irritability; epidemic abortions and sharp drop of milk production. Sub-clinical infection: weak kids; stillbirths; prolonged calving intervals; sterility in buck and infertility in doe; requires more services per conception	Vomiting, diarrhoea and abdominal pain with high rise of temperature; Meningitis; intense hepatitis with jaundice	Direct or indirect contact with urine Contaminated tissues and soil Consumption of contaminated food/water
Campylobacteriosis	*Campylobacter jejuni*	Abortion; Stillbirths and weak kids	Diarrhoea; Vomiting; Abdominal pain; Occasional abortions; Endocarditis	Ingestion of contaminated grass/food or consumption of contaminated water
Chlamydiosis	*Chlamydia abortus*	Stillbirths and abortions in doe; Epididymitis in buck; Sometimes severe respiratory infection like pneumonia and conjunctivitis	Flu-like symptoms with pneumonia; Abortions	Direct contact with aborted fetal materials and placental fluids; Venereal transmission during seasonal mating; Sometimes kids get infected through consumption of doe milk (Nietfeld, 2001)

Continued

Table 1.1. Continued

Disease	Aetiological agent	Clinical signs in goats	Clinical signs in humans	Major transmission route
Listeriosis	*Listeria monocytogenes*	Dull and depressed condition; Anorexia with high rise of temperature; Uncoordinated movements; Salivation; Facial paralysis and, in extreme condition, circling movements; Vestibular ataxia	Septicaemic condition with meningoencephalitis; Abortions	Ingestion of leftover foods or vegetable wastes from the markets/roadsides in free-ranging goats (Barman *et al.*, 2020); Ingestion of spoiled hay/silage/ green fodder in stall-fed goats
Q fever	*Coxiella burnetii*	Abortions; Stillbirths; Birth of weak kids; Haemoglobinuria Haemolytic anaemia; Jaundice	High fever; Nausea; Vomiting; Diarrhoea; Abortion Endocarditis Chronic fatigue syndrome	Aerosols of body fluids, especially amniotic body fluids of infected aborted goats (Porter *et al.*, 2011); Consumption of contaminated forage from pastures; Tick bites
Salmonellosis	*Salmonella* spp. and serotypes	Abortion; Diarrhoea; Fever; Arthritis	Severe vomiting with diarrhoea; Fever; Abdominal pain	Consumption of water and food contaminated with bacteria
Staphylococcal infection	*Staphylococcus aureus*	Red hot swelling of the mammary glands with discharge of pus-like milk/watery milk; Pustule formation on the skin with pruritis	Vomiting; Diarrhoea; Abdominal pain; Oral or cutaneous skin lesions	Direct contact with infected animals; During milking through milker's hand
Pasteurellosis	*Pasteurella multocida* *Mannheimia haemolytica* *Bibersteinia trehalosi*	Fever; Listlessness; Poor appetite; Polyarthritis in young kids; Fibrinonecrotic pneumonia	Severe pneumonia; Fever; Abscess formation	Oro-nasal transmission
Tuberculosis	*Mycobacterium bovis* *Mycobacterium caprae*	Respiratory distress Pneumonia Excessive coughing Lower respiratory tract disease syndrome; Lymphadenitis Mastitis	Coughing; Excessive weight loss within short periods of time; Night sweating; Loss of appetite; Lymphadenitis	Ingestion and inhalation of causal bacteria; Close contact with infected/carrier animals

Continued

Table 1.1. Continued

Disease	Aetiological agent	Clinical signs in goats	Clinical signs in humans	Major transmission route
Erysipelas	*Erysipelothrix rhusiopathiae*	Cutaneous form: cyanotic skin lesion on non-hairy parts; Systemic form: polyarthritis with lameness, endocarditis	Erythematous condition; Arthritis; Generalized septicaemic condition	Transmitted to gastrointestinal tract of goat through intake of contaminated food or water (To and Nagai, 2007)
VIRAL ZOONOSES				
Contagious ecthyma/Orf	Parapoxvirus	First erythematous spots appear in the lips, gingiva, tongue, labia, nostrils, testis and toes, further spots developed into papules, vesicles and ultimately developed into pustules with ulcerative exudates (Bala *et al.*, 2019); High mortality in young kids due to long starvation with inability to swallow	Skin lesions like papules start on hands, arms and nose of human beings which then progresses into severe pustular dermatitis lesions (Ma *et al.*, 2022)	Direct contact with infected animals; Through milk and saliva of the infected doe to young kids (Ma *et al.*, 2022)
Rabies	Family: *Rhabdoviridae* Genus: *Lyssavirus*	Changes in behaviour including: Depression Somnolence Auricular hyperesthesia; Opisthotonus episodes and severe ataxia (Moreira *et al.*, 2018); Anorexia; Change in voice; Death	First stage – Fever, discomfort, headache; Second stage – confusion, agitation, anxiety; Third or terminal stage - delirium, abnormal behaviour, hallucinations, hydrophobia (fear of water) and insomnia (CDC, 2021)	Bite by infected animals
Rift Valley fever	Family: *Bunyaviridae* Genus: *Phlebovirus*	High fever; Nasal and ocular secretions in adult goats Haemorrhagic diarrhoea; Vomiting; Abdominal pain; Lasting prostration; Dysagalactia; Jaundice; High rate of abortions/abortion storms; High mortality rate in kids (Ikegami and Makino, 2011)	Fever; Headache; Muscular pain; Photophobia; Haemorrhagic fever that progresses to jaundice; Death	By different mosquito bites (*Aedes*, *Culex* and *Anopheles*); Close contact with infected animals Infection can occur by inhaling aerosols of infectious body fluids (Kwasnik *et al.*, 2021)

Continued

Table 1.1. Continued

Disease	Aetiological agent	Clinical signs in goats	Clinical signs in humans	Major transmission route
Vesicular stomatitis	*Vesiculovirus*	Blisters on tongue, gingiva, mammary glands, coronary bands; High rise of temperature	Fever; Muscular pain; Headache; Rashes on the palm and fingertips	Close contact with infected animals/fomites/feed utensils
PROTOZOAL ZOONOSES				
Toxoplasmosis	*Toxoplasma gondii*	Fetal death and mummification; Abortion; Stillbirth and neonatal death	Fever; Swelling of the superficial lymph nodes; Headache; Muscular pain; Abortion	Horizontal transmission occurs through the ingestion of food or water contaminated with sporulated oocysts of the parasite (Tzanidakis *et al.*, 2012); Congenital transplacental transmission helps maintenance and dissemination of the infection in goat flocks (Dubey, 2010)
Giardiasis	*Giardia duodenalis*	Asymptomatic; Reduction in growth rate; Poor feed conversion ratio and persistent diarrhoea	Diarrhoea with abdominal cramp; General weakness with anorexia	Consumption of food/water contaminated with infective cysts
PARASITIC ZOONOSES				
Hydatidosis	*Echinococcus granulosus*	Swollen abdomen Progressive weakness; Anaemia; Inappetence with persistent diarrhoea	Formation of hydatid cyst in liver/kidney; Abdominal pain with severe respiratory distress	Ingestion of cysts/cystic larvae through feed and water
NON-VIRAL ACELLULAR ZOONOSES				
Bovine spongiform encephalopathy (mad cow disease)	Prion protein	Intense pruritis; Extreme reaction to external stimuli; Changes in fleece colour; Progressive ataxia	Ataxia with progressive nervousness; Memory loss with changes of personality	Consumption of contaminated food/meal

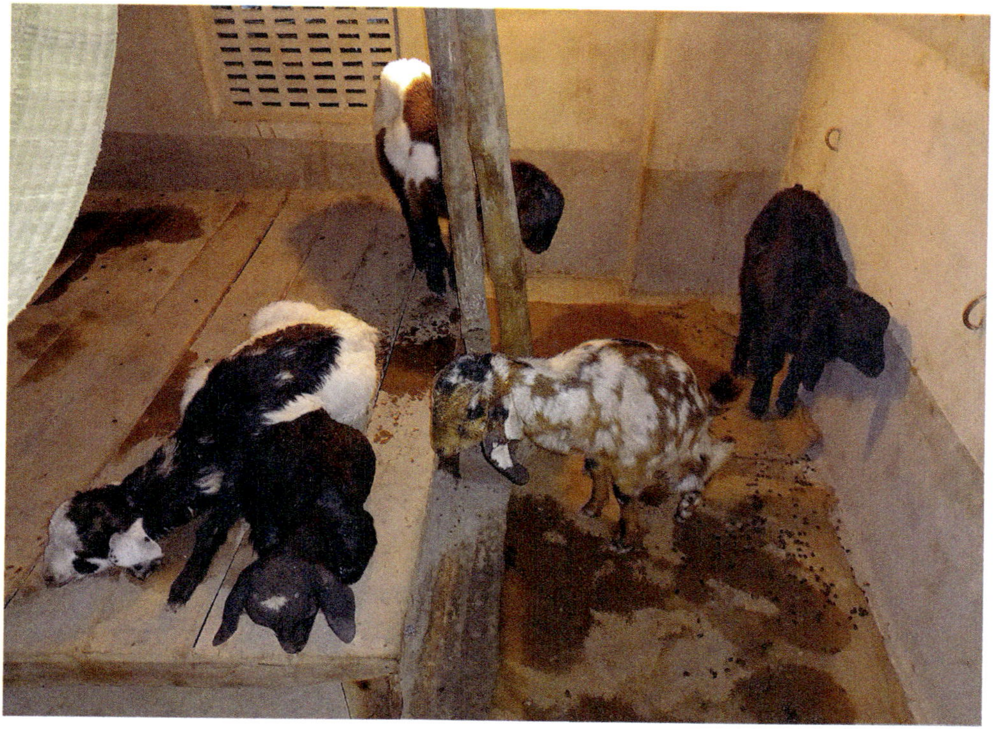

Fig. 1.6. Shelter for goats. (Author's own image.)

prevalence, incidence, morbidity, mortality and economic loss even if it is difficult to put a number on it (Meslin, 2006). Zoonoses have a significant impact on human life and well-being. The obstacles faced by the afflicted people have a severe effect on their capacity to perform well at work and, consequently, provide for their families. These circumstances are regularly observed in developing Asian and African countries. The affected people are sometimes kept apart from the rest of the population, which makes them more vulnerable to mental health problems. The treatment of bacterial zoonoses can be adversely affected by antibiotic resistance, which is a problem for world health. Patients with illnesses brought on by resistant microorganisms require specialized care and costly medications and they generally place a strain on the healthcare system, particularly in the developing countries of Asia and Africa. Zoonotic disease-related animal mortality can result in significant financial losses for any nation's livestock industry. Animal health and productivity can still suffer even if no animals die. More than 70% of animal products may be lost as a result. The decreased availability of high-protein foods of animal origin has an impact on human health and nutrition (Arámbulo and Thakur, 1992). Zoonotic diseases like toxoplasmosis, leptospirosis, chlamydiosis and brucellosis can cause infertility, abortions and poor progeny. Farmers and the entire nation may suffer significant financial losses as a result. The worldwide transportation of animals, animal products (meat, milk and eggs) and by-products like keratin and bonemeal can be hampered by zoonotic diseases, including BSE, avian influenza and anthrax. The measures necessary for the control and eradication of zoonoses, such as surveillance, diagnosis, isolation and quarantine, restrictions on animal transportation, treatment and vaccination programmes, inspection of meat and milk and biosecurity, have a significant negative impact on the economy. Zoonotic outbreaks had an overall economic impact of more than US$120 billion between 1995 and 2008 (Cascio *et al.*,

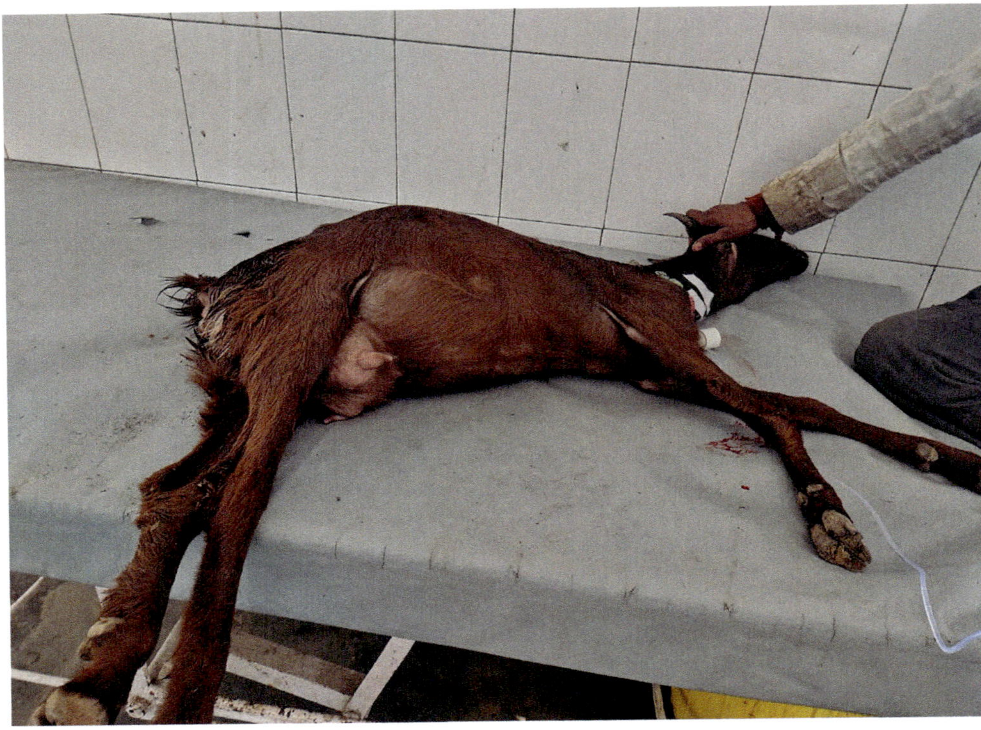

Fig. 1.7. A goat in treatment. (Author's own image.)

2011). The economic costs of zoonotic illnesses were high in the UK (Bennett and Ijpelaar, 2005). *Campylobacter* spp., *Salmonella* (non-typhoidal), *Escherichia coli* VTEC O157, *Listeria monocytogenes* and norovirus were some of the severe foodborne pathogens that caused major economic losses in the UK in 2007 (Martins *et al.*, 2015) (Fig. 1.8). In addition, outbreaks of zoonotic foodborne infections caused significant economic losses in other nations. For instance, salmonella contamination in Ireland's pig products has resulted in a significant economic loss (Martins *et al.*, 2015). The World Bank estimated that outbreaks that affected sheep and beef caused Australia's livestock sector to lose 16% of its value (World Bank, 2012).

Milk is a balanced diet for human beings and it supports the growth of pathogenic organisms. Mastitic milk is a potent reservoir of many pathogenic microorganisms, like *Staphylococcus* spp., *Streptococcus* spp. *E. coli*, *Listeria* spp., *Camphylobacter* spp., *Yersenia* spp. and *Salmonella* spp. (Hameed, 2006). According to Gilmour and Havey (1990), infected milk is the main source of enterotoxigenic *Staphylococcus aureus* of animal origin. It produces some heat-resistant enterotoxins that cause nausea, vomiting and abdominal cramps in human beings and are responsible for staphylococcal food-poisoning outbreaks (Kluytmans *et al.*, 1997). Mastitic milk is also a potent source of *Streptococcus agalactiae*, which is a most common factor of invasive infections in neonates as well as in adults (Schuchat, 2001). Several food-poisoning outbreaks occur through consumption of the milk of cattle with infected udders (Osteras, 1999). This mastitic milk is unsuitable for human consumption and may result in staphylococcal toxaemia, sore throat, scarlet fever and severe gastroenteritis (Radostits *et al.*, 2007). Another public health concern regarding mastitis is antibiotic residues in milk due to extensive use of antibiotics in the treatment and control of the disease. The presence of these antibiotic residues in milk and its products leads to severe allergic manifestations in sensitive individuals. It has been estimated

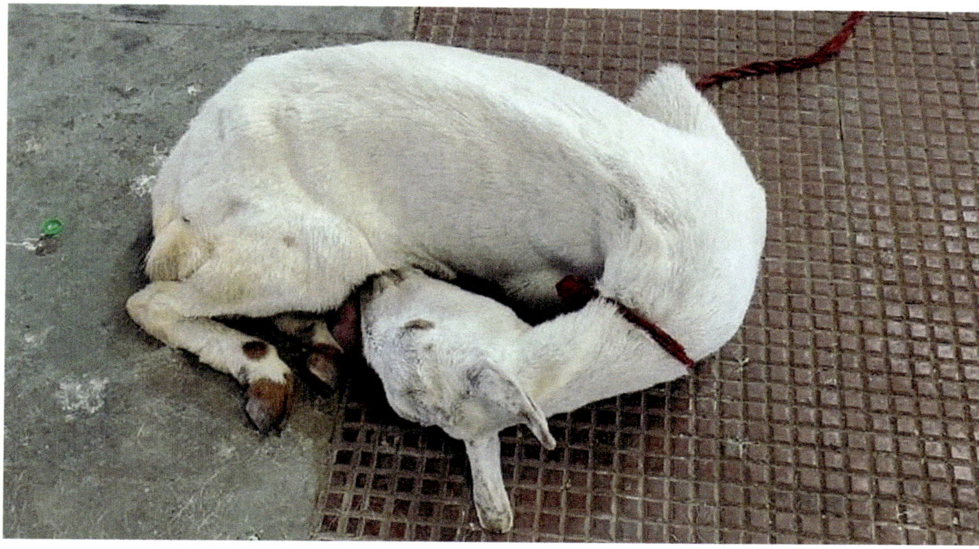

Fig. 1.8. Listeriosis in a goat. (Author's own image.)

that one in ten individuals will be sensitive to this antibiotic residue (Sharma and Malik, 2002). It also causes dermatitis, undesirable side reactions and development of antibiotic-resistant pathogenic gut flora in human beings (Adesiyun, 1994).

Bovine mastitis is one of the important production diseases of growing dairy sectors which directly or indirectly affect the economy for farmers as well as the economy of countries. Mastitis is known as the most costly disease of dairy animals and estimated annual losses are about US$184 per cow (Cremonesi *et al.*, 2006). These include low milk production (70%), discarding of milk (9%), medicine costs, veterinarian costs (7%) and increased labour costs (National Mastitis Council, 1998; Bhikane and Kawitkar, 2000). According to the first report on mastitis-induced loss in India, there was an annual loss of Rs. 52.9 crore (Dhanda and Sethi, 1962), which increased to Rs. 1607.20 crore by the year 1994 (Singh and Singh, 1994) (crore = 10 million). According to Dua (2001), this loss increased to Rs. 6053.21 crore annually, including Rs. 2646.0 crore and Rs. 1723.32 crore for subclinical mastitis in cattle and buffalo, respectively, and due to clinical mastitis Rs. 987.60 and 696.29 crore, respectively. It is a matter of public health concern that antibiotic residues have an undesirable effect on humans. Mastitis control programmes also increase the economic loss by the use of chemical disinfectants, antiseptics and herbal teat-dips (Maiti *et al.*, 2004).

The severe acute respiratory syndrome (SARS) outbreak, which had a negative influence on several sectors of the economy, including the tourism industry, is significant. SARS had a serious negative impact on the economies of Singapore, China, Hong Kong, Taiwan and India (Keusch *et al.*, 2009). In addition, the highly virulent avian influenza outbreak severely reduced travel to Mexico, causing that country to suffer economic losses (Rassy and Smith, 2013). India also experienced financial losses as a result of the 1994 plague outbreak's restrictions on travel (Keusch *et al.*, 2009). In addition, the outbreak of highly virulent avian influenza caused Chile to experience significant economic losses (Wright, 2004). The shutdown of poultry export markets during the outbreak of highly pathogenic avian influenza resulted in significant economic losses for many countries in the European Union (Keusch *et al.*, 2009).

One of the significant emerging zoonoses is bovine spongiform encephalopathy (BSE). Most European nations forbade the importation of British beef when BSE outbreaks occurred in the UK. Extensive control measures, such as the slaughter of all at-risk animals and the culling of all infected cattle, came at an astronomical cost (Burroughs *et al.*, 2002). Toronto, in Canada, suffered a 0.5% GDP loss as a result of the BSE outbreak. Numerous nations prohibited trade with Canada once the disease was found in millions of animals (Mitura and Di Piétro, 2004). Numerous nations banned imports of American beef after BSE was discovered in the United States in 2003, resulting in significant economic damages (Coffey *et al.*, 2005).

Other economically significant zoonoses include brucellosis. Annual economic losses due to bovine brucellosis were reported in Kenya (FAO, 2020), Argentina (Samartino, 2002) and Nigeria (Ajogi, 1998). The most recent COVID-19 outbreak has had a big effect on the world economy. All societal sectors, including those in the fields of health and education, finance, travel and hospitality, and sports, have been greatly impacted by COVID-19 (Ozili and Arun, 2023). The pandemic is expected to cause the travel industry to lose a sizeable amount of money (Ozili and Arun, 2023). According to estimates, millions of people would experience extreme poverty as a result of the stagnant growth caused by the pandemic (World Bank, 2023).

1.5 Conclusion

Compared with other farm animal species, small ruminants such as goats pose a significant risk of transmitting zoonotic diseases to humans. There are other circumstances where this risk can grow even more. The risk of spreading *C. burnetii* or *C. abortus* increases during kidding, and the organisms can be spread by aerosols. Goat farms should be avoided during parturition, especially by pregnant women. The likelihood that humans will acquire zoonotic diseases transmitted by goats varies greatly, depending on both the disease and human behaviour. The risk can be decreased in part by providing training to those who are exposed. The farmer introduces and implements biosecurity measures on the farm as the first step in this educational process. Treatment or prophylactic measures against a zoonotic agent are to be encouraged among the farmers as well as goat breeders. This is only conceivable if people who own animals that have zoonotic diseases are not stigmatized and if the community, rather than just the farmer, pays for the monitoring and control efforts.

References

Adesiyun, A.A. (1994) Bacteriological quality and associated public health risk of pre-processed bovine milk in trinidad. *International Journal of Food Microbiology* 21, 253–261.

Ajogi, I. (1998) Settling the nomads in Wase and Wawa-Zange grazing reserves in the Sudan Savannah zone of Nigeria IV: Strategies for the control of bovine brucellosis. *Nigerian Veterinary Journal* 19, 40–48.

Arámbulo, P.V. III and Thakur, A.S. (1992) Impact of zoonoses in tropical America. *Annals of the New York Academy of Sciences* 653, 6–18.

Bae, S.E. and Son, H.S. (2011) Classification of viral zoonosis through receptor pattern analysis. *BMC Bioinformatics* 12, 96.

Bala, J.A., Balakrishnan, K.N., Abdullah, A.A., Adamu, L., Bin Noorzahari, M.S. *et al.* (2019) An association of orf virus infection among sheep and goats with herd health programme in Terengganu state, Eastern region of the Peninsular Malaysia. *BMC Veterinary Research* 15, 250.

Barman, N.N., Nath, A.J., Doley, S., Begum, S.A., Kakati, P. *et al.* (2020) Listeriosis in a peri-urban area: Cultural and molecular characterization of *Listeria monocytogenes* isolated from encephalitic goats. *Veterinary World* 13(9), 1743–1749.

Bennett, R. and Ijpelaar, J. (2005) Updated estimates of the costs associated with thirty-four endemic livestock diseases in Great Britain: A note. *Journal of Agricultural Economics* 56, 135–144.

Berri, M., Rousset, E., Champion, J.L., Aricau-Bouvery, N., Russo, P. *et al.* (2003) Ovine manure used as a garden fertilizer as a suspected source of human Q fever. *Veterinary Record* 153, 269–270.

Bhikane, A.V. and Kawitkar, S.B. (2000) *Hand Book for Veterinary Clinician*, 5th edn. Venkatesh Books, Udgir, India.

Blasco, J.M. and Molina-Flores, B. (2011) Control and eradication of *Brucella melitensis* infection in sheep and goats. *Veterinary Clinics: Food Animal Practice* 27, 95–104.

Bothe, F., Eibach, R., Runge, M., Fischer, S.F. and Ganter, M. (2013) Q fever infections in humans after caesarean of a goat. In: *Proceedings of the 8th International Sheep Veterinary Congress*, New Zealand Veterinary Association, p. 167.

Burroughs, T., Knobler, S. and Lederberg, J. (eds) (2002) *The Emergence of Zoonotic Diseases: Understanding the Impact on Animal and Human Health: Workshop Summary*. National Academy Press, Washington, DC.

Cascio, A., Bosilkovski, M., Rodriguez-Morales, A.J. and Pappas, G. (2011) The socio-ecology of zoonotic infections. *Clinical Microbiology and Infection* 17, 336–342.

CDC (2021) One Health Zoonotic Disease Prioritization (OHZDP). Available at: https://www.cdc.gov/onehealth/what-we-do/zoonotic-disease-prioritization/index.html (accessed 12 February 2023).

Chomel, B.B. (2009) Zoonoses. In: *Encyclopedia of Microbiology*, 3rd edn. Elsevier Inc., University of California, Davis, California, pp. 820–829.

Coffey, B., Mintert, J., Fox, S., Schroeder, T. and Valentin, L. (2005) *Economic Impact of BSE on the US Beef Industry: Product Value Losses, Regulatory Costs and Consumer Reactions*. Kansas State University, Manhattan, Kansas.

Cremonesi, P., Castiglioni, B., Malferrai, G., Biunno, I., Vimercati, C. *et al*. (2006) Technical note: Improved method for rapid DNA extraction of mastitis pathogens directly from milk. *Journal of Dairy Science* 89, 163–169.

Dhanda, M.R. and Sethi, M.S. (1962) *Investigation of Mastitis in India*. ICAR Res. Series No. 35, New Delhi, India.

Dua, K. (2001) Incidence aetiology and estimated loss due to mastitis in india – An update. *Indian Dairyman* 53, 41–48.

Dubey, J.P. (2010) *Toxoplasmosis of Animals and Humans*, 2nd edn. CRC Press, Boca Raton, Florida.

Eibach, R., Bothe, F., Runge, M., Fischer, S.F., Philipp, W. *et al*. (2012) Q fever: Baseline monitoring of a sheep and a goat flock associated with human infections. *Epidemiology and Infection* 140, 1939–1949.

Food and Agriculture Organization of the United Nations (FAO) (2020) The Monetary Impact of Zoonotic Diseases on Society, Evidence from Three Zoonoses in Kenya. Available at: http://www.fao.org/3/i8968en/I8968EN.pdf

Ganter, M. (2015) Zoonotic risks from small ruminants. *Veterinary Microbiology* 181(1–2), 53–65.

Gilmour, A. and Havey, J. (1990) Staphylococci in milk and milk products. *Society for Applied Bacteriology Symposium Series* 19, 147–166.

Goel, A.K. (2015) Anthrax: A disease of biowarfare and public health importance. *World Journal of Clinical Cases* 3, 20–33.

Grace, D., Mutua, F., Ochungo, P., Kruska, R., Jones, K. *et al*. (2012) Mapping of poverty and likely zoonoses hotspots. In: *Zoonoses Project 4*. Report to the UK Department for International Development. International Livestock Research Institute, Nairobi, Kenya.

Hameed, K.G.A. (2006) Association of BoLA-DRB3 polymorphism with occurrence of mastitis caused by *Staphylococcus aureus* and *Streptococcus agalactiae*. PhD thesis, Polish Academy of Sciences Institute of Genetics and Animal Breeding, Jastrzębiec.

Hubálek, Z. (2003) Emerging human infectious diseases: Anthroponoses, zoonoses, and sapronoses. *Emerging Infectious Diseases* 9(3), 403–404.

Hull, N.C. and Schumaker, B.A. (2018) Comparisons of brucellosis between human and veterinary medicine. *Infection Ecology & Epidemiology* 8, 1–12.

Ikegami, T. and Makino, S. (2011) The pathogenesis of Rift Valley fever. *Viruses* 3, 493–519.

Keusch, G.T., Pappaioanou, M., Gonzalez, M.C., Scott, K.A. and Tsai, P. (eds) (2009) *Sustaining Global Surveillance and Response to Emerging Zoonotic Diseases*. National Research Council (US) Committee on Achieving Sustainable Global Capacity for Surveillance and Response to Emerging Diseases of Zoonotic Origin. The National Academies Press, Washington, DC.

Klous, G., Huss, A., Heederik, D.J. and Coutinho, R.A. (2016) Human–livestock contacts and their relationship to transmission of zoonotic pathogens, a systematic review of literature. *One Health* 2, 65–76.

Kluytmans, J., Vanbelkuma, A. and Verbrugh, H. (1997) Nasal carriage of *Staphylococcus aureus*: Epidemiology, underlying mechanisms, and associated risks. *Clinical Microbiology Review* 10, 505–520.

Kwasnik, M., Rozek, W. and Rola, J. (2021) Rift valley fever – a growing threat to humans and animals. *Journal of Veterinary Research* 65(1), 7–14.

Ma, W., Pang, M., Lei, X., Wang, Z., Feng, H. *et al.* (2022) Orf virus detection in the saliva and milk of dairy goats. *Frontiers in Microbiology* 13, 1–8.

Maiti, S.K., Sharma, N. and Koley, K.M. (2004) Efficacy of post milking herbal teat dip in the control of mastitis in cows. *Veterinary Practice* 5(2), 105–106.

Martins, S., Häsler, B. and Rushton, J. (2015) Economic aspects of zoonoses: Impact of zoonoses on the food industry. In: Sing, A. (ed.) *Zoonoses – Infections Affecting Humans and Animals*. Springer, Dordrecht, Netherlands, pp. 1107–1126.

McNeill, W.H. (1976) *Plagues and People*. Anchor Press, New York.

Meslin, F.X. (2006) Impact of zoonoses on human health. *Veterinaria Italiana* 42, 369–379.

Mitura, V. and Di Piétro, L. (2004) *Canada's beef cattle sector and the impact of BSE on farm family income 2000–2003*. Agriculture and Rural Working Paper Series Working Paper no.69. Canada Statistics, Agricultural Division, Ottawa, Ontario, Canada.

Morand, S., McIntyre, K.M. and Baylis, M. (2014) Domesticated animals and human infectious diseases of zoonotic origins: Domestication time matters. *Infection, Genetics and Evolution* 24, 76–81.

Moreira, I.L., De Sousa, D.E.R., Ferreira-Junior, J.A., De Castro, M.B., Fino, T.C.M. *et al.* (2018) Paralytic rabies in a goat. *BMC Veterinary Research* 14(1), 338.

National Mastitis Council (1998) Current concepts in bovine mastitis, 4th edn. National Mastitis Council, Madison, Wisconsin.

Nettleton, P.F., Gilray, J.A., Yirrell, D.L., Scott, G.R. and Reid, H.W. (1996) Natural transmission of orf virus from clinically normal ewes to orf-naive sheep. *Veterinary Record* 139, 364–366.

Nietfeld, J.C. (2001) Chlamydial infections in small ruminants. *Veterinary Clinics of North America: Food Animal Practice* 17(2), 301–314.

Nougairede, A., Fossati, C., Salez, N., Cohen-Bacrie, S., Ninove, L. *et al.* (2013) Sheep-to-human transmission of Orf virus during Eid al-Adha religious practices, France. *Emerging Infectious Diseases* 19, 102–105.

Osteras, O. (1999) Use of SCC as a guidance tool. *Buskap* 2, 54–55.

Ozili, P.K. and Arun, T. (2023) Spillover of COVID-19: Impact on the global economy. In: Akkucuk, U. (ed.) *Managing Inflation and Supply Chain Disruptions in the Global Economy*. IGI Global. DOI: 10.4018/978-1-6684-5876-1.ch004.

Pearce-Duvet, J.M. (2006) The origin of human pathogens: Evaluating the role of agriculture and domestic animals in the evolution of human disease. *Biological Reviews* 81, 369–382.

Porter, S.R., Czaplicki, G., Mainil, J., Guatteo, R. and Saegerman, C. (2011) Q fever: Current state of knowledge and perspectives of research of a neglected zoonosis. *International Journal of Microbiology* 1–22.

Radostits, O., Gay, C., Hinchchiff, K. and Constable, P.A. (2007) *Text Book of the Disease of Cattle, Sheep, Pigs and Goats*. Baillière Tindall.

Rassy, D. and Smith, R.D. (2013) The economic impact of H1N1 on Mexico's tourist and pork sectors. *Health Economics* 22, 824–834.

Rodolakis, A. (2014) Zoonoses in goats: How to control them. *Small Ruminant Research* 121, 12–20.

Roest, H.I.J., Tilburg, J.J.H.C., Van der Hoeck, W., Vellema, P., Van Zijderveld, F.G. *et al.* (2011) The Q fever epidemic in the Netherlands: History, onset, response and reflection. *Epidemiology and Infection* 139, 1–12.

Runge, M., Binder, A., Schotte, U. and Ganter, M. (2012) Investigations concerning the prevalence of *Coxiella burnetii* and *Chlamydia abortus* in sheep in correlation with management systems and abortion rate in Lower Saxony in 2004. *Berliner und Münchener Tierärztliche Wochenschrift* 125, 138–143.

Samad, M.A. (2011) Public health threat caused by zoonotic diseases in Bangladesh. *Bangladesh Journal of Veterinary Medicine* 9, 95–120.

Samartino, L.E. (2002) Brucellosis in Argentina. *Veterinary Microbiology* 90, 71–80.

Schuchat, A. (2001) Group B streptococcal disease: From trials and tribulations to triumph and trepidation. *Clinical Infectious Diseases* 33, 751–756.

Sharma, M. and Malik, R.K. (2002) Recent approaches in mastitis therapy. *Indian Dairyman* 54(6), 51–62.

Singh, P.J. and Singh, K.B. (1994) A study of economic losses due to mastitis in india. *Indian Journal of Dairy Science* 47(4), 265–272.
Thompson, A. and Kutz, S. (2019) Introduction to the special issue on'Emerging zoonoses and wildlife'. *International Journal of Parasitology: Parasites and Wildlife* 9, 322.
Tissot-Dupont, H., Amadei, M.A., Nezri, M. and Raoult, D. (2004) Wind in November, Q fever in December. *Emerging Infectious Diseases* 10, 1264–1269.
To, H. and Nagai, S. (2007) Genetic and antigenic diversity of the surface protective antigen proteins of *Erysipelothrix rhusiopathiae*. *Clinical and Vaccine Immunology* 14, 813–820.
Tzanidakis, N., Maksimov, P., Conraths, F.J., Kiossis, E., Brozos, C. *et al.* (2012) *Toxoplasma gondii* in sheep and goats: Seroprevalence and potential risk factors under dairy husbandry practices. *Veterinary Parasitology* 190, 340–348.
World Bank (2012) *People, Pathogens and Our Planet: The Economics of One Health*. World Bank, Washington, DC. Available at: http://documents.worldbank.org/curated/en/2012/06/16360943/peoplepathogensplanet-economics-one-health
World Bank (2023) *The Global Economic Outlook during the COVID-19 Pandemic: A Changed World*. World Bank, Washington, DC. Available at: https://www.worldbank.org/en/news/feature/2020/06/08/the-global-economic-outlook-during-the-covid-19-pandemic-a-changed-world
World Health Organization (2020) WHO Health Topic Page: Zoonoses. Available at: https://www.who.int/topics/zoonoses/en/ (accessed 12 February 2023).
Wright, C. (2004) The avian influenza outbreak in Chile. *Poultry International (February)* 34–39.

2 Main Global Challenges of Controlling Zoonotic Diseases

Nishant Patel*, J.B. Nayak, Sonali Thakur, M.N. Brahmbhatt and J.H. Chaudhary

Department of Veterinary Public Health and Epidemiology, College of Veterinary Science and Animal Husbandry, Kamdhenu University, Anand, Gujarat, India

Abstract

Controlling zoonotic diseases, which are infections that can be transmitted between animals and humans, poses a multifaceted global challenge. These diseases, such as Ebola, COVID-19 and Zika, have the potential to cause devastating pandemics and significant public health threats. Several key challenges are impeding effective control efforts. First, zoonotic diseases often originate in wildlife, making early detection and monitoring complex. Surveillance and timely reporting of potential outbreaks are hindered by limited resources and infrastructure in many regions. Secondly, the globalization of trade and travel accelerates the spread of zoonotic pathogens, demanding international cooperation. Coordination across borders is essential for effective response strategies. Thirdly, socioeconomic factors, like urbanization and deforestation, increase human–wildlife interactions, raising the risk of zoonotic spillover. Adequate funding and policies to address these root causes are necessary. Lastly, there is a need for research and development of vaccines, diagnostics and treatments for emerging zoonotic diseases. Addressing these challenges requires a concerted global effort that involves governments, health organizations, scientists and communities to enhance preparedness and response to zoonotic threats.

Keywords: zoonotic diseases, global health, disease surveillance, international cooperation, pandemic preparedness

2.1 Introduction

Throughout human history, animals have played a significant role in our evolution. Early humans domesticated animals for various purposes, such as food, transportation, agriculture, security and even recreation. This resulted in increased contact between humans and animals, leading to the transmission of diseases from animals to humans and vice versa. The 21st century is the age of globalization, urbanization and industrialization (Negrón, 2019). As these all took hold, there was a need for mass breeding of animals for food, sports and other recreational activities (Coker *et al.*, 2011). Technological advancements and faster communication also meant that humans, animals and animal products could move across the globe quickly, potentially carrying infections with them (Machalaba *et al.*, 2021). This globalization has created new challenges in preventing and controlling the spread of zoonotic diseases. The interconnectedness of human, animal and environmental health

*Corresponding author: patelnishant582@gmail.com

DOI: 10.1079/ 9781800622852.0002

highlights the need for a One Health approach to address the burden of zoonotic diseases. This approach emphasizes collaboration and coordination among various sectors and disciplines to promote the health and well-being of all (Krishnasamy *et al.*, 2018).

As stated in Chapter 1, the World Health Organization (WHO) defines zoonotic diseases as 'diseases and infections which are naturally transmitted between vertebrate animals and humans'; the term zoonosis comes from the Greek words *zoon*, meaning 'animal', and *nosos*, meaning 'disease'. Zoonotic diseases have been a concern for humans throughout history, and some of the most devastating pandemics in history have been caused by zoonotic diseases (Grace *et al.*, 2012). These are caused by either bacteria, viruses, fungi or parasites. These can be transmitted to humans through a variety of ways, including direct contact with infected animals or their bodily fluids, consumption of contaminated food or water, or exposure to contaminated environmental sources such as soil or air (Jones *et al.*, 2008). The risk of transmission can be higher in certain populations, such as people who work closely with animals or those who live in areas with a high incidence of zoonotic diseases. Zoonotic diseases are a major public health concern because they can cause serious illness and even death in humans (Hampson *et al.*, 2015). In addition, zoonotic diseases can spread quickly and easily, making them difficult to contain. For example, the predictions suggest that the global human population will constantly increase and reach almost 10 billion by 2050 (Holden *et al.*, 2016). The World Organisation for Animal Health (WOAH, formerly OIE) suggests that 60% of pathogens that cause human diseases originate from domestic animals or wildlife (Rahman *et al.*, 2020). A wide range of emerging and re-emerging infectious diseases has become a major threat to human health, approximately 75% of which are zoonoses. Zoonotic diseases in South-east Asia can be classified into three categories: emerging, re-emerging and endemic (Dong and Soong, 2021).

- **Emerging zoonotic diseases:** Infectious diseases that are newly recognized, or previously known but have recently increased in incidence or geographical range, or have the potential to do so soon; e.g. COVID-19, Middle East Respiratory Syndrome (MERS), Ebola, Zika virus disease (Han *et al.*, 2019).
- **Re-emerging zoonotic diseases:** Infectious diseases that were previously under control but have recently resurfaced and increased in incidence or geographic range; e.g. Rift Valley fever (RVF), avian influenza, Lyme disease (Halliday *et al.*, 2017).
- **Endemic zoonotic diseases:** Diseases that are constantly present in a particular region or population; e.g. rabies, brucellosis, leptospirosis, anthrax (Hattendorf *et al.*, 2017).

2.2 Historical Burden of Zoonotic Diseases

Zoonotic diseases have been known to humans for thousands of years. The ancient Egyptians, Greeks and Romans recognized the risk of diseases transmitted from animals to humans and took measures to prevent them (Head *et al.*, 2019). However, the understanding of the transmission of zoonotic diseases remained limited until the late 19th century when Louis Pasteur discovered the first vaccine for rabies (Heaton, 2020). Since then, numerous outbreaks of zoonotic diseases have occurred throughout history, including major pandemics caused by zoonotic pathogens such as smallpox, influenza and cholera (Hattendorf *et al.*, 2017). In the Middle Ages, the Black Death, caused by the bacterium *Yersinia pestis* and transmitted by fleas, killed an estimated 75–200 million people in Europe, Asia and Africa (Kaniewski and Marriner, 2020). In the 20th century, zoonotic diseases continued to pose a significant threat to human health. The Spanish flu pandemic of 1918–1919, caused by the H1N1 influenza virus, which was believed to have originated from birds, was responsible for the deaths of an estimated 50 million people worldwide (Nickol and Kindrachuk, 2019).

Other notable zoonotic disease outbreaks in the 20th century include the 1957–1958 Asian flu pandemic, caused by the H2N2 influenza virus, and the 2002–2003 SARS outbreak, caused by the SARS-CoV virus (Gagnon *et al.*, 2018). Zoonotic diseases have also affected animal populations throughout history. The rinderpest virus, a disease that affects cattle and other cloven-hoofed animals, devastated livestock populations in Europe and Asia in the 18th and 19th centuries, leading to famine and social unrest (Jones and Koolmees, 2022). In addition to these major pandemics, zoonotic diseases have also had a significant impact on human health in many parts of the world. For example, malaria, transmitted by mosquitoes, is responsible for an estimated 400,000 deaths annually, mostly in sub-Saharan Africa (Al-Awadhi *et al.*, 2021). Other zoonotic diseases that have a significant impact on human health include rabies, dengue fever and Lyme disease (Wallace *et al.*, 2017).

2.3 Current Burden of Zoonotic Diseases

Despite advances in medical research and public health measures, zoonotic diseases continue to pose a significant threat to global health. According to the WHO, approximately 60% of all infectious diseases in humans are zoonotic, and 75% of emerging infectious diseases are zoonotic (Dong and Soong, 2021). The current global burden of zoonotic diseases includes both endemic and epidemic diseases. For example, according to the European Food Safety Authority (EFSA), the most frequent zoonoses in 2020 in the EU were campylobacteriosis, salmonellosis, Shiga-toxic *Escherichia coli* (STEC) infections, yersiniosis, listeriosis and tularaemia, each reaching more than 1000 human cases requiring hospitalization (Aggarwal and Ramachandran, 2020). Meanwhile, the Centre for Diseases Control (CDC) in the USA suggests prioritizing the following diseases and pathogens with zoonotic properties: influenza, salmonellosis, West Nile virus, plague, emerging coronaviruses, Middle East respiratory syndrome (MERS-CoV)), rabies (Lyssavirus), brucellosis (*Brucella* species) and Lyme disease (*Borrelia burgdorferi*) (Harper *et al.*, 2021). Leptospirosis is responsible for an estimated 1 million human cases and 60,000 deaths each year, mostly in developing countries (Mayfield *et al.*, 2018). Around 500,000 cases of brucellosis in humans are reported worldwide each year. However, the true incidence is estimated to be 5–12.5 million cases annually, mostly in developing countries (Rushton *et al.*, 2018).

In India, there are several zoonotic diseases that pose a significant public health threat. These include rabies, brucellosis, toxoplasmosis, cysticercosis, echinococcosis, Japanese encephalitis (JE), plague, leptospirosis, scrub typhus, nipah, trypanosomiasis, Kyasanur forest disease and Crimean–Congo haemorrhagic fever (European Centre for Disease Prevention and Control, 2017). According to the Central Bureau of Health Intelligence (CBHI), there were provisional reports of 110 cases of rabies, 1674 cases of JE, 14,971 cases of H1N1, 57,813 cases of chikungunya, 4380 cases of kala-azar and 101,192 cases of dengue fever during the year 2018 (Gibb *et al.*, 2020a, b). These diseases have significant impacts on human health, causing illness, death and economic losses (Taylor, 2001). To address the burden of zoonotic diseases, there is a need for a coordinated One Health approach that involves collaboration among multiple sectors and disciplines, including public health, veterinary health and environmental health.

2.4 Importance of Controlling Zoonotic Diseases

Controlling zoonotic diseases is essential for protecting human and animal health, preventing the spread of infectious diseases and reducing the risk of pandemics (Semenza *et al.*, 2012). The importance of controlling zoonotic diseases cannot be overstated. Many zoonotic diseases cause severe illness, disability, or death in humans. For example, the Ebola virus, which is transmitted to humans through contact with infected animals, has a mortality rate of up to 90% (Alexander *et al.*, 2015). Similarly, the H5N1 strain of avian influenza has a mortality rate of over 50% in humans (Avelin *et al.*, 2022). There are several reasons why controlling zoonotic diseases is important, including the following.

2.4.1 Protection of human health

Zoonotic diseases pose a significant threat to human health, as they can cause serious illness and even death. Many zoonotic diseases, such as rabies, Lyme disease and West Nile virus, can be prevented through vaccination, proper hygiene and effective control of animal populations. By controlling zoonotic diseases, we can protect human health and reduce the burden of infectious diseases (Libera *et al.*, 2022).

2.4.2 Prevention of animal diseases

Zoonotic diseases not only affect human health but also pose a threat to animal health. Controlling zoonotic diseases can help prevent outbreaks of infectious diseases in animals and reduce the risk of transmission to humans. This is particularly important for animals that are raised for food production, as zoonotic diseases can have significant economic consequences for farmers and the food industry (Thornton *et al.*, 2022).

2.4.3 Reduced risk of pandemics

Zoonotic diseases are a significant risk factor for pandemics, as they can rapidly spread from animals to humans and between humans. For example, COVID-19 is thought to have originated from bats and was transmitted to humans through an intermediate host, likely a pangolin. By controlling zoonotic diseases, we can reduce the risk of future pandemics and protect global health security (Bernstein *et al.*, 2022).

2.4.4 Conservation of wildlife

Many zoonotic diseases can affect wildlife populations, which can have ecological implications. By controlling these diseases, we can help to protect wildlife and maintain biodiversity (Hassell *et al.*, 2017).

2.4.5 Economic benefits

Outbreaks of zoonotic diseases can cause disruptions to global trade, tourism and agriculture, leading to significant economic losses. The 2002–2003 outbreak of SARS is estimated to have cost the global economy over US$40 billion (Munikannaian *et al.*, 2022). Controlling zoonotic diseases can reduce the economic burden of infectious diseases on healthcare systems, reduce the cost of treatment and lost productivity, and support sustainable agriculture and food production (Mazzeo *et al.*, 2022).

2.5 Global Challenges of Controlling Zoonotic Diseases

Preventing and controlling zoonotic diseases is a crucial public health issue that requires the collaboration of various sectors, including medical and veterinary fields. It is not possible for the health sector alone to address all the factors involved in controlling these diseases (Kock *et al.*, 2021). The success of reducing the impact of zoonotic diseases on public health depends on cooperation and collaboration between medical and veterinary sectors, including sharing information, organizing surveillance systems and providing common training for staff (Awaidy and Al Hashami, 2020). Some of the challenges that make controlling zoonotic diseases difficult include the following.

2.5.1 Globalization

Globalization is a significant challenge to controlling zoonotic diseases. As travel, trade and transportation have become more interconnected, the movement of people, animals and animal products across borders has increased (Chala and Hamde, 2021). This has resulted in the rapid spread of zoonotic diseases across different regions and continents. The global movement of livestock and wildlife, as well as animal products, has facilitated the spread of zoonotic diseases such as avian influenza, Ebola and COVID-19. Additionally, globalization has increased the risk of zoonotic diseases emerging in new areas, where they may not have been previously present (Khater, 2018).

2.5.2 Lack of awareness and understanding

Lack of awareness and understanding about zoonotic diseases is a significant challenge in preventing and controlling these diseases. Unfortunately, many people are unaware of the risks associated with zoonotic diseases. It is possible that they do not understand how zoonotic diseases spread or what the symptoms are, caused by insufficient education and communication. Additionally, there may be cultural and language barriers that prevent effective communication about zoonotic diseases. This lack of awareness can lead to people not taking the necessary precautions to protect themselves and their families from these illnesses (Kelly *et al.*, 2018).

2.5.3 Limited resources and poor infrastructure

Many low- and middle-income countries (LMICs) lack the resources and infrastructure necessary to detect, respond to and control zoonotic disease outbreaks (Seimenis and Battelli, 2018). They have limited resources for disease surveillance, prevention and control. Poor infrastructure, such as inadequate sanitation and waste management systems, can also contribute to the spread of zoonotic diseases. Diseases such as anthrax, bovine tuberculosis and rabies are, for the most part, successfully managed in high-income countries but persist in LMICs, causing billions of cases and millions of deaths annually (Madhav *et al.*, 2018). Inadequate surveillance in remote rural areas can cause delayed detection and ineffective response to disease outbreaks, increasing the risk of pandemics due to latent amplification, regional and global travel and animal trade (Ghai *et al.*, 2022). Many countries have a shortage of skilled personnel, including epidemiologists, veterinarians and laboratory technicians, who are essential for the detection, diagnosis and control of zoonotic diseases. There is often a lack of sharing of data between countries and between sectors, which can hinder the early detection and response to zoonotic diseases. There is also a lack of resources for research and development of new diagnostic tests, treatments and vaccines for zoonotic diseases. This can limit the availability of effective tools for controlling outbreaks (Hernández-Castellano *et al.*, 2019).

2.5.4 Limited access to healthcare

Many people in LMICs have limited access to healthcare, which makes it difficult to diagnose and treat zoonotic diseases. Without access to healthcare services, individuals may not be aware of the risk factors for zoonotic diseases or how to prevent them. Additionally, those who do become infected may not seek medical care, allowing the disease to spread further. This is particularly problematic for zoonotic diseases that have the potential to cause outbreaks, such as Ebola and COVID-19. The health sector alone can only detect and treat cases of zoonotic disease among humans. The prevention or elimination of zoonotic diseases requires long-term actions from the veterinary sector to decrease incidence among disease hosts and reduce or interrupt transmission. This requires high-level commitment between the health sector and veterinary sector to implement common control programmes (Kheirallah *et al.*, 2021). Healthcare workers in many countries may not receive adequate training and education on zoonotic diseases, leading to delayed diagnosis and poor management of cases. This can also increase the risk of healthcare workers becoming infected and transmitting the disease to others. This can lead to delays in seeking treatment, misdiagnosis and inappropriate use of antibiotics, which can lead to the development of drug-resistant strains of zoonotic pathogens (WHO, 2018). Vaccination is an effective way to prevent the spread of zoonotic diseases, but in many countries the vaccination coverage is low due to a lack of resources, limited access to vaccines and vaccine hesitancy among some communities (Gibb *et al.*, 2020a, b).

2.5.5 Climate change

Climate change can affect the distribution and prevalence of zoonotic diseases, as it can alter the distribution and abundance of disease vectors and hosts (Zhang *et al.*, 2022). Climate change can also alter the timing and intensity of disease outbreaks, making it difficult to predict and control their spread. As temperatures rise and rainfall patterns change, the geographical range of many vector-borne diseases, such as malaria and dengue fever, is expanding (Watts *et al.*, 2018). This increases the risk of these diseases spreading to new areas and populations. Additionally, changing weather patterns can affect the availability of food and water sources for animals, leading to changes in their behaviour and migration patterns, which can increase the risk of zoonotic disease transmission (Lake and Barker, 2018).

2.5.6 Antimicrobial resistance (AMR)

The emergence of antimicrobial resistance (AMR) can make it difficult to treat zoonotic diseases, particularly in regions where antibiotics are overused or misused. According to the WHO, AMR is one of the top ten global public health threats facing humanity, with misuse and overuse of antimicrobials as the main drivers for the development of drug-resistant pathogens (Cassini *et al.*, 2019). The overuse and misuse of antimicrobial drugs in animals, agriculture and human medicine can contribute to the emergence and spread of AMR in zoonotic pathogens (Maugeri *et al.*, 2022).

2.5.7 Poor biosecurity measures

Poor biosecurity measures are contributing to the spread of zoonotic diseases around the globe in several ways. They can lead to the spread of zoonotic diseases through contact with animals (Huber *et al.*, 2022). For example, when animals are not kept in secure enclosures, they can encounter humans and other animals, allowing for the transmission of zoonotic diseases. Additionally, when animals are not vaccinated or treated for parasites, they can become carriers of zoonotic diseases, which can then be spread to humans and other animals (Indrawan and Daryanto, 2020). Poor biosecurity measures can lead to the spread of zoonotic diseases through contact with contaminated food or water. For example, when food and water sources are not properly stored or handled, they can become contaminated with zoonotic pathogens, which can then be spread to humans and other animals. Spread of zoonotic diseases can also occur through contact with contaminated surfaces and contaminated air (Robertson, 2020). Overall, poor biosecurity measures are contributing to the spread of zoonotic diseases around the globe by allowing for the transmission of zoonotic pathogens through contact with animals, contaminated food or water, contaminated surfaces and contaminated air (Bayot and Limaiem, 2023).

2.5.8 Wildlife trade

The wildlife trade for human consumption, driven by domestic and international demand, can lead to population declines of species, even to extinction, whereas zoonotic spillovers can lead to pandemics (Borsky *et al.*, 2020). The illegal wildlife trade is a multibillion-dollar industry that involves the capture, transportation and sale of live animals, as well as their body parts and products. This trade brings humans into close contact with wild animals that may harbour new and dangerous pathogens (Shivaprakash *et al.*, 2021). For example, the SARS-CoV-2 virus that causes COVID-19 is believed to have originated in bats and was transmitted to humans through an intermediate host, possibly a pangolin, at a wildlife market in China (Borzée *et al.*, 2020).

2.5.9 Uncoordinated and inefficient international efforts to fight zoonotic diseases

Zoonotic disease outbreaks are transboundary in nature and the control of these diseases requires coordinated efforts across countries and regions. The lack of international cooperation and coordination can hinder efforts to control zoonotic diseases and increase the risk of disease transmission (Kulikowski, 2021).

To address the rapid spread of zoonotic diseases, it is essential to implement policies that promote sustainable land use, protect wildlife habitats and regulate the trade and consumption of wildlife. Improved surveillance and early detection systems can also help identify and contain outbreaks before they become global pandemics. Additionally, addressing the root causes of zoonotic diseases, such as climate change and unsustainable agriculture practices, can help prevent future outbreaks and protect public health.

2.6 Global Challenges to Control Zoonotic Diseases Using the One Health Approach

Zoonotic diseases – infectious agents shared between animals and people – are a formidable challenge in One Health.

2.6.1 One Health approach

The One Health approach recognizes the interconnectedness of human, animal and environmental health and seeks to promote collaboration and coordination across sectors to prevent and control zoonotic diseases (Kelly *et al.*, 2020). The approach emphasizes the need for multidisciplinary collaboration among different sectors, including health, agriculture, environment and wildlife conservation, to address the challenges of zoonotic diseases. According to The One Health Global Network, the aim of One Health is to 'improve health and well-being through the prevention of risks and the mitigation of effects of crises that originate at the interface between humans, animals and their various environments' (Acharya *et al.*, 2020).

The One Health approach recognizes that zoonotic diseases are not only a health issue but also an environmental and social issue. Internationally, the Tripartite organizations, namely the Food and Agriculture Organization of the United Nations (FAO), the World Organisation for Animal Health (WOAH) and World Health Organization (WHO), have exemplified using a multisectoral, One Health approach through mandated inter-agency collaboration, and endorsement of One Health to facilitate sustained collaboration for zoonotic disease control at the local, subnational, national, regional and international levels through the guide, *Taking a Multisectoral, One Health Approach: A Tripartite Guide to Addressing Zoonotic Diseases in Countries* (hereafter the Tripartite Zoonoses Guide, or TZG) (European Food Safety Authority *et al.*, 2023). But there are several global challenges to controlling zoonotic diseases using the One Health approach, including the following.

- **Lack of political will and investment:** Despite the growing recognition of the importance of One Health, many governments and organizations have not made the necessary investments in One Health approaches. This can limit the effectiveness of One Health interventions and programmes.
- **Limited capacity and resources:** Many countries, particularly those in low-income settings, lack the capacity and resources to implement One Health approaches. This can limit the ability of these countries to detect and respond to zoonotic disease outbreaks.
- **Fragmentation of health systems:** The One Health approach requires collaboration across multiple sectors, including public health, animal health and environmental health. However, health systems are often fragmented, making it difficult to implement effective One Health programmes.
- **Lack of data and surveillance:** Effective zoonotic disease surveillance and response require high-quality data from multiple sources. Many countries lack the necessary data and surveillance systems to effectively monitor and control zoonotic diseases.
- **Cultural and behavioural factors:** Cultural and behavioural factors can influence the transmission of zoonotic diseases, such as the consumption of bushmeat or the use of traditional medicine. Addressing these factors requires a multifaceted

approach that involves community engagement and education.

2.7 Risk Assessment and Risk Management of Zoonotic Diseases

Effective risk assessment and management are critical to controlling the spread of zoonotic diseases. Here we will explore the principles of risk assessment and management as they relate to zoonotic diseases, including the identification of potential sources of exposure, risk communication and the role of surveillance and response systems (Belay *et al.*, 2017).

2.7.1 Risk assessment

A risk assessment involves the identification of potential hazards, the likelihood of those hazards occurring and the potential consequences of those hazards (Dzingirai *et al.*, 2017). Some steps to conduct a risk assessment of zoonotic diseases are as follows.

1. **Hazard identification:** This step involves identifying the zoonotic diseases that can be transmitted to humans from animals. This includes identifying the animal reservoirs, modes of transmission and factors that can contribute to the transmission. To identify potential sources of exposure, it is important to understand the ecology of the pathogen and the behaviour of the host and reservoir species.
2. **Exposure assessment:** This step involves determining the extent of exposure to the zoonotic disease. This includes identifying the population at risk, the frequency and duration of exposure and the routes of exposure.
3. **Hazard characterization:** This step involves assessing the severity of the zoonotic disease. This includes identifying the health effects, such as morbidity and mortality rates, and the impact on public health.
4. **Risk characterization:** This step involves combining the results of the hazard identification, exposure assessment and hazard characterization to determine the overall risk associated with the zoonotic disease.

2.7.2 Risk management of zoonotic diseases

Risk management is the process of identifying, assessing and controlling risks associated with zoonotic diseases (Keesing and Ostfeld, 2021). The following are the steps involved in risk management

- **Identification and prioritization of risks:** Conduct a risk assessment to identify and prioritize the risks associated with zoonotic diseases. This includes evaluating the likelihood and potential impact of disease transmission, as well as identifying vulnerable populations (Ng and Sargeant, 2013).
- **Risk communication of zoonotic diseases:** This step involves communicating the risks associated with zoonotic diseases to the public, healthcare professionals and other stakeholders. This includes providing information on the potential hazards, the methods of transmission and the strategies for prevention and control. Risk communication should be clear, concise and accessible to all members of the public, including those with limited literacy or language skills (Clarke, 2009).
- **Risk reduction of zoonotic diseases:** This step involves implementing measures to reduce the risk of zoonotic diseases. This includes measures such as vaccination, quarantine and disinfection (Narrod *et al.*, 2012).
- **Risk monitoring and evaluation of zoonotic diseases:** This step involves monitoring the effectiveness of the risk management strategies and evaluating the outcomes. This includes tracking the incidence of zoonotic diseases, assessing the effectiveness of prevention and control measures and adjusting the strategies as needed. For zoonoses control activities, data are generally aggregated and tabulated, but rarely analysed or interpreted (De La Rocque *et al.*, 2019).
- **Educating the public:** Educating the public about the risks associated with zoonotic diseases and how to prevent transmission can be done through public awareness campaigns, public health messaging

and targeted education programmes for high-risk populations.

2.7.3 Risk management of zoonotic diseases: surveillance and response systems

Risk management involves the implementation of strategies to reduce or eliminate those risks. Surveillance and response systems are critical to the effective management of zoonotic diseases (Hay and McCauley, 2018). Surveillance involves the collection and analysis of data on the occurrence and distribution of zoonotic diseases, including information on the number and location of cases, the demographic characteristics of affected individuals and the potential sources of exposure (Zinsstag *et al.*, 2020). Response systems involve the implementation of measures to control the spread of the disease, including the isolation and treatment of infected individuals, the quarantine of exposed individuals and the implementation of public health measures to reduce the risk of transmission (Li *et al.*, 2021). Response systems should also include mechanisms for the rapid detection and reporting of outbreaks, as well as the development of contingency plans for responding to outbreaks in different settings (Burke *et al.*, 2012).

Effective risk assessment and management are critical to the control and prevention of zoonotic diseases. Identifying potential sources of exposure, communicating risks to the public and implementing surveillance and response systems are all important components of effective risk management strategies (Wendt *et al.*, 2015). By implementing these strategies, we can reduce the burden of zoonotic diseases on human and animal health, economies and ecosystems. Zoonotic diseases can be transmitted from animals to humans, and they represent a significant threat to public health (Zinsstag *et al.*, 2020). The COVID-19 pandemic has shown us how devastating a zoonotic disease outbreak can be. The risk of zoonotic diseases can be minimized through risk assessment and management strategies. In this chapter, we discuss the risk assessment and management of zoonotic diseases (IOM and NRC, 2009).

2.8 Strategies for Overcoming Global Challenges

Zoonotic diseases continue to pose a significant global challenge, but there are strategies that can be implemented to overcome them. Strategies for strengthening zoonosis prevention and control need to focus on enhancing political commitment, identifying the most appropriate control interventions and ensuring collaboration among all relevant stakeholders (Conraths *et al.*, 2011). Intersectoral cooperation is fundamental for controlling zoonoses. However, processes involved in planning and implementation of intersectoral actions are complex. Each country must develop its own strategy and approaches for intersectoral action (Conrad *et al.*, 2013) (Fig. 2.1).

2.8.1 Improved surveillance and diagnostic capacity

Surveillance is key to detecting and responding to outbreaks of zoonotic diseases (Lefrancois *et al.*, 2010). Improving surveillance systems to monitor both animal and human populations for signs of disease can help identify outbreaks before they become widespread. This includes the use of diagnostic tests, such as polymerase chain reaction (PCR) assays, to detect pathogens in both animal and human populations. Early detection and response are key to controlling the spread of zoonotic diseases (Kulkarni *et al.*, 2015). Disease reporting from clinical and veterinary diagnostic laboratories is a crucial element in public health surveillance, particularly in prevention of outbreaks of emerging and re-emerging zoonoses (Dar *et al.*, 2013).

2.8.2 Increased public awareness and education

Education and awareness are essential for reducing the risk of zoonotic disease transmission (Hasanov *et al.*, 2018). Raising public awareness about zoonotic diseases and how they are transmitted can help individuals take steps to protect themselves and their communities. Education programmes can also help reduce

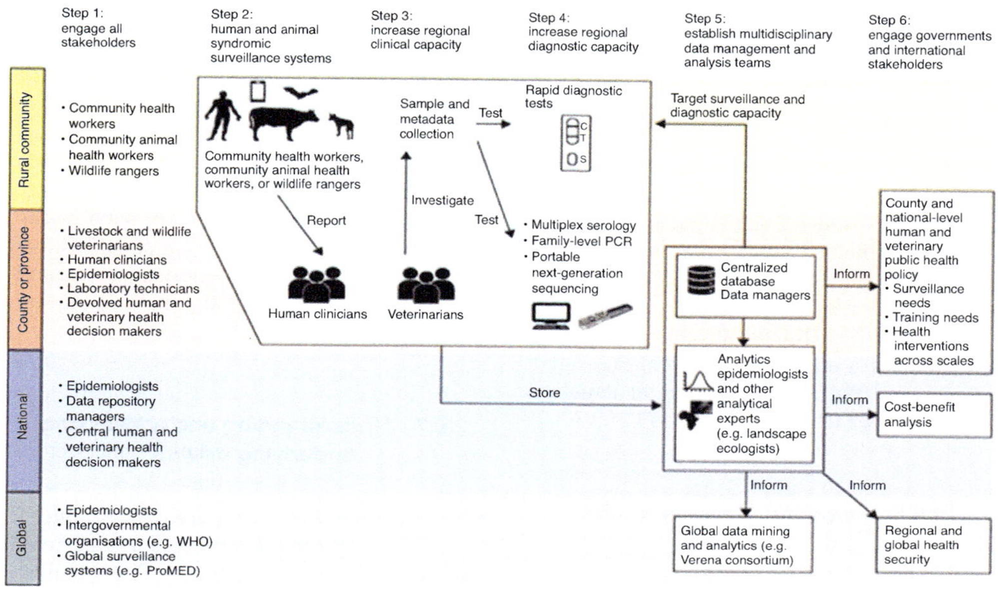

Fig. 2.1. Monitoring zoonotic diseases in remote rural areas using a framework that can be integrated into existing surveillance systems. (Author's own image.)

the demand for wildlife products and promote more sustainable agricultural practices. Education can be provided through schools, community centres and social media platforms to reach a wide audience (Ogdee *et al.*, 2016). Communities need to be actively involved in the decision-making process and in implementing strategies to control or eliminate diseases of animal origin. Health education programmes should be developed for individual target groups (such as, children, women, consumers, opinion leaders and schoolteachers). Appropriately prepared materials, such as pamphlets and posters, can be used to communicate information on diseases to local communities and to encourage them to adopt healthy lifestyles. It is particularly important to reach livestock producers, as they are key players in efforts to control zoonoses (Hasanov *et al.*, 2018).

2.8.3 Enhanced biosecurity measures

Biosecurity measures refer to the various practices and measures aimed at minimizing the risk of infectious diseases spreading. Biosecurity measures can include strict hygiene protocols, isolation of infected animals and the use of protective gear for animal handlers. These measures can help prevent the spread of zoonotic diseases and protect both human and animal health (Indrawan and Daryanto, 2020).

2.8.4 Increased regulatory frameworks

Governments can play a key role in regulating wildlife trade, agricultural practices and other factors that contribute to the spread of zoonotic diseases. Strengthening regulatory frameworks can help ensure that these practices are sustainable and do not contribute to disease transmission. Governments can also work with international organizations to develop and enforce regulations that reduce the risk of zoonotic disease transmission (Farnese, 2013). The pressing challenge for the national programmes is to develop and enhance surveillance of outbreaks of emerging and re-emerging diseases and to monitor changes in the incidence and geographical distribution of these diseases. Mechanisms for cooperation with private medical and veterinary sectors must be developed for collection of the essential information. The Convention on the Conservation of Migratory Species of Wild Animals Scientific Council agreed in November 2011 to create an expert working group on migratory species and public health, including zoonoses linked to the wildlife trade (Coker *et al.*, 2011). These initiatives combined could potentially be used as a starting point to launch the policy relevant science platform for pandemic prevention, which could be like the Intergovernmental Science-Policy Platform on Biodiversity and Ecosystem Services and the Intergovernmental Panel on Climate Change (Hassell *et al.*, 2017).

2.8.5 Investing in research and development

Continued research and development into zoonotic diseases and their transmission can help identify new interventions and control strategies (Carlson *et al.*, 2021). This includes developing new vaccines, treatments and diagnostic tools, as well as improving our understanding of the underlying biology and ecology of these diseases. Research can be funded through public and private sources to support the development of new interventions and control strategies. Management and communication skills of zoonoses control staff need to be strengthened through educational training, and control staff must be better represented in key policy-making positions (Sekar et al., 2011). It is important that the educational curricula for veterinary and health professions be reviewed and developed on a regional basis, with emphasis on specific problems of a geographical region. In addition, the national programmes need to encourage interdisciplinary, cost-effective, problem-oriented research relevant to their needs (Tacconelli *et al.*, 2018).

2.8.6 Increased global collaboration

Zoonotic diseases do not respect borders and so it is crucial to promote global collaboration and information sharing. This includes collaborating on disease surveillance, sharing research findings and coordinating responses to outbreaks. The WHO can play a key role in facilitating this collaboration by bringing together researchers, policy makers and public health experts from around the world (Jones *et al.*, 2008). An additional challenge is to keep the activities of the national programme in pace with new developments in society, such as the introduction of novel food products of animal origin, changes in production systems and changes in sources of animal protein (Hampson *et al.*, 2015).

2.8.7 Understanding and addressing underlying drivers

Addressing the underlying drivers of zoonotic disease transmission is crucial for long-term control (Dzingirai *et al.*, 2017). This includes addressing issues such as habitat destruction, unsustainable agricultural practices and climate change, which can all contribute to the emergence and spread of zoonotic diseases. Governments can work with local communities and international organizations to address these underlying drivers and promote sustainable practices (Li *et al.*, 2021). Sustainable land-use planning can help to reduce the risk of zoonotic disease emergence and transmission by addressing some of the underlying drivers, including habitat destruction, wildlife trade and animal agriculture (Plowright *et al.*, 2021) (Fig. 2.2).

2.8.8 Adopting a one health approach

The One Health approach recognizes the interconnectedness of human, animal and environmental health. Promoting One Health approaches can help prevent and control zoonotic diseases by improving collaboration and communication between different sectors. The Generalized One Health Framework (GOHF) provides recommendations for how to use a One Health approach to improve multisectoral collaboration and thereby enhance the prevention and control of zoonotic diseases (Hattendorf *et al.*, 2017). It was developed primarily for use by governmental officials in public health,

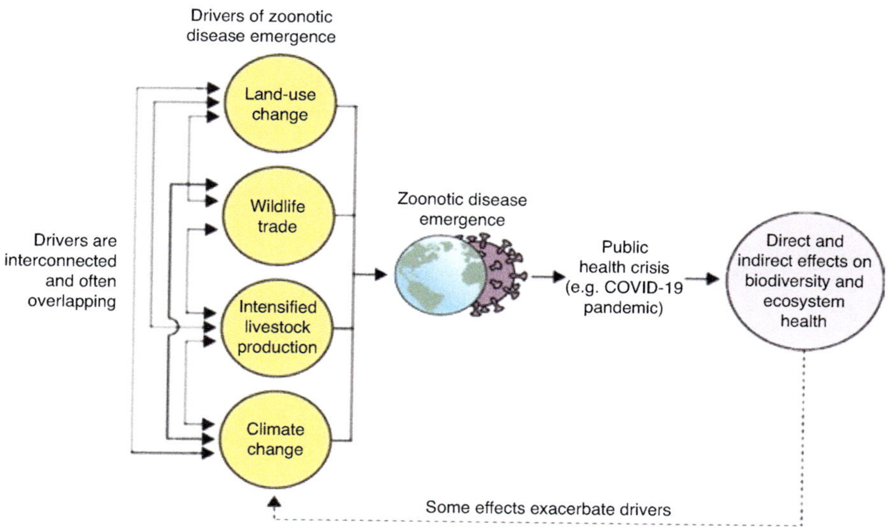

Fig. 2.2. Feedback loops associated with zoonotic disease emergence. (Author's own image.)

animal health, or environment sectors working on One Health and zoonotic disease programming at local, subnational, national, or international levels. The GOHF presents the following series of five steps and corresponding activities, which provide structure for how countries may develop capacity to coordinate zoonotic disease programming across sectors (Machalaba *et al.*, 2021).

- **Engagement:** To establish an initial One Health collaborations platform that brings together representatives from the human health, animal health and environmental sectors to work collaboratively around zoonotic disease control. This platform should develop a clear mandate, establish working groups and develop an action plan including:
  - establishing One Health interest by identifying and engaging stakeholders
  - identifying and engaging stakeholders
  - prioritizing zoonotic diseases
  - establishing sustained government support for One Health.
- **Assessment:** To understand limitations and disparities in resources within the One Health system and/or relevant One Health sectors. Areas of strengths and weakness in each sector relevant to the One Health system or zoonotic disease programme are identified by:
  - mapping infrastructure
  - establishing baseline information on the status of current activities, such as the burden of the zoonotic disease and its epidemiological situation
  - conducting gap analysis to identify gaps in current capacity within and between sectors responsible for managing the system or programme
  - completing economic assessments.
- **Planning:** To develop plans and protocols that include and leverage all relevant One Health sectors. It outlines the priorities, goals and objectives of the One Health Coordination Platform. The plan should be developed through a participatory process and should involve input from all relevant stakeholders including:
  - developing a multisectoral, One Health strategic plan
  - developing action plans for priority zoonotic diseases.

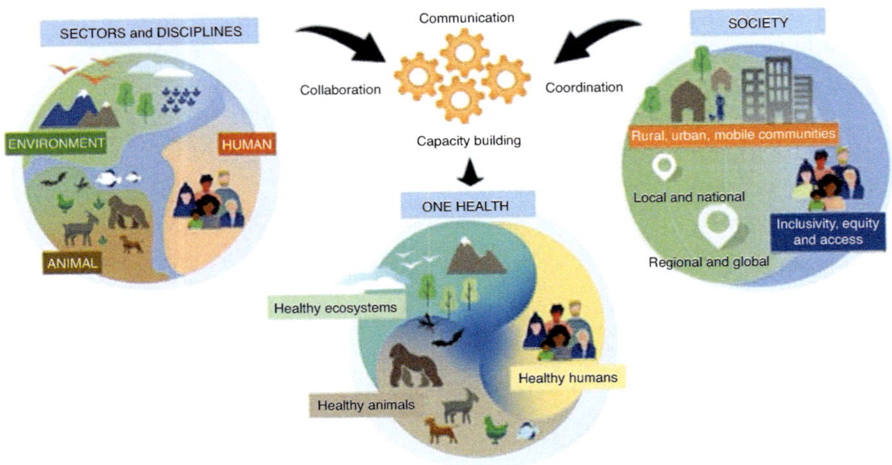

Fig. 2.3. A system for a collaborative, coordinated and communicative approach to One Health across sectors. (Author's own image.)

- **Implementation:** Implementation of programmes that use a One Health approach by:
  - soliciting, acquiring and allocating resources
  - implementing plans, protocols and procedures.
- **Monitoring and evaluation:** To identify successes and improve upon weaknesses of One Health systems and/or programmes by:
  - Monitoring and evaluating systems and/or programmes to track implementation outputs and systematically evaluating the successes, challenges, scope and scale of programmes (Fig. 2.3).

By implementing these strategies, we can work to overcome the global challenges posed by zoonotic diseases and improve the health and well-being of both animal and human populations around the world. The primary challenge for effective implementation of zoonoses control is to establish an effective veterinary public health system with well-trained staff in the broad areas of public health and preventive medicine. These strategies require a multisectoral approach that involves collaboration between governments, international organizations, researchers and local communities. Through sustained effort and investment, we can reduce the risk of zoonotic disease transmission and prevent future pandemics.

2.9 Global Governance and Policies for Zoonotic Diseases

Global health threats such as zoonotic diseases require government, international organizations and other stakeholders to coordinate and collaborate. Policy and governance at the global level are crucial for preventing and controlling zoonotic diseases. In this part we will show how international organizations, national governments and the private sector influence global governance and policies for zoonotic diseases (Galaz *et al.*, 2017).

2.9.1 Global governance

Global governance for zoonotic diseases involves the development and implementation of policies, regulations and standards at the international, regional and national levels (Figuié, 2014). International organizations play a critical role in the governance and management of zoonotic diseases. The following are the key stakeholders involved in global governance for zoonotic diseases.

- **The World Health Organization (WHO):** The WHO is the United Nations specialized agency for health. They are responsible for setting norms and standards, providing technical assistance and coordinating global health efforts.
- **The Food and Agriculture Organization (FAO):** The FAO is a specialized agency of the United Nations responsible for leading international efforts to defeat hunger and improve food security.
- **The World Organisation for Animal Health** (**WOAH**): The WOAH (formerly OIE) is an intergovernmental organization responsible for improving animal health worldwide, including the prevention and control of zoonotic diseases.
- **The United Nations Environment Programme (UNEP):** The UNEP is the United Nations agency responsible for promoting sustainable development and protecting the environment.

2.9.2 National governments

National governments also play an important role in the governance and management of zoonotic diseases. Each country has its own policies and guidelines for the prevention and control of zoonotic diseases, which are often based on the recommendations of international organizations such as WHO and FAO (Bardosh *et al.*, 2017). National governments are responsible for implementing policies and guidelines for the prevention and control of zoonotic diseases, as well as providing resources for research, surveillance and response systems. National governments may also work with other countries to share information and resources, particularly during outbreaks or epidemics (Belay *et al.*, 2017). National programmes need to strengthen their laboratory components to serve for the routine confirmation of clinical syndromes and for rapid confirmation of the causative agent in outbreaks.

2.9.3 Private sector

The private sector also plays an important role in the governance and management of zoonotic diseases. The private sector includes businesses involved in agriculture, food production and processing, pharmaceuticals and other industries that are involved in the prevention and control of zoonotic diseases (Donadeu *et al.*, 2019). Private sector companies may develop new vaccines, diagnostic tools and treatments for zoonotic diseases, as well as implementing measures to prevent the spread of disease within their own operations. Private sector companies may also work with national governments and international organizations to develop policies and guidelines for the prevention and control of zoonotic diseases (Head *et al.*, 2019).

2.9.4 Global policies

The following are the key global policies for zoonotic diseases.

- **International Health Regulations (2005):** The International Health Regulations (IHR) is a legally binding agreement among 196 countries that aims to prevent and respond to public health emergencies of international concern. The IHR require countries to develop core capacities to detect, assess and report public health events.
- **Global Health Security Agenda (GHSA):** The GHSA is a partnership of countries, international organizations and other stakeholders that aims to strengthen global health security and prevent, detect and respond to infectious disease threats. The GHSA focuses on implementing the IHR core capacities, improving laboratory systems and strengthening disease surveillance.
- **One Health:** The One Health approach recognizes that human health, animal health and environmental health are interconnected and that zoonotic diseases can only be effectively addressed through a multisectoral approach. The One Health approach involves collaboration between

the health sector, animal health sector and environmental sector to prevent, detect and respond to zoonotic diseases.

- **Sustainable Development Goals (SDGs):** The SDGs are a set of 17 goals adopted by the United Nations in 2015 that aim to end poverty, protect the planet and ensure prosperity for all. The SDGs are relevant to zoonotic diseases as they address issues such as food security, sustainable agriculture and environmental protection, which are key factors in the emergence and transmission of zoonotic diseases.

Effective global governance and policies for zoonotic diseases play a critical role in preventing and controlling these diseases. The development and implementation of policies, regulations and standards at the international, regional and national levels, along with collaboration between the health sector, animal health sector and environmental sector, are essential in addressing this global health threat. By working together and implementing evidence-based policies and guidelines, we can reduce the burden of zoonotic diseases on human and animal health, economies and ecosystems.

2.10 Case Studies of Zoonotic Diseases

These case studies illustrate the devastating impact of zoonotic diseases on public health and the need for effective measures to prevent and control these diseases. They also highlight the importance of collaboration between the health sector, animal health sector, and environmental sector in addressing these threats (Mishra *et al.*, 2021).

2.10.1 Ebola virus disease (EVD)

Ebola virus disease (EVD) is a severe, often fatal, disease in humans and non-human primates caused by the Ebola virus. The virus is transmitted to people from wild animals, such as fruit bats, and spreads through human-to-human transmission. The 2014–2016 outbreak of EVD in West Africa was the largest and most complex outbreak of the disease in history, with more than 28,000 cases and 11,000 deaths reported (Alexander *et al.*, 2015). The outbreak was caused by a new strain of Ebola virus, which was transmitted to humans through contact with infected animals, such as fruit bats and primates, and through human-to-human transmission. The outbreak was exacerbated by weak health systems and a lack of preparedness for an outbreak of this magnitude. The response to the outbreak involved a range of measures, including isolation of cases, contact tracing, safe burial practices and community engagement (Tomori and Kolawole, 2021).

2.10.2 Avian influenza (H5N1)

Avian influenza (H5N1) is a highly contagious zoonotic disease that primarily affects birds but can also infect humans. The virus is transmitted to humans through direct contact with infected birds or their droppings, or through contact with contaminated surfaces. The disease can cause severe respiratory illness and has a high mortality rate in humans. The first human cases of H5N1 were reported in Hong Kong in 1997 and the virus has since spread to other countries (Nickol and Kindrachuk, 2019). The disease has caused sporadic outbreaks in humans, with the most severe outbreak occurring in 2006, when more than 100 cases were reported in several countries. The response to the outbreaks has involved measures such as culling of infected birds, vaccination of poultry and public awareness campaigns (Gagnon *et al.*, 2018).

2.10.3 COVID-19

COVID-19 is a zoonotic disease caused by the SARS-CoV-2 virus. The virus is believed to have originated from bats and was transmitted to humans through an intermediate host, possibly a pangolin, in a wet market in Wuhan, China (Heaton, 2020). The disease has since spread rapidly across the globe, with more than 200 million cases and 4 million deaths reported as of September 2021 (Wang *et al.*, 2021). The response to the COVID-19 pandemic has involved a range of measures, including lockdowns, travel restrictions, mask mandates and vaccination campaigns. The pandemic has highlighted the importance of preparedness and response measures for zoonotic diseases and the need for global collaboration in addressing these threats (Maugeri *et al.*, 2022).

2.11 Conclusion

Zoonoses pose a significant threat to global public health and it is imperative to take proactive measures to prevent and control their spread. This requires a coordinated effort from different sectors, including human health, animal health and environmental health, as well as international organizations such as the WHO, FAO and OIE/WOAH. To effectively monitor and control zoonotic diseases, there is a need to integrate human and animal health concerns into a new public health agenda. Intersectoral collaboration is critical to the implementation of successful zoonosis control programmes and coordination structures need to be put in place to provide technical and administrative support to enhance these efforts. In addition, education and communication are crucial for the prevention and control of zoonoses. Raising awareness of the risks associated with these diseases, emphasizing the importance of seeking medical attention and tailoring public health campaigns to the cultural and linguistic needs of different communities can help limit the spread of zoonoses. Investing in laboratory infrastructure, training staff to respond to outbreaks and strengthening surveillance systems for early detection of outbreaks are also critical to containing the spread of zoonoses. Finally, promoting a One Health approach emphasizes the interconnectedness of human, animal and environmental health and recognizes the need for collaboration between different sectors to prevent and control zoonotic diseases. By working together and taking proactive measures, we can prevent and control zoonotic diseases and reduce the risk of future pandemics, ultimately protecting public health worldwide.

References

Acharya, K.P., Acharya, N., Phuyal, S., Upadhyaya, M. and Lasee, S. (2020) One-health approach: A best possible way to control rabies. *One Health* 10, 100161. DOI: 10.1016/j.onehlt.2020.100161.

Aggarwal, D. and Ramachandran, A. (2020) One health approach to address zoonotic diseases. *Indian Journal of Community Medicine* 45(Suppl. 1), S6–S8. DOI: 10.4103/ijcm.IJCM_398_19.

Al-Awadhi, M., Ahmad, S. and Iqbal, J. (2021) Current status and the epidemiology of malaria in the middle east region and beyond. *Microorganisms* 9(2), 338. DOI: 10.3390/microorganisms9020338.

Alexander, K.A., Sanderson, C.E., Marathe, M., Lewis, B.L., Rivers, C.M. *et al.* (2015) What factors might have led to the emergence of Ebola in West Africa? *PLoS Neglected Tropical Diseases* 9(6), e0003652. DOI: 10.1371/journal.pntd.0003652.

Avelin, V., Sissonen, S., Julkunen, I. and Oesterlund, P. (2022) Inactivation efficacy of H5N1 avian influenza virus by commonly used sample preparation reagents for safe laboratory practices. *Journal of Virological Methods* 304, 114527. DOI: 10.1016/j.jviromet.2022.114527.

Awaidy, S.A. and Al Hashami, H. (2020) Zoonotic diseases in Oman: Successes, challenges, and future directions. *Vector-Borne and Zoonotic Diseases* 20(1), 1–9. DOI: 10.1089/vbz.2019.2458.

Bardosh, K.L., Scoones, J.C., Grace, D., Kalema-Zikusoka, G., Jones, K.E. *et al.* (2017) Engaging research with policy and action: What are the challenges of responding to zoonotic disease in Africa? *Philosophical Transactions of the Royal Society B: Biological Sciences* 372(1725), 20160172. DOI: 10.1098/rstb.2016.0172.

Bayot, M. and Limaiem, F. (2023) *Biosafety Guidelines*. StatPearls Publishing, Treasure Island, Florida. Available at: https://www.ncbi.nlm.nih.gov/books/NBK537210

Belay, E.D., Kile, J.C., Hall, A.J., Barton-Behravesh, C., Parsons, M.B. *et al.* (2017) Zoonotic disease programs for enhancing global health security. *Emerging Infectious Diseases* 23(Suppl. 1), S65. DOI: 10.3201/eid2313.170544.

Bernstein, A.S., Ando, A.W., Loch-Temzelides, T., Vale, M.M., Li, B.V. *et al*. (2022) The costs and benefits of primary prevention of zoonotic pandemics. *Science Advances* 8(5), eabl4183. DOI: 10.1126/sciadv.abl4183.

Borsky, S., Hennighausen, H., Leiter, A. and Williges, K. (2020) CITES and the zoonotic disease content in international wildlife trade. *Environmental and Resource Economics* 76, 1001–1017. DOI: 10.1007/s10640-020-00456-7.

Borzée, A., McNeely, J., Magellan, K., Miller, J.R., Porter, L. *et al*. (2020) COVID-19 highlights the need for more effective wildlife trade legislation. *Trends in Ecology & Evolution* 35(12), 1052–1055. DOI: 10.1016/j.tree.2020.10.001.

Burke, R.L., Kronmann, K.C., Daniels, C.C., Meyers, M., Byarugaba, D.K. *et al*. (2012) A review of zoonotic disease surveillance supported by the armed forces health surveillance center. *Zoonoses and Public Health* 59(3), 164–175. DOI: 10.1111/j.1863-2378.2011.01440.x.

Carlson, C.J., Farrell, M.J., Grange, Z., Han, B.A., Mollentze, N. *et al*. (2021) The future of zoonotic risk prediction. *Philosophical Transactions of the Royal Society B* 376(1837), 20200358. DOI: 10.1098/rstb.2020.0358.

Cassini, A., Högberg, L.D., Plachouras, D., Quattrocchi, A., Hoxha, A. *et al*. (2019) Attributable deaths and disability-adjusted life-years caused by infections with antibiotic-resistant bacteria in the EU and the European economic area in 2015: A population-level modelling analysis. *The Lancet Infectious Diseases* 19(1), 56–66. DOI: 10.1016/S1473-3099(18)30605-4.

Chala, B. and Hamde, F. (2021) Emerging and re-emerging vector-borne infectious diseases and the challenges for control: A review. *Frontiers in Public Health* 9, 715759. DOI: 10.3389/fpubh.2021.715759.

Clarke, C. (2009) Seeking and processing information about zoonotic disease risk: A proposed framework. *Human Dimensions of Wildlife* 14(5), 314–325. DOI: 10.1080/10871200903096155.

Coker, R., Rushton, J., Mounier-Jack, S., Karimuribo, E., Lutumba, P. *et al*. (2011) Towards a conceptual framework to support one-health research for policy on emerging zoonoses. *The Lancet Infectious Diseases* 11(4), 326–331. DOI: 10.1016/S1473-3099(10)70312-1.

Conrad, P.A., Meek, L.A. and Dumit, J. (2013) Operationalizing a one health approach to global health challenges. *Comparative Immunology, Microbiology and Infectious Diseases* 36(3), 211–216. DOI: 10.1016/j.cimid.2013.03.006.

Conraths, F.J., Schwabenbauer, K., Vallat, B., Meslin, F.X., Füssel, A.E. *et al*. (2011) Animal health in the 21st century – a global challenge. *Preventive Veterinary Medicine* 102(2), 93–97. DOI: 10.1016/j.prevetmed.2011.04.003.

Dar, O., McIntyre, S., Hogarth, S. and Heymann, D. (2013) Rift valley fever and a new paradigm of research and development for zoonotic disease control. *Emerging Infectious Diseases* 19(2), 189. DOI: 10.3201/eid1902.120941.

De La Rocque, S., Caya, F., El Idrissi, A.H., Mumford, L., Belot, G. *et al*. (2019) One health operations: A critical component in the international health regulations monitoring and evaluation framework. *Revue Scientifique et Technique de l'OIE* 38(1), 303–314. DOI: 10.20506/rst.38.1.2962.

Donadeu, M., Nwankpa, N., Abela-Ridder, B. and Dungu, B. (2019) Strategies to increase adoption of animal vaccines by smallholder farmers with focus on neglected diseases and marginalized populations. *PLoS Neglected Tropical Diseases* 13(2), e0006989. DOI: 10.1371/journal.pntd.0006989.

Dong, X. and Soong, L. (2021) Emerging and re-emerging zoonoses are major and global challenges for public health. *Zoonoses* 1(1), e999. DOI: 10.15212/ZOONOSES-2021-0001.

Dzingirai, V., Bett, B., Bukachi, S., Lawson, E., Mangwanya, L. *et al*. (2017) Zoonotic diseases: Who gets sick, and why? explorations from Africa. *Critical Public Health* 27(1), 97–110. DOI: 10.1080/09581596.2016.1187260.

European Centre for Disease Prevention and Control (ECDC) (2017) Antimicrobial resistance surveillance in Europe 2015. *Annual Report of the European Antimicrobial Resistance Surveillance Network (EARS-Net),* Stockholm, Sweden.

European Food Safety Authority (EFSA), Berezowski, J., De Balogh, K., Dórea, F.C., Ruegg, S. *et al* (2023) Coordinated surveillance system under the one health approach for cross-border pathogens that threaten the union – options for sustainable surveillance strategies for priority pathogens. *EFSA Journal* 21(3), e07882. DOI: 10.2903/j.efsa.2023.7882.

Farnese, P.L. (2013) Searching for wildlife: A critique of Canada's regulatory response to emerging zoonotic diseases. *Queen's Law Journal* 39, 471.

Figuié, M. (2014) Towards a global governance of risks: International health organisations and the surveillance of emerging infectious diseases. *Journal of Risk Research* 17(4), 469–483. DOI: 10.1080/13669877.2012.761277.

Gagnon, A., Acosta, E., Hallman, S., Bourbeau, R., Dillon, L.Y. *et al.* (2018) Pandemic paradox: Early life H2N2 pandemic influenza infection enhanced susceptibility to death during the 2009 H1N1 pandemic. *MBio* 9(1), e02091-17. DOI: 10.1128/mBio.02091-17.

Galaz, V., Tallberg, J., Boin, A., Ituarte-Lima, C., Hey, E. *et al.* (2017) Global governance dimensions of globally networked risks: The state of the art in social science research. *Risk, Hazards & Crisis in Public Policy* 8(1), 4–27. DOI: 10.1002/rhc3.12108.

Ghai, R.R., Wallace, R.M., Kile, J.C., Shoemaker, T.R., Vieira, A.R. *et al.* (2022) A generalizable one health framework for the control of zoonotic diseases. *Scientific Reports* 12(1), 8588. DOI: 10.1038/s41598-022-12619-1.

Gibb, R., Franklinos, L.H., Redding, D.W. and Jones, K.E. (2020b) Ecosystem perspectives are needed to manage zoonotic risks in a changing climate. *BMJ* 371, m3389. DOI: 10.1136/bmj.m3389.

Gibb, R., Redding, D.W., Chin, K.Q., Donnelly, C.A., Blackburn, T.M. *et al.* (2020a) Zoonotic host diversity increases in human-dominated ecosystems. *Nature* 584(7821), 398–402. DOI: 10.1038/s4158%206-020-2562-8.

Grace, D., Gilbert, J., Randolph, T. and Kang'ethe, E. (2012) The multiple burdens of zoonotic disease and an ecohealth approach to their assessment. *Tropical Animal Health and Production* 44, 67–73. DOI: 10.1007/s11250-012-0209-y.

Halliday, J.E., Hampson, K., Hanley, N., Lembo, T., Sharp, J.P. *et al.* (2017) Driving improvements in emerging disease surveillance through locally relevant capacity strengthening. *Science* 357(6347), 146–148. DOI: 10.1126/science.aam8332.

Hampson, K., Coudeville, L., Lembo, T., Sambo, M., Kieffer, A. *et al.* (2015) Correction: Estimating the global burden of endemic canine rabies. *PLoS Neglected Tropical Diseases* 9(5), e0003786. DOI: 10.1371/journal.pntd.0003786.

Han, B.A., Majumdar, S., Calmon, F.P., Glicksberg, B.S., Horesh, R. *et al.* (2019) Confronting data sparsity to identify potential sources of Zika virus spillover infection among primates. *Epidemics* 27, 59–65. DOI: 10.1016/j.epidem.2019.01.005.

Harper, S.L., Cunsolo, A., Babujee, A., Coggins, S., Aguilar, M.D. *et al.* (2021) Climate change and health in North America: Literature review protocol. *Systematic Reviews* 10(1), 1–13. DOI: 10.1186/s13643-020-01543-y.

Hasanov, E., Zeynalova, S., Geleishvili, M., Maes, E., Tongren, E. *et al.* (2018) Assessing the impact of public education on a preventable zoonotic disease: Rabies. *Epidemiology & Infection* 146(2), 227–235. DOI: 10.1017/S0950268817002850.

Hassell, J.M., Begon, M., Ward, M.J. and Fevre, E.M. (2017) Urbanization and disease emergence: Dynamics at the wildlife-livestock-human interface. *Trends in Ecology & Evolution* 32, 55–67. DOI: 10.1016/j.tree.2016.09.012.

Hattendorf, J., Bardosh, K.L. and Zinsstag, J. (2017) One health and its practical implications for surveillance of endemic zoonotic diseases in resource limited settings. *Acta Tropica* 165, 268–273. DOI: 10.1016/j.actatropica.2016.10.009.

Hay, A.J. and McCauley, J.W. (2018) The WHO Global Influenza Surveillance and Response System (GISRS) – a future perspective. *Influenza and Other Respiratory Viruses* 12(5), 551–557. DOI: 10.1111/irv.12565.

Head, J.R., Vos, A., Blanton, J., Müller, T., Chipman, R. *et al.* (2019) Environmental distribution of certain modified live-virus vaccines with a high safety profile presents a low-risk, high-reward to control zoonotic diseases. *Scientific Reports* 9(1), 1–12. DOI: 10.1038/s41598-019-42714-9.

Heaton, P.M. (2020) The covid-19 vaccine-development multiverse. *New England Journal of Medicine* 383(20), 1986–1988. DOI: 10.1056/NEJMe2025111.

Hernández-Castellano, L.E., Nally, J.E., Lindahl, J., Wanapat, M., Alhidary, I.A. *et al.* (2019) Dairy science and health in the tropics: Challenges and opportunities for the next decades. *Tropical Animal Health and Production* 51, 1009–1017. DOI: 10.1007/s11250-019-01866-6.

Holden, B.A., Fricke, T.R., Wilson, D.A., Jong, M., Naidoo, K.S. *et al.* (2016) Global prevalence of myopia and high myopia and temporal trends from 2000 through 2050. *Ophthalmology* 123(5), 1036–1042. DOI: 10.1016/j.ophtha.2016.01.006.

Huber, N., Andraud, M., Sassu, E.L., Prigge, C., Zoche-Golob, V. *et al.* (2022) What is a biosecurity measure? A definition proposal for animal production and linked processing operations. *One Health* 100433. DOI: 10.1016/j.onehlt.2022.100433.

Indrawan, D. and Daryanto, A. (2020) Food control and biosecurity roles in the global value chain: Supporting producers or safeguarding consumers? In: *IOP Conference Series: Earth and Environmental Science*, Vol. 519. IOP Publishing, Bristol, UK, p. 012040. DOI: 10.1088/1755-1315/519/1/012040.

IOM (Institute of Medicine) and NRC (National Research Council) (2009) Making the case for zoonotic disease surveillance. In: Keusch, G.T., Pappaioanou, M., Gonzalez, M.C., Scott, K.A. and Tsai, P. (eds) *Sustaining Global Surveillance and Response to Emerging Zoonotic Diseases*. National Academies Press, Washington, DC.

Jones, K.E., Patel, N.G., Levy, M.A., Storeygard, A., Balk, D. *et al.* (2008) Global trends in emerging infectious diseases. *Nature* 451(7181), 990–993. DOI: 10.1038/nature06536.

Jones, S.D. and Koolmees, P.A. (2022) *A Concise History of Veterinary Medicine*. Cambridge University Press, Cambridge, UK.

Kaniewski, D. and Marriner, N. (2020) Conflicts and the spread of plagues in pre-industrial Europe. *Humanities and Social Sciences Communications* 7(1), 1–10. DOI: 10.1057/s41599-020-00661-1.

Keesing, F. and Ostfeld, R.S. (2021) Impacts of biodiversity and biodiversity loss on zoonotic diseases. *Proceedings of the National Academy of Sciences* 118(17), e2023540118. DOI: 10.1073/pnas.2023540118.

Kelly, T.R., Bunn, D.A., Joshi, N.P., Grooms, D., Devkota, D. *et al.* (2018) Awareness and practices relating to zoonotic diseases among smallholder farmers in Nepal. *EcoHealth* 15, 656–669. DOI: 10.1007/s10393-018-1343-4.

Kelly, T.R., Machalaba, C., Karesh, W.B., Crook, P.Z., Gilardi, K. *et al.* (2020) Implementing one health approaches to confront emerging and re-emerging zoonotic disease threats: Lessons from PREDICT. *One Health Outlook* 2, 1–7. DOI: 10.1186/s42522-019-0007-9.

Khater, H.F. (2018) Introductory chapter: The globalization of mosquito-borne diseases and their ecofriendly control. In: *From Local to Global Impact of Mosquitoes*. IntechOpen, London.

Kheirallah, K.A., Al-Mistarehi, A.H., Alsawalha, L., Hijazeen, Z., Mahrous, H. *et al.* (2021) Prioritizing zoonotic diseases utilizing the one health approach: Jordan's experience. *One Health* 13, 100262. DOI: 10.1016/j.onehlt.2021.100262.

Kock, R., Michel, A.L., Yeboah-Manu, D., Azhar, E.I., Torrelles, J.B. *et al.* (2021) Zoonotic tuberculosis – the changing landscape. *International Journal of Infectious Diseases* 113, S68–S72. DOI: 10.1016/j.ijid.2021.02.091.

Krishnasamy, V., Behravesh, C.B., Varela, K., Goryoka, G., Oussayef, N. *et al.* (2018) Using a multisectoral one health approach to prioritize zoonotic diseases in the United States. *Open Forum Infectious Diseases* 5(Suppl. 1), S244. DOI: 10.1093/ofid/ofy210.683.

Kulikowski, C.A. (2021) Pandemics: Historically slow 'learning curve' leading to biomedical informatics and vaccine breakthroughs. *Yearbook of Medical Informatics* 30(1), 290–301. DOI: 10.1055/s-0041-1726482.

Kulkarni, M.A., Berrang-Ford, L., Buck, P.A., Drebot, M.A., Lindsay, L.R. *et al.* (2015) Major emerging vector-borne zoonotic diseases of public health importance in Canada. *Emerging Microbes & Infections* 4(1), 1–7. DOI: 10.1038/emi.2015.33.

Lake, I.R. and Barker, G.C. (2018) Climate change, foodborne pathogens and illness in higher-income countries. *Current Environmental Health Reports* 5, 187–196. DOI: 10.1007/s40572-018-0189-9.

Lefrancois, T., Petit-Sinturel, M., Kalloo, M., Shaw, J., Herbert-Hackshaw, K. *et al.* (2010) CaribVET: A model for surveillance of zoonotic diseases. *International Journal of Infectious Diseases* 14(1), e185.

Li, H., Chen, Y., Machalaba, C.C., Tang, H., Chmura, A.A. *et al.* (2021) Wild animal and zoonotic disease risk management and regulation in China: Examining gaps and one health opportunities in scope, mandates, and monitoring systems. *One Health* 13, 100301. DOI: 10.1016/j.onehlt.2021.100301.

Libera, K., Konieczny, K., Grabska, J., Szopka, W., Augustyniak, A. *et al.* (2022) Selected livestock-associated zoonoses as a growing challenge for public health. *Infectious Disease Reports* 14(1), 63–81. DOI: 10.3390/idr14010008.

Machalaba, C., Raufman, J., Anyamba, A., Berrian, A.M., Berthe, F.C. *et al.* (2021) Applying a one health approach in global health and medicine: Enhancing involvement of medical schools and global health centers. *Annals of Global Health* 87(1). DOI: 10.5334/aogh.2647.

Madhav, N., Oppenheim, B., Gallivan, M., Mulembakani, P., Rubin, E. *et al.* (2018) Pandemics: risks, impacts, and mitigation. In: Jamison, D.T., Gelband, H. and Horton, S. (eds) *Disease Control Priorities: Improving*

Health and Reducing Poverty, 3rd edn. International Bank for Reconstruction and Development / The World Bank, Washington, DC, pp. 315–345. DOI: 10.1596/978-1-4648-0527-1_ch17.

Maugeri, A., Barchitta, M., Basile, G. and Agodi, A. (2022) How COVID-19 has influenced public interest in antimicrobials, antimicrobial resistance and related preventive measures: A google trends analysis of Italian data. *Antibiotics* 11(3), 379. DOI: 10.3390/antibiotics11030379.

Mayfield, H.J., Smith, C.S., Lowry, J.H., Watson, C.H., Baker, M.G. *et al.* (2018) Predictive risk mapping of an environmentally driven infectious disease using spatial Bayesian networks: A case study of leptospirosis in Fiji. *PLoS Neglected Tropical Diseases* 12(10), e0006857. DOI: 10.1371/journal.pntd.0006857.

Mazzeo, A., Tremonte, P., Lombardi, S.J., Caturano, C., Correra, A. *et al.* (2022) From the intersection of food-borne zoonoses and EU green policies to an In-embryo one health financial model. *Foods* 11(18), 2736. DOI: 10.3390/foods11182736.

Mishra, J., Mishra, P. and Arora, N.K. (2021) Linkages between environmental issues and zoonotic diseases: With reference to COVID-19 pandemic. *Environmental Sustainability* 4(3), 455–467. DOI: 10.1007/s42398-021-00165-x.

Munikannaian, R., Upendra, R.S. and Nagar, S.S. (2022) Significance of *in silico* approaches in finding novel biomolecules challenging newly emerging, resurging, deliberately emerging global outbreaks. *Eurasia Proceedings of Science Technology Engineering and Mathematics* 20, 134–141. DOI: 10.55549/epstem.1222685.

Narrod, C., Zinsstag, J. and Tiongco, M. (2012) A one health framework for estimating the economic costs of zoonotic diseases on society. *EcoHealth* 9, 150–162. DOI: 10.1007/s10393-012-0747-9.

Negrón, M.E., Kharod, G.A., Bower, W.A. and Walke, H. (2019) Notes from the field: Human Brucella abortus RB51 infections caused by consumption of unpasteurized domestic dairy products – United States, 2017–2019. *Morbidity and Mortality Weekly Report* 68(7), 185. DOI: 10.15585/mmwr.mm6807a6.

Ng, V. and Sargeant, J.M. (2013) A quantitative approach to the prioritization of zoonotic diseases in North America: A health professionals' perspective. *PloS ONE* 8(8), e72172. DOI: 10.1371/journal.pone.0072172.

Nickol, M.E. and Kindrachuk, J. (2019) A year of terror and a century of reflection: Perspectives on the great influenza pandemic of 1918–1919. *BMC Infectious Diseases* 19, 1–10. DOI: 10.1186/s12879-019-3750-8.

Ogdee, J.L., Henke, S.E. and Wester, D.B. (2016) Lack of human awareness and the need for increased public education regarding the zoonotic parasite, *Baylisascaris procyonis*. *Human–Wildlife Interactions* 10(2), 12. DOI: 10.26077/d0ks-qq16.

Plowright, R.K., Reaser, J.K., Locke, H., Woodley, S.J., Patz, J.A. *et al.* (2021) Land use-induced spillover: A call to action to safeguard environmental, animal, and human health. *The Lancet Planetary Health* 5(4), e237–e245. DOI: 10.1016/S2542-5196(21)00031-0.

Rahman, M.T., Sobur, M.A., Islam, M.S., levy, S., Hossain, M.J. *et al.* (2020) Zoonotic diseases: Etiology, impact, and control. *Microorganisms* 8(9), 1405. DOI: 10.3390/microorganisms8091405.

Robertson, I.D. (2020) Disease control, prevention and on-farm biosecurity: The role of veterinary epidemiology. *Engineering* 6(1), 20–25. DOI: 10.1016/j.eng.2019.10.004.

Rushton, J., Bruce, M., Bellet, C., Torgerson, P., Shaw, A. *et al.* (2018) Initiation of global burden of animal diseases programme. *The Lancet* 392(10147), 538–540. DOI: 10.1016/S0140-6736(18)31472-7.

Seimenis, A. and Battelli, G. (2018) Main challenges in the control of zoonoses and related foodborne diseases in the south Mediterranean and middle east region. *Veterinaria Italiana* 54(2), 97–106. DOI: 10.12834/VetIt.1340.7765.1.

Sekar, N., Shah, N.K., Abbas, S.S., Kakkar, M., and Roadmap to Combat Zoonoses in India (RCZI) Initiative (2011) Research options for controlling zoonotic disease in india, 2010–2015. *PloS ONE* 6(2), e17120. DOI: 10.1371/journal.pone.0017120.

Semenza, J.C., Herbst, S., Rechenburg, A., Suk, J.E., Höser, C. *et al.* (2012) Climate change impact assessment of food-and waterborne diseases. *Critical Reviews in Environmental Science and Technology* 42(8), 857–890. DOI: 10.1080/10643389.2010.534706.

Shivaprakash, K.N., Sen, S., Paul, S., Kiesecker, J.M. and Bawa, K.S. (2021) Mammals, wildlife trade, and the next global pandemic. *Current Biology* 31(16), 3671–3677. DOI: 10.1016/j.cub.2021.06.006.

Tacconelli, E., Carrara, E., Savoldi, A., Harbarth, S., Mendelson, M. *et al.* (2018) Discovery, research, and development of new antibiotics: The WHO priority list of antibiotic-resistant bacteria and tuberculosis. *The Lancet Infectious Diseases* 18(3), 318–327. DOI: 10.1016/S1473-3099(17)30753-3.

Taylor, L.H., Latham, S.M. and Woolhouse, M.E. (2001) Risk factors for human disease emergence. *Philosophical Transactions of the Royal Society of London. Series B: Biological Sciences* 356(1411), 983–989. DOI: 10.1098/rstb.2001.0888.

Thornton, P., Nelson, G., Mayberry, D. and Herrero, M. (2022) Impacts of heat stress on global cattle production during the 21st century: A modelling study. *The Lancet Planetary Health* 6(3), e192–e201. DOI: 10.1016/S2542-5196(22)00002-X.

Tomori, O. and Kolawole, M.O. (2021) Ebola virus disease: Current vaccine solutions. *Current Opinion in Immunology* 71, 27–33. DOI: 10.1016/j.coi.2021.03.008.

Wallace, R.M., Undurraga, E.A., Blanton, J.D., Cleaton, J. and Franka, R. (2017) Elimination of dog-mediated human rabies deaths by 2030: Needs assessment and alternatives for progress based on dog vaccination. *Frontiers in Veterinary Science* 4, 9. DOI: 10.3389/fvets.2017.00009.

Wang, C., Wang, Z., Wang, G., Lau, J.Y., Zhang, K. and Li, W. (2021) COVID-19 in early 2021: current status and looking forward. *Signal Transduction and Targeted Therapy* 6(1), 114. DOI: 10.1038/s41392-021-00527-1.

Watts, N., Amann, M., Ayeb-Karlsson, S., Belesova, K., Bouley, T. *et al.* (2018) The lancet countdown on health and climate change: From 25 years of inaction to a global transformation for public health. *The Lancet* 391(10120), 581–630. DOI: 10.1016/S0140-6736(17)32464-9.

Wendt, A., Kreienbrock, L. and Campe, A. (2015) Zoonotic disease surveillance–inventory of systems integrating human and animal disease information. *Zoonoses and Public Health* 62(1), 61–74. DOI: 10.1111/zph.12120.

WHO (2018) *Managing epidemics: Key facts about major deadly diseases*. World Health Organization, Geneva.

Zhang, L., Rohr, J., Cui, R., Xin, Y., Han, L. *et al.* (2022) Biological invasions facilitate zoonotic disease emergences. *Nature Communications* 13(1), 1762. DOI: 10.1038/s41467-022-29378-2.

Zinsstag, J., Utzinger, J., Probst-Hensch, N., Shan, L. and Zhou, X.N. (2020) Towards integrated surveillance-response systems for the prevention of future pandemics. *Infectious Diseases of Poverty* 9(5), 87–92. DOI: 10.1186/s40249-020-00757-5.

3 Deliberate Releases of Biological Agents of Zoonosis

Nishant Patel*, Sonali Thakur, J.B. Nayak, J.H. Chaudhary and M.N. Brahmbhatt

Department of Veterinary Public Health and Epidemiology, College of Veterinary Science and Animal Husbandry, Kamdhenu University, Anand, Gujarat

Abstract

Deliberate releases of zoonotic biological agents, a subset of bioterrorism, represent a grave threat to global health and security. Zoonotic agents are those capable of causing diseases in both animals and humans, and their use in a deliberate act poses unique challenges. This chapter discusses the key aspects of this emerging concern. Such deliberate releases, often involving pathogens like anthrax or avian influenza, have the potential to cause widespread harm, disrupt economies and instil fear. They exploit the interconnected nature of our modern world, where zoonotic diseases can quickly cross borders. The consequences of such acts may strain healthcare systems and challenge public health responses. Preventing and mitigating deliberate releases of zoonotic agents require international collaboration, intelligence sharing and rigorous security measures for laboratories handling such pathogens. Moreover, raising awareness among healthcare professionals, public health agencies and law enforcement is essential to enhance early detection and response capabilities. As this threat evolves, a proactive and coordinated global effort is vital to safeguard against deliberate zoonotic releases, ensuring the health and security of populations worldwide.

Keywords: bioterrorism, zoonotic agents, deliberate releases, biological threats, security, preparedness

3.1 Introduction

Throughout history, warfare has evolved from the use of cavalry, chariots, swords, daggers and arrows to modern systems such as ammunition, tanks, and missiles. In the contemporary era, there has been a shift towards the utilization of bioweapons, which are considered the most terrifying form of weapons of mass destruction. This is because the costs associated with developing a biological weapons programme are significantly lower than those of a nuclear weapons programme, leading to concerns that they could become the weapon of choice for those with limited resources (Pal *et al.*, 2017). Bioterrorism is a deliberate act that involves the use of microorganisms, viruses, infectious substances, or biological products that may be created through biotechnology or naturally occurring sources (Sandbrink, 2022). The purpose of this act is to cause harm, such as death or disease, to any living organism

*Corresponding author: patelnishant582@gmail.com

DOI: 10.1079/ 9781800622852.0003

including plants, humans and other animals, with the aim of influencing government actions or intimidating civilian populations (Noah *et al.*, 2002). Such an attack could be carried out by individuals, groups, or state actors, and the consequences could be catastrophic (Tumbarski, 2020).

The emergence of zoonotic diseases and their potential use in bioterrorism pose significant threats to public health and global security. Zoonotic diseases can be intentionally or unintentionally released into populations, causing widespread illness and death. Intentional release of zoonotic diseases as a bioterrorism weapon is a growing concern, as advances in biotechnology and genetic engineering have made it possible to modify pathogens to enhance their virulence, spread ability and resistance to treatment (Beeching *et al.*, 2002). In addition to the direct impact on public health, the intentional release of zoonotic diseases could have significant economic and social consequences. The disruption of global trade and travel could lead to severe economic losses, while the fear and panic associated with a bioterrorist attack could undermine social cohesion and stability (Dembek *et al.*, 2007).

Preventing the intentional release of zoonotic diseases as a bioterrorism weapon requires a coordinated international effort, including improved surveillance and monitoring of biological threats, increased biosecurity measures and enhanced preparedness and response capabilities (Pavlin *et al.*, 2002). Efforts to prevent the emergence of zoonotic diseases and control their spread can also contribute to reducing the risk of their intentional use as a bioterrorism weapon. Overall, the emergence of zoonotic diseases and their potential use in bioterrorism pose significant challenges to global health and security. Addressing these challenges requires a comprehensive approach that involves cooperation among governments, international organizations, and the scientific community (Jiskani, 2020).

A biological agent is a microorganism (bacteria, viruses, fungi, or toxins produced by these organisms) capable of harming or killing humans (Solodoukhina, 2011). Today, zoonotic diseases are a potential bioterrorism threat, and there are concerns that terrorist organizations and rogue states may be developing or acquiring zoonotic pathogens for use as biological weapons (Ryan, 2008). To understand the threat of deliberate release of zoonotic diseases, it is important to first understand the nature of zoonotic diseases themselves. Zoonotic diseases are those that are transmitted between animals and humans, either through direct contact with infected animals or through vectors such as ticks or mosquitoes, and include deadly pathogens as Ebola, SARS and avian influenza (Gori and Tomar, 2020). Some of the biological agents of zoonosis that are commonly used as weapons include anthrax, smallpox, botulism and plague. Zoonotic diseases are considered attractive for use as bioweapons because they are easily transmissible and can be lethal to humans and animals (Pappas *et al.*, 2006). They can cause widespread illness and death, and they can also disrupt social and economic activities. The development and use of biological agents are illegal under international law, and there are strict regulations governing the possession and use of these agents (Pal *et al.*, 2017). In this chapter, we explore the link between biological agents, zoonotic diseases and their impact on public health and global security.

3.2 Historical Overview of Biological Weapons

3.2.1 Bioweapons: Their history and use

The use of zoonotic diseases as biological weapons dates back centuries, but it was not until the 20th century that the technology to weaponize biological agents became more sophisticated (Oliveira *et al.*, 2020). Historically, since ancient and medieval times, many efforts for spread of infectious diseases during wars have been made, using human and animal carcasses, drinking water pollution and other ways having devastating impacts on the enemy (Carus, 2017). The following is a detailed overview of their historical use.

1. **400 BC:** Scythian archers infected their arrows by dipping them in decomposing bodies or in blood mixed with manure.
2. **300–200 BC:** Kautilya's *Arthashastra* talked about use of poison as part of war tactics,

as prevalent in all Puranic wars described in the Hindu scriptures of Ancient India. It also talked about Visha Kanyas, women whose blood and bodily fluids were purportedly poisonous to other humans.

3. For centuries, primitive tribes in Amazonia have used poison dart frogs to coat their arrowheads with toxin. Homer described the use of poisoned spears and arrows in his epic poems, speaking of 'black blood', which is commonly associated with snake bite and poisoned wounds.
4. **1155:** The Holy Roman Emperor Barbarossa poisoned water wells with human bodies (Tortona, Italy).
5. **Siege of Caffa (1346):** During the siege of Caffa, the Mongol army catapulted the bodies of plague-infected individuals over the city walls, causing an outbreak of the disease among the population. In this period, more than 24 million people died.
6. **1495:** The Spanish mixed wine with blood of leprosy patients to sell to their French foes (Naples, Italy).
7. **1650:** The Polish fired saliva from rabid dogs towards their enemies.
8. **French and Indian War (1754–1763):** The British forces gave smallpox-infected blankets to Native Americans to weaken them.
9. **1797:** Napoleon flooded the plains around Mantua, Italy, to enhance the spread of malaria.
10. **1863:** Confederates sold clothing from yellow fever and smallpox patients to Union troops (USA).
11. **First World War (1914–1918):** Both the Allies and the Central Powers conducted research on biological weapons. In the First World War the Germans developed anthrax, glanders, cholera and a wheat fungus. The French were also involved in development of bioweapons.
12. **Second World War (1939–1945):** Japan conducted extensive research on biological weapons and used anthrax, cholera and plague against Chinese civilians and soldiers, resulting in the deaths of thousands.
13. **Cold War (1945–1991):** Both the United States and the Soviet Union conducted research on biological weapons and stockpiled them, but there was no evidence of their actual use.
14. **Anthrax attacks (2001):** In the after math of the 9/11 terrorist attacks in the United States, letters containing anthrax spores were sent to various individuals and organizations in the United States, resulting in the deaths of five people and the infection of 17 others.

3.2.2 History of zoonotic diseases

Zoonotic diseases have been responsible for some of the deadliest pandemics in human history (Bobdey and Ray, 2020). Here are some examples of their historical use.

1. **Plague of Athens (430 BC):** The plague of Athens is believed to have been caused by the bacterium *Yersinia pestis*, which is transmitted by fleas that infest rats. The outbreak resulted in the deaths of an estimated 100,000 people, including the Athenian leader Pericles.
2. **Black Death (1347–1351):** The Black Death was caused by the same bacterium that caused the plague of Athens. It is estimated to have killed between 75 million and 200 million people in Eurasia, making it one of the deadliest pandemics in human history.
3. **Smallpox (16th–18th centuries):** Smallpox was introduced to the Americas by European colonizers and resulted in the deaths of millions of Native Americans, who had no natural immunity to the disease.
4. **HIV/AIDS (1980s–present):** HIV is believed to have originated from a type of chimpanzee in central Africa. The virus crossed over to humans through the hunting and consumption of infected animals.
5. **COVID-19 pandemic (2019–present):** The COVID-19 pandemic is caused by the SARS-CoV-2 virus, which is believed to have originated in bats and crossed over to humans through an intermediate animal host, possibly a pangolin.

3.2.3 Current state of biological weapons programmes worldwide

The current state of biological weapons programmes worldwide is a topic of ongoing concern and debate among experts and policy makers. While many countries have signed and ratified the Biological Weapons Convention (BWC) and pledged not to engage in the development, production, or stockpiling of biological weapons, there are persistent concerns about the potential for illicit biological weapons programmes to emerge or for existing programmes to be expanded (Gross and McGoey, 2015). The following provides a detailed overview of the current state of biological weapons programmes worldwide.

1. **Countries with declared biological weapons programmes:** A small number of countries have officially declared biological weapons programmes in the past, including the former Soviet Union, Iraq and North Korea (Park, 2016). The Soviet Union declared an offensive biological weapons programme in 1972, and while it claimed to have dismantled the programme in the 1990s, there are concerns that some capabilities may still exist. Iraq admitted to having a biological weapons programme in the 1980s and 1990s but claimed to have destroyed it before the 2003 invasion by the United States. North Korea has been suspected of having a biological weapons programme for several decades, and recent reports suggest that it may be expanding its capabilities (Nie, 2020).
2. **Countries suspected of having biological weapons programmes:** Several countries are suspected of having biological weapons programmes but have not officially declared them. These include Iran, Syria and Russia. In recent years, there have been allegations that Russia may be violating the BWC by conducting research and development on biological agents for military purposes (Leitenberg, 2020).
3. **Dual-use research:** The potential for dual-use research, where legitimate scientific research could be used for both peaceful and military purposes, is also a concern. Advances in biotechnology have made it easier and cheaper to manipulate and synthesize genetic material, which could be used to create new and dangerous biological agents (Beedham and Davies, 2020). There have been instances where legitimate scientific research has been misused, such as the case of Bruce Ivins, who used his position as a government scientist to develop anthrax spores that were used in the 2001 anthrax attacks in the United States (Oltmann, 2015).
4. **Non-state actors:** The threat of use of biological weapons by non-state actors, such as terrorist groups or individuals, is also a concern. While it may be more difficult for these actors to acquire the expertise and resources needed to produce sophisticated biological weapons, the potential for the use of simpler, but still deadly, agents such as anthrax or ricin remains a concern (Hammes, 2019).

While the use of biological weapons has decreased in recent years, the threat of their use by state or non-state actors remains a serious concern. The threat posed by dual-use research and the potential for non-state actors to acquire and use biological weapons further complicates the landscape. Ongoing international efforts to strengthen the implementation of the BWC, promote transparency and confidence-building measures, and prevent the misuse of biotechnology are critical to mitigating these threats.

3.3 Zoonotic Diseases and Their Potential as Biological Weapons

Zoonotic diseases are primarily seen as a threat to public health but there are also concerns about their potential as biological weapons. Several zoonotic diseases, such as anthrax, plague and tularaemia, have been weaponized in the past and used in biowarfare. Other zoonotic diseases, such as Ebola and Marburg virus, have been identified as potential bioterrorism agents due to their high mortality rates and ability to spread rapidly (Lotfy, 2015). Zoonotic diseases have the potential to be used as biological weapons due to their ability to cause widespread illness and death. This potential threat has become increasingly recognized in recent years, as advances in biotechnology have made it easier to manipulate and weaponize microorganisms (Goel, 2015).

3.3.1 What are zoonotic diseases and how do they spread?

Zoonotic diseases are illnesses caused by pathogens (such as bacteria, viruses, fungi, or parasites) that can be transmitted from animals to humans. These diseases can spread in various ways, depending on the specific pathogen and the type of contact between humans and infected animals (Pile *et al.*, 2020). According to the United Nations (UN), efforts to develop delivery devices for assassinations or sabotage operations, including a variety of sprays, brushes and injection systems as well as means for contaminating food and clothing, have also been documented (Uchejeso *et al.*, 2021). It is possible to purposefully release a zoonotic disease through a variety of methods, including infecting food or water supplies, releasing infected animals, or using aerosolized agents. Different delivery systems such as missiles, bombs, grenades and rockets as well as spray-tanks mounted on aircraft, vehicles and boats have been created under the programmes for bioweapons development (Bielecka-Oder, 2018).

Some common ways that zoonotic diseases can spread include the following.

1. **Direct contact:** Zoonotic diseases can be transmitted through direct contact with an infected animal, such as through bites or scratches. Examples of diseases that can be spread this way include rabies, Lyme disease and psittacosis.
2. **Indirect contact:** Zoonotic diseases can also be transmitted through indirect contact with contaminated materials, such as through exposure to animal faeces or urine, contaminated water or soil, or contaminated food or water. Examples of diseases that can be spread this way include salmonellosis, *E. coli* infections and leptospirosis.
3. **Vector-borne transmission:** Some zoonotic diseases are spread by insects or other arthropods, known as vectors, that can carry and transmit the pathogens from animals to humans. Examples of diseases that can be spread this way include West Nile virus, Zika virus and Lyme disease.
4. **Airborne transmission:** Zoonotic diseases can also be spread through the air, such as through inhalation of airborne pathogens or through contact with airborne particles. Examples of diseases that can be spread this way include avian influenza and hantavirus.
5. **Foodborne transmission:** Zoonotic diseases can also be transmitted through contaminated food, or through water that has been contaminated by animal faeces, urine, or other bodily fluids. Contaminating food is a popular method of terrorizing civilian populations during wartime or due to different motivations – economic (targeted to financially impact a specific commercial entity or industry unit), political (making a statement, influencing the outcome of an election, forcing a particular political outcome), or various malicious incitements (Tumbarski, 2020). Examples of diseases that can be spread this way include infections caused by *Salmonella*, *Clostridium* and *Campylobacter*.

The use of zoonotic diseases as biological weapons raises many ethical and practical concerns. Unlike other types of biological weapons, zoonotic diseases are naturally occurring, making it difficult to differentiate between a deliberate release and a natural outbreak (Pile *et al.*, 2020). This can complicate efforts to respond to an outbreak and may make it more difficult to identify and hold accountable those responsible for a deliberate release. Furthermore, zoonotic diseases are often associated with animal populations, making it challenging to prevent outbreaks in the natural environment. Efforts to prevent the spread of zoonotic diseases as biological weapons may require significant changes in the way animals are raised, traded and consumed (Novossiolova *et al.*, 2022). This can be difficult to implement in areas where traditional practices are deeply ingrained and where access to healthcare and veterinary services is limited.

3.3.2 Antecedents of zoonotic diseases and their impact on humans and animals

There are many zoonotic diseases that can affect both humans and animals. Each of these diseases has unique characteristics that make them potentially useful as biological weapons. Some examples of zoonotic diseases that have been studied for their potential as biological weapons include anthrax, Ebola virus, plague, brucellosis, Rift Valley fever (RVF), Q fever and tularaemia (Basu and Sandhu, 2021).

Antecedents of zoonoses

1. **Anthrax:** Anthrax is a disease caused by the bacterium *Bacillus anthracis*. The spores of this bacterium can survive for long periods of time in the environment and can be easily disseminated through the air. Inhaling anthrax spores can cause severe respiratory illness, and the disease can also be spread through contact with contaminated animal products (Doganay and Demiraslan, 2015). The use of anthrax as a biological weapon is not new – it has been used in the past by both state and non-state actors. In 2001, anthrax spores were sent through the mail in the United States, resulting in 22 cases of anthrax and five deaths (Blatny, 2022).
2. **Ebola virus:** Ebola virus is a highly infectious virus that causes severe haemorrhagic fever. It is transmitted through contact with the bodily fluids of infected animals or humans. The disease is characterized by symptoms such as fever, vomiting and haemorrhage, and can have a high mortality rate. While the use of Ebola virus as a biological weapon has not been documented, some experts believe that it could be a potential threat due to its high lethality and ability to cause fear and panic (Gunaratne, 2015).
3. **Plague:** Plague is a disease caused by the bacterium *Yersinia pestis*. It is primarily spread through the bites of infected fleas that live on rodents. The disease can cause severe respiratory illness or bubonic plague, which is characterized by painful swelling of lymph nodes. Plague has been used as a biological weapon in the past, including during the Second World War by the Japanese army (Guillemin, 2016). In recent years, there have been concerns about the potential for the bacterium to be used as a bioterrorism agent (Ansari *et al.*, 2020).
4. **Q fever:** Q fever is caused by the bacterium *Coxiella burnetii* and can be transmitted through contact with infected animals or their products, such as livestock or wool. It can cause fever, fatigue and muscle pain in humans, and can lead to chronic illness if left untreated. It can also cause reproductive problems in animals (Tagesu, 2019).
5. **Tularaemia:** Tularaemia is caused by the bacterium *Francisella tularensis* and can be transmitted through contact with infected animals, such as rabbits or rodents, or their products. It can cause fever, headache and muscle aches in humans, and can be fatal in severe cases. It can also cause illness and death in animals (Hirschmann, 2018).
6. **Brucellosis:** Brucellosis is caused by the bacterium *Brucella* and can be transmitted through contact with infected animals or their products, such as unpasteurized milk. It can cause fever, fatigue and muscle pain in humans, and can lead to chronic illness if left untreated. It can also cause reproductive problems in animals (El-Sayed and Awad, 2018).
7. **RVF:** RVF is caused by a virus that is transmitted by mosquitoes and can cause severe illness in humans and animals, including fever, muscle pain and bleeding. In severe cases, it can lead to blindness, encephalitis, or death (Islam *et al.*, 2022).

Impact of zoonoses

1. **Impact on public health:** The impact of biological agents and zoonotic diseases on public health can be significant. They can cause widespread illness and death, and they can also have long-term effects on the health of individuals who have been infected (Ryan, 2008). In addition, the outbreak of a zoonotic disease can have significant economic consequences. For example, the COVID-19 pandemic has led to the closure of businesses, loss of jobs and a significant economic downturn in many countries. In addition to the immediate health impact,

there could be long-term effects on public health, such as an increased risk of developing chronic illnesses or disabilities (Park, 2016).

2. **Impact on animal health:** Zoonotic diseases could also have a significant impact on animal health. In addition to the direct impact on infected animals, there could be significant economic impacts on the agriculture and livestock industries. The outbreak of a zoonotic disease could result in the culling of large numbers of animals, loss of income for farmers and ranchers and disruptions to the food supply chain (Kim *et al.*, 2018).
3. **Psychological impact:** The use of zoonotic diseases as bioterrorism agents could also have a significant psychological impact on both human and animal populations. Fear, anxiety and trauma could lead to long-term mental health issues for those affected and could also result in social and economic disruption (Ellison, 2022).
4. **Impact on global security:** The use of zoonotic agents in bioterrorism can lead to political instability and conflict between nations. The response to such an attack could be influenced by geopolitical tensions and could impact diplomatic relations between countries (Nie, 2020)

3.3.3 Attractive qualities of zoonotic diseases as biological weapons

There are several characteristics that make zoonotic diseases attractive as potential biological weapons (Cong and Elsheikha, 2021).

1. **Easy accessibility:** Many zoonotic pathogens are readily available in nature, making them relatively easy to obtain compared with other biological weapons. For example, anthrax spores can be found in soil and hantavirus can be found in rodent populations.
2. **Ease of transmission:** Zoonotic diseases can easily spread through populations, especially in urban areas where people live near each other. This can result in a rapid spread of the disease, making it difficult to contain and control.
3. **High virulence:** Many zoonotic diseases are highly virulent and can cause severe illness or death in humans. This makes them effective weapons for causing mass casualties and panic.
4. **Limited treatment options:** Many zoonotic diseases have limited treatment options, which can increase the impact of a biological attack. For example, there are no specific treatments for hantavirus and those for Ebola virus infections are limited.
5. **Fear and panic:** Zoonotic diseases are often associated with high levels of fear and panic, due to their potential to cause widespread illness and death. A biological attack using a zoonotic pathogen could cause significant social and economic disruption, as well as political instability.
6. **High morbidity and mortality rates:** Many zoonotic diseases have a high mortality rate, meaning that they can cause severe illness and death in a significant portion of infected individuals. Diseases like Ebola and Marburg virus can have mortality rates of up to 90%. As biological weapons, the high mortality rate of zoonotic diseases makes them attractive because they can cause significant damage to human populations.
7. **Person-to-person transmission:** Some zoonotic diseases can be transmitted from person to person, which means they can spread quickly through a population. This makes them attractive as bioweapons because they have the potential to cause a rapid and widespread outbreak.
8. **Long incubation period:** Some zoonotic diseases have a long incubation period, which means it can take several days or even weeks for symptoms to appear. This makes them attractive as bioweapons because they can be difficult to detect and control.
9. **Potential for genetic modification:** Some zoonotic diseases can be genetically modified to increase their virulence or make them more resistant to treatment. This makes them even more attractive as potential biological weapons. With genetic modification, zoonotic diseases can be

tailored to target specific populations or to cause even more severe illness and death.

10. **Difficulty in diagnosis:** Zoonotic diseases are often difficult to detect, especially in the early stages of infection. This is because the symptoms of these diseases can be like those of other illnesses. As a biological weapon, the difficulty of detecting zoonotic diseases makes them attractive because it can delay the response time of public health officials and allow the disease to spread further.

Due to these factors, zoonotic diseases are considered attractive as biological weapons by both state and non-state actors. These characteristics make zoonotic diseases a serious threat to public health and safety and underscore the importance of ongoing research and development of countermeasures to prevent and respond to potential biological attacks.

3.4 Threat of Deliberate Release of Zoonotic Diseases

The threat of deliberate release of zoonotic diseases is a growing concern in today's world. Deliberate release of zoonotic diseases can occur in several ways. One way is through bioterrorism, where terrorists intentionally release a zoonotic disease with the aim of causing harm to a population or destabilizing a country. Another way is through laboratory accidents or negligence, where a zoonotic disease is accidentally released from a laboratory that is studying the disease (Valdes and Valdes, 2022). The consequences of a deliberate release of a zoonotic disease can be catastrophic. To mitigate the threat of deliberate release of zoonotic diseases, there are several measures that can be taken. These include improving surveillance and detection systems for zoonotic diseases, enhancing biosecurity measures in laboratories and other facilities that handle these pathogens and increasing collaboration and information sharing among public health agencies and international organizations (Frinking *et al.*, 2017). Additionally, investing in research and development of new vaccines, therapeutics and diagnostic tools can help to reduce the impact of zoonotic diseases, whether they are released intentionally or accidentally (Uchejeso *et al.*, 2021).

3.4.1 Risks associated with the deliberate release of zoonotic diseases

The deliberate release of zoonotic diseases poses significant risks to public health, global security and social and economic stability. These risks include the rapid transmission of the disease to humans, the severity of the disease, difficulties in containing the disease, panic and social unrest, economic disruption, political instability, increased strain on healthcare systems and disruption of global trade and travel (Cardoen *et al.*, 2017). Here are some of the potential risks associated with deliberate release of zoonotic diseases.

1. **Widespread illness and death:** A deliberate release could result in widespread illness and death, especially in populations that are not immune to the disease.
2. **Economic disruption:** An outbreak of a zoonotic disease could lead to widespread economic disruption, as people avoid travel and public gatherings. This could lead to losses in industries such as tourism and hospitality.
3. **Social disruption:** The fear and uncertainty caused by a deliberate release of a zoonotic disease could lead to panic and social unrest. People may hoard essential supplies or take other extreme measures to protect themselves and their families.
4. **Increased strain on healthcare systems:** A large outbreak of a zoonotic disease could overwhelm healthcare systems, leading to shortages of medical supplies and personnel.
5. **Political instability:** A deliberate release of a zoonotic disease could lead to political instability, especially in countries that are already experiencing social and political tensions. This could lead to further destabilization and even conflict.
6. **Disruption of global trade and travel:** An outbreak of a zoonotic disease could lead to disruptions in global trade and travel, as countries impose restrictions to prevent the spread of the disease.

7. **Potential for bioterrorism arms race:** A deliberate release of a zoonotic disease could lead to a global arms race in bioterrorism, as countries and non-state actors seek to develop their own biological weapons capabilities in response.

To mitigate these risks, it is important to invest in public health infrastructure and surveillance systems, improve biosecurity measures in laboratories and enhance international collaboration and information sharing. Additionally, research and development of vaccines, therapeutics and diagnostic tools can help to reduce the impact of zoonotic diseases, whether they are intentionally or accidentally released (Serrano *et al.*, 2019).

3.4.2 Political and terrorist motives for an attack, with examples

The potential motives for a deliberate release of zoonotic diseases can be varied and complex, ranging from terrorism to political gain, personal beliefs and ideological differences. Some may seek to cause harm or chaos, while others may be motivated by a desire to gain power, influence, or control. Understanding the possible motives can help to inform efforts to prevent and respond to intentional acts of disease release (Yeh *et al.*, 2012).

1. **Terrorism:** One of the most discussed motives for the deliberate release of zoonotic diseases is terrorism. A terrorist organization may use the release of a disease to cause mass panic, disrupt public life and create a sense of insecurity among the population. The goal may be to undermine public confidence in the government or to advance an ideological agenda (Roberge, 2019).
2. **Political gain:** In some cases, individuals or groups may seek to use the release of a disease to gain political power or influence. This could involve targeting a particular group or community to exploit existing tensions or to create new ones. Alternatively, a government or political party may use the release of a disease as a pretext for increased surveillance, restrictions on civil liberties, or other measures that consolidate power (Beall *et al.*, 2021).
3. **Personal beliefs:** Some individuals or groups may be motivated by personal beliefs, such as a desire to harm animals or to disrupt the food supply chain. Such individuals may not necessarily have a political agenda but may be acting out of a desire to advance their own interests or ideologies (Gerhold and Jessup, 2013).
4. **Ideological differences:** Finally, some individuals or groups may be motivated by ideological differences or religious beliefs. For example, a group may view the release of a disease to punish those who do not share their beliefs or to advance a particular religious or political agenda (Etukudoh *et al.*, 2020).

Overall, the potential motives for a deliberate release of zoonotic diseases are varied and complex and may involve a range of factors such as political ideology, personal beliefs and the desire for power or control. Understanding these motives is important for developing effective strategies to prevent and respond to intentional acts of disease release.

3.4.3 Challenges in responding to zoonotic diseases intentionally released

Detecting and responding to a deliberate release of a zoonotic disease poses significant challenges, due to factors such as the stealthy nature of bioterrorism, the potential for rapid and widespread transmission and the need for a coordinated response across multiple sectors and jurisdictions (Pappas *et al.*, 2006). These challenges require a comprehensive and integrated approach that includes surveillance, early warning systems and strong partnerships between public health agencies, law enforcement and other stakeholders (WHO, 2002).

1. **Difficulty in distinguishing natural outbreaks from bioterrorism:** Zoonotic diseases can occur naturally and it can be difficult to distinguish between a natural outbreak and a deliberate release of a disease as a bioterrorism attack.

2. **Stealthy nature of bioterrorism:** Attackers may use sophisticated methods to avoid detection, such as disguising the release as a natural outbreak or using a low-profile release method that goes unnoticed.
3. **Limited resources:** Many public health systems have limited resources and capacity to respond to an outbreak of a zoonotic disease, especially if the outbreak is deliberate and on a large scale. This can result in delays in response, insufficient treatment options and inadequate surveillance.
4. **Limited surveillance and early warning systems:** Many countries have limited surveillance and early warning systems for zoonotic diseases, which can make it difficult to detect and respond to an outbreak in a timely manner.
5. **Limited diagnostic capabilities:** Many zoonotic diseases have limited diagnostic capabilities, which can make it difficult to quickly identify the disease and confirm that it is a deliberate release.
6. **Limited treatment options:** Many zoonotic diseases have limited treatment options, which can make it difficult to respond effectively to an outbreak and limit the spread of the disease.
7. **Global interconnectedness:** The global interconnectedness of travel and trade can facilitate the spread of zoonotic diseases, making it difficult to contain an outbreak once it has begun.
8. **Sociopolitical factors:** Sociopolitical factors such as distrust of government, civil unrest and lack of cooperation between countries can make it difficult to effectively detect and respond to a deliberate release of a zoonotic disease.

3.5 Biodefence and Biosafety

Biodefence and biosafety are two related fields that focus on the prevention, detection and response to biological threats, whether they are naturally occurring outbreaks or intentional bioterrorism attacks (Tian and Zheng, 2014). Both biodefence and biosafety are critical components of public health and national security, as they aim to protect populations from the spread of infectious diseases and mitigate the potential consequences of biological attacks (Sutton, 2014).

Biodefence refers to the protection against biological agents (such as viruses, bacteria, toxins and fungi) that could be used in bioterrorism attacks or outbreaks of naturally occurring infectious diseases (DiEuliis *et al.*, 2019). Biodefence measures include developing vaccines, diagnostics and therapeutics, as well as enhancing biosafety and biosecurity measures in research laboratories and other high-risk environments to prevent accidental or intentional releases of biological agents (Jonsson *et al.*, 2013). Biodefence measures aimed at preventing deliberate releases of zoonotic pathogens include the development of early warning systems and surveillance programmes to detect the presence of potential biological threats and the implementation of biosecurity protocols to prevent unauthorized access to high-risk facilities or materials (Khalil *et al.*, 2015).

Biosafety, on the other hand, refers to the practices and protocols that ensure the safe handling, storage and disposal of biological agents in research laboratories and other settings where exposure to these agents could pose a risk to human health (Mordini, 2016). Biosafety measures include the use of personal protective equipment, the proper handling and disposal of infectious materials and the maintenance of physical and procedural barriers to prevent the release of infectious agents. Biosafety measures also involve regular training and education for laboratory workers to ensure proper adherence to safety protocols (Burnette, 2021).

In the event of a deliberate release of a zoonotic pathogen, biodefence and biosafety measures would be critical in containing the outbreak and minimizing its impact. The primary goal of biodefence is to prevent and mitigate the impact of biological threats, including deliberate releases of zoonotic pathogens (Canyon and Ryan, 2023). This involves a range of activities, including the following.

1. **Monitoring:** Biodefence experts monitor animal populations for the emergence of new infectious diseases, as well as the monitoring of human populations for unusual disease outbreaks.

2. **Risk assessment:** Biodefence experts evaluate the risk posed by different zoonotic pathogens, based on factors such as their virulence, transmissibility and availability.
3. **Preparedness planning:** Biodefence experts develop plans and procedures for responding to a deliberate release of a zoonotic pathogen, including identifying and containing the outbreak, providing medical treatment to those affected and communicating with the public.
4. **Research and development:** Biodefence experts work to develop new vaccines, treatments and diagnostic tools to detect and respond to outbreaks of zoonotic pathogens.
5. **International cooperation:** Biodefence experts work with international partners to share information and resources to prevent and respond to outbreaks of zoonotic pathogens. Collaboration and coordination among government agencies, public health organizations and research institutions are necessary for the implementation of effective biodefence and biosafety measures to encourage the development and implementation of best practices and standards (Berger *et al.*, 2018).
6. **Biosafety measures:** Biosafety measures are used to prevent accidental or intentional releases of infectious agents in research laboratories and other high-risk settings. Regular training and education for laboratory workers is essential to ensure proper adherence to safety protocols and to prevent the accidental release of pathogens (Gronvall *et al.*, 2021).

3.5.1 Preventing accidental releases and insider threats via biosafety and biosecurity

Biosafety and biosecurity are essential components of the overall management of infectious disease agents and other biological materials that are used in research laboratories, medical facilities and other settings. These measures are designed to prevent accidental releases and insider threats, which could have significant public health and security implications (Finley *et al.*, 2016). The importance of biosafety and biosecurity in preventing accidental releases and insider threats cannot be overstated. Accidental releases of infectious agents can result in serious public health consequences, including disease outbreaks and fatalities (Linkous *et al.*, 2021). For example, in 1978, an accidental release of smallpox virus from a research laboratory in the United Kingdom resulted in the deaths of three people (Rutjes *et al.*, 2023). Therefore, a strong biosafety programme is essential to prevent accidental releases. In the event of an accidental release of a biological agent, a biosafety programme should have procedures in place to detect and contain the release, alert authorities and initiate appropriate measures to prevent the spread of the agent. Insider threats also pose a significant risk, as individuals with authorized access to biological materials may intentionally or unintentionally release infectious agents or toxins (Peng *et al.*, 2018). The threat of insider attacks has increased in recent years, as advances in biotechnology have made it easier to create and manipulate biological agents. The use of biosecurity measures can help prevent insider threats by controlling access to biological agents and toxins and monitoring personnel with access to these materials (Ishaque *et al.*, 2021).

To address these risks, a comprehensive biosafety and biosecurity programme must be established that includes policies, procedures and training to prevent accidental releases and insider threats. The programme should be designed to address the specific risks associated with the infectious agents or toxins being handled, as well as the laboratory or facility in which they are being used (Linkous *et al.*, 2021). The programme should also be regularly reviewed and updated to ensure that it remains effective in preventing accidental releases and insider threats. Biosafety and biosecurity are critical components of preventing accidental releases and insider threats in laboratory and other settings. A comprehensive biosafety and biosecurity programme including policies, procedures and training should be designed to address the specific risks associated with biological agents and toxins and should be regularly reviewed and updated to ensure that it remains effective (Peng *et al.*, 2018).

3.5.2 Biodefence and biosafety challenges

While biodefence and biosafety have made significant progress in protecting against biological threats, there are still several challenges and gaps that need to be addressed (Linkous *et al.*, 2021). Some of the major challenges and gaps in biodefence and biosafety include the following.

1. **Complex zoonotic disease transmission dynamics:** Zoonotic diseases are often transmitted through complex and multifactorial pathways that involve humans, animals and the environment. This makes it difficult to identify and control the sources of infection.
2. **Limited understanding of zoonotic disease ecology:** The ecology of zoonotic diseases is poorly understood, making it challenging to predict and prevent the emergence and re-emergence of these diseases.
3. **Limited surveillance and reporting of zoonotic diseases:** The surveillance and reporting of zoonotic diseases are critical for early detection and control of outbreaks. Surveillance and reporting systems for zoonotic diseases are often limited or non-existent in many countries.
4. **Inadequate laboratory capacity for zoonotic disease diagnosis:** Laboratory capacity for the diagnosis of zoonotic diseases is often inadequate, leading to delays in diagnosis and treatment. There is a need for more investment in laboratory capacity to enhance the speed and accuracy of zoonotic disease diagnosis.
5. **Limited access to vaccines and therapeutics:** Vaccines and therapeutics are critical for the prevention and treatment of zoonotic diseases. However, access to these interventions is often limited, particularly in low- and middle-income countries. This limits the ability to prevent and treat zoonotic disease outbreaks, leading to increased morbidity and mortality.
6. **Fragmented international response to zoonotic disease outbreaks:** Zoonotic disease outbreaks often require an international response to effectively control and prevent their spread. but the international response to zoonotic disease outbreaks is often fragmented, with limited coordination and communication between countries and organizations.
7. **Lack of international standards:** There is a lack of international standards and guidelines for biosafety and biosecurity, which can make it challenging to ensure consistent practices across different countries and regions.
8. **Funding constraints:** Biodefence and biosafety require substantial investments in infrastructure, training and research. Funding constraints can limit the resources available for these activities, compromising preparedness and response capabilities.

Addressing these challenges and gaps in the biodefence and biosafety of zoonoses requires a comprehensive approach that involves improving our understanding of zoonotic disease ecology, enhancing surveillance and reporting systems, investing in laboratory capacity, increasing access to vaccines and therapeutics and improving international coordination and communication (Etukudoh *et al.*, 2020).

3.6 Preventing Deliberate Release of Zoonotic Diseases

Preventing deliberate release of zoonotic diseases is a crucial component of global health security. While zoonotic diseases can occur naturally, the risk of deliberate release of these pathogens by individuals or groups with malicious intent is a growing concern. One of the key strategies for preventing the deliberate release of zoonotic diseases is strengthening laboratory biosafety and biosecurity (Etukudoh *et al.*, 2020).

3.6.1 The role of organizations and governments in preventing the development and use of biological weapons

International organizations and governments play a critical role in preventing the development and use of these weapons through various measures, including the establishment of legal frameworks, international treaties and initiatives to promote transparency and accountability. The World Health Organization (WHO) is responsible for coordinating global efforts to prevent the spread of infectious diseases, including zoonotic diseases that have the potential to be used as biological weapons (Gronvall, 2017). The WHO promotes biosafety and biosecurity measures in laboratories and provides technical assistance to countries in implementing these measures. The WHO also plays a leading role in the development and implementation of international treaties and agreements to prevent the development and use of biological weapons (van Lenteren *et al.*, 2018). The Biological Weapons Convention (BWC) is one such international treaty that prohibits the development, production, stockpiling and use of biological weapons. The UN Security Council has the mandate to prevent the development and use of weapons of mass destruction, including biological weapons (Bailey, 2016). National governments also play a critical role in preventing the development and use of biological weapons. Governments are responsible for establishing national regulations and guidelines for biosafety and biosecurity in laboratories, implementing international treaties and agreements related to the prevention of biological weapons and enforcing sanctions against individuals or countries that violate these regulations, guidelines, treaties, or agreements. Governments also have a responsibility to provide funding for research and development of new diagnostic tools and treatments for zoonotic diseases and other potential biological weapons agents (Ellison, 2022).

3.6.2 Biosecurity and safety techniques to prevent insider threats to laboratories

Improving biosafety and biosecurity in laboratories is essential to prevent accidental releases and insider threats. Here are some of the key strategies that can be employed to improve biosafety and biosecurity in laboratories.

1. **Risk assessment:** Conducting risk assessments is a crucial step in identifying potential hazards and assessing the risk of accidents or deliberate actions. Regular risk assessments can help identify gaps in laboratory safety and security protocols and provide an opportunity for improvement.
2. **Personnel training and education:** This involves providing regular training and education to laboratory staff on biosafety and biosecurity protocols, including the proper handling and disposal of hazardous materials, emergency procedures and reporting of any safety or security incidents.
3. **Facility design and engineering:** The design and engineering of laboratory facilities can impact the safety and security of the laboratory. Implementing measures such as the use of physical barriers, secure access controls and surveillance systems can help prevent unauthorized access to laboratory facilities.
4. **Physical security measures:** Physical security measures, such as access control systems, video surveillance and alarms, can be implemented to prevent unauthorized access to laboratory areas and equipment. Physical security measures can help prevent insider threats by limiting access to sensitive areas and ensuring that only authorized personnel have access to hazardous materials.
5. **Containment equipment:** Appropriate containment equipment, such as biosafety cabinets, autoclaves and waste disposal systems, can be used to prevent accidental releases of hazardous materials. Containment equipment can help prevent accidental releases by providing an additional layer of protection for laboratory staff and the environment (Bailey, 2016).
6. **Quality management systems:** Quality management systems, such as ISO 9001 or ISO 17025, can be implemented to ensure that laboratory procedures and processes are standardized, and that quality is maintained. Quality management systems can help prevent accidental releases by ensuring that laboratory staff follow standard operating procedures and that all laboratory equipment is properly maintained and calibrated (Mukherjee, 2019).
7. **Compliance with regulations and standards:** National and international regulations and standards related to biosafety and biosecurity include the

WHO's 'Laboratory Biosafety Manual', the Centres for Disease Control and Prevention's 'Biosafety in Microbiological and Biomedical Laboratories', and the International Organization for Standardization's ISO 15189 (Trump, 2017).

8. **Implementation of safety protocols:** Implementing safety protocols, such as decontamination procedures, proper waste management and emergency response plans, can help prevent accidents and mitigate the impact of incidents that do occur.
9. **Regular audits and inspections:** Conducting regular audits and inspections of laboratory facilities can help identify areas for improvement and ensure compliance with biosafety and biosecurity regulations and guidelines.
10. **Communication and transparency:** Promoting a culture of open communication and transparency can help prevent accidents and insider threats by encouraging laboratory personnel to report potential safety and security concerns.

3.6.3 Importance of surveillance and early detection systems for zoonotic diseases

Surveillance and early detection systems are crucial for preventing the deliberate release of zoonotic diseases. Surveillance and early detection systems involve the systematic monitoring of animal and human populations for signs of disease outbreaks (Woods *et al.*, 2019). These systems allow for the early identification and response to outbreaks of zoonotic diseases, which can help prevent the spread of disease and limit the potential for intentional release. There are several key components of effective surveillance and early detection systems, including the following (Rodríguez-Prieto *et al.*, 2015).

1. **Animal and human health monitoring:** Monitoring animal and human populations for signs of disease outbreaks, including symptoms and laboratory test results. This requires a coordinated effort between veterinary and human health professionals, as well as close collaboration with local communities.
2. **Laboratory capacity:** Maintaining a robust laboratory network capable of quickly and accurately diagnosing zoonotic diseases. This includes the development and distribution of diagnostic tests and protocols, as well as the training of laboratory staff.
3. **Data sharing and analysis:** Sharing information on disease outbreaks and trends across national and international borders, as well as analysing this data to identify emerging threats and prioritize interventions.
4. **Risk assessments:** Conducting regular risk assessments to identify potential threats and vulnerabilities, and developing targeted interventions to address these risks.
5. **Rapid response capacity:** Maintaining the capacity to respond rapidly to disease outbreaks, including the deployment of medical supplies, personnel and other resources.

Effective surveillance and early detection systems require close coordination between veterinary and human health professionals, laboratory networks and local communities. Regular risk assessments should be conducted to identify potential threats and vulnerabilities, and targeted interventions should be developed to address these risks. Information on disease outbreaks and trends should be shared across national and international borders and analysed to identify emerging threats and prioritize interventions. This requires building a network of partnerships between different stakeholders, including governments, international organizations and local communities.

3.6.4 Legislation and rules of governments for handling biological agents

The handling of biological agents is regulated by governments around the world through legislation and rules designed to prevent the accidental release of dangerous pathogens and the intentional use of biological weapons. These regulations cover a range of activities, including possession, use and transfer of biological agents and toxins. Here, we discuss some of the key legislation and government rules related to the handling of biological agents (WHO, 2020).

Biological Weapons Convention (BWC)

The BWC is a multilateral disarmament treaty that prohibits the development, production and stockpiling of biological weapons. It was signed in 1972 and entered into force in 1975. The BWC aims to promote global peace and security by preventing the use of biological agents as weapons of mass destruction (Leach, 2021). Under the BWC, signatory countries are required to establish and maintain effective national measures to prevent the spread of biological weapons. This includes implementing regulations to control the production, transfer and use of biological agents, as well as providing transparency and confidence-building measures to promote trust and prevent violations (Abdul Majid *et al.*, 2016).

National Select Agent Program (NSAP)

The National Select Agent Program (NSAP) is a United States government programme that regulates the possession, use and transfer of biological agents and toxins that have the potential to pose a severe threat to public health and safety (Wurtz *et al.*, 2016). The NSAP was established in response to concerns about the potential use of biological agents as weapons of mass destruction. Entities that possess or use select agents and toxins are subject to registration, inspection and oversight by federal agencies, including the Centres for Disease Control and Prevention (CDC) and the US Department of Agriculture (USDA). The NSAP was established in response to the 2001 anthrax attacks and is administered by the CDC and the Animal and Plant Health Inspection Service (APHIS) (Walper *et al.*, 2018).

Laboratory Biosafety Guidelines

The Laboratory Biosafety Guidelines are a set of international standards developed by the WHO, which provide guidance on the safe handling of biological agents in laboratories. The guidelines outline the minimum requirements for laboratory facilities, equipment and procedures to ensure the safety of laboratory workers and prevent the accidental release of dangerous pathogens (Kaufer *et al.*, 2020). The Laboratory Biosafety Guidelines are widely recognized as a critical component of laboratory biosafety programmes. They are intended to provide a framework for the development of national biosafety regulations and guidelines, as well as to guide the safe handling of biological agents in laboratories around the world (Pastorino *et al.*, 2017).

National legislation

Many countries have their own legislation and rules governing the handling of biological agents. For example, in the United States, the Federal Select Agent Program regulates the possession, use and transfer of select agents and toxins. In Canada, the Human Pathogens and Toxins Act regulates the possession, handling and transfer of human pathogens and toxins (Wurtz *et al.*, 2016).

Institutional Biosafety Committees (IBCs)

International Biosafety Committees (IBCs) are committees established by research institutions to oversee research involving biological agents. IBCs are responsible for ensuring that research is conducted safely and in compliance with biosafety regulations (Ahuja, 2018).

Export controls

Many countries have established export controls on biological agents to prevent the spread of biological weapons technology. These controls may include licensing requirements and restrictions on the transfer of biological agents to certain countries or organizations.

Criminal penalties

Some countries have established criminal penalties for the illegal possession or use of biological agents. These penalties may include fines, imprisonment, or both.

3.7 Responding to a Deliberate Release of Zoonotic Diseases

The response to a deliberate release of a zoonotic disease would require close collaboration between public health agencies, law enforcement and other government agencies. It would also require the cooperation of the public to follow recommendations for reducing the spread of the disease, such as social distancing, wearing masks and getting vaccinated (Bloom and Cadarette, 2019). Preparedness is key in responding to a deliberate release of zoonotic diseases. Public health agencies should have plans in place to respond to outbreaks of infectious diseases, including procedures for identifying and isolating infected individuals, distributing vaccines and treatments and communicating with the public about the outbreak. Overall, responding to a deliberate release of zoonotic diseases is a complex and challenging task that requires a coordinated and rapid response from multiple stakeholders (Cardoen *et al.*, 2017).

3.7.1 Reaction to intentional release of zoonotic diseases

In the event of a deliberate release of a zoonotic disease, a coordinated response is necessary to minimize the spread of the disease and protect public health (Valdes and Valdes, 2022). The following steps should be taken.

1. **Early detection and alert system:** The first step in responding to a deliberate release of a zoonotic disease is to have an early detection and alert system in place. This includes surveillance systems, laboratory testing capabilities and public health reporting requirements.
2. **Activation of emergency response plan:** In the event of a suspected or confirmed deliberate release of a zoonotic disease, the emergency response plan should be activated immediately. This plan should be comprehensive and include a coordinated response among public health agencies, law enforcement, emergency management and other stakeholders.
3. **Containment and quarantine measures:** The initial response should focus on containing the spread of the disease and implementing quarantine measures to limit further transmission. This includes isolating infected individuals, identifying and tracing contacts and restricting travel and movement.
4. **Treatment and management of cases:** Appropriate medical care and support should be provided, as well as ensuring adequate supplies of medications and other resources.
5. **Communication and public education:** Accurate and timely information should be provided to the public, including information about the disease, how to prevent transmission and the status of the outbreak.
6. **Investigation and prosecution:** In the aftermath of a deliberate release, law enforcement agencies should conduct a thorough investigation to identify the perpetrator and prevent future attacks. Prosecution of those responsible is also an important deterrent to future attacks.
7. **Recovery and restoration:** Once the outbreak is under control, efforts should focus on recovery and restoration of affected communities. This includes supporting those who have been impacted by the outbreak, restoring public confidence in public health systems and ensuring that critical infrastructure is restored.

3.7.2 Coordination and effectiveness challenges in responding to zoonotic diseases

Responding to an outbreak of a zoonotic disease can be challenging due to several factors (Buregyeya *et al.*, 2020). Some of the challenges include the following.

1. **Limited knowledge of the disease:** Zoonotic diseases are caused by pathogens that are often unknown and can be challenging to diagnose and treat.
2. **Delayed detection:** Early detection is crucial to controlling the spread of an outbreak. However, detecting zoonotic diseases can be challenging due to their unpredictable nature and the need for a strong surveillance system.
3. **Lack of coordination:** Responding to an outbreak requires collaboration between

multiple agencies and stakeholders, such as public health departments, animal health departments and the community. Lack of coordination can lead to confusion and delays in implementing control measures.

4. **Limited resources:** Response efforts require adequate resources, including funding, trained personnel and equipment. In many cases, these resources may be limited, particularly in low- and middle-income countries.
5. **Stigma and misinformation:** Mis information and stigma surrounding zoonotic diseases can lead to fear and panic, hindering effective response efforts.
6. **Animal–human interface:** Many zoonotic diseases are transmitted from animals to humans. Addressing this interface requires a One Health approach that involves collaboration between human and animal health sectors, which can be challenging to achieve.

3.7.3 Interaction between international organizations, governments and the public

Effective communication and collaboration between international organizations, governments and the public is crucial in the response to a zoonotic disease outbreak. International organizations such as the WHO work with national governments, academia, non-governmental and philanthropic organizations and regional and international partners to prevent and manage zoonotic threats and their public health, social and economic impacts. This involves fostering cross-sectoral collaboration at the human–animal–environment interface among the different relevant sectors at regional, national and international levels (Berger *et al.*, 2018). The WHO also works to develop capacity and promote practical, evidence-based and cost-effective tools and mechanisms for zoonoses prevention, surveillance and detection through reporting, epidemiological and laboratory investigation, risk assessment and control and assisting countries in their implementation (Meier *et al.*, 2017).

Effective communication and collaboration between governments and the public is also important in the response to a zoonotic disease outbreak. Governments should provide timely and accurate information to the public about the outbreak, including the risks and measures being taken to control its spread (Hilderink and de Winter, 2021). The public should also be educated on how to protect themselves and their families from zoonotic diseases, such as washing hands after being around animals and avoiding contact with sick animals. The effective sharing of information and coordination of efforts can help minimize the impact of the outbreak and reduce the risk of future outbreaks (Isiko *et al.*, 2017). Below are some of the ways in which communication and collaboration can help in the deliberation of a zoonotic disease.

1. **Early detection:** Early detection of an outbreak is critical to containing its spread. Effective communication between international organizations and governments can facilitate the sharing of information about potential outbreaks and enable rapid response measures.
2. **Coordinated response:** In the event of an outbreak, governments can work together to deploy response measures, including the identification and isolation of infected individuals, contact tracing and the deployment of medical supplies and personnel.
3. **Resource sharing:** In many cases, low-income countries may not have the resources to respond effectively to an outbreak. International organizations and governments can share resources, including funding, equipment and personnel, to bolster response efforts in affected countries.
4. **Public awareness:** Effective communication with the public is essential in raising awareness about the outbreak, its causes, symptoms and prevention measures. Governments can disseminate information about the outbreak through various channels, including social media, TV and radio.
5. **Research and development:** Collaboration between international organizations, governments and research institutions can help accelerate research and development efforts

for vaccines and treatments for unknown or newly engineered pathogens.

3.8 International Response and Cooperation

The use of biological weapons is a serious threat to international security, and the international community has developed several mechanisms to respond and cooperate in addressing this issue (Wurtz *et al.*, 2016).

3.8.1 International frameworks and agreements for preventing biological weapons

The evolution of international efforts to control biological weapons and zoonotic diseases has been shaped by the recognition of the potentially catastrophic consequences of their misuse or uncontrolled spread (Heymann *et al.*, 2015). The following are some of the key developments.

Geneva Protocol (1925)

The Geneva Protocol was the first international agreement that prohibited the use of biological and chemical weapons in warfare. The Protocol was drawn up and signed at a conference that was held in Geneva under the auspices of the League of Nations from 4 May to 17 June 1925, and it entered into force on 8 February 1928 (Guillemin, 2017).

Biological Weapons Convention (1972)

The BWC effectively prohibits the development, production, acquisition, transfer, stockpiling and use of biological and toxin weapons. It was the first multilateral disarmament treaty banning an entire category of weapons of mass destruction (WMD). It was signed by 108 countries and entered into force in 1975 (Goldblat, 2020). The BWC has reached almost universal membership with 185 States Parties and four Signatory States. It is the key international treaty governing the use of biological weapons. The BWC has established a few mechanisms to promote international cooperation and response in the event of a biological weapons attack (Elyasa, 2021). These include the following.

1. **Confidence-Building measures (CBMs):** The BWC requires states to submit annual declarations on their activities related to biological weapons. This includes information on facilities, research and development activities and other relevant data. This transparency builds trust among states and enables early detection of potential biological weapons programmes.
2. **Verification:** The BWC does not include formal verification procedures, but the States Parties have established an ad hoc group to develop a protocol for verifying compliance with the treaty. The protocol would provide for on-site inspections and other measures to ensure compliance with the treaty.
3. **Assistance and cooperation:** The BWC requires states to assist each other in investigating and responding to incidents involving biological weapons. The treaty also calls for international cooperation in areas such as scientific and technical cooperation, public health and emergency response.

Chemical Weapons Convention (CWC)

Although not specifically targeting biological weapons, the Chemical Weapons Convention (CWC) is an important international treaty that prohibits the development, production, stockpiling and use of chemical weapons. It requires member states to destroy their chemical weapons stockpiles and production facilities, and to allow for inspections to verify compliance (Frinking *et al.*, 2017).

BWC review conferences (1980–2016)

The BWC holds review conferences every 5 years to assess the implementation of the convention and to identify areas for improvement. The 2016 review conference adopted a final declaration that reaffirmed the importance of the convention and called for strengthened measures to prevent the misuse of biological agents (Gibbons, 2018).

UN Security Council resolution 1540 (2004)

In resolution 1540 (2004), the UN Security Council decided that all States shall refrain from providing any form of support to non-State actors that attempt to develop, acquire, manufacture, possess, transport, transfer or use nuclear, chemical or biological weapons and their means of delivery, in particular for terrorist purposes (Gronvall *et al.*, 2021). The resolution requires all States to adopt and enforce appropriate laws to this effect as well as other effective measures to prevent the proliferation of these weapons and their means of delivery to non-State actors, for terrorist purposes (Finley *et al.*, 2016).

Global Health Security Agenda (2014)

The Global Health Security Agenda is a partnership of over 50 countries, international organizations and non-governmental organizations that aims to prevent, detect and respond to infectious disease outbreaks. It focuses on building public health capacity, strengthening surveillance systems and enhancing communication and coordination among countries (Gostin *et al.*, 2015). It also includes efforts to prevent and control zoonotic diseases. It promotes collaboration among different sectors, including public health, agriculture and wildlife conservation, to identify and address the root causes of zoonotic disease outbreaks (Linkous *et al.*, 2021).

Australia Group

The Australia Group is an informal arrangement among 42 countries that aims to prevent the spread of chemical and biological weapons. It was established in 1985 and has developed a list of controlled items that require export authorization. Member states also share information and coordinate their export controls to prevent the proliferation of these weapons (Fidler, 2020).

International Health Regulations (1969)

The International Health Regulations (IHR) is a legally binding international agreement that requires countries to report outbreaks of certain diseases to the WHO. The IHR was revised in 2005 to include additional diseases and to improve the global response to public health emergencies (Gostin and Katz, 2016). It aims to prevent the international spread of disease and other health threats, including those caused by biological weapons. The IHR requires member states to report any public health emergencies of international concern and to take measures to prevent the spread of disease (Heymann *et al.*, 2015).

The Global Outbreak Alert and Response Network (2000)

The Global Outbreak Alert and Response Network (GOARN) is guided by a steering committee that consists of up to 20 representatives from participating institutions and networks. An operational support team (OST) based at WHO headquarters coordinates and conducts the day-to-day activities of the network. The network at the global level has expanded to include over 300 partner institutions, including government agencies, universities, laboratories, non-governmental organizations, international organizations and a range of related networks in specialist areas and diseases (Basu and Sandhu, 2021). The GOARN assists in increasing global health security through:

- rapidly detecting, verifying and responding to outbreaks of emerging infectious diseases with potential for international spread;
- ensuring that the requisite technical support reaches affected areas immediately; and
- providing support for long-term epidemic preparedness and capacity-building.

One Health (2004)

One Health is an approach that recognizes the interconnectedness of human, animal and environmental health. It promotes collaboration among different sectors, including public health, veterinary medicine and environmental science, to address zoonotic diseases and other health threats (Buregyeya *et al.*, 2020).

The Pandemic Influenza Preparedness (PIP) Framework (2011)

The Pandemic Influenza Preparedness (PIP) Framework brings together member states, industry, other stakeholders and the WHO to implement a global approach to pandemic influenza preparedness and response. Its key goals include: (i) to improve and strengthen the sharing of influenza viruses with human pandemic potential; and (ii) to increase the access of developing countries to vaccines and other pandemic-related supplies. It came into effect on 24 May 2011 when it was unanimously adopted by the 64th World Health Assembly (2011) (Rourke, 2019).

Global action plans

In 2015, the WHO developed a Global Health Security Agenda (GHSA) to improve the world's ability to prevent, detect and respond to infectious disease threats. One of the GHSA's targets is to enhance zoonotic disease surveillance and response, and several countries have developed their own national action plans to address this issue (Wurtz *et al.*, 2016).

Vaccine development

In addition to surveillance and response, efforts are also under way to develop vaccines for zoonotic diseases. For example, there are currently vaccines available for some zoonotic diseases such as rabies, and research is under way to develop vaccines for diseases such as Ebola and COVID-19 (Rashmi and Madhavi, 2021).

3.8.2 Role of international organizations in responding to deliberate releases of zoonotic pathogens

International organizations play a critical role in monitoring and responding to outbreaks of deliberate releases of zoonotic pathogens. These organizations have a variety of roles, from collecting and analysing data on disease outbreaks to coordinating response efforts among different countries and stakeholders. One of the most important international organizations involved in monitoring and responding to disease outbreaks is the WHO (WHO, 2002). The Food and Agriculture Organization (FAO) and World Organisation for Animal Health (WOAH) are also important international organizations involved in monitoring and responding to outbreaks of zoonotic pathogens. The FAO focuses on food security and agricultural development, and works to prevent and control animal diseases that can affect human health (Vasconcelos Gioia *et al.*, 2021). The WOAH, on the other hand, focuses specifically on animal health and welfare and has a role in preventing and controlling the spread of zoonotic diseases (Kim *et al.*, 2023). In addition to these organizations, other international bodies, such as the UN and the International Committee of the Red Cross (ICRC), have a role in responding to outbreaks of deliberate releases of zoonotic pathogens. The UN has various agencies, including the UN Office for the Coordination of Humanitarian Affairs (OCHA) and the UN Development Programme (UNDP), that provide support and assistance during public health emergencies (Nie, 2020). The ICRC provides humanitarian assistance during conflicts, including medical care and support for the most vulnerable populations. International organizations play a crucial role in monitoring and responding to outbreaks of deliberate releases of zoonotic pathogens. These organizations provide technical expertise, coordinate response efforts and work to build capacity in countries to detect and respond to outbreaks. Collaboration and coordination among international organizations is essential for an effective response to these outbreaks and for preventing their spread on a global scale (Singh *et al.*, 2020).

3.9 Case Studies of the Deliberate Release of Zoonotic Diseases

There have been several notable cases in recent history that demonstrate the potential for intentional use of zoonotic pathogens as weapons.

1. **Anthrax attacks in the United States:** One of the most well-known cases occurred in the United States in 2001, when letters containing anthrax spores were sent to media organizations and politicians. The attack resulted in five deaths and multiple infections, and the anthrax was traced back to a government laboratory. The perpetrator, Bruce Ivins, a microbiologist at the laboratory, committed suicide before being

charged. The anthrax attack highlighted the potential for bioterrorism using zoonotic pathogens (Goel, 2015).

2. **Sarin gas in Japan:** Another case occurred in Japan in 1995, when members of the Aum Shinrikyo cult released sarin gas on the Tokyo subway system. Although sarin is not a zoonotic pathogen, the incident highlighted the potential for non-conventional weapons to cause widespread harm. The Aum Shinrikyo cult had also experimented with anthrax and botulinum toxin as potential bioweapons (Pal *et al.*, 2017).
3. **Ricin attack in the United States:** In 2013, letters containing ricin, a toxin derived from the castor bean plant, were sent to several government officials, including the President of the United States. The letters were intercepted, and no one was harmed, but the incident highlighted the potential for the use of naturally occurring toxins as weapons (Jiskani, 2020).
4. **Foot-and-mouth disease outbreak in the United Kingdom:** In 2001, an outbreak of foot-and-mouth disease, a highly contagious viral disease affecting cloven-hoofed animals, occurred in the United Kingdom. The outbreak resulted in the culling of millions of animals, costing billions of dollars in economic losses. Although the cause of the outbreak was not determined to be deliberate, the incident highlighted the potential for the use of zoonotic diseases as weapons of economic sabotage (Flora and Pachauri, 2019).
5. **SARS outbreak in Taiwan:** In 2003, an outbreak of severe acute respiratory syndrome (SARS) occurred in Asia, with China being the epicentre of the outbreak. While the outbreak was not intentionally caused, it highlighted the potential for infectious diseases to spread rapidly and widely. The response to the SARS outbreak led to the development of the IHR, which are designed to strengthen global health security and prevent the international spread of disease (Beedham and Davies, 2020).

These cases illustrate the potential for intentional use of zoonotic pathogens as weapons and the need for continued vigilance and preparedness to prevent and respond to such incidents. Effective disease surveillance and response systems, international cooperation and strengthened regulations and enforcement mechanisms are all necessary to prevent and mitigate the effects of deliberate zoonotic pathogen releases (Pile *et al.*, 2020).

3.10 Future Directions

Preventing and responding to deliberate releases of zoonotic diseases is an ongoing challenge that requires continuous improvement and adaptation to new threats. Some of the future directions that can be taken to prevent and respond to deliberate releases of zoonotic diseases include the following.

1. **Strengthening global bio surveillance:** Enhancing global bio surveillance networks can improve early detection of emerging and re-emerging zoonotic diseases, allowing for rapid responses to potential threats.
2. **Investing in innovative technologies:** Advancements in diagnostic tools, genetic sequencing and other biotechnologies can improve our ability to detect and respond to zoonotic diseases. With the advancement of technology, new tools and techniques have been developed to detect and respond to outbreaks more effectively. Significant improvements have been made recently in many areas, including genomics, monitoring and vaccine research, which can enhance the response to planned releases of zoonotic diseases. Additionally, emerging technologies such as nanotechnology, artificial intelligence and machine learning can be utilized to develop more effective vaccines and treatment methods. These technologies can analyse vast amounts of data from various sources, such as social media, news reports and health records, to identify potential outbreaks early. This approach has been used successfully in predicting the spread of influenza and COVID-19.
3. **Improving collaboration and coordination:** Increased collaboration and coordination between public health agencies, researchers and other stakeholders can help

to identify potential threats and develop effective response plans.

4. **Developing and implementing national and international guidelines:** Developing and implementing guidelines for the safe and secure handling of zoonotic pathogens can help to prevent deliberate releases and ensure that biological materials are handled safely.
5. **Promoting transparency and trust:** Promoting transparency and trust between countries and organizations can help to reduce the risk of malicious use of zoonotic pathogens. Sharing information about potential threats and outbreaks can help prevent the spread of diseases and aid in their response.
6. **Strengthening health systems:** Strengthening health systems can improve preparedness and response capacity to zoonotic diseases, ensuring that necessary resources are available to respond quickly and effectively to outbreaks.
7. **Addressing root causes of zoonotic diseases:** Addressing the root causes of zoonotic diseases, such as deforestation, climate change and illegal wildlife trade, can help to reduce the risk of zoonotic disease emergence.
8. **Increasing public awareness and education:** Educating the public on the importance of proper hygiene, vaccination and reporting of suspicious symptoms can help identify and control outbreaks early. Therefore, continued investment in public education and awareness campaigns is crucial in ensuring the safety and security of individuals and society.

3.11 Conclusion

Preventing the deliberate release of zoonotic diseases is of critical importance to safeguard public health and global security. The urgency of preventing deliberate releases of zoonotic agents stems from the potential for such events to cause widespread and devastating public health consequences. Zoonotic agents are viruses, bacteria, parasites, or fungi that can be transmitted from animals to humans, and they have the potential to cause pandemics if they are released deliberately. The deliberate release of zoonotic diseases, through either bioterrorism or biocrime, poses a significant threat to human populations. Such an act can cause widespread illness and death, disrupt social and economic activities, and create panic and fear among people. In recent years, there have been concerns about the possibility of bioterrorism using zoonotic agents, as advances in biotechnology have made it easier for individuals or groups to manipulate these agents to increase their virulence or make them resistant to treatments. Moreover, many zoonotic agents are highly contagious, making them particularly dangerous if they are released in populated areas. There is also a possibility that the release of zoonotic diseases can have long-term consequences for public health, since it can be difficult to control the spread of these diseases and to treat them once they have spread.

Preventing the deliberate release of zoonotic agents requires a multifaceted approach, including monitoring and surveillance of animal populations, strict regulation of laboratory research and strong international cooperation to prevent illicit trade in biological materials. Additionally, public awareness and education about the risks of bioterrorism are essential to help prevent intentional releases and to respond effectively in the event of an attack. Overall, the prevention of deliberate releases of zoonotic agents is crucial to protect public health and global security. It requires the collaboration and commitment of governments, scientific communities and the public to ensure that appropriate measures are in place to prevent and respond to any potential threat.

The need for increased international cooperation and investment in prevention and response efforts has become increasingly urgent due to the global threat of pandemics caused by zoonotic diseases. The spread of zoonotic diseases is a global issue that requires coordinated efforts from multiple countries and international organizations to prevent, detect and respond to outbreaks effectively. Increased investment in prevention and response efforts is essential to develop new vaccines, diagnostics and treatments for emerging diseases and to enhance global preparedness and response capacity. Furthermore, international cooperation is necessary to support the implementation of effective prevention and response strategies, including improved surveillance and early detection systems, enhanced laboratory capacity and rapid response to outbreaks.

In addition to the public health benefits, investing in global prevention and response efforts has economic and social benefits. By preventing the spread of zoonotic diseases, it reduces the economic and social disruption caused by pandemics and helps to protect the livelihoods of individuals and communities. In summary, increased international cooperation and investment in prevention and response efforts are necessary to combat the global threat of zoonotic diseases. It requires a collaborative effort from governments, international organizations, and the private sector to ensure a coordinated response to the challenges of emerging infectious diseases.

References

Abdul Majid, M., Abdullah, N.A., Mohd Noor, S.N. and Gan, C.K. (2016) The principle of integration in International Sustainable Development Law (ISDL) with reference to the Biological Weapons Convention (BWC). *Sustainability* 8(2), 166. DOI: 10.3390/su8020166.

Ahuja, V. (2018) Regulation of emerging gene technologies in India. *BMC Proceedings* 12(8), 5–11.

Ansari, I., Grier, G. and Byers, M. (2020) Deliberate release: Plague – a review. *Journal of Biosafety and Biosecurity* 2(1), 10–22. DOI: 10.1016/j.jobb.2020.02.001.

Bailey, S. (2016) *The UN Security Council and Human Rights*. Springer.

Basu, A. and Sandhu, H. (2021) International conventions & one health. *The Indian Journal of Medical Research* 153(3), 253–255. DOI: 10.4103/ijmr.IJMR_644_21.

Beall, J.M., Casola, W.R., Peterson, M.N., Larson, L.R., Carr, W.A. *et al*. (2021) Cultural cognition and ideological framing influence communication about zoonotic disease in the era of COVID-19. *Frontiers in Communication* 6, 645692. DOI: 10.3389/fcomm.2021.645692.

Beeching, N.J., Dance, D.A., Miller, A.R. and Spencer, R.C. (2002) Biological warfare and bioterrorism. *BMJ* 324(7333), 336–339. DOI: 10.1136/bmj.324.7333.336.

Beedham, R.J. and Davies, C.H. (2020) The UK biological-warfare program: dual-use contributions to the field of aerobiology. *The Nonproliferation Review* 27(4–6), 309–322. DOI: 10.1080/10736700.2020.1823621.

Berger, K.M., DiEuliis, D., Meyer, C. and Rao, V. (2018) Roadmap for biosecurity and biodefense policy in the United States. *Journal of Health Security*.

Bielecka-Oder, A. (2018) Safety and security regulations against biological threats. In: Radosavljevic, V., Banjari, I. and Belojevic, G. (eds) *Defence Against Bioterrorism: Methods for Prevention and Control*. Springer, Dordrecht, Netherlands, pp. 151–176.

Blatny, J.M. (2022) Biological threats. In: Biggins, P.D.E. and Chana, D. (eds) *CBRNE: Challenges in the 21st Century*. Springer International Publishing, Cham, Switzerland, pp. 47–78.

Bloom, D.E. and Cadarette, D. (2019) Infectious disease threats in the twenty-first century: Strengthening the global response. *Frontiers in Immunology* 10, 549. DOI: 10.3389/fimmu.2019.00549.

Bobdey, S. and Ray, S. (2020) Going viral – covid-19 impact assessment: A perspective beyond clinical practice. *Journal of Marine Medical Society* 22(1), 9. DOI: 10.4103/jmms.jmms_12_20.

Buregyeya, E., Atusingwize, E., Nsamba, P., Musoke, D., Naigaga, I. *et al*. (2020) Operationalizing the one health approach in Uganda: Challenges and opportunities. *Journal of Epidemiology and Global Health* 10(4), 250–257. DOI: 10.2991/jegh.k.200825.001.

Burnette, R.N. (2021) Redefining biosecurity by application in global health, biodefense, and developing technologies. In: Burnett, R.N. (ed.) *Applied Biosecurity: Global Health, Biodefense, and Developing Technologies*. Springer International, Cham, Switzerland, pp. 1–12.

Canyon, D. and Ryan, B. (2023) National biodefense strategies in Southeast Asian states. *Security Nexus* 24.

Cardoen, S., De Clercq, K., Vanholme, L., De Winter, P., Thiry, E. *et al*. (2017) Preparedness activities and research needs in addressing emerging infectious animal and zoonotic diseases. *Revue Scientifique et Technique. Office International des Epizooties* 36(2), 557–568. DOI: 10.20506/rst.36.2.2674.

Carus, W.S. (2017) *A Short History of Biological Warfare: From Pre-History to the 21st Century*. CSWMD Occasional Paper 12. National Defense University Press, Washington, DC.

Cong, W. and Elsheikha, H.M. (2021) Focus: Zoonotic disease: Biology, epidemiology, clinical features, diagnosis, and treatment of selected fish-borne parasitic zoonoses. *The Yale Journal of Biology and Medicine* 94(2), 297.

Dembek, Z.F., Kortepeter, M.G. and Pavlin, J.A. (2007) Discernment between deliberate and natural infectious disease outbreaks. *Epidemiology & Infection* 135(3), 353–371. DOI: 10.1017/S0950268806007011.

DiEuliis, D., Rao, V., Billings, E.A., Meyer, C.B. and Berger, K. (2019) Biodefense policy analysis – a systems-based approach. *Health Security* 17(2), 83–99. DOI: 10.1089/hs.2018.0082.

Doganay, M. and Demiraslan, H. (2015) Human anthrax as a re-emerging disease. *Recent Patents on Anti-Infective Drug Discovery* 10(1), 10–29.

Ellison, D.H. (2022) *Handbook of Chemical and Biological Warfare Agents, Volume 2: Nonlethal Chemical Agents and Biological Warfare Agents*. CRC Press, Boca Raton, Florida.

El-Sayed, A. and Awad, W. (2018) Brucellosis: Evolution and expected comeback. *International Journal of Veterinary Science and Medicine* 6(sup.1), S31–S35. DOI: 10.1016/j.ijvsm.2018.01.008.

Elyasa, Y. (2021) Bioterrorism: The development and its regulations according to the international law. *Lampung Journal of International Law* 3(1), 29–40. DOI: 10.25041/lajil.v3i1.2103.

Etukudoh, N.S., Ejinaka, O., Obeta, U., Utibe, E., Lote-Nwaru, I. *et al.* (2020) Zoonotic and parasitic agents in bioterrorism. *Journal of Infectious Diseases and Travel Medicine* 4(2), 000139. DOI: 10.23880/jidtm-16000139.

Fidler, D. (2020) Nuclear, chemical and biological terrorism in international law. In: Saul, B. (ed.) *Research Handbook on International Law and Terrorism*, 2nd edn. Edward Elgar Publishing, Cheltenham, UK, pp. 80–96.

Finley, M.R., Astuto-Gribble, L.M. and Brass, V.H. (2016) *Biosafety and Biosecurity in Veterinary Laboratories*. Sandia National Lab. (SNL-NM), Albuquerque, New Mexico.

Flora, S.J.S. and Pachauri, V. (eds) (2019) *Handbook on Biological Warfare Preparedness*. Academic Press.

Frinking, E., Sinning, P., Bontje, E., della, C.F. and Abdalla, M. (2017) *The Increasing Threat of Biological Weapons: Handle with Sufficient and Proportionate Care*. The Hague Centre for Strategic Studies, The Hague, Netherlands.

Gerhold, R.W. and Jessup, D.A. (2013) Zoonotic diseases associated with free-roaming cats. *Zoonoses and Public Health* 60(3), 189–195. DOI: 10.1111/j.1863-2378.2012.01522.x.

Gibbons, R.D. (2018) The humanitarian turn in nuclear disarmament and the treaty on the prohibition of nuclear weapons. *The Nonproliferation Review* 25(1–2), 11–36. DOI: 10.1080/10736700.2018.1486960.

Goel, A.K. (2015) Anthrax: A disease of biowarfare and public health importance. *World Journal of Clinical Cases* 3(1), 20–33. DOI: 10.12998/wjcc.v3.i1.20.

Goldblat, J. (2020) The biological disarmament convention. In: Carlton, D. and Schaerf, C. (eds) *The Dynamics of the Arms Race*. Routledge, Abingdon, UK, pp. 170–177.

Gori, S. and Tomar, A.S. (2020) Bioterrorism & biodefense: An environmental and public health preparedness. *Rupkatha Journal on Interdisciplinary Studies in Humanities* 12(2), 1–15. DOI: 10.21659/rupkatha.v12n2.13.

Gostin, L.O. and Katz, R. (2016) The international health regulations: The governing framework for global health security. *The Milbank Quarterly* 94(2), 264–313. DOI: 10.1111/1468-0009.12186.

Gostin, L.O., DeBartolo, M.C. and Friedman, E.A. (2015) The international health regulations 10 years on: The governing framework for global health security. *The Lancet* 386(10009), 2222–2226. DOI: 10.1016/S0140-6736(15)00948-4.

Gronvall, G.K. (2017) Prevention of the development or use of biological weapons. *Health Security* 15(1), 36–37. DOI: 10.1089/hs.2016.0096.

Gronvall, G.K., Trotochaud, M., Hosangadi, D., Inglesby, T.V. and Cicero, A. (2021) *United States–India Strategic Dialogue on Biosecurity: Report from the Seventh Dialogue Session, Focused on COVID-19 Responses in India and the United States: Lessons Learned and Path Forward*. Johns Hopkins Bloomberg School of Public Health. Center for Health Security, Baltimore, Maryland.

Gross, M. and McGoey, L. (eds) (2015) *Routledge International Handbook of Ignorance Studies*. Routledge.

Guillemin, J. (2016) Crossing the normative barrier: Japan's biological warfare in China in World War II. In: Lentzos, F. (ed.) *Biological Threats in the 21st Century: The Politics, People, Science and Historical Roots*. Imperial College Press, London, pp. 17–40. DOI: 10.1142/9781783269488_0002.

Guillemin, J. (2017) The 1925 Geneva protocol: China's CBW charges against Japan at the Tokyo war crimes tribunal. In: Friedrich, B., Hoffmann, D., Renn, J., Schmaltz, F. and Wolf, M. (eds) *One Hundred Years of Chemical Warfare: Research, Deployment, Consequences*. Springer International, Cham, Switzerland, pp. 273–286. DOI: 10.1007/978-3-319-51664-6_15.

Gunaratne, N.D. (2015) The Ebola virus and the threat of bioterrorism. *Fletcher Forum of World Affairs* 39, 63.

Hammes, T.X. (2019) *Technology converges; non-state actors benefit*. Governance in an Emerging New World, no. 319. Hoover Institution, Stanford University, California. Available at: https://www.hoover.org/research/technologyconverges-non-state-actors-benefit#

Heymann, D.L., Chen, L., Takemi, K., Fidler, D.P., Tappero, J.W. *et al*. (2015) Global health security: The wider lessons from the West African Ebola virus disease epidemic. *The Lancet* 385(9980), 1884–1901. DOI: 10.1016/S0140-6736(15)60858-3.

Hilderink, M.H. and de Winter, I.I. (2021) No need to beat around the bushmeat – The role of wildlife trade and conservation initiatives in the emergence of zoonotic diseases. *Heliyon* 7(7), e07692. DOI: 10.1016/j.heliyon.2021.e07692.

Hirschmann, J.V. (2018) From squirrels to biological weapons: The early history of tularemia. *The American Journal of the Medical Sciences* 356(4), 319–328. DOI: 10.1016/j.amjms.2018.06.006.

Ishaque, S., Asrhad, A., Haider, M.A. and Fatima, F. (2021) Biosafety and biosecurity of lab and hospital acquired infections. *Biological and Clinical Sciences Research Journal* 2021(1). DOI: 10.54112/bcsrj.v2021i1.55.

Isiko, J., Khaitsa, M.L., Ekiri, A. and Sischo, W. (2017) Engaging intergovernmental organizations in the training of students on global animal health, public health and food security. *The Pan African Medical Journal* 27, 12. DOI: 10.11604/pamj.supp.2017.27.4.12368].

Islam, K., Carlsson, M., Enquist, P.A., Qian, W., Marttila, M. *et al*. (2022) Structural modifications and biological evaluations of rift valley fever virus inhibitors identified from chemical library screening. *ACS Omega* 7(8), 6854–6868. DOI: 10.1021/acsomega.1c06513.

Jiskani, S.A. (2020) Bioterrorism – are we ready to face another biological war? *Asian Journal of Allied Health Sciences* 72–83. DOI: 10.52229/ajahs.v5i2.632.

Jonsson, C.B., Cole, K.S., Roy, C.J., Perlin, D.S. and Byrne, G. (2013) Challenges and practices in building and implementing biosafety and biosecurity programs to enable basic and translational research with select agents. *Journal of Bioterrorism & Biodefense* 15, 12634–12634. DOI: 10.4172/2157-2526.S3-015.

Kaufer, A.M., Theis, T., Lau, K.A., Gray, J.L. and Rawlinson, W.D. (2020) Laboratory biosafety measures involving SARS-CoV-2 and the classification as a risk group 3 biological agent. *Pathology* 52(7), 790–795. DOI: 10.1016/j.pathol.2020.09.006.

Khalil, A., Tanveer, F. and Shinwari, Z.K. (2015) Pakistan's bio-preparedness with regard to biosecurity, biodefense strategies and policy measures. *Journal of Bioterrorism & Biodefense* 6(132), 1000132. DOI: 10.4127/2157-2526.1000132.

Kim, K.H., Kabir, E. and Jahan, S.A. (2018) Airborne bioaerosols and their impact on human health. *Journal of Environmental Sciences* 67, 23–35. DOI: 10.1016/j.jes.2017.08.027.

Kim, Y., Jones, B.A., Pfeiffer, D.U., Marrana, M., Simmons, H.L. *et al*. (2023) Risk of rinderpest virus re-introduction 10-years post-eradication. *Preventive Veterinary Medicine* 213, 105867. DOI: 10.1016/j.prevetmed.2023.105867.

Leach, B. (2021) Necessary measures: Synthetic biology & the biological weapons convention. *Stanford Technology Law Review* 25, 141.

Leitenberg, M. (2020) False allegations of biological-weapons use from Putin's Russia. *The Nonproliferation Review* 27(4–6), 425–442. DOI: 10.1080/10736700.2021.1964755.

Linkous, B., Burnette, R.N. and Dittrich, S. (2021) Biodefense promotes biosecurity through threat reduction programs and global health security. In: Burnette, R.N. (ed.) *Applied Biosecurity: Global Health, Biodefense, and Developing Technologies*. Springer International, Cham, Switzerland, pp. 51–71.

Lotfy, W.M. (2015) Plague in Egypt: Disease biology, history and contemporary analysis: A minireview. *Journal of Advanced Research* 6(4), 549–554. DOI: 10.1016/j.jare.2013.11.002.

Meier, B.M., Tureski, K., Bockh, E., Carr, D., Ayala, A. *et al*. (2017) Examining national public health law to realize the global health security agenda. *Medical Law Review* 25(2), 240–269. DOI: 10.1093/medlaw/fwx020.

Mordini, E. (2016) The biodefense field. *Bioethics* 30(6), 382. DOI: 10.1111/bioe.12269.

Mukherjee, P.K. (2019) *Quality Control and Evaluation of Herbal Drugs: Evaluating Natural Products and Traditional Medicine*. Elsevier.

Nie, J.B. (2020) In the shadow of biological warfare: Conspiracy theories on the origins of COVID-19 and enhancing global governance of biosafety as a matter of urgency. *Journal of Bioethical Inquiry* 17(4), 567–574. DOI: 10.1007/s11673-020-10025-8.

Noah, D.L., Huebner, K.D., Darling, R.G. and Waeckerle, J.F. (2002) The history and threat of biological warfare and terrorism. *Emergency Medicine Clinics* 20(2), 255–271. DOI: 10.1016/S0733-8627(01)00002-5.

Novossiolova, T., Dando, M. and Shang, L. (2022) Strengthening the web of prevention against chemical and biological weapons. (Video).

Oliveira, M., Mason-Buck, G., Ballard, D., Branicki, W. and Amorim, A. (2020) Biowarfare, bioterrorism and biocrime: A historical overview on microbial harmful applications. Forensic Science International 314, 110366. DOI: 10.1016/j.forsciint.2020.110366.

Oltmann, S. (2015) Dual use research: Investigation across multiple science disciplines. *Science and Engineering Ethics* 21, 327–341. DOI: 10.1007/s11948-014-9535-y.

Pal, M., Tsegaye, M., Girzaw, F., Bedada, H., Godishala, V. *et al.* (2017) An overview on biological weapons and bioterrorism. *American Journal of Biomedical Research* 5(2), 24–34. DOI: 10.12691/ajbr-5-2-2.

Pappas, G., Panagopoulou, P., Christou, L. and Akritidis, N. (2006) Biological weapons: Brucella as a biological weapon. *Cellular and Molecular Life Sciences* 63, 2229–2236. DOI: 10.1007/s00018-006-6311-4.

Park, S.Y. (2016) North korea's military policy under the Kim Jong-un regime. *Journal of Asian Public Policy* 9(1), 57–74. DOI: 10.1080/17516234.2015.1122718.

Pastorino, B., de Lamballerie, X. and Charrel, R. (2017) Biosafety and biosecurity in European containment level 3 laboratories: Focus on french recent progress and essential requirements. *Frontiers in Public Health* 5, 121. DOI: 10.3389/fpubh.2017.00121.

Pavlin, J.A., Witt, C.J., Noah, D.L. and Timoney, P.J. (2002) Bioterrorism and equids. *Clinical Techniques in Equine Practice* 1(2), 109–115. DOI: 10.1053/ctep.2002.34239.

Peng, H., Bilal, M. and Iqbal, H.M. (2018) Improved biosafety and biosecurity measures and/or strategies to tackle laboratory-acquired infections and related risks. *International Journal of Environmental Research and Public Health* 15(12), 2697. DOI: 10.3390/ijerph15122697.

Pile, J.C., Malone, J.D., Eitzen, E.M. and Friedlander, A.M. (2020) Anthrax as a potential biological warfare agent. In: McBride, D. (ed.) *Bioterrorism: The History of a Crisis in American Society*. Routledge, pp. 133–138. DOI: 10.1001/archinte.158.5.429.

Rashmi, P. and Madhavi, B.L.R. (2021) Vaccine development and delivery strategies – A glimpse. *Journal of Vaccines and Immunology* 7(1), 004–008. DOI: 10.17352/jvi.000038.

Roberge, L.F. (2019) Agrobioterrorism. In: Singh, S.K. and Kuhn, J.H. (eds) *Defense Against Biological Attacks*, Vol. II. Springer Nature, Cham, Switzerland, pp. 359–383.

Rodríguez-Prieto, V., Vicente-Rubiano, M., Sánchez-Matamoros, A., Rubio-Guerri, C., Melero, M. *et al.* (2015) Systematic review of surveillance systems and methods for early detection of exotic, new and re-emerging diseases in animal populations. *Epidemiology & Infection* 143(10), 2018–2042. DOI: 10.1017/S095026881400212X.

Rourke, M.F. (2019) Access by design, benefits if convenient: A closer look at the pandemic influenza preparedness framework's standard material transfer agreements. *The Milbank Quarterly* 97(1), 91–112. DOI: 10.1111/1468-0009.12364.

Rutjes, S.A., Vennis, I.M., Wagner, E., Maisaia, V. and Peintner, L. (2023) Biosafety and biosecurity challenges during the COVID-19 pandemic and beyond. *Frontiers in Bioengineering and Biotechnology* 11, 1117316. DOI: 10.3389/fbioe.2023.1117316.

Ryan, C.P. (2008) Zoonoses likely to be used in bioterrorism. *Public Health Reports* 123(3), 276–281.

Sandbrink, J., Ahuja, J., Swett, J., Koblentz, G. and Standley, C. (2022) Mitigating biosecurity challenges associated with zoonotic risk prediction. *Preprint, Available at SSRN 4035760*.

Serrano, I., Gomes, D., Ramilo, D., Rebelo, M.T., da Fonseca, I.P. *et al.* (2019) An overview of zoonotic disease outbreaks and its forensic management over time. *Journal of Forensic Sciences* 64(5), 1304–1311. DOI: 10.1111/1556-4029.14034.

Singh, M.R., Singh, D., Kanwar, J. and Chauhan, N.S. (2020) *Advances and Avenues in the Development of Novel Carriers for Bioactives and Biological Agents*. Academic Press.

Solodoukhina, D. (2011) Food safety and bioterrorism from public health perspective. In: Hefnawy, M. (ed.) *Advances in Food Protection: Focus on Food Safety and Defense*. Springer, Dordrecht, Netherlands, pp. 17–25. DOI: 10.1007/978-94-007-1100-6_2.

Sutton, V. (2014) *Biosecurity Law and Policy: Biosecurity, Biosafety and Biodefense Law*. Vargas Publishing, Lubbock, Texas.

Tagesu, T. (2019) Q fever in small ruminants and its public health importance. *Journal of Dairy and Veterinary Science* 9, 555752. DOI: 10.19080/JDVS.2019.09.555752.

Tian, D. and Zheng, T. (2014) Comparison and analysis of biological agent category lists based on biosafety and biodefense. *PloS ONE* 9(6), e101163. DOI: 10.1371/journal.pone.0101163.

Trump, B.D. (2017) Synthetic biology regulation and governance: Lessons from TAPIC for the United States, European Union, and Singapore. *Health Policy* 121(11), 1139–1146. DOI: 10.1016/j.healthpol.2017.07.010.

Tumbarski, Y.D. (2020) Foodborne zoonotic agents and their food bioterrorism potential: A review. *Bulgarian Journal of Veterinary Medicine* 23(2), 147–159. DOI: 10.15547/bjvm.2232.

Uchejeso, O., Etukudoh, N., Chukwudimma, O., Ogechukwu, E. and Amadi, K. (2021) Coronavirus: The biological threat of our time. *Journal of Current Emergency Medicine Reports* 1(1), 1–7.

Valdes, J.J. and Valdes, E.R. (2022) Biological agents: Threat and response. In: Masys, A.J. (ed.) *Handbook of Security Science*. Springer International, Cham, Switzerland, pp. 739–769.

van Lenteren, J.C., Bolckmans, K., Köhl, J., Ravensberg, W.J. and Urbaneja, A. (2018) Biological control using invertebrates and microorganisms: Plenty of new opportunities. *BioControl* 63, 39–59. DOI: 10.1007/s10526-017-9801-4.

Vasconcelos Gioia, G., Lamielle, G., Aguanno, R., ElMasry, I., Mouillé, B. *et al.* (2021) Informing resilience building: FAO's Surveillance Evaluation Tool (SET) biothreat detection module will help assess national capacities to detect agro-terrorism and agro-crime. *One Health Outlook* 3, 1–13. DOI: 10.1186/s42522-021-00045-8.

Walper, S.A., Lasarte Aragonés, G., Sapsford, K.E., Brown, C.W. III, Rowland, C.E. *et al.* (2018) Detecting biothreat agents: From current diagnostics to developing sensor technologies. *ACS Sensors* 3(10), 1894–2024. DOI: 10.1021/acssensors.8b00420.

WHO (2002) *Preparedness for the deliberate use of biological agents: A rational approach to the unthinkable (No. WHO/CDS/CSR/EPH/2002.16)*. World Health Organization, Geneva.

WHO (2020) *Laboratory biosafety guidance related to coronavirus disease (COVID-19): Interim guidance, 13 May 2020 (No. WHO/WPE/GIH/2020.3)*. World Health Organization, Geneva.

Woods, R., Reiss, A., Cox-Witton, K., Grillo, T. and Peters, A. (2019) The importance of wildlife disease monitoring as part of global surveillance for zoonotic diseases: The role of Australia. *Tropical Medicine and Infectious Disease* 4(1), 29. DOI: 10.3390/tropicalmed4010029.

Wurtz, N., Papa, A., Hukic, M., Di Caro, A., Leparc-Goffart, I. *et al.* (2016) Survey of laboratory-acquired infections around the world in biosafety level 3 and 4 laboratories. *European Journal of Clinical Microbiology & Infectious Diseases* 35, 1247–1258. DOI: 10.1007/s10096-016-2657-1.

Yeh, J.Y., Park, J.Y., Cho, Y.S. and Cho, I.S. (2012) Animal biowarfare research: Historical perspective and potential future attacks. *Zoonoses and Public Health* 59(8), 536–544. DOI: 10.1111/j.1863-2378.2012.01505.x.

4 Surveillance of Veterinary and Human Health in Pertaining Risk Analysis of Zoonoses Throughout the Globe

Barkha Sharma[1*] **and Isha Agrawal**[2]
[1]Department of Veterinary Epidemiology, College of Veterinary Sciences, DUVASU, Mathura, India; [2]Department of Pathobiology, College of Veterinary Medicine, University of Illinois, Urbana-Champaign, USA

Abstract
Recently, we all have witnessed the widespread devastating effects of many emerging and remerging infectious disease which have taken us by surprise and created havoc in both human and animal populations all over the world. Be it COVID-19 or lumpy skin disease, Zika virus or Ebola haemorrhagic fever, each of these diseases has impacted the world tremendously and challenged our capacity to detect the threat in advance and strengthen our monitoring and surveillance network. These outbreaks have given additional impetus to the need for cross-sector engagement as exemplified by the widespread endorsement of the One Health movement by leading international agencies like the Food and Agriculture Organization (FAO), World Organisation for Animal Health (WOAH), World Health Organization (WHO) and successive national governments globally. It is high time we realized the need for multisectoral, multinational collaboration to combat the increasing threat of diseases. Factors for disease emergence are varied. Climate change, burgeoning human populations, increasing wildlife–human interaction, increasing international trade and globalization, and non-judicious use of drugs are a few of the most prominent factors causing emergence and re-emergence of infectious diseases. Various organizations are working all over the globe towards achieving this goal but the road ahead is too long and bumpy. There is a need for a multi-pronged, diversified approach to develop disease management policies involving various sectors of governments and science-stream experts. Early warning systems, disease monitoring and surveillance capacity should be continuously improved and real-time disease status information should be shared all across the globe, because an outbreak of any disease at one place is bound to affect the health of populations in other parts of the world. This chapter shares information regarding the various disease monitoring and surveillance approaches and networks operational all over the world and what further needs to be done to achieve a safer world without disease.

Keywords: zoonoses, One Health, WHO, surveillance, emerging and remerging diseases

4.1 Introduction

During the past few decades, we have witnessed the emergence and re-emergence of so many diseases and global health threats arising from unique and complex interactions of human, animal and environmental factors. Severe acute respiratory syndrome (SARS) was the first pandemic of the millennium, originating from South China in 2002 and quickly spreading all over the world.

*Corresponding author: barkha16vet@gmail.com

 The Handbook of Zoonotic Diseases of Goats (ed. T. Rana)
DOI: 10.1079/ 9781800622852.0004

Almost 60% of all the currently known infectious diseases affecting humans are zoonotic in nature, with nearly three-quarters having a wildlife reservoir (Kruse *et al.*, 2004; Jones *et al.*, 2008; Cutler *et al.*, 2010). Around 75% of emerging infectious diseases are zoonotic. Over 30 new human pathogens have been identified in the past three decades, 75% of which are of animal origin. Rift Valley fever (RVF), SARS, influenza A (H1N1), yellow fever, avian influenza (H5N1 and H7N9 subtypes), West Nile fever, the Middle East respiratory syndrome (MERS-COV) and the dreaded SARS-CoV2 are a few examples. Small rodents, lagomorphs and wild birds are all known to carry zoonotic pathogens and effectively contribute to the global spread of emerging infectious diseases (EIDs).

These diseases are responsible for the staggering statistics of nearly 2.5 billion human illnesses and 2.7 million deaths annually along with unfathomable economic losses. A zoonosis like rabies alone causes more than 59,000 deaths and an economic loss of US$8.6 billion per year all over the world. The 2014 Ebola virus epidemic claimed around 11,316 deaths and economic losses of US$2.2 billion. The economic impact of highly pathogenic avian influenza (HPAI) in South-east Asia was more than US$60 billion and that of bovine spongiform encephalitis (BSE) was more than US$10 billion. Since 1980, a new disease has emerged on average every 7 months. There is absolutely no way to predict when or where the next new zoonotic pathogen will emerge or what its ultimate importance might be.

Infectious diseases also lead to compromised health and disability, accounting for losses of nearly 30% of all 4.9 billion disability-adjusted life years (DALYs) and 25% of all the deaths worldwide (Fauci *et al.*, 2005), causing immense economic losses to governments due to the associated cost of deaths, hospitalization and inabilities.

Zoonoses can be in the form of either endemics already widespread in many geographical areas or epidemics having spatial and temporal distribution. They can be newly emerging, or previously existing but regaining grounds (re-emerging zoonoses), or transboundary animal diseases (TADs), which are highly contagious animal diseases with high socioeconomic impact that can spread extremely quickly across national borders, causing many more deaths in their wake.

In a world where 40% of total agricultural output comes from the livestock sector, which directly or indirectly supports the livelihood and food security of almost 1.3 billion people, these emerging infectious diseases are becoming a great cause for concern. Strong surveillance in remote rural areas of low- and middle-income countries (LMICs) have served as hotspots for various emerging zoonotic diseases, so it is also essential to provide early warning of emerging zoonotic diseases.

Reasons for the emergence and re-emergence of these diseases are myriad. Changing landscape and land usage, changing life patterns, burgeoning population, globalization, international travel and trade are a few such causes. Wet markets, trade of wildlife, bushmeat hunting and poaching leading to aetiological agents of wildlife diseases adapting themselves to cause disease in humans have also been considered to be a major cause of infectious disease emergence. As food production, manufacturing and marketing are now global, infectious agents can be disseminated from the original point of processing and packaging to locations thousands of miles away (Hulebak *et al.*, 2013). A multitude of factors, from climate change, to population displacement into novel ecosystems, social norms such as possession of companion animals and husbandry practices, are radically expanding the contact points and evolutionary pressures for zoonotic pathogens. The continued growth in international trade of animals and animal products has become a sensitive issue for both developed and developing countries by posing the risk of the spread of animal and human pathogens whilst at the same time being an essential activity to ensure worldwide food security and food safety.

4.2 One Health Approach for Effective Zoonoses Surveillance and Control

It has become clear that the source of most human diseases is animals. In disregard for this knowledge, we still continue to have a predominantly human-centric public health approach as evidenced by repeated epidemics and pandemics from Ebola to Middle East respiratory syndrome

(MERS), to SARS-CoV-2. Animal reservoirs present within or around the human populations have been responsible for the majority of high-consequence infectious diseases that have led to nearly 1500 epidemics and pandemics across all countries in the past decade. SARS-COV-2 virus with its ability to move in and out of multiple mammalian species, including humans, has shown us that new approaches are necessary to detect high-consequence zoonotic pathogens. Countries such as the UK, USA and Australia maintain strict livestock public health systems; however, the broader landscape of relapsing–remitting infectious disease interactions between animals and humans at all scales of analysis has not been integrated effectively into preparedness for domestic pandemic threats. The fact that medical and veterinary communities should be synergistic collaborators in outbreak response has been largely neglected.

The One Health approach is a viable strategy for managing zoonotic disease and should be made an integral element of the global health security architecture. It provides an opportunity to shift from silo-based functioning towards a shared-umbrella approach to handle zoonotic diseases at human, animal and environment interfaces in a much more efficient way. Real-time sharing of valuable information between all the stakeholders is the key to effective and prompt diagnosis and management of zoonotic diseases. Syndromic surveillance (reporting of disease indicators) and One Health approaches may form effective surveillance systems in rural communities. Enhanced capacity for early detection of any such emerging zoonoses is the most crucial step towards controlling and preventing any further outbreaks. Cross-sectional engagement emphasis by leading international agencies like the World Health Organization (WHO), the World Organisation for Animal Health (WOAH), Food and Agriculture Organization (FAO), etc. is proof of this.

4.3 Need for Disease Surveillance, Risk Analysis and Mitigation

The term surveillance was first used during the 19th century and came from the French word *surveiller*, meaning 'to oversee or to watch', and indicated keeping a watch over a group of people during the French Revolution. Later on, this term has been widely used by epidemiologists and other health professionals to mean keeping an eye on disease outbreaks and other health-related events in human and animal populations. Although the terms monitoring and surveillance have been used interchangeably when describing the need for watchfulness over a disease situation, they are different and should be used appropriately.

- **Disease monitoring** focuses on identifying a specific disease or group of diseases to ascertain changes in prevalence and to determine the rate and direction of disease spread. It lacks an action to prevent or control the health problem that is being monitored.
- **Disease surveillance** is a more intense form of monitoring that includes analysing the obtained information and subsequently taking corrective action.

Disease surveillance forms an integral part of any disease control programme since it enables early predictions, rapid forecast, identification and prevention of transboundary threats and in-time corrective action. Effective and sustainable disease surveillance systems need to be sensitive, specific, timely and representative. A small lapse in this entire process makes disease prevention, control and risk mitigation much more difficult. Sharing of accurate surveillance data of humans and animals can substantially improve public health through rapid and timely detection of diseases before they cause havoc, as shown in Kenya. Good-quality authentic data are the basis of a robust disease monitoring and surveillance system (MO&SS) with the ultimate goal of developing an effective disease control programme and intervention strategies to reduce the frequency of a specific disease (Christensen, 2001). Data can be either primary, gathered actively through actual field surveys (active surveillance), or secondary, collected for other purposes (passive surveillance). Different goals and requirements need different surveillance methods. Currently there has been a broad interest in certain aspects of disease surveillance such as risk-based surveillance, genomic surveillance, spatio-temporal visualization and analysis of surveillance data. Animals can serve as sentinels for bioterrorist or natural infectious disease epidemics (sentinel surveillance). Surveillance systems can also contribute to the identification of disease priorities at national and subnational levels and lead to the prompt recognition of emerging disease problems. Participatory epidemiological methods and community health networks are beginning to be integrated as part of routine disease reporting systems.

4.4 Information and Reporting Systems and Health Networks

As in most other technical and management fields, collection of relevant and authentic real-time information is the key to effective disease surveillance. The major goal of a modern disease information and reporting system is to provide such information from the field, in a processed and usable form for national policy makers and field staff, enabling them to devise and implement appropriate actions for effective disease control. An information system provides a platform to exchange relevant information between interested users. Such systems play an important role in surveillance of endemic diseases and fulfilling international reporting needs. They provide information for the economic assessment of diseases, and their control, and monitor the technical efficacy of control programmes, along with monitoring productivity and managing laboratory data.

Various disease information systems are operational throughout the world. Computerized veterinary information systems have a history dating back to the mid-1960s (Hutton, 1969).

4.5 International Disease Monitoring and Surveillance

Epidemics and outbreaks of infectious diseases anywhere in the world can be potential international public health emergencies requiring immediate and comprehensive multidisciplinary responses at a global level. The current requirements are to share the latest knowledge and knowhow with poorer regions of the world, strengthen primary care services and health systems and devise common international laws for enforcing strategies to tackle outbreaks of such infectious diseases effectively. Integrated surveillance for zoonoses is uncommon. Only 19% of zoonoses surveillance systems cover humans and animals (Day *et al.*, 2012). As there is no single institution with the ability to guarantee health safety worldwide, collaboration by international agencies, national governments and individuals with special expertise is important. Several global disease surveillance systems and their networks have been instituted primarily for detecting either human outbreaks of emerging zoonotic diseases or animal outbreaks of animal diseases. These have focused primarily on diseases such as human immunodeficiency virus/acquired immunodeficiency syndrome (HIV/AIDS), tuberculosis (TB), malaria, cholera, vaccine-preventable diseases and those causing high morbidity and mortality. Major stakeholders in this field are the WOAH, WHO and FAO (these three are collectively known as International Technical Agencies or the Tripartite organizations) and the World Trade Organization (WTO). They are continuously making conscious efforts to put health on the agenda of all policy and decision makers and encouraging them to tackle health issues using an integrated approach. They have emphasized the integration of national disease surveillance systems with international systems for better and more effective prevention of diseases from spreading across the national borders (WOAH and FAO, 2004). They have standardized and implemented legally binding instruments and voluntary norms for the protection and promotion of health in the context of globalization. In 2019, the Tripartite organizations developed the Tripartite Zoonoses Guide (TZG) to provide guidance for addressing zoonotic diseases at global level.

The Program for Monitoring Emerging Diseases (ProMED-mail) was one of the first online disease reporting systems; it was introduced globally in 1994 after the success of the internet and is part of the International Society for Infectious Diseases (ISID) in Boston, Massachusetts. Its main intent is to assist local, national and international organizations by worldwide dissemination of information on outbreaks of emerging infectious diseases and toxins of humans, animals and crop plants and the threat posed by their potential use for bioterrorism. It has reported several emerging diseases for the first time, including outbreaks of Ebola virus in Zaire (1995), West Nile in the USA (1999), SARS in China (2002) and H5N1 avian influenza in Indonesia (2003).

4.6 World Health Organization (WHO)

The first fully empowered international agency of the United Nations (UN) in the field of global public health (incorporating the Office International d'Hygiene Publique and the League of Nations), the WHO came into force on 7 April 1948, the day that is celebrated every year as World Health Day. The WHO was the first agency to work for the international promotion of health, with initial priority areas being malaria, TB, sexually transmitted diseases (STDs), maternal and childcare, and nutritional and environmental hygiene. In 1977, it adopted the ambitious goal of 'Health for All'. The WHO Global Influenza Programme (GIP) is the oldest disease surveillance and control programme. Eradication of smallpox in 1979 was the first WHO victory. It started its Global Polio Eradication initiative in 1988 and its Stop TB and Measles initiatives in 2000 and 2001, respectively. The WHO assists affected countries by providing technical expertise and supplies and by promoting national and international programmes for the control of diseases like rabies, anthrax, leptospirosis, RVF and toxoplasmosis. In 2006, the WHO launched the Foodborne Disease Burden Epidemiology Reference Group (FERG) to build a framework estimating the global burden of foodborne disease. It has developed integrated global alert and response systems for epidemics and other public health systems, like the Global Outbreak Alert and Response Network (GOARN) and the Global Public Health Intelligence Network (GPHIN) in collaboration with the Public Health Agency of Canada. In 1992, a London-based database, the Advanced Veterinary Information System (AVIS), was established with the help of FAO and OIE (the OIE is now known as the WOAH) for the control of animal diseases. The WHO Global Salm-Surv (GSS) is a growing international surveillance system for *Salmonella* and other major foodborne pathogens. The WHO International Health Regulations (IHR-2005) and Global Health Security Agenda (GHSA) are a step in the right direction for enhanced laboratory capacity and surveillance for possible zoonotic disease outbreaks. The GHSA, launched in 2014, is a growing partnership of more than 50 nations, and non-government stakeholders and international organizations.

4.6.1 International Health Regulations (IHR-2005)

The IHR is an international treaty, legally binding on 196 countries, including the 194 WHO member states, adopted by the WHO in 2005 (coming into force on 15 June 2007) to fulfil the need for a better disease surveillance and response tool at a global level. IHR-2005 has tried to establish a global surveillance system which focuses on detection and containment of public health emergencies of international concern (PHEIC) at the source itself. It requires all 194 WHO member states to set up a National Focal Point (NFP) to be in regular touch with the WHO in order to strengthen their capacities for disease detection, assessment, reporting and response.

4.6.2 Global Early Warning and Response System (GLEWS)

The Tripartite (the WHO, FAO and OIE/WOAH) Global Early Warning and Response System (GLEWS) has a multidisciplinary approach to perform global animal disease surveillance, risk assessment and disease intelligence. It supports member countries to collect and manage disease information systems and to support early warning systems (EWSs) at local, regional and national levels.

4.7 Food and Agriculture Organization (FAO)

The FAO of the United Nations is a Rome-based UN agency established on 16 October 1945 with a mandate to fight hunger, malnutrition and extreme poverty. In September 2012, the priorities were expanded to include joint action on progressive control of TADs like foot-and-mouth disease (FMD), goat plague (PPR) (*peste de petits ruminants*) and RVF, establishment of regional animal health centres, and joint work on food safety and wildlife diseases, and aquatic diseases and aquaculture. The FAO and WOAH aim to provide a system for efficient exchange of disease information, so that every member country of the WOAH and/or FAO can be ready in advance for any disease outbreak that threatens their borders.

4.7.1 Animal Genomics for Animal Health (AGAH)

The FAO's Animal Health Service includes Animal Genomics for Animal Health (AGAH), which mainly assists member countries in controlling animal diseases along with improving livestock production, reinforcing networks of reference laboratories for specific diseases and promoting the application of biotechnology for disease diagnosis and vaccine production. AGAH has played a major role in prevention, diagnosis and control of diseases such as FMD, trypanosomiasis, African swine fever (ASF), RVF and screwworm (through the Screwworm Emergency Centre (SECNA) in North Africa).

4.7.2 Emergency Prevention System (EMPRES)

The Emergency Prevention System (EMPRES) against transboundary animal and plant pests and diseases is an FAO initiative, established in 1994 for the surveillance and control of livestock epidemics like rinderpest (RP) initially but now FMD, contagious bovine pleuropneumonia (CBPP), PPR, etc. It prepares prevention and prediction models, disseminates warning messages and implements risk communication. The EMPRES Global Animal Disease Information System (EMPRES-i) is a web-based application that feeds information to the GLEWS for major transboundary animal diseases, including zoonoses. OpenFlu DB is an open database for accurate surveillance of influenza virus, linked with EMPRESi. EMAi is an Event Mobile Application for improved disease reporting and communication in Uganda (since 2013), Mali (since 2015) and Zanzibar (United Republic of Tanzania) (since 2016).

4.7.3 European Commission for the control of FMD (EuFMD)

An autonomous body within FAO, with headquarters in Rome, EuFMD was founded in 1954 in response to the widespread epidemics of FMD in Europe in the early 1950s. It collects and disseminates information on foot-and-mouth disease outbreaks to member countries to diagnose, control and prevent the disease. It also registers available virus stocks for use in vaccine production.

4.7.4 Global Framework for the progressive control of Transboundary Animal Diseases (GF-TADs)

GF-TADS is a joint FAO and OIE (now the WOAH) initiative started in 2004, with the WHO as a partner for the zoonoses, to address the spread of TADs. It works by developing global and regional early warning systems, enabling new research for sustained effects on disease management at molecular and ecological level and promoting safe trade in livestock and animal products at all levels.

4.8 The World Organisation for Animal Health (WOAH)

The WOAH is an intergovernmental organization, originally established as the Office International des Epizooties (OIE) in 1924 as an aftermath of a rinderpest outbreak in 1920 in Belgium from Indian zebu cattle destined for Brazil which were transiting via the port of Antwerp, reintroducing the cattle plague to Europe. In 2003, it became the World Organisation for Animal Health, but retained the original OIE acronym until 2022, when it became known as the WOAH.

Since its inception, it has been instrumental in providing recent authentic information on animal disease situation (TADs and zoonoses included), surveillance and control throughout the world, harmonizing regulations and setting standards for trade in animals and animal products among member countries (Blajan and Chillaud, 1991; Bruckner, 2009). Member states are required to submit timely reports regarding status of OIE/WOAH listed diseases in their territories. A twinning programme links the OIE/WOAH reference laboratories (RLs) and collaborating centres (CCs) to selected local laboratories to develop local competence in disease diagnostics up to the OIE/WOAH standards, making them self-sufficient to provide support to other countries. These laboratories may apply to become an RL or CC themselves.

Although the WOAH's major emphasis is on global regulation of animal diseases and zoonoses, it also works towards achieving the goals of the Convention on Biological Diversity (CBD) along with FAO and various other organizations. It has introduced the concept of zoning the disease-free areas within an infected country, to facilitate the trade in animals and animal products from that country.

4.8.1 International standard setting activities of the WOAH

The WTO Agreement on the Application of Sanitary and Phytosanitary Measures (the SPS Agreement 1995) aims to minimize the negative effects of health restrictions on international trade. It recognizes the 'three sisters' consisting of the WOAH, International Plant Protection Convention (IPPC) and the Codex Alimentarius Commission (CAC) as the international standard-setting body for the sanitary safety of international trade in animals and animal products. The standards are included in various OIE/WOAH publications such as the *Terrestrial Animal Health Code*, the *Aquatic Animal Health Code*, the *Manual of Diagnostic Tests and Vaccines for Terrestrial Animals* and the *Manual of Diagnostic Tests for Aquatic Animals*.

4.8.2 World Animal Health Information System and Database (WAHIS and WAHID) interface and GLEWS

The World Animal Health Information System (WAHIS) is an internet-based computer system to process and share real-time data on the status of OIE/WOAH listed animal diseases in member countries with the international community (Cirkel, 2010; Kshirsagar *et al.*, 2013). It replaced the former OIE/WOAH web interface named Handistatus II System in 2006.

WAHIS has two components: the early warning system (EWS), which informs the international community of relevant epidemiological events; and the monitoring system (MS), which monitors WOAH listed diseases over real time.

OIE/WOAH, together with the WHO and FAO, also established the internet-based GLEWS to share information on disease outbreaks and epidemiological analysis of major animal diseases and zoonoses. The GLEWS initiative does not duplicate the work done by WAHIS and WAHID (Domenech *et al.*, 2006).

4.8.3 Other joint activities

WAHIS and WAHID are supported in their endeavours by services rendered by smaller disease-tracking initiatives such as ProMED, Emerging Health Threat Forum (EHTF), the Global Infections Diseases Epidemiology Network (GIDEON), Animal Health and Emerging Animal Diseases (AHEAD), the Food Safety Network (FSnet) and Agriculture Network (AGnet), etc. (Burgos and Otte, 2009), along with the Centers for Disease Control and Prevention, located in USA (USCDC) and in Europe (ECDC).

The FAO and WOAH have developed their programmes and activities to address the problem of controlling transboundary and emerging diseases. These organizations generate authentic and reliable information on animal health and productivity which can be utilized by various regional and global agencies towards achieving the goal of a disease-free world. The FAO, WOAH and WHO have long-standing experience in direct collaboration regarding disease control and surveillance. In 2019, the

Tripartite organization – the FAO, WHO and WOAH – developed the Tripartite Zoonoses Guide (TZG) to provide baseline guidance for addressing zoonotic diseases. The need for wildlife health surveillance has also been stressed by many international organizations and a European wildlife health network was set up in February 2010 as the EWDA (European Wildlife Disease Association) Network for Wildlife Health Surveillance in Europe (Kuiken *et al.*, 2011).

The Generalized One Health Framework (GOHF), developed by experts at the USCDC and FAO, provides recommendations for how to use a One Health approach to improve multisector collaboration and to enhance the prevention and control of zoonotic disease.

4.9 The World Trade Organization (WTO)

One of the most significant outcomes of the Uruguay Round (the last of a series of multilateral negotiations known as the 'trade rounds') of the 1980s and early 1990s was the transformation of the General Agreement on Tariffs and Trade (GATT, 1948–1994) into the WTO and the signing in 1994 of the Application of Sanitary and Phytosanitary Measures Agreement (known as the SPS Agreement), with the aim to minimize the negative effects of health restrictions on international trade. This Agreement recognizes the international standards adopted by the WOAH in matters of animal health and zoonoses and those adopted by the CAC ('the Commission') in matters of food safety and it is essential for international trade in animal and animal products.

4.10 Disease Monitoring and Surveillance at Regional and Sub-Regional Level

Disease monitoring and surveillance at sub-regional and regional levels are quite challenging, because the reasons, requirements and the aptitude for dealing with disease at a regional level requires an entirely different and participatory approach. Regional health networks cover a wider geographical area than a single country (Dufour and Hendrikx, 2009) and show a bottom-up approach as they connect local, national and transnational surveillance along with top-down global and larger regional systems through horizontal cooperation across the borders and sectors.

Major international organizations have initiated various regional entities addressing the specific regional needs in different regions of the world. FAO was probably the first international organization to realize the requirement for a regional approach to combat diseases at regional level. The OIE (now the WOAH) followed suit and recommended strong regional coordination and cooperation between countries of a particular region.

- The 62nd session of the OIE in 1994 included the Regional Strategy for Control of Animal Diseases (**RESCAD**) to prevent, control or eradicate the great epizootics, major zoonoses, etc.
- The FAO has initiated the Middle and Near East Regional Animal Production and Health Project (**MINEADEP**), the Pan African Rinderpest Campaign (**PARC**), the West Asian RP Eradication Campaign (**WAREC**), the Screwworm Emergency Centre in North Africa (**SECNA**) and the Regional Animal Disease Surveillance and Control Network (**RADISCON**). The Association of South-east Asian Nations (**ASEAN**) and South Asian Association for Regional Cooperation (**SAARC**) in Asia and the Caribbean Animal Health Network (**CaribVET**) (Abreu *et al.*, 2011) are also striving towards achieving a similar goal of animal disease control in Asia and the Caribbean, respectively.
- **RADISCON** *for North Africa, the Middle East and the Arab Peninsula* was founded in 1996 as a joint project of FAO and the International Fund for Agricultural Development (**IFAD**) to promote animal disease surveillance in *North Africa* and the Middle East.
- Founded in 1962, the Canadian Animal Health Emergency Management (**CAHEM**) strategy has 52 member countries divided under six regions representing East, Central and Southern Africa, West Africa,

Australasia/Oceania, Canada/Caribbean and UK/Mediterranean.

- In 2009, the Nuclear Threat Initiative (**NTI**) launched a Connecting Organizations for Regional Disease Surveillance (**CORDS**), a global non-governmental alliance to link regional and sub-regional infectious disease networks. In all, six sub-regional networks (EAIDSNet, SACIDS, SEEHN, APEIR, MECIDS and MBDS) came together to form CORDS. Its main purpose is to speed up the capabilities of all CORDS network members by combining the strengths of all networks of the area in order to boost the global surveillance against various infectious diseases of humans and animals. It further supports the mandate of the FAO, WHO and OIE/WOAH to improve the vision of global health security. Its vision is a world united against infectious diseases.
- The Global Infectious Diseases Epidemiology Network (**GIDEON**) is a web-based program for diagnosis and informatics in infectious diseases.
- The USAID Emerging Pandemic Threats (**EPT**) program (**PREDICT**) was launched in 2009 to enhance global capacity to identify threats of zoonotic viral pandemics at wildlife–human interfaces. It became the largest zoonotic virus surveillance project worldwide, establishing infrastructure and expertise required for the operation of pandemic threat surveillance and diagnostics to support the One Health Workforce (**OHW**). The huge success of EPT led to the launch of **EPT2**, which aims to: discover diseases of known and unknown origin; minimize the possibility of disease outbreaks by reducing human activities that promote disease spillover; boost national readiness; and ultimately reduce the repercussions of novel zoonotic pathogen emergence.
- The Agriculture Research Centre for Institute Development (**CIRAD**) (Centre de coopération internationale en recherche agronomique pour le developpement) is a French agricultural research and international cooperation organization for the sustainable development of more than 100 tropical and Mediterranean countries.

4.10.1 North, Central and South America

The Conference of Research Workers in Animal Health (**CRWAD**) is a non-profit organization, based in South Dakota, USA. It was established in 1920 with the sole purpose of discussing and disseminating research advances in animal diseases.

Zoonotic disease surveillance in the USA usually comes under the aegis of Centers for Disease Control and Prevention (**CDC**) and the Council of State and Territorial Epidemiologists (**CSTE**). Both collectively administer the national Notifiable Disease Surveillance System (**NDSS**), which is a common platform to share relevant information regarding the occurrence and spread of state-reportable and nationally notifiable infectious between public health practitioners at local, state and national levels to support disease prevention and control. The list of nationally notifiable diseases is routinely updated based on the need to respond to emerging priorities. CDC's National Center for Emerging and Zoonotic Infectious Diseases (**NCEZID**) is responsible for fighting against zoonotic infections. Wildlife disease surveillance and research in the USA is the responsibility of the US Geological Survey (**USGS**) in collaboration with the US Association of Fish and Wildlife Agencies (**USFWS**). The USGS is in the process of developing a national wildlife disease database. The National Wildlife Health Center (**NWHC**) in Wisconsin is a BSL-3 laboratory dedicated to wildlife surveillance.

Apart from this, the United States Department of Agriculture (USDA) Animal Plant Health Inspection Services – Veterinary Services (**APHIS–vs**) and the Centers of Epidemiology and Animal Health (**CEAH**) are also engaged in keeping tabs on the zoonotic disease situation in the USA. The National Animal Health Monitoring System (**NAHMS**) initiated by USDA–APHIS in 1983 is a national-level, macroscale system, designed to collect, analyse and disseminate data on animal health management and productivity across the USA.

- In 1980, the International Clinical Epidemiology Network (**INCLEN**), a unique global network of clinical epidemiologists, biostatisticians, health social scientists, health economists and other health professionals, was established by The Rockefeller Foundation for collaborative, interdisciplinary, evidence-based research on high-priority health problems, including both communicable and non-communicable diseases, promotion of healthcare and efficient use of resources.

- **Pulse-Net** is a nationwide foodborne disease surveillance system in the USA.
- The Inter-American Cooperation Group on Animal Health (Gruppo Interamericano de Coordinación Salud Animal) (**GICSA**) is a platform to exchange information, avoid duplication and promote complementary support of specific activities. It comprises the Pan American Health Organization, the Pan American Zoonoses Center, the Pan American FMD Center, OIE/WOAH and the Regional International Organization for Plant Protection and Animal Plant Health.
- The Pan American Health Organization (**PAHO**), created in 1902, works to promote and coordinate efforts of American countries to control the spread of infectious diseases and also supports veterinary public health services concerning zoonoses and sanitary inspection of livestock and fishery products. The Pan American Center for FMD and VPH (**PANAFTOSA/VPH**) is a specialized PAHO centre for prevention, control and elimination of zoonoses, improvement of food safety and eradication of FMD.
- The Inter-American Institute for Cooperation on Agriculture (**IICA**) provides technical assistance to veterinary services through regional mechanisms such as the Inter-American Laboratories Network, Animal and Plant Health Information and Monitoring Network and the Caribbean Animal and Plant Health Information Network.
- The Regional International Organization for Plant Protection and Animal Health (Organismo Internacional Regional de Sanidad Agropecuoría) (**OIRSA**) works to improve plant and animal health and quarantine services and to develop and coordinate programmes for prevention, control and eradication of diseases in its member countries – Belize, Costa Rica, Dominican Republic, El Salvador, Guatemala, Honduras, Mexico, Nicaragua and Panama.
- The Caribbean Animal Health Network (**CaribVet**) was created in 2006 to establish a consensus in the national veterinary services of all Caribbean countries and territories in order to improve animal and veterinary public health within the region (Abreu *et al.*, 2011).

4.10.2 Africa

Animal disease surveillance programmes within the African Continent are facilitated by the OIE (WOAH), FAO, European Union (**EU**), Organisation of African Unity/Inter-African Bureau for Animal Resources (**OUA/IBAR**) and regional organizations such as the Southern African Development Coordination Conference (**SADCC**) and the Southern African Regional Commission for the Conservation and Utilisation of the Soil (**SARCUSS**).

- The Inter-African Bureau for Animal Resources (**IBAR**) is based at Nairobi, Kenya, and is a technical branch of the Organisation of African Unity (**OAU**) (since replaced by the African Union (**AU**)) dealing with livestock in Africa. It periodically issues the *Bulletin of Animal Health and Animal Production*, which contains technical and scientific articles concerning disease control, research and animal production. It also issues monthly animal health statistics providing the status of the major contagious diseases in Africa.
- The Pan African Programme for the Control of Epizootics (**PACE**) was a 5-year programme (1999–2004) coordinated by OAU/IBAR to establish low-cost national and continental epidemiological surveillance networks for animal diseases.
- The Southern African Centre for Disease Surveillance (**SACIDS**) consists of Tanzania, Mozambique, Zambia, Democratic Republic of the Congo and South Africa. It works to improve the capacity of African countries to detect, identify and monitor infectious diseases affecting humans and animals.

- The East African Integrated Disease Surveillance Network (**EAIDSNet**) is an intergovernmental collaboration consisting of five East African countries, including Rwanda, Uganda, Kenya, Tanzania and Burundi. It is responsible for prevention and control of both human and animal diseases under the One Health concept and consolidation of disease surveillance in the region.

4.10.3 Asia

The Animal Production and Health Commission for Asia and Pacific (**APHCA**) **was** established by FAO at the 60th session of the FAO Council. Its headquarters are at Bangkok. Based on the concept of Technical Cooperation among Developing Countries (**TCDC**), it aims to develop strategies to solve important problems in livestock agriculture. The APHCA also maintains semen and vaccine banks. Its publication includes a monthly magazine known as *Asian Livestock*.

The ASEAN is an association of ten South-east Asian nations. Under its Committee on Food, Agriculture and Forestry (**ASEAN-COFAF**), it has the mechanism to endorse the disease-free status of a member country or a part of it. In the past, some parts of territories in Malaysia and the Philippines have been endorsed as FMD-free by the ASEAN.

- The Middle East Consortium on Infectious Disease Surveillance (**MECIDS**), initiated in 2003, comprises Israel, the Palestinian Authority and Jordan. In 2009, it coordinated efforts against the dreaded H1N1 influenza A outbreak in these countries. The **Middle East Regional Veterinary Information System Project** is a disease control project with Egypt, Israel, the Palestinian Authority and Jordan as its members. There is a direct exchange of official disease notification to the OIE/WOAH.
- The Pacific Public Health Surveillance Network (**PPHSN**), also known as the Asian Partnership on Emerging Infectious Disease Research (**APEIR**), is a multi-country, multisectoral, multidisciplinary research partnership launched initially in 2006 for regional collaboration in influenza research. It later expanded its scope to include all emerging infectious diseases. It includes Cambodia, China, Indonesia, Laos, Thailand and Vietnam.
- The South-east Asia and China FMD (**SEACFMD**) campaign is a programme to increase productivity and economic output of the livestock of this region by controlling and eradicating FMD.
- The **One Health Network** South-east Asia platform has been established with the support of the European Union to promote collaboration, networking and sharing between South-east Asian One Health programmes. It presently has two programmes: LACANET and ComAcross. **LACANET** (Lao PDR–Cambodia One Health Surveillance and Laboratory Network) is a joint Cambodia and Laos effort to improve zoonotic disease detection and surveillance, promoting regional and national collaborations. **ComAcross** in Thailand, Cambodia and Laos is aimed at assembling a multidisciplinary framework to address complex One Health problems and to improve integration between public health, animal health, agriculture and livestock, ecology, environmental science, social science and engineering.
- The Mekong Basin Disease Surveillance Network (**MBDS**) is one of the oldest successful self-organized infectious disease surveillance networks, comprising six countries (Cambodia, China, Lao PDR, Myanmar, Thailand and Vietnam) of the Mekong Basin Area in Asia, which is considered to be a hotspot for the emergence of new emerging diseases.

In India, the One Health Consortium (**IOHN**) has been launched by the Ministry of Science and Technology constituting 27 premier healthcare institutes with an aim to study the prevalence of selected zoonotic diseases and transboundary animal diseases and subsequent risk analysis to provide early warnings to the stakeholders. USAID is also doing commendable work in collaboration with the CDC, FAO, WHO and other partners in India to stop disease outbreaks by closing gaps in the early detection of threats. USAID is working to strengthen India's capacity to detect early threats, prevent and reduce disease outbreaks and respond with a rapid, coordinated effort to save lives. It also aims to fight antimicrobial resistance and to promote the One Health Initiative in India to strengthen and operationalize the intersectoral collaboration between the human health, animal health and food sectors.

4.10.4 Europe

The European Centre for Disease Prevention and Control (**ECDC**) is facilitating interdisciplinary collaboration and assessing public health needs for the integration of microbial genotyping data into surveillance and epidemic preparedness at European level.

The Mediterranean Network of Animal Health (**REMESA**) is an association of ten western Mediterranean nations, established in 2009 for improving coordination between the countries in prevention of and fighting against diseases like rabies, brucellosis, bluetongue (BT), sheep pox, tuberculosis, FMD, avian influenza (AI), leishmaniasis, RVF and African horse sickness (AHS). Four other technical sub-networks have been established to assist the activities of REMESA. These are the Animal Health Laboratories Network (**RELABSA**), the Veterinary Epidemio-surveillance Network (**REPIVET**), the Animal Health Communication Network (**RECOMSA**) and the Animal Health Socioeconomics and Production Systems Network (**RESEPSA**).

The South Eastern Europe Health Network (**SEEHN**) is a political and institutional forum set up in 2001 by the governments of Albania, Bosnia and Herzegovina, Bulgaria, Croatia, Montenegro, Republic of Moldova, Romania, Serbia and the former Yugoslav Republic of Macedonia to promote health in the region. Israel joined the network in 2011 as its tenth member. Technical support to SEEHN's various health projects is provided by Europe.

4.11 Conclusion

In the light of recent global outbreaks of diseases, an effective surveillance system that can detect disease emergence in human or animal populations anywhere in the world at the earliest time possible and is global in scope is the need of the moment (Dufour and Hendrikx, 2009).

There are numerous obstacles to the creation of health-supporting environments. Disease surveillance faces many of the problems encountered by surveillance efforts for human disease, including lack of clear case definitions, fragmented and paper-based information systems, and conflicting governance and regulatory authorities, apart from inadequate resources, frail diagnostic infrastructure and knowhow and lack of specific government policies and legal framework for surveillance.

To ensure the achievement of an effective global disease monitoring and surveillance and a prompt response to any sort of emergency, many national and international organizations and agencies are actively working in consortium, with the aim of securing knowledge and communications about animal disease occurrence, spread, prevention and control. They regularly generate authentic data regarding disease surveillance that are shared by various governments, which is essential for the continued development of epidemiological methodology, as well as for production, dissemination and application of scientific results to enable control and eradication of animal disease problems. Much more openness and collaboration than currently exist are needed to fully achieve these goals.

In many countries, health remains the concern of a single ministry rather than a goal to which each sector or ministry should contribute in a coordinated manner. Similarly, traditional boundaries between governmental and non-governmental organizations, and between the public and the private sector, hinder the development of strategies and policies. Thus there is a need of a multipronged, diversified approach to develop disease management policies involving various sectors of governments and science-stream experts.

Although human surveillance systems have identified a number of zoonotic disease outbreaks in humans, these global systems have yet to be adequate in detecting infections in animal populations early enough to prevent transmission from animal to human populations. Unfortunately, because disease surveillance efforts in livestock, poultry and wildlife typically have been under-resourced even more than disease surveillance in human populations, it is frequently the detection of disease outbreaks in humans that has led to the detection of disease outbreaks in animal populations rather than the reverse.

Acronyms

This table shows (in alphabetical order) the many acronyms used in this chapter, along with their definitions.

ACRONYM	DEFINITION
AGAH	Animal Genomics for Animal Health
AGnet	Agriculture Network
AHEAD	Animal Health and Emerging Animal Diseases
AHEM	*see* CAHEM
AHS	African horse sickness
AI	avian influenza
APEIR	Asian Partnership on Emerging Infectious Disease Research
APHCA	Animal Production and Health Commission for Asia and Pacific
APHIS-VS	Animal and Plant Health Inspection Service – Veterinary Services
ASEAN	Association of South-east Asian Nations
ASEAN-COFAF	ASEAN Committee on Food, Agriculture and Forestry
ASF	African swine fever
AU	African Union
AVIS	Advanced Veterinary Information System
BSE	bovine spongiform encephalitis
BSL	biosafety level
BT	blue tongue
CAC	Codex Alimentarius Commission
CAHEM	Canadian Animal Health Emergency Management (*in 52 countries*)
CaribVET	Caribbean Animal Health Network
CBD	Convention on Biological Diversity
CBPP	contagious bovine pleuropneumonia
CCs	collaborating centres
CDC	Centers for Disease Control and Prevention
CEAH	Center for Epidemiology and Animal Health
CIRAD	Centre de coopération internationale en recherche agronomique pour le developpement (= Agricultural Research Centre for International Development)
CORDS	Connecting Organizations for Regional Disease Surveillance
CRWAD	Conference of Research Workers in Animal Health
CSTE	Council of State and Territorial Epidemiologists
DALYs	disability-adjusted life years
EAIDSnet	East African Integrated Disease Surveillance Network
ECDC	European Centre for Disease Prevention and Control
EHTF	Emerging Health Threat Forum
EID	emerging infectious disease
EIOS	Epidemic Intelligence from Open Sources
EMAi	Event Mobile Application

Continued

ACRONYM	DEFINITION
EMPRES	Emergency Prevention System
EPT	emerging pandemic threats
EU	European Union
EWDA	European Wildlife Disease Association
EWS	early warning system
FAO	Food and Agriculture Organization (UN)
FERG	Foodborne Disease Burden Epidemiology Reference Group
FMD	foot-and-mouth disease
FSnet	Food Safety Network
GATT	General Agreement on Tariffs and Trade
GF-TADs	Global Framework (for the progressive control of) Transboundary Animal Diseases
GHSA	Global Health Security Agenda
GICSA	Grupo Interamericano de Coordinación Salud Animal = Inter-American Group for Cooperation in Animal Health
GIDEON	Global Infectious Diseases Epidemiology Network
GIP	Global Influenza Programme (WHO)
GLEWS	Global Early Warning and Response System (FAO, OIE, WHO)
GOARN	Global Outbreak Alert and Response Network
GOHF	Generalized One Health Framework
GPHIN	Global Public Health Intelligence Network
GSS	Global Salm-Surv (WHO)
H1N1	Influenza A virus
H5N1	(avian influenza A subtype)
H7N9	(avian influenza A subtype)
HIV/AIDS	human immunodeficiency virus / acquired immunodeficiency syndrome
HPAI	highly pathogenic avian influenza
IBAR	Inter African Bureau for Animal Resources
IFAD	International Fund for Agricultural Development
IHR	International Health Regulations
IICA	Inter-American Institution for Cooperation on Agriculture
INCLEN	International Clinical Epidemiology Network
IOHN	India One Health Network
IPPC	International Plant Protection Convention
ISID	International Society for Infectious Diseases
LACANET	Lao PDR-Cambodia One Health Surveillance and Laboratory Network
LMICs	low- and middle-income countries
LSD	lumpy skin disease
MBDS	Mekong Basin Disease Surveillance Network
MECIDS	Middle East Consortium on Infectious Disease Surveillance
MECRVIS	Middle East Consortium Regional Veterinary Information System project

Continued

ACRONYM	DEFINITION
MERS	Middle East respiratory syndrome
MERS-COV	Middle East respiratory syndrome coronavirus
MINEADEP	Middle and Near East Regional Animal Production and Health Project
MO&SS	monitoring and surveillance system
MS	monitoring system
NAHMS	National Animal Health Monitoring System
NCEZID	National Center for Emerging and Zoonotic Infectious Diseases
NDSS	Notifiable Disease Surveillance System
NFP	National Focal Point
NTT	Nuclear Threat Initiative
NWHC	National Wildlife Health Center
OAU	Organization of African Unity
OHW	One Health Workforce
OIE	Office International des Epizooties<now WOAH>
OIRSA	Organismo Internacional Regional de Sanidad Agropecuoria (= Regional International Organization for Plant Protection and Animal Health)
PACE	Pan African Programme for the Control of Epizootics
PAHO	Pan American Health Organization
PANAFTOSA	Pan American Center for Foot-and-Mouth Disease and Veterinary Public Health
PARC	Pan African Rinderpest Campaign
PHEIC	public health emergencies of international concern
PPHSN	Pacific Public Health Surveillance Network
PPR	peste des petits ruminants (= goat plague)
PREDICT	USAID Emerging Pandemic Threats (EPT) program
ProMED	Program for Monitoring Emerging Diseases
RADISCON	Regional Animal Disease Surveillance and Control Network
RECOMSA	REMESA Communication Network
RELABSA	REMESA Laboratories Network
REMESA	REseau MEditerranéen de Santé Animale (= Mediterranean Network of Animal Health). Four thematic sub-networks: laboratories (RELABSA), epidemiology (REPIVET), communication (RECOMSA) and socioeconomics (RESEPSA)
REPIVET	REMESA Veterinary Epidemio-surveillance Network
RESCAD	Regional Strategy for Control of Animal Diseases
RESEPSA	REMESA Socioeconomics and Production Systems Network
RLs	reference laboratories
RP	rinderpest
RVF	Rift Valley fever
SAARC	South Asian Association for Regional Cooperation
SACIDS	Southern African Centre for Disease Surveillance
SADCC	Southern African Development Coordination Conference

Continued

ACRONYM	DEFINITION
SARCCUS	Southern African Regional Commission for the Conservation and Utilization of the Soil
SARS	severe acute respiratory syndrome
SARS-CoV-2	severe acute respiratory syndrome coronavirus 2
SEACFMD	South-east Asia and China FMD campaign
SEAOHN	South-east Asia One Health Network
SECNA	Screwworm Emergency Centre in North Africa
SEEHN	South Eastern Europe Health Network
SPS	Sanitary and Phytosanitary Agreement
STDs	sexually transmitted diseases
TADs	transboundary animal diseases
TB	tuberculosis
TCDC	Technical Cooperation among Developing Countries
TZG	Tripartite Zoonoses Guide
UN	United Nations
USAID	United States Agency for International Development
USCDC	United States Centers for Disease Control
USDA	United States Department of Agriculture
USFWS	United States Association of Fish and Wildlife Agencies
USGS	United States Geological Survey
WAHID	World Animal Health Information Database
WAHIS	World Animal Health Information System
WAREC	West Asian RP Eradication Campaign
WHO	World Health Organization
WOAH	World Organisation for Animal Health (*formerly OIE*)
WTO	World Trade Organization

References

Abreu, M.I.P., Guitian, J., Herbert-Hackshaw, K., Pradel, J., Biurnex, L. *et al.* (2011) Developing a disease preventive strategy in the caribbean: The importance of assessing animal health-related risks at required level. *Revue scientifique et technique – Office international des épizooties* 30(3), 725–731.

Blajan, L. and Chillaud, T. (1991) The OIE world animal disease information system. *Revue scientifique et technique* 10(1), 51–87.

Bruckner, G.K. (2009) The role of the world organisation of animal health (OIE) to facilitate the international trade in animals and animal products. *Ondenstepoort Journal of Veterinary Research* 76(1), 141–146.

Burgos, S. and Otte, J. (2009) *Animal Health in the 21st Century: Challenges and Opportunities*. Pro-Poor Livestock Policy Initiative: A Living from Livestock Research Report, FAO, Rome.

Christensen, J. (2001) Epidemiological concepts regarding disease monitoring and surveillance. *Acta Veterinaria Scandinavica* 94, 11–16.

Cirkel, K. (2010) *Epidemiological Surveillance System*. World Organization of Animal Health and Food and Agriculture Organization of UN, Rome.

Cutler, S., Fooks, A. and Van der Poel, W. (2010) Public health threat of new, reemerging, and neglected zoonoses in the industrialized world. *Emerging Infectious Diseases* 16, 1–7.

Day, M.J., Breitschwerdt, E., Cleaveland, S., Karkare, U., Khanna, C. *et al.* (2012) Surveillance of zoonotic infectious diseases transmitted by small companion animals. *Emerging Infectious Diseases* 18, 12. DOI: 10.3201/eid1812.120664.

Domenech, J., Lubroth, L., Eddi, C., Martin, V. and Roger, F. (2006) Reginal and international approaches on prevention and control of animal transboundary and emerging diseases. *Annals of the New York Academy of Sciences* 1081, 90–107.
Dufour, B. and Hendrikx, P. (2009) *Epidemiological Surveillance in Animal Health*, 2nd edn. Food and Agriculture Organization (FAO), Rome.
Fauci, A., Touchette, N. and Folkers, G. (2005) Emerging infectious diseases: A 10-year perspective from the National Institute of Allergy and infectious diseases. *Emerging Infectious Diseases* 11, 519–525.
Hulebak, K., Rodricks, J. and Smith DeWall, C. (2013) Integration of animal health, food, pathogens and food borne disease surveillance in the Americas. *Revue scientifique et technique – Office international des épizooties* 32(2), 529–538.
Hutton, N.E. (1969) Veterinary medical information systems. MSc Thesis, Iowa State University.
Jones, K.E., Patel, N.G., Levy, M.A., Storeygard, A., Balk, D. *et al*. (2008) Global trends in emerging infectious diseases. *Nature* 451(7181), 990–993.
Kruse, H., Kirkemo, A. and Handeland, K. (2004) Wildlife as source of zoonotic infections. *Emerging Infectious Diseases* 10, 2067–2072.
Kshirsagar, D.P., Savalia, C.V., Kalyani, I.H.., Kumar, R. and Nayak, D.N. (2013) Disease alerts and forecasting of zoonotic diseases: An overview. *Veterinary World* 6(11), 889–896.
Kuiken, T., Ryser-Degiorgis, M.P., Gavier-Widen, D. and Gortazar, C. (2011) Establishing a European network for wildlife health surveillance. *Revue scientifique et technique – Office international des épizooties* 30(3), 755–761.
WOAH and FAO (2004) Report of the WHO/FAO/OIE Joint Consultation on Emerging Zoonotic Diseases. World Health Organization (WHO), Food and Agriculture Organization of the United Nations (FAO) and World Organisation for Animal Health (WOAH/OIE). Available at: https://www.oie.int/doc/ged/D5681.PDF

5 The Global Burden of Zoonotic Diseases and Public Health Impact Assessment

Simant Kumar Nanda*, Rajesh Kumar Sahu and Dwarikanath Mohanty
Fisheries and Animal Resources and Development Department, Government of Odisha, Bhubaneswar, India

Abstract
Zoonoses, animal farming and food safety are all interconnected topics in as much as they all directly impact human health and well-being. In the past 30 years, there has been an average of one annual discovery of emerging infectious diseases. Zoonotic diseases constitute about 70% of them. They pose major health threats and lead to complex scientific study and policy challenges necessitating new social, cultural and political norms essential for devising successful control outcomes. For global trade expansion and travel, zoonotic diseases are real threats to global trade, travel and tourism. In daily life situations, humans face new health challenges due to the human, animal and environmental interface. To overcome these threats and issues, the need for collaborative action and multisectoral coordination at all levels has become paramount. The basis of this inter-sector collaboration depends upon enhancement of inter-personnel and inter-organizational interaction – the more the better. The application of the 'One Health' and 'One World' concept has been recognized as a critical need by World Health Organization (WHO), World Organisation for Animal Health (OIE, now WOAH) and Food and Agriculture Organization (FAO) as the preferred approach to address global health issues. Health education and risk reduction, communication and social mobilization can be major determinants in overall environmental health issues.

Keywords: wildlife, One Health, vector, diseases, livestock

5.1 Introduction

Life began on Earth millions of years ago and all the creatures on it evolved through the ages sharing the same ecosystem, with *Homo sapiens* at the top of the tree of evolution and considered the most intelligent amongst all of them. In pursuit of their own welfare, human activity has increased each passing day with catastrophic consequences – beginning with impacts on the ecosystem, climate change and emergence of new pathogens affecting both humans and animals. With material and intellectual progress, the whole world has become a global community and the threat to life has also increased, necessitating the 'One Health and One World' philosophy. Anything occurring in one part of the world could impact the entire humankind. That is a big lesson we learnt from the COVID-19 pandemic, which originated from China and engulfed the whole world like wildfire. The world economy has been shattered and countries are fighting to overcome the subsequent doldrums.

*Corresponding author: drsimantkumarnanda@gmail.com

DOI: 10.1079/ 9781800622852.0005

5.2 Zoonoses

The modern world faces multiple challenges, many of which are health related. Zoonoses are one of them. The question is: why so? Humans and animals have shared common living spaces from time immemorial. With the advancement of civilization and because of demographic increases, civil society and human habitation have gradually encroached upon forested areas and wildlife habitats for multiple purposes, like cultivation, housing, industrial farming, major industrial activity, irrigation projects and mining, throwing the entire ecosystem out of gear. The proximity of humans to animals, including wildlife, became closer than ever before. It is but natural that many animal diseases, which are referred to as 'zoonotic', have jumped to humans over time, with emerging ones being added each year to the list in most developing and underdeveloped countries.

What is 'zoonoses' for our purposes? An expert WHO Committee defined zoonoses as 'diseases and infections that are naturally transmitted between vertebrate animals and man' (Sherikar, 2005). The word 'zoonoses' is derived from the Greek word *zoo*, which means animals, and *noses* as diseases. Zoonoses may be classified as: (i) endemic zoonoses, which are present in many places where many people and animals get affected; (ii) epidemic zoonoses, which are sporadic in temporal and spatial distribution; and (iii) emerging and re-emerging zoonoses, which appear in a population or were already present and may rapidly increase in incidence. It is estimated that more than 60% of the 1700 infectious diseases globally reported in people are of animal origin. The WHO (2023) reported that 'over 30 new human pathogens have been detected in the last three decades, 75% of which have originated from animals'. Today's symptoms of an unknown disease may become a disease reality of tomorrow, starting from sporadic phenomena in rural areas and reaching global portions to emerge as public health emergencies (Budke *et al.*, 2011). That is how the behavioural pattern of diseases and epidemiological picture have been changing fast globally in recent times. The pathogens include novel viruses. They are major public health threats around the world due to our coexistence with animals in agriculture, intensive domestic animal farming, indiscriminate use of antibiotics, consumption of meat of wild animals, companion animals and also sharing the same ecosystem, which has become more frequent due to habitat degradation, land-use changes and increased trans-boundary movement of humans, pet animals and the animal products trade. Sometimes it so happens that the world battles to save life and livelihood.

The zoonotic nature of a pathogen has been unequivocally considered to be an independent factor that increases its potential for emergence or re-emergence. 'Emerging' means the appearance of a newly recognized or newly evolved pathogen or the appearance of a known pathogen in a geographical area where it has not been found earlier. 'Re-emerging' diseases are from known pathogens whose incidence is reported again in a given geographical area (Grace *et al.*, 2011). Zoonotic infections can cause serious ill health and economic losses in humans as well as in domesticated animals. The challenge in assessing the burden of a zoonotic infection is that most of the approaches will estimate the impact of the infection in one species at a particular period, whereas some approaches are applicable to measure human health impact and not applicable to animal health impact assessment. To overcome this challenge, researchers have endeavoured to assess the burden of these infections in both non-monetary and monetary terms (Narrod *et al.*, 2012).

'Disease burden' is the impact of a disease on society measured by financial cost, mortality, morbidity, or other indicators. It holds true for zoonotic diseases. Calculating the total burden in monetary terms has the advantage that there may be substantial health loss both in humans and animals that can be calculated in unitary figures. Monetary costs include loss of productivity, income and livelihood, and increased treatment cost in individual households. However, the absolute cost of treatment and convalescence of human patients is higher in high-income countries compared with low-income countries, due to variations in medical and wage costs. Thus a disease in a wealthy country may have a higher financial burden for the same disease compared with a low-income country even if the latter has a much higher incidence (Abegunde *et al.*, 2007).

5.2.1 Zoonoses as public health threat

Why should zoonotic diseases be a cause of global concern and why should their burden vis-à-vis public health impact need to be assessed? It is necessary to quantify their effect on the economy and human welfare globally, because these diseases tend to cause morbidity, mortality and loss of productivity in both human and animal populations. For instance, we cannot turn our eyes away from the COVID-19 pandemic and its immediate aftermath. Some other examples are rabies and brucellosis as test cases, amongst many others. World Rabies Day is celebrated globally on 28 September to mark the anniversary of the death of the legendary Louis Pasteur, whose invention of anti-rabies vaccine saved millions of lives. To rein in the menace of rabies, some governments have designed and operated animal birth control (ABC) programmes to control populations of stray dogs, who are the main reservoir of the rabies virus. This apart, zoonoses can also cause disruptions in livestock production, affecting agricultural operation dependent on working animals, and the trading of animal food products, leading to adverse impact on the livelihoods of millions of farmers (Karesh *et al.*, 2012).

Zoonoses can be classified according to the aetiological agent – viral, bacterial, parasitic, mycotic (fungal) or unconventional (prions) – which can cause different types of illness in humans and animals ranging from mild to serious in nature and even death. Therefore, zoonoses have become an important cause of hospitalization. Adding to the woes, there are some newly appearing or re-emerging zoonoses that are capable of occurring and spreading rapidly to new geographical regions in devastating proportions. Examples include Rift Valley fever (RVF), severe acute respiratory syndrome (SARS), pandemic H1N1 influenza, yellow fever, avian influenza (H5N1 and H7N9), West Nile virus, MERS-CoV and the recent COVID-19 pandemic. The latter, caused by SARS-CoV-2, has been classified as a zoonotic disease, though no animal reservoir has yet been found. However, it has been suggested that COVID-19 should be classified as an 'emerging infectious disease' (EID) of probable animal origin (Haider *et al.*, 2020).

Since March 2020, concerns over COVID-19 have dominated the world, with fresh reports in Chinese cities. The world is slowly moving to the endemic phase, which means that COVID-19 is becoming a manageable infectious disease. This is as the result of large-scale vaccination of vulnerable populations. It is a big concern in Japan, Thailand and across Europe and North America. Human-to-human transmission is very limited but if H5N1 manages to mutate in a way that sustains human-to-human transmission it will be very difficult to fight it within human populations. The WHO estimates avian flu to have a 60% fatality rate in humans as compared with around 1% to 3% in COVID-19. The reports are worth pondering.

It is imperative to describe the origin and subsequent spillover of COVID-19, its impact on human life, national and global economy, livelihood and economy of several countries worldwide. Initially several people were presumably exposed to the coronavirus at a seafood market in China but only a few out of the many samples collected from surfaces and cages in the market tested positive for SARS-CoV-2; no virus was isolated directly from animals and no animal reservoir was detected. The subject is as complex as it was at the beginning of the pandemic. However, the virus has been detected in domestic cats, dogs and ferrets, as well as captive lions, tigers, deer and mice, confirming zooanthroponosis. Other than the circumstantial evidence of zoonotic cases in mink farms in the Netherlands, no cases of natural transmission from wild or domestic animals have been confirmed. Has the virus jumped from humans to animals, which can be termed as reverse zoonosis? As the SARS-CoV-2 virus and COVID-19 do not fully meet the WHO definition of zoonoses, they can be classified as emerging infectious diseases (EIDs) until the viruses are established to have animal origin. EIDs are currently defined as diseases that have newly appeared in a population, or existed but are rapidly increasing in incidence and geographical range.

Parasitic zoonoses are a cause of concern in the tropical countries where most of the world's poor live. Helminthes (nematodes), trematodes, cestodes, pentastomids and protozoa are major causes of parasitic diseases (Krauss *et al.*, 2003). A number of factors are responsible for emergence of such diseases, including overpopulation, disruption of habitat due to war, mass migration due to natural calamities, manmade disasters, migration of populations into urban areas, inadequate food and water supplies and changes in land-use patterns displacing animal populations. Some diseases such as schistosomosis, cysticercosis, echinococcosis (*Echinococcus multilocularis*), *Toxocara canis*, hookworm infection, leishmaniasis, trypanosomosis, cryptosporidiosis, etc. have parasitic zoonotic importance.

Another focal point is transmission and dissemination of zoonotic diseases to humans from reservoir animals, including wildlife. Bacterial and viral zoonotic infections are a stream of endless, ever-expanding entities with variable consequences. Rabies is mainly transmitted by the bite of a rabid dog and exceptionally as a rare spillover from wildlife. Humans may contract zoonotic diseases either through direct contact with animals or by indirect routes such as vector-borne infection or environmental and food pathogens. Outbreaks of SARS and avian influenza (AI) have shown that the viruses responsible do have the potential to adapt to human hosts. Not only this, but also experience of past decades has amply demonstrated that many previously unknown human infectious diseases have emerged from animal reservoirs, such as human immunodeficiency virus (HIV) (originally a virus harboured by chimpanzees in Africa), Ebola virus, West Nile virus, Nipah virus, hantavirus, etc. At the beginning of the present century it was estimated that more than 75% of human diseases are caused by pathogens originating from animals or animal products. The pathogens may be viruses, bacteria, parasites or prions. Considering the complex scenario of the large number and range of reservoir hosts, their proximity to human population and the nature of the pathogens, effective surveillance, prevention and control of zoonotic diseases has become a real challenge to public health particularly in developing and underdeveloped country (Pal, 2013). The concept of the 'One Health and One World' approach may play a defining role to counter and combat emerging and re-emerging zoonotic diseases. But predicting them may be difficult according to their geographical origin, as these regions and the pathogens are constantly evolving, like human behaviour in the affected areas. Potential risk factors include routes of transmission of pathogens from animals that include food- and waterborne diseases and direct or indirect (vector-borne). Overall zoonotic disease outbreaks are often characteristically dynamic and unpredictable, being strongly influenced by environmental factors.

Zoonotic diseases are caused by a wide range of pathogens. Based on aetiology, zoonoses are classified as: (i) bacterial zoonoses (such as anthrax, salmonellosis, tuberculosis, Lyme disease, brucellosis and plague); (ii) viral zoonoses (such as rabies, acquired immune deficiency syndrome (AIDS), Ebola and avian influenza); (iii) parasitic zoonoses (such as trichinosis, toxoplasmosis, trematodosis, giardiasis, malaria and echinococcosis); (iv) fungal zoonoses (such as ringworm); (v) rickettsial zoonoses (Q fever); (vi) chlamydial zoonoses (psittacosis); (vii) mycoplasma zoonoses (mycoplasma pneumonia); (viii) protozoal zoonoses; and (ix) diseases caused by acellular non-viral pathogenic agents (such as transmissible spongiform encephalopathies, including mad cow disease) (Table 5.1).

Domestic animals play a significant role in the transmission of various diseases to humans and in many cases they work as amplifiers of pathogens emerging from wild animals. The positive association between domestic animals and humans in influencing pathogen diversity was first hypothesized long ago. Nearly 60% of human infectious diseases come from vertebrate animals. Direct human contact with animals has expanded with the introduction of domestication of different animals. The possible transmission patterns of zoonotic bacteria, virus, parasites, or fungi are through direct contact, ingestion, inhalation, conjunctiva or bites (Kuchenmüller *et al.*, 2013) (Table 5.2).

5.2.2 Importance of public health in management of zoonotic diseases in 'One Health' concept

Numerous zoonotic diseases cause morbidity, mortality and productivity losses in both humans and animal populations. In endemic areas there are big societal impacts of zoonotic diseases. Estimates of monetary impact and disease burden provide essential evidence-based

Table 5.1. Important zoonotic diseases and their hosts.

Group	Hosts	Zoonotic diseases
Companion animals	Cat	Toxoplasmosis, Q fever, variant Creutzfeldt-Jakob disease, *Capnocytophaga canimorsus*, plague, bartonellosis
	Dog	Q fever, rabies, leptospirosis, *Capnocytophaga canimorsus*
	Horse	Tuberculosis, glanders
Livestock	Cattle	Q fever, Creutzfeldt-Jacob disease, Crimean–Congo haemorrhagic fever, tuberculosis, leptospirosis, RVF, brucellosis
	Pig	Toxoplasmosis, Japanese encephalitis, campylobacteriosis, tuberculosis, streptococcosis, tularaemia, brucellosis, leptospirosis, zoonotic influenza
	Sheep/Goat	Toxoplasmosis, Q fever, RVF, tularaemia, brucellosis
	Deer	Q fever, tuberculosis, human granulocytotropic anaplasmosis, leptospirosis
Poultry	Poultry	Campylobacteriosis, chlamydiosis, salmonellosis, influenza (avian flu)
Wild birds	Waterfowl	Influenza, Japanese encephalitis, Q fever, West Nile fever, Eastern equine encephalitis, chlamydiosis
Aquatic	Fish	Leptospirosis
Arthropod	Insects	Campylobacteriosis

Table 5.2. Transmission routes of zoonotic diseases.

Transmission routes	Zoonotic diseases
Airborne	Influenza, tuberculosis, Q fever
Physical contact	Influenza, Q fever
Bite	Rabies, pasturellosis
Faecal matter	Toxoplasma, ancylostoma, *E. coli*, salmonellosis
Infected carcass handling	CCHF, anthrax, streptococcosis, Q fever
Food	Toxoplasma, campylobacteriosis
Water	Leptospirosis, tularaemia
Vector	West Nile fever, Japanese encephalitis, Lyme disease

data for conducting cost–benefit and cost–utility analyses, which can contribute to securing political will and financial and technical resources (Grace *et al.*, 2011). To overcome this challenge a number of large-scale attempts besides individual researches have been initiated to assess the burden of these infections in both non-monetary and monetary terms. Non-monetary assessment can include measures of mortality, morbidity (which often includes reduction in productivity in animals) and health-adjusted life year (HALY) measures, which include the quality-adjusted life year (QALY) and the disability-adjusted life year (DALY). Monetary assessment of these conditions should include both direct and indirect costs associated with disease, which overall comprises one health loss (Murray, 1994).

The One Health concept has gained wide acclaim and acceptance across different regions to fight the menace of zoonotic diseases. It is a collaborative, multisectoral and multidisciplinary approach involving local, regional, national and global players with a mission to achieve overall well-being and optimal health outcomes between humans, animals, plants and their ecosystem. The players could be disease detectives, laboratory technicians, physicians, veterinarians and environmentalists working together to keep everyone safe. The concept is gaining ground in India, though not as fast as in the United States or other developed countries. The first and foremost objective of the One Health concept is saving lives and concurrent misery and connecting and bonding human, animal and environmental health in view of rapidly emerging climate change. Every year millions of people get sick due to the spread of diseases between animals and people. The Centers for Disease Control and Prevention (CDC), which works in the USA and around the world to protect human, animal and environmental health, recognizes the connection between the health of animals (including pets, livestock and wildlife) and our shared environment as consequential for human survival (Fig. 5.1).

5.2.3 Objectives of the one health approach

- Educate rural youth in agricultural spheres by working with multiple partners, making them aware about preventing the spread of diseases shared between people and animals.
- One Health teams, once formed, can be the first responders in an outbreak in a community to pinpoint the source of the illness.
- Respond to outbreaks and public health emergencies.
- Ensure public–private partnership leading to Zoonoses Coalitions to develop evidence-based recommendations to prevent diseases for pet owners, breeders and stores.
- The One Health office can share messages about how to stay healthy on websites, having appropriate captions.
- Organize One Health zoonotic disease prioritization workshops.
- Identify a country's top five diseases to get One Health approbation.
- Develop strategies to tackle newly prioritized zoonotic diseases and vaccination.

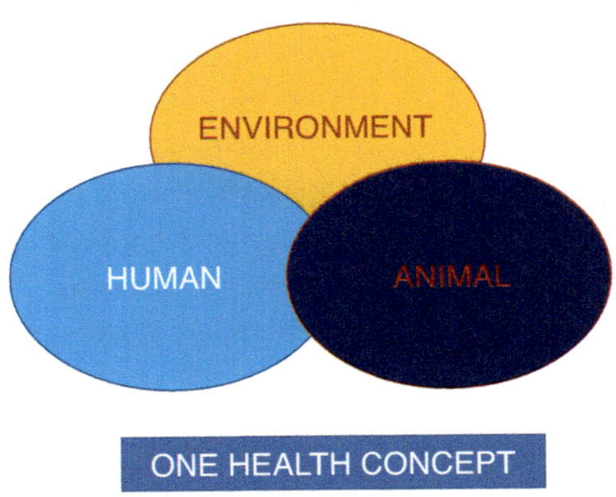

Fig. 5.1. The One Health concept in combating infectious diseases. (Author's own image.)

- Build more laboratories with better capacity; conduct surveillance; plan outbreak response and preparedness activities.

5.2.4 Important facts to know

In a changing world, zoonotic diseases represent a major public health challenge, previously underestimated and not well understood although we lived in close relationship with domestic animals in agriculture and peri-domestic animals as companions, and in natural environments with wild animals in the forested regions of the world. It is desirable to know how and why our relationship with animals is important. Animals provide many benefits to people. They provide food, fibre, livelihood, travel, sport, companionship, education in life sciences as experimental animals, drug evaluation and standardization, science and research, and production of vaccines and antiserum. Through our association in either urban or rural settings we come into contact with them knowingly or unknowingly. However, during our interface with them in various settings we mostly remain unaware of harmful pathogens that might jump from them to us and cause illnesses – which are known as zoonotic diseases. Therefore, people must know, as a public health safety measure, the source and routes of transmission of germs from animals to the human body (Collins and Wall, 2004).

- **Direct contact:** Coming into frequent contact with animals, which may be common or routine. In the process one may come into contact with the saliva, blood, urine, mucus, faeces, or other body discharges of an infected animal, for example by petting or touching animals, and from bites and scratches (especially playful children). Veterinarians, para-vets and zoo animal handlers are the most vulnerable group.
- **Indirect contact:** Coming into contact with areas where animals live and roam, or objects or surfaces that have been contaminated with pathogens. These may be, for example, aquariums, tank water, pet habitats, chicken farms, barns, plants and soil, pet-food plates and drinking water bowls.
- **Vector-borne:** Being bitten by ticks, or by insects like mosquitoes, haematophagous (blood-sucking) flies and fleas and by vermin.
- **Foodborne:** Eating contaminated and improperly cooked meat and eggs or drinking something such as unpasteurized (raw) milk, or eating raw fruits and vegetables that are contaminated with faeces/urine of infected animals. These are considered unsafe.
- **Waterborne:** Drinking or coming into contact with water that has been contaminated with faeces of infected animals.

5.2.5 Who is at a higher risk of serious illnesses from zoonotic disease?

Anyone can get sick from zoonotic disease, irrespective of race, creed, age or health status. However, some are more at risk than others because of occupational hazards – people like wool sorters, animal traders, zookeepers and those with professional obligation (veterinarians). Children below 5 years of age, or adults with weakened immune systems, or who are pregnant, ill-nourished, etc. are equally vulnerable.

5.2.6 Minimal steps necessary to avoid zoonotic diseases

Standard operational procedures (SOPs) include the following.

- Wash hands with soap or use alcohol-based sanitizer (60%) and running water immediately after touching or being in proximity with animals (even if having not touched any animals).
- Use face masks whenever desired or possible and stay safe around pets.
- Be aware of zoonotic diseases both at home and away from home (e.g. zoos).
- Avoid bites and scratches from animals, especially in the case of playful children.

- Prevent breeding of mosquitoes, flies, ticks, fleas and prevent bites from mosquitoes, ticks and fleas.
- Maintain safe distance, avoid crowding and adopt SOPs when attending sick animals.
- Prohibit marketing of sick chickens or pigs in case of avian flu (AI) and swine flu; and ban the consumption of contaminated food of animal origin.

5.3 Zoonoses as a Global Concern

According to WHO reports, zoonoses comprise a large percentage of all newly identified infectious diseases as well as many existing ones. All of them fall into this category, with the exception of HIV, which began as a zoonotic pathogen but later mutated as a human strain. Other zoonoses can cause recurring outbreaks, such as Ebola virus disease and salmonellosis. Other novel viruses like COVID-19 have the potential to cause global pandemics and may continue for much longer periods if appropriate preventive measures are not taken.

In humans, both direct and indirect losses due to zoonoses should include monetary assessment of the disease burden. Direct burdens include costs associated with resources spent for healthcare (e.g. diagnostics, medications, surgical treatment). Indirect costs include burdens on resources, loss in earning, extra cost on unavoidable transportation, loss of life and higher spending during convalescence and aftercare (Narrod *et al.*, 2012).

Animal-associated monetary losses can also be divided into direct and indirect costs. Direct costs can stem from monetary losses due to condemnation of an infected carcass or parts thereof. For example, the condemnation of a pig carcass heavily infected with *T. solium* cysticerci or the condemnation of a sheep liver infected with cystic echinococcosis are direct costs. Indirect costs would encompass other disease-related production losses. For example, lower carcass weight linked to reduced bodyweight gain, poor hide value, decreased milk production and suboptimal fecundity due to cystic echinococcosis infection in a sheep. Even though estimates of these losses are sometimes uncertain and have very little available data, studies incorporating estimates of indirect costs for livestock-associated losses have shown that these losses are likely to be significant. For example, monetary losses associated with cystic echinococcosis in Spanish livestock contributed to an estimated 10.4% of cystic echinococcosis total costs, with indirect costs contributing 10.3% and direct costs contributing only 0.12% of losses (Benner *et al.*, 2010). Likewise, the non-monetary estimates of disease burden, an estimate of monetary losses, due to echinococcosis, was performed in China for Shiqu County (Budke *et al.*, 2011).

5.3.1 Important zoonotic diseases in India and other countries recognized by the World Health Organization

The list includes plague, Nipah virus outbreaks, Ebola haemorrhagic fever, Zika virus, coronavirus (COVID-19), rabies, swine flu, Q fever, *Salmonella* and *E. coli* infections, streptococcal sepsis, brucellosis, anthrax, bovine tuberculosis, glanders, avian flu (AI), toxoplasmosis, cysticercosis, echinococcosis, Japanese encephalitis, bovine spongiform encephalopathy (BSE) (mad cow disease) due to abnormal prion in feed, leptospirosis, trypanosomosis, Kyasanur forest disease (KFD), Crimean–Congo haemorrhagic fever (CCHF), blastomycosis, psittacosis (chlamydial infection), histoplasmosis, coccidiomycosis, cat scratch disease (bartonellosis), toxocariasis) ringworm (dermatophytosis) and trichinellosis. Foot-and-mouth disease (FMD) of cloven-footed animals is often encountered in India, though it has been eradicated from some developed countries. The question is: does FMD have any human consequence? Simultaneously it should not be confused with hand, foot and mouth disease, which is a mild, contagious viral infection recently reported in humans and common in young children.

Table 5.3 lists some important outbreaks of emerging zoonotic diseases over the past five decades.

Table 5.3. Aetiological agents of some important outbreaks of emerging zoonotic diseases. (Author's own table.)

Year	Zoonotic pathogens
1976	*Cryptosporidium parvum*
1976	*Yersinia enterocolotica*
1977	*Campylobacter jejuni*
1978	Korean haemorrhagic fever
1994	Hendravirus
1996	Prion
1998	Nipay
1999	West Nile fever
2003	SARS
2014	Ebola

5.3.2 Antibacterial resistance as a complicating factor in the control and prevention of zoonoses and the WHO response

The answer to the question, 'Does FMD have any human consequence?' is probably 'yes'. Antimicrobial resistance is a zoonotic health threat. The perception of zoonosis having an emerging link to antibiotic-resistant bacteria (ARB) has become potent, with zoonotic pathogens causing severe infections in human population worldwide as well as a growing concern under the One Health approach. As in humans, indiscriminate and higher use of antibiotics in animal treatment is a very common practice with the result that emergence and spread of resistant bacteria has become very risky worldwide (Elelu *et al.*, 2019). Additionally, widespread use of antibiotics to raise farm animals and poultry for quicker feed conversion and growth has substantially added to the emergence of ARBs. Such resistant bacteria may be passed on to humans via the food chain or by direct animal contact. For example, increasing prevalence of resistance to antimicrobial drugs such as fluoroquinolones and third-generation cephalosporins, which are important for treatment of infections caused by enteric pathogens, has significant public health implications. Therefore, for controlling the spread of drug-resistant bacterial strains, the collaboration of multidisciplinary teams of mammalogists, ecologists, entomologists, epidemiologists, ornithologists, farming communities, veterinary, medical and public health personnel is required.

To prevent and manage zoonotic threats arising out of human and animal environment interface over several centuries, efforts have been made to develop inter-sectoral collaborations in relevant sectors at various levels (Torgerson and Macpherson, 2011). In view of this emerging situation, the WHO in collaboration with the FAO and OIE (WOAH) on the Global Early Warning System (GLEWS) for major animal diseases are eager to develop strategies to strengthen capacity-building to combat all possible angles of zoonoses as a part of the One Health approach. The joint system builds on the added value by combining and coordinating the technical 'know-how and do-how' to assist countries and people, especially in the developing and underdeveloped countries. These include risk assessment, management and data sharing and, most importantly, surveillance, detection by laboratory investigation, forecasting, reporting, warning and prevention to combat animal disease threats.

5.3.3 Looking ahead: how the one health approach makes us better prepared

The One Health approach plays a significant role in the prevention and control of zoonoses. New and re-emerging zoonoses have evolved throughout the past decades as a result of highly increased interdependence of humans on animals and their products, as well as close association. About 60% of human disease-causing pathogens are multihost pathogens which are characterized by their movement across different species. A total of 335 emerging infectious diseases were identified between 1940 and 2004. Agriculture, livestock production, aquaculture and food safety practices are intimately linked with the prevention and control of zoonoses through the One Health approach, which was conceptualized to accelerate biomedical research discoveries, increase public health efficacy and expand scientific knowledge, higher technical medical education and clinical care. Human behavioural changes with continued encroachment of people and livestock into wildlife habitats has prompted a multifaceted need to study the ecology of bats, for example.

The One Health concept has been successful in replacing the disease-centred approach to zoonoses with a system-based approach that aligns multiple disciplines from grassroots level to a higher plane for attaining optimal wellness of people and animals as well as the environment. The need to employ the One Health approach is illustrated in the case of H5N1 avian influenza, where there was a lack of addressing the complex dynamics of zoonotic diseases. It is the approach, disease surveillance, monitoring, management of case strategy and eradication through collaborative action between veterinarians, ecologists and public health experts that may have yielded a more rapid resolution to combat any outbreak. The application of the One Health approach has been recognized as a critical need by international organizations as well as being the preferred approach to address global health issues. It has gained momentum and now encompasses zoonotic infections, food safety and even health delivery systems from door to door. In recent times the concept has been expanded to encompass the health, balance and sustainability of the world's ecosystems. Collaboration between veterinary, medical and public health professionals to understand the ecological interactions, ecological interface and reactions to flux in a system can help a clearer understanding of global climate change, which always has an impact on humans, animals and the environment. These issues can intensify the importance of interdisciplinary and collaborative research and, further, they have great impact on the sustainability of human race.

5.4 Impact of Zoonoses on Human Health and Economy

We do not have to look far back regarding the impact of zoonotic diseases on human health and economy. The corona pandemic since 2020 is enough of an indicator. Earlier SARS and MERS had caused severe mortality and morbidity in countries from where these were reported. Socioeconomic losses from zoonoses are difficult to quantify, unlike human diseases, because the costs of labour, damage to livelihood, trade of animals and animal products, and sufferings of farming communities cannot be measured in terms of loss of work capacity, loss of earning, clinical implications, burden and interference with family life (in the case of migrant labourers) and potential malnutrition of already poor and malnourished population. This is especially true for underdeveloped regions. Workplaces were shut down, office hours curtailed and attendance in offices restricted. All these had direct impacts on production and the economy. However, sometimes some good comes out of evil. 'Work from Home' was an innovative idea and became a common practice in many establishments during the COVID-19 pandemic.

5.4.1 Direct and indirect loss

Many of the zoonotic diseases cause serious illness with high mortality rates. Some others, but not those belonging to fulminant types like tuberculosis and brucellosis, result in considerable morbidity and prove to be silent killers unless detected and diagnosed early. Clinically, febrile conditions generally include loss of capacity to work, which results in loss of earning. This is manifested in working-class people. If not treated in time, it leads to clinical complications. In addition to clinical effects, the presence of zoonoses in a community has untold economic repercussions in the shape of cost of treatment, diagnostics and healthcare services which the poor can hardly bear, unless there is provision of health insurance. Hospitalization may also disrupt patterns of family life. All such factors lead to malnutrition and lowering of immunity levels of large numbers of people. Periods of convalescence increase the demand for nutritious food and better care. It adds an extra burden on poorly nourished families. School-going children may drop out, leading to disruption of education, as happened in the current corona pandemic. Besides loss of human efficiency and work hours, the overall impact of zoonotic diseases in terms of the gross domestic product (GDP) and national economy of any country is enormous. Zoonotic livestock diseases have direct consequences for a country's economic development, as about 80% of rural populations depend upon livestock for their livelihood. Zoonoses adversely impact livestock health and productivity, resulting in lowered production of milk, meat, eggs and wool and reduced draught power in working animals. There are several instances when entire flocks of poultry have been destroyed to prevent the spread of avian flu virus to other areas and also probable infection in humans. Affected animals or poultry consume less feed during illness, which ultimately affects feed production and marketing. There is also wastage of feed during illness. At the community level, the presence of animal diseases may be detrimental to human habitation. Prevalence of zoonotic diseases in an area also impacts traditional food markets of animal origin, leading to great financial hardship for traders who depend upon trading animals and animal products as their only means of livelihood (Christou, 2011). International animal trade and travel of people is either greatly restricted or stopped. The latter has adverse repercussions on the tourism, travel and hotel industries. Expenditure incurred to control zoonotic diseases is often huge, in addition to healthcare services provided at public cost (Fig. 5.2).

5.4.2 COVID-19 pandemic and its aftermath

COVID-19, which apparently is a zoonotic disease, has had long and consequential effects on global health and economy that do not seem to die down. Over the past 2 years researchers have focused on the long-term effects of the disease. Whereas the symptoms of COVID-19 are well known, much less is known about what happens after recovery. While most people recover and return to normal health (Haider *et al.*, 2020), some patients can exhibit an array of symptoms for weeks or months post recovery. The WHO has warned about the devastating 'long Covid' situation and persisting symptoms that could have long-term impacts on health and productivity. It has been observed that 5% of people who have been sick with the virus have not recovered at all by 6–18 months after COVID infection.

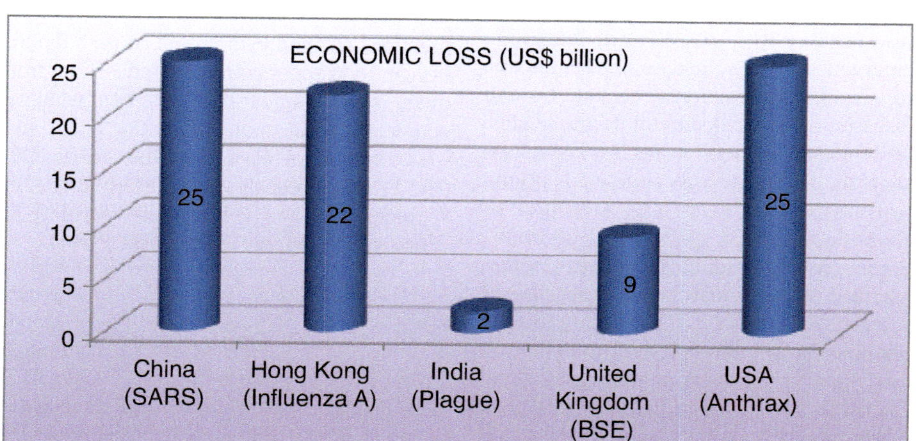

Fig. 5.2. Economic loss due to emerging and re-emerging diseases. (Author's own image.)

5.5 Messages and Key Takeaways

Messages and key takeaways from zoonotic disease outbreaks and preventing the next outbreak by breaking the chain of transmission include the following.

- De-risking food systems. It is accepted that the COVID-19 outbreak originated from a Wuhan animal food market in China and became a pandemic.
- There needs to be greater urgency in handling the emerging situations. As diseases are emerging more frequently than ever before, rapid action is necessary to fill the gaps in scientific knowledge and enable fast-tracking development of knowledge and tools to help governments, the health sector, local authorities and other stakeholders to reduce the risk of future pandemics.
- There also needs to be rapid assessment and exploration of the risk of emerging zoonotic diseases from domesticated animals and wildlife.
- Assessment of the scope of the problem is needed. As nearly 60% of infectious diseases in humans have animal origin and as some 75% 'jump species' from other species due to unsustainable human activities, prediction of outbreak frequencies has become imperative based on outcomes of how people source and grow food, and how they trade and consume animal food (Collins and Wall, 2004).
- As our environment is being altered very fast, biodiversity also is affected, leading to emergence of new infectious diseases due to complex interactions between human diseases, domesticated animals and wildlife and the environment. It has become necessary to determine the source of origin, transmission pathways and amplifiers of zoonotic diseases.
- Some seven human-mediated factors ascribed to act as drivers for emergence of zoonotic diseases are: (i) increasing human demand for animal food due to change in food habit; (ii) unsustainable agricultural intensification meaning industrial livestock production practices; (iii) increased use and exploitation of wildlife; (iv) increased unsustainable land use and over-exploitation of natural resources and industrialization; (v) international travel, transportation and animal trade; (vi) changes in food supply; and (vii) climate change.

Primary biosecurity measures based on a risk assessment are applicable in different farming enterprises or environments that will reduce the incidence of most zoonotic agents. The World Trade Organization (WTO) agreement for the application of sanitary and phyto-sanitary measures requires scientifically based data. The main elements of this agreement are risk analysis, regionalization, harmonization, equivalence and transparency. Two of these elements, namely risk analysis and regionalization, are dependent on epidemiological surveillance. This may provide a basis for practical application in regard to export and import of animals and animal products.

5.6 Zoonotic Disease Impact and Cost

In the past, the world has endured the impact and cost associated with zoonotic diseases but nothing can be compared with the impact of the COVID-19 pandemic. The greatest burden was borne by the poor, with loss of livelihood and daily earning as wage earners, monetary loss, healthcare expenses associated with mental health problems, death of dear and near ones, psychological trauma, post-illness morbidity and other untold miseries. The monetary loss incurred by the developed countries was higher, due to loss of trade and burgeoning inflation. The pandemic could cause a dip in the hunger-index poor countries. India has a hunger index of 107 out of 121 countries, which may deteriorate if adequate preventive public health measures are not taken under the One Health and One World approach where veterinarians, environmentalists and collaborative partners have definitive roles to play (Kiedrowski, 2014).

5.7 Policy Options

The WHO, FAO, WOAH (OIE), International Livestock Research Institute (ILRI) and the World Environmentalist Group recommended ten policy response options to reduce the risk of future zoonotic pandemics and to 'build back better', as follows: (i) raise awareness of health and environment risks; (ii) improve health governance, including by engaging environmental stakeholders; (iii) expand scientific inquiry into the environmental dimensions of zoonotic diseases; (iv) ensure full cost financial accounting of the societal impacts of disease; (v) enhance monitoring and regulation of food systems using risk-based approaches; (vi) phase out unsustainable agricultural practices; (vii) develop and implement stronger biosecurity measures; (viii) strengthen animal health (including wildlife health services); (ix) capacity building among health stakeholders to incorporate environmental dimensions of health; and (x) mainstream and implement One Health approaches.

It needs to be remembered that human, animal and environmental health are intricately and intrinsically linked (Parkes, 1987), that biosafety of all the living creatures inhabiting 'Mother Earth' is paramount and that no one can act in isolation and afford to be careless.

References

Abegunde, D.O., Mathers, C.D., Adam, T., Ortegon, M. and Strong, K. (2007) The burden and costs of chronic diseases in low-income and middle-income countries. *The Lancet* 370(9603), 1929–1938.

Benner, C., Carabin, H., Sánchez-Serrano, L.P., Budke, C.M. and Carmena, D. (2010) Analysis of the economic impact of cystic echinococcosis in Spain. *Bulletin of the World Health Organization* 88, 49–57B.

Budke, C.M., Carabin, H. and Torgerson, P.R. (2011) Health impact assessment and burden of zoonotic diseases. In: Palmer, S.R., Soulsby, L., Torgerson, P.R. and Brown, D.W.G. (eds) *Oxford Textbook of Zoonoses. Biology, Clinical Practice, and Public Health Control*. Oxford University Press, Oxford, UK, pp. 30–37.

Christou, L. (2011) The global burden of bacterial and viral zoonotic infections. *Clinical Microbiology and Infection* 17(3), 326–330.

Collins, J.D. and Wall, P.G. (2004) Food safety and animal production systems: Controlling zoonoses at farm level. *Revue Scientifique et Technique-Office International des Épizooties* 23(2), 685–700.

Elelu, N., Aiyedun, J.O., Mohammed, I.G., Oludairo, O.O., Odetokun, I.A. *et al.* (2019) Neglected zoonotic diseases in Nigeria: Role of the public health veterinarian. *Pan African Medical Journal* 32(1), 36.

Grace, D., Gilbert, J., Lapar, M.L., Unger, F., Fèvre, S. *et al.* (2011) Zoonotic emerging infectious disease in selected countries in Southeast Asia: Insights from ecohealth. *Ecohealth* 8(1), 55–62.

Haider, N., Rothman-Ostrow, P., Osman, A.Y., Arruda, L.B., Macfarlane-Berry, L. *et al.* (2020) COVID-19 – zoonosis or emerging infectious disease? *Frontiers in Public Health* 8, 596944.

Karesh, W.B., Dobson, A., Lloyd-Smith, J.O., Lubroth, J., Dixon, M.A. *et al.* (2012) Ecology of zoonoses: Natural and unnatural histories. *The Lancet* 380(9857), 1936–1945.

Kiedrowski, L.M. (2014) The one world/one health concept applied in the field, laboratory, and hospital. Doctoral dissertation, North Dakota State University.

Krauss, H., Weber, A., Appel, M., Isenberg, H.D., Schiefer, H.G. *et al.* (2003) *Zoonoses: Infectious Diseases Transmissible from Animals to Humans*, 3rd edn. American Society of Microbiology Press, Washington, DC.

Kuchenmüller, T., Abela-Ridder, B., Corrigan, T. and Tritscher, A. (2013) World Health Organization initiative to estimate the global burden of foodborne diseases. *Revue Scientifique et Technique (International Office of Epizootics)* 32(2), 459–467.

Murray, C.J. (1994) Quantifying the burden of disease: The technical basis for disability-adjusted life years. *Bulletin of the World Health Organization* 72(3), 429.

Narrod, C., Zinsstag, J. and Tiongco, M. (2012) A one health framework for estimating the economic costs of zoonotic diseases on society. *EcoHealth* 9(2), 150–162.

Pal, M. (2013) Public health concern due to emerging and re-emerging zoonoses. *International Journal of Livestock Research* 3(1), 56–62.

Parkes, P. (1987) Livestock symbolism and pastoral ideology among the Kafirs of the Hindu Kush. *Man* 22, 637–660.

Sherikar, A.T., Bachchil, V.N. and Thapliyal, D.C. (2005) *Text Book of Elements of Veterinary Public Health*. ICAR, New Delhi, India.

Torgerson, P.R. and Macpherson, C.N. (2011) The socioeconomic burden of parasitic zoonoses: Global trends. *Veterinary Parasitology* 182(1), 79–95.

WHO (2023) 5 things to know about One Health in the WHO European Region. News release, World Health Organization, Geneva. Available at: https://www.who.int/europe/news/item/23-03-2023-5-things-to-know-about-one-health-in-the-who-european-region

6 Antimicrobial Resistance: Consequence of Animal Use of Antibiotics

Jinu Manoj[1]*, Manoj Kumar Singh[2], Indu Panchal[3] and Z.B. Dubal[4]
[1]College Central Laboratory, Lala LajPat Rai University of Veterinary and Animal Sciences, Hisar, Haryana, India; [2]College of Veterinary and Animal Sciences, Sardar Vallabhbhai Patel University of Agriculture and Technology, Meerut, Uttar Pradesh, India; [3]College of Dairy Sciences, Lala LajPat Rai University of Veterinary and Animal Sciences, Hisar, Haryana, India; [4]Division of Veterinary Public Health, ICAR-Indian Veterinary Research Institute, Izatnagar, Bareilly, Uttar Pradesh, India

Abstract

Antibiotic abuse and overuse in food animals fosters the development and dissemination of antibiotic-resistant strains. Antimicrobial resistance (AMR) has detrimental repercussions for the environment, food animals, agriculture and healthcare systems. The resistant bacteria of public health importance, like *Escherichia coli*, *Klebsiella pneumoniae*, *Salmonella* spp., *Staphylococcus aureus* and *Campylobacter* spp., can be transmitted to humans through food, water, soil or manure. Animal wastes as manure also promote the horizontal transmission of genes. The use of antibiotics in aquaculture contributes to antibiotic accumulation in water bodies. Failure to follow drug withdrawal periods in food animals leads to antibiotic residues in the products, which raises concerns about the safety of consumers. Antibiotic alternatives are urgently needed for animal production and health, which may include plant-based compounds, bacteriophages, probiotics, antimicrobial peptides and proteins. Several surveillance programmes have been initiated to combat AMR. Understanding the contributions of all the sectors of the One Health concept along with antimicrobial stewardship is crucial in the fight against AMR.

Keywords: antibiotic resistance, antibiotic alternatives, livestock, One Health, stewardship

6.1 Introduction

Antibiotics are substances produced by microorganisms that selectively inhibit or kill the growth of other microorganisms. The discovery of antibiotics was a boon in the medical field, revolutionizing modern medicine and changing the therapeutic paradigm. However, when Sir Alexander Fleming received the Nobel Prize in 1928 for discovering penicillin, he predicted the dangers of antibiotic misuse (Devasahayam *et al.*, 2010; Sharma *et al.*, 2018).

According to the data of the Food and Agriculture Organization (FAO), the global demand for animal protein is rising every year. Subsequently, to meet this increasing demand antibiotics are frequently employed for raising food animals, mostly to boost their growth. Antimicrobial resistance (AMR) is one of the most important public health threats to humanity (WHO, 2021). Antimicrobial resistance refers

*Corresponding author: drjinumanoj@gmail.com

DOI: 10.1079/ 9781800622852.0006

to a microorganism's capacity not to respond to a drug to which it was previously found to be sensitive. The resilient bacterial subpopulations adapt this trait for their survival and selection. Although it is a phenomenon of natural evolution, antimicrobial overuse, misuse, poor infection control practices and poor hygienic and sanitary measures contribute to its acceleration (Sharma *et al.*, 2018).

6.2 AMR and Health Implications

Globally, an estimated 700,000 human deaths are attributable to resistant pathogens each year. In the USA, AMR causes 35,000 mortalities and 2.8 million infections each year (CDC, 2019). Bacteria that are not treated properly can mutate and become resistant to antibiotic treatment. The resistance genes can spread to other bacteria, making them resistant as well. Humans and animals both use antibiotics. Use of the same class of antibiotics for humans and for food-producing animals increases the emergence of resistant pathogens. AMR against antibiotics for use in farm animals has implications for human health. Once resilient, these microorganisms can reach humans through contact with the animals, contaminated food or environment. This results in infection that cannot be treated with currently available medications and requires the use of newer and potentially more expensive antibiotics. The confluence of elements, including a deficient healthcare system, income growth, a heavy disease burden and low-cost, unregulated antibiotic sales, has produced the perfect environment for a sharp increase in antibiotic-resistant infections in India. India has some of the highest non-prescription carbapenem sales worldwide, which contributes to the rise in carbapenem resistance in Gram-negative bacteria (Laxminarayan and Chaudhury, 2016).

6.3 Antimicrobial Usage in Animals

The health and productivity of animals are usually met through the use of antibiotics in the livestock sector either as prophylactic, metaphylactic or therapeutic agents. Antimicrobial growth promoters (AGPs) are administered to animals in sub-therapeutic doses to modify the intestinal microbiota and kill specific pathogenic intestinal bacteria. AGPs increase animal performance by lowering bacterial and host competition for nutrients. As a result, they improve the performance and growth rate of animals. Low doses of antibiotics have been included in animals' basic feed to control potential enteropathogens like *Salmonella* serovars and *Clostridium* species (Ma *et al.*, 2021). Intense cost-effective animal husbandry practices forced producers to increase the use of antimicrobials in food animals. These procedures posed a serious risk to public health by facilitating the spread of pathogens that are resistant to antibiotics in both humans and livestock. The abuse and overuse of antibiotics as well as their agricultural application in the feed of livestock for the purposes of promoting growth, preventing sickness and boosting feed capacity can be the reasons for the rising rate of AMR.

According to estimates, the average worldwide annual demand for antimicrobials for animal products was 148 mg/kg for chicken, 45 mg/kg for beef and 172 mg/kg for pork (Ma *et al.*, 2021). An approximate 80% of all antibiotics used in the USA were for animals raised for food. Cattle and pigs were the animals with the highest consumption of medically significant drugs, estimated as 42 and 39%, respectively, of the 6653 tonnes of antibiotics sold in the USA in 2018. Cattle and chickens consumed the most (61 and 25%, respectively) of the 6096 tonnes of non-medically essential antimicrobial medications in the same year. The most common medically significant antimicrobials being used for food animals that year were tetracyclines (66%), penicillins (12%) and macrolides (8%) (FDA, 2019).

The World Bank estimates that the reduction in global gross domestic product (GDP) by 2050 will range from 3.8% in the worst case to 1.1% in the best case with little impact from AMR. By 2030, this will result in a US$3.4 trillion annual shortfall. A conservative estimate of the amount of antibiotics used worldwide in livestock in 2010 was 63,200 tonnes (t) and the estimated increase in consumption is to 200,235t by 2030. It is estimated that antimicrobial consumption may rise by 67% from 2010 to 2030. Approximately 3% of the world's antimicrobials used in food animals are consumed in India. Animal population growth accounts for two-thirds of the increase, while the transition from extensive to intense farming accounts for the final one-third (van Boeckel *et al.*, 2014; Mutua *et al.*, 2020).

6.4 Mechanism of AMR

There are several factors involved in the development of AMR, including the indiscriminate use, improper dose and regime of the antibiotic. Antibiotics are commonly used in conditions where there is no necessity for them. Poor hygienic and sanitary practices also contribute to antimicrobial resistance. The pathogens that develop a resistant mechanism have the opportunity to multiply again and also to contaminate the environment.

There have been five main methods used by bacteria for resistance (Fig. 6.1).

1. Pathogens reduce the ability of the active ingredient to enter the cell, preventing it from reaching its target site.
2. General or specific signal transduction expels the antimicrobial agent from the cell.
3. The inactivation of antibiotics.
4. By modifying the antimicrobial agents.
5. By modifying the target sites within the bacteria.

Based on the genetic basis of resistance, antibiotic resistance in bacteria can be broadly divided into intrinsic resistance and extrinsic or acquired resistance. Intrinsic resistance is encoded in the chromosome and cannot be horizontally transmitted. Through the use of mobile genetic elements like plasmids, transposases and integrases, horizontal gene transfer (HGT) takes place between various bacterial species. HGT makes a sizeable contribution to the quick spread of resistance. Veterinarians, farmworkers and slaughterhouse employees are easily exposed to resistant bacteria through their routine contact with diseased animals. The acquired resistance can be spread horizontally

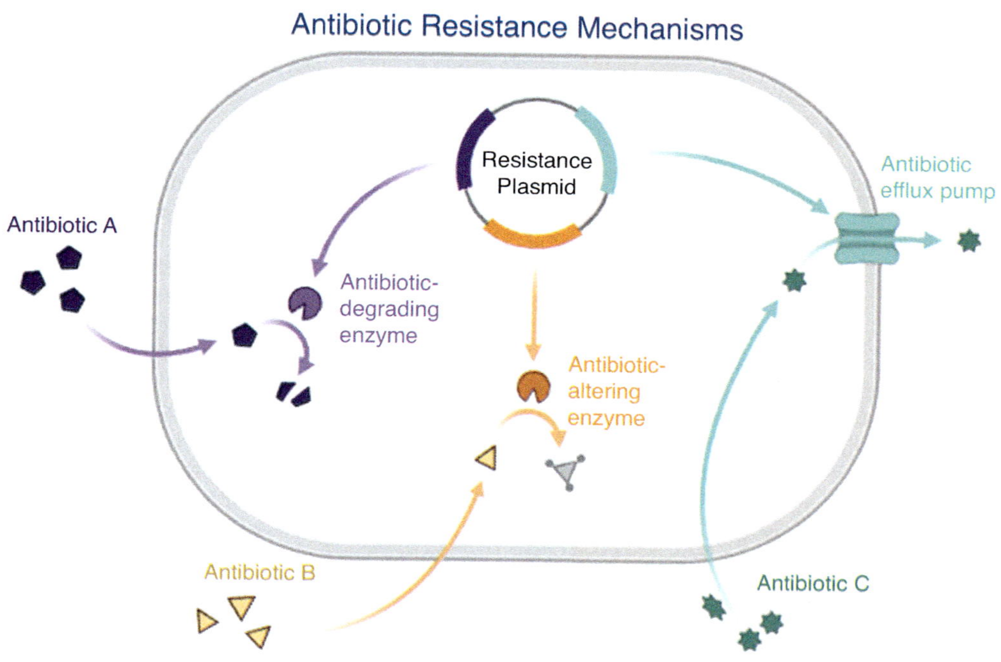

Fig. 6.1. Mechanisms of antibiotic resistance. (Author's own image.)

among bacteria and is present in some strains of a species of bacterium that is typically susceptible towards the antibiotic of interest. Acquired resistances are caused by transferable resistance genes that are acquired either from donors or by the development of mutations in the organism's own DNA that eventually result in resistance to the associated antibiotic. Plasmids or (conjugative) transposable elements may be able to spread acquired antibiotic resistances caused by exogenous DNA acquisition to different bacterial species or genera. Mutations in housekeeping chromosomal genes that result in acquired antibiotic resistance most likely represent a negligible risk of horizontal dissemination. (Vankerckhoven *et al.*, 2008; Ma *et al.*, 2021).

Multiple drug resistance (MDR) is the lack of susceptibility of microbes to at least one agent in three or more chemical classes of antibiotics like beta-lactam, aminoglycoside or macrolide. MDR in bacteria may be generated by one of two mechanisms. First, these bacteria may accumulate multiple genes, each coding for resistance to a single drug, within a single cell. This accumulation occurs typically on resistance plasmids. Secondly, MDR may also occur by the increased expression of genes that code for multidrug efflux pumps, extruding a wide range of drugs.

6.5 AMR in the Veterinary Sector

Drug resistance is brought on by the indiscriminate utilization of antibiotics, endangering the health of both humans and animals. Animal health is significantly impacted by AMR in food animals and it may also be linked to infections that are resistant to treatment in people. Antibiotic use in food animals over an extended period of time fosters the development and dissemination of resistant strains. Animals may transmit resistant bacteria to humans either directly or indirectly through food, water, soil or manure.

Since 1980, several feed formulations containing antibiotics were allowed to be used in animals raised for food. Many such feed formulations are used in India, especially in the livestock and poultry sectors. This results in excretion of large amounts of active antibiotics and their metabolites through faeces, milk, meat and their products (Jechalke *et al.*, 2014). There were several reports of antibiotic residues in foods of animal and poultry origin from all over the globe, including India (Vishnuraj *et al.*, 2016). These antibiotic residues then enter into human and animal guts, soil, water and the environment and affect the natural microbiota. The AMR genes are then easily transmitted through mobile genetic elements like plasmids and transposon to unexposed groups of organisms.

The antibiotic contamination and the development of possibly resistant bacteria are also brought on by the use of animal waste as a fertilizer. Also, the nutrients in the manure promote horizontal transmission of genes among the various species. Asia has the highest global aquaculture production. Fish and many other aquaculture products have been found to contain many antimicrobials. Chicken and pig manures are frequently used to retain the fertility of fish farms for the purpose of promoting fish growth because of the substantial amount of antibiotics present in livestock manure. These antibiotics would eventually get into different water structures and contaminate wild fish and other aquaculture products. The presence of chloramphenicol, norfloxacin, ciprofloxacin and enrofloxacin have been reported in marine fish (Ma *et al.*, 2021). The use in aquaculture of antibiotics like oxytetracycline, ormetoprim and sulfadimethoxine also contributed to antibiotic accumulation. Usually, fish do not efficiently metabolize antibiotic medications and instead expel them in the active state into the environment, leading to the emergence of AMR in microbial populations.

Numerous antimicrobial-resistant bacteria of public health importance have been noticed in broilers and laying hens. Third-generation cephalosporin-resistant *Escherichia coli* and *Klebsiella pneumoniae* were estimated to be responsible for 4.6–6.4 million bloodstream infections caused by drug-resistant WHO priority pathogens, while carbapenem-resistant pathogens were responsible for 0.4–0.5 million. Since 1995, ciprofloxacin-resistant *Campylobacter* has emerged as a result of the widespread use of fluoroquinolone antibiotics, particularly in the production of poultry. This strain was later found in the breast flesh of killed birds. Vancomycin resistance is thought to be promoted by the antibiotic avoparcin, which is used to enhance growth in livestock. In Europe, vancomycin-resistant *Enterococcus faecalis* was still widely distributed in poultry. According to certain *in vivo* transfer experiments, the *vanA* gene was found in transposon Tn1546, which suggests it can be transmitted between enterococci that are adapted for humans and animals. Also found in a transferable element, the *vanM* gene might be transferred through conjugation. Comparable VRE strains have been found in humans and farm animals, suggesting that some of these strains may be capable of becoming accustomed to food animals and disseminate infectious diseases to humans (Ahmed and Baptiste, 2018).

Chickens can act as reservoirs for a range of foodborne infections. The two predominant species, *Campylobacter jejuni* and *Campylobacter coli*, are major cause of foodborne bacterial gastroenteritis in humans. *Campylobacter* is transmitted to human beings mainly through contaminated foods of animal origin, particularly unpasteurized milk and milk products, and raw or undercooked poultry meat. Therefore, chicken is considered as the primary source of infection to humans with a very low dose of infection, i.e. 500 organisms. Once infected, it will be well adopted by the intestinal tract (Kaakoush *et al.*, 2015). *Campylobacter* isolates were found to be moderately to highly sensitive against tetracycline and fluoroquinolones in earlier years, but later showed increasing resistance trends (Kanaan *et al.*, 2022). However, Khan *et al.* (2018) reported that 59.4% of isolates were resistant to tetracycline, though they reported much less resistance against fluoroquinolone (FQ) and erythromycin (6.9–8.9%). In contrast, 92.3% resistance to erythromycin was observed for *Campylobacter* isolates from Chennai in Tamil Nadu (Elango *et al.*, 2009).

There are several reports worldwide describing fluoroquinolone-resistant *Campylobacter* infections in humans. It is possible for the FQ-resistant *Campylobacter* population to eventually infiltrate avian intestines and spread to humans through tainted chicken meat. In the USA, nalidixic acid-resistant *Campylobacter* spp. increased from 1.3% in 1992 to 10.2% in 1998 (Smith and Coast, 2013). *Campylobacter* isolates from pets showed resistance to aztreonam, penicillin, ampicillin, amoxycillin, streptomycin, lincomycin and oxytetracycline (Verma *et al.*, 2014).

Several countries have reported finding antimicrobial resistance among Gram-negative bacteria isolated from chickens that had been slaughtered and sold for consumption, and from free-range chickens. *E. coli* consistently exhibited higher levels of antimicrobial resistance than the other Enterobacteriaceae. Ampicillin, amoxicillin, tetracycline and doxycycline all had median levels of resistance that were >70%. Ceftiofur, a broad-spectrum antibiotic in the cephalosporin group, is used as a prophylactic measure in piglets to prevent diarrhoea, septicaemia, arthritis and meningitis. The extended spectrum beta lactamases (ESBLs) producing *E. coli* emerged because of the use of cephalosporins in livestock and transmitted to humans via contaminated food and water (Nhung *et al.*, 2017). During the 1990s, colistin, also called polymyxin E, has been utilized to treat MDR Gram-negative infections, particularly those Enterobacteriaceae that produce carbapenemase. Colistin was used as a preventive measure and a growth enhancer in pigs until it was banned from usage in humans owing to its nephrotoxic effects. *E. coli* and *K. pneumonia*, a significant human pathogen that causes infections in hospitals and the population, have now developed resistance to beta lactamases (Behera and Mathur, 2011).

Tetracycline is used as a growth promoter and therapeutic in cattle; beta-lactams, cephalosporin and macrolides are used to cure diseases and boost growth; and peptidomimetics are used as growth promoters in poultry. Tetracycline resistance genes are frequently found in various transferable elements such as integrons and plasmids. Tetracycline resistance in bacteria can occur through ribosome protection and efflux pumps as well as enzymatic inactivation of antibiotics (Meade *et al.*, 2017).

Many bacterial diseases related to dairy animals are listed in India and some of them are held responsible for outbreaks of diseases in dairy animals. Among bacterial diseases, salmonellosis and mastitis are the major diseases associated with dairy animals. Antibiotics are commonly used for the treatment of salmonellosis, mastitis and other bacterial diseases. At present, the introduction of large commercial farming and improved production and profitability in the dairy sector has led to emergence of antimicrobial-resistant pathogens in farm environments. Primarily due to uncontrolled use of antibiotics, large-scale AMR has been developed in pathogens of dairy husbandry origin.

The antibiotic-resistant bacteria and their antibiotic-resistance genes cause resistance to the main classes of antibiotics that are used for therapeutics in mastitis. Amoxycillin plus sulbactam, ceftriaxone, enrofloxacin, gentamicin, ceftiofur and cefquinome are being used predominantly for the treatment of mastitis due to *Staphylococcus aureus* in livestock. Emergence of methicillin-resistant *Staphylococcus aureus* (MRSA) in bovine mastitis is a matter of concern for animal health and the dairy industry. The MRSA isolates discovered from chickens, pigs and cows had the same *mecA* gene as that of human isolates. Human ciprofloxacin-resistant isolates of *E. coli* have a linkage to poultry. *Salmonella* isolates from humans and chicken strains were significantly less resistant to antibiotics after temporary discontinuation of ceftiofur injection into eggs and chickens (Ma *et al.*, 2021).

6.6 Significance of Antibiotic Sensitivity Tests

Drug resistance can be detected using special laboratory tests which test the bacteria for sensitivity to the drugs or detect resistance patterns. The antimicrobial susceptibility test (AST) provides an *in vitro* measure of susceptibility and resistance by determining the concentration of drug required to inhibit an organism to a specified degree, the minimum inhibitory concentration (MIC). Antibiotic sensitivity testing is used to measure the sensitivity of microbes such as bacteria to antibiotics. The test results may indicate the bacteria to be completely susceptible (S) or resistant (R) to the bacteria or have intermediate (I) susceptibility for the antibiotic (Fig. 6.2). The AST profiling is performed in phenotypic- and genotypic-based methods. There are two standards accepted for clinical laboratory AST testing: those established by the Clinical Laboratory Standards Institute (CLSI) and those established by the European Committee on Antimicrobial Susceptibility Testing (EUCAST). Most of the Clinical Microbiology Laboratories report their AST results according to CLSI guidelines. Nowadays, more and more laboratories prefer the guideline that has been published by EUCAST. In Indian laboratories, CLSI breakpoints for reporting AST are usually followed.

Tests for antimicrobial susceptibility are usually carried out in cases when there has been a failure or poor response towards the first line of therapy in the field conditions. Veterinarians prefer to employ new-generation antibiotics for the treatment of refractory mastitis. However, because of their high cost and potential unaffordability to farmers, these medications may

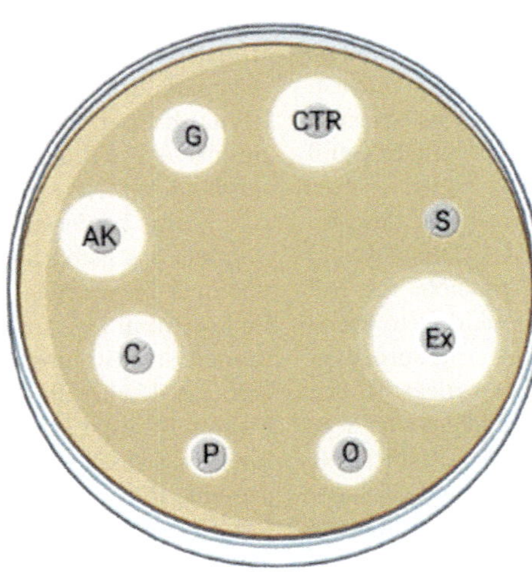

Fig. 6.2. Antibiotic sensitivity test (phenotypic method). (Author's own image.)

only be used as a last resort to treat serious human infections. Moreover, their use may promote the development of resistance, limiting their potential future applications in human health. The treatment of sick animals is not always left to qualified veterinarians; sometimes farmers treat the animals themselves. Farmers make the decisions regarding when they should handle antibiotics because extension networks are not yet completely formed. Antibiotics can be purchased over the counter with or without a prescription. Farmers choose treatments that provide them with immediate results and they base their decisions on the options available, their prior experiences using the medication to treat illnesses that are similar and guidance from vets, feed stores and colleagues. There have also been reports of drug access through cooperatives, feed stores and milk vendors. Critically important antibiotics are frequently utilized in aquaculture and animal husbandry. The consequences of improperly discarding milk of infected and medicated cows, which may lead to environmental contamination, are also unknown to farmers (Sharma *et al.*, 2022).

AMR has detrimental repercussions for the environment, food animals, agriculture and healthcare systems. AMR to broad-spectrum antibiotics like fluoroquinolones and third-generation cephalosporins has been reported in more than 70% of cases in Gram-negative bacteria like *E. coli*, *K. pneumoniae* and *Acinetobacter baumannii* and in more than 50% of cases in *Pseudomonas aeruginosa*. MRSA is the most prevalent among Gram-positive bacteria (Roshan *et al.*, 2022).

Antimicrobial residues have been found in food of animal origin from various parts of world, indicating a widespread use of antimicrobials among animals. The lack of written plans for treating sick animals and the keeping of records of antibiotic treatments, as well as the owner's own administration, make it difficult to predict the actual values of its use in dairy farms in India (Sharma *et al.*, 2018). The presence of antibiotic residues in dairy products is a major issue. Antibiotics residue in milk was first detected in the 1960s and has been found with an increasing trend since then. In milk, β-lactam is the most prevalent contaminant, followed by tetracyclines, fluoroquinolones, sulfonamides and aminoglycosides (Sachi *et al.*, 2019; Behera *et al.*, 2023). Failure to follow drug withdrawal periods in food animals leads to residues in the products and raises concerns about the safety of consumers. Antibiotic residue limits have been defined and items that exceed them should be disposed of, while taking precautions to minimize the likelihood of environmental contamination.

6.7 Mitigation Methods for AMR

AMR remains a grave issue for public health. It has an impact on human, animal and environmental health. Understanding the contributions of all the sectors of the One Health concept is crucial for the fight against AMR. One Health emphasizes the role of the interdependence of humans, animals and environment for achieving health for all (Fig. 6.3). It encourages cooperation among all these sectors for attaining One Health. Various strategies are designed for this mission, involving relevant organizations. AMR in the environment has received little attention so far. Reduction in antibiotic consumption in both agriculture and aquaculture sectors will help to reduce the number of AMR bacteria in the environment.

To protect public health, the European Union outlawed the use of smaller concentrations of antimicrobial growth promoters in livestock feed, because prolonged exposure to this low-dose antibiotic could cause bacteria to develop resistance, due to selective pressure. In many countries, including India, this restriction has not been put into place where antibiotics are regularly and widely used for farming purposes. Administration of quinolones in aquaculture was prohibited in several industrialized countries because AMR to one kind of quinolone often develops into resistance to all kinds of this class of antibiotics (Martinez, 2009). Besides these, the optimum and appropriate use of antibiotics is essential. The most important thing is to protect ourselves, our livestock and our environment through proper sanitation and hygiene.

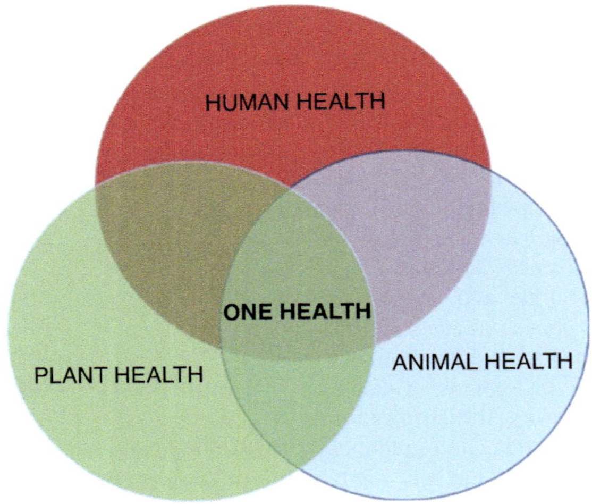

Fig. 6.3. One Health Concept. (Author's own image.)

6.8 Alternatives to Antibiotics

Antibiotic alternatives are urgently needed for animal production and health. The most effective alternatives are plant-based compounds, bacteriophages, probiotics and antimicrobial peptides and proteins (Sharma *et al.*, 2018). In our opinion, development of herbal preparations against resistant pathogens will be more meaningful than the synthetic antibiotics. In the ruminant, pig and poultry sectors, phytochemicals have been employed as natural growth boosters. Many herbs and spices have been used in poultry for their potential as AGP substitutes, including black cumin, cinnamon, coriander, garlic, marjoram, rosemary, oregano, thyme and yarrow. Using avian lymphocytes and macrophages, researchers have examined the immune-stimulating abilities of herbal medicines such as mustard, dandelion and safflower.

In place of antibiotics, nanoparticles are being employed more frequently to target microorganisms. Utilization of the nanoparticles in antibacterial vaccines to prevent bacterial infections, bacterial identification techniques for microbial diagnostics, antibiotic carriers to cure diseases and antibacterial coating materials for medical implants and pharmaceuticals to enhance wound healing and reduce the risk of infection are extensively studied. The antibacterial mechanisms of these nanoparticles include metal ion release, oxidative stress induction and non-oxidative mechanisms (Wang *et al.*, 2017).

Antibiotic therapy may be replaced by the use of bacteriophages to treat infections brought on by bacteria that are multidrug-resistant. Phage therapy might serve as an alternative kind of treatment for diseases that are found in chicken farms. Phage therapy was used for systemic infection in chickens due to *Salmonella enterica*, *Campylobacter jejuni*, *E. coli* and *Clostridium perfringens*. Research on the application of phage therapy to manage mastitis in bovine species and respiratory diseases in pigs was conducted (Loponte *et al.*, 2021). Following proper husbandry techniques can help animals experience fewer clinical illnesses and reduce the demand for antibiotics. It is necessary to investigate methods for increasing animal production without relying on antibiotic use. A vibrant ethnoveterinary medical culture exists in India and this should be considered for practical utility for combating AMR.

Vaccines as a legitimate therapeutic alternative to antibiotics have garnered considerable attention, due to their unique properties and mode of action. Also, the development of resistance is not observed among vaccines. The administration of vaccines in the livestock sector is preferred instead of antibiotic use for preventive purposes (Sharma *et al.*, 2018).

6.9 Activities at International and National Level

Surveillance of AMR is equally important to combat the problem. Several international and national surveillance programmes have been initiated all over the world. The international surveillance programmes include the Global Antimicrobial Resistance Surveillance System (GLASS), NNIS System/National Healthcare Safety Network (NHSN), Alexander Project, Hospitals in Europe Link for Infection Control through Surveillance (HELICS), Tracking Resistance in the United States Today (TRUST), SENTRY Antimicrobial Surveillance Program, Meropenem Yearly Susceptibility Test Information Collection (MYSTIC) Program, European Antimicrobial Resistance Surveillance System (EARSS), Prospective Resistant Organism Tracking and Epidemiology for the Ketolide Telithromycin (PROTEKT), ECO·SENS Project, Surveillance of Antimicrobial Use and Antimicrobial Resistance in ICUs (SARI), Gonococcal Antimicrobial Surveillance Programme (GASP), European Surveillance of Antimicrobial Consumption Network (ESAC-Net) and European Antimicrobial Resistance Surveillance Network (EARS-Net). The World Health Organization (WHO) Global Action Plan provides a number of methods that nations could employ to reduce the risk, such as raising awareness and knowledge of AMR through effective communication, education and training. According to the WHO's recommendations, it is necessary to limit the administration of highest priority and critically important antibiotics in animals.

The Government of India also initiated the Indian Network for Surveillance of Antimicrobial Resistance (INSAR), Antimicrobial Resistance Surveillance Research Network (AMRSN), National Action Plan on Antimicrobial Resistance (NAP-AMR), Indian Network for Fishery and Animals Antimicrobial Resistance (INFAAR) and National Programme on Containment of Antimicrobial Resistance programmes to combat AMR.

India has a number of laws governing the administration of antibiotics on animals used for food production, but enforcement and compliance are problems. There are wide ranges of challenges to reduce the occurrence of antimicrobial resistance, despite India's National Policy for Containment of Antimicrobial Resistance. There were several approaches to combat AMR in India, including the following.

1. Control and regulations regarding the unauthorized sale of antibiotics and their improper use in the agriculture, aquaculture and human sectors.
2. Development of SOP/standard recommendations for treating prevalent pathogenic diseases.
3. Public awareness of the impact of AMR on human and animal health through social media, pamphlets, radio talks and extension activities.
4. Maintaining personal hygiene by nutritious and adequate diet, regular exercise, yoga, meditation, banning tobacco and alcohol, avoiding junk foods and regular consumption of fruit will help personal protection by improving immunity and health.
5. Cleanliness of house, kitchen, surroundings and our environment. Good public health measures like improved sanitation and hygiene practices, increased immunization coverage, quick response to outbreaks and promotion of ayurvedic and many other holistic mechanisms of healing will decrease dependence on antibiotics and prevent the emergence of resistant microbes.
6. Continuous surveillance of AMR pathogens for monitoring resistance in humans, animals and aquaculture is necessary.

6.10 Antimicrobial Stewardship

Asia has less advanced antimicrobial stewardship, which is thought to be the primary cause of AMR in India. Antimicrobial stewardship is defined as a set of coordinated actions aimed at enhancing and evaluating the proper use of antimicrobial agents by encouraging the choice of suitable antimicrobial drug regimens, including dosing, duration of therapy and route of administration. It alludes to a series of steps that encourage the prudent use of antibiotics.

Multidisciplinary teams that include skilled doctors, microbiologists, pharmacists, infectious disease experts and epidemiologists carry out stewardship programmes.

Although initially created for health professionals, it is crucial for veterinarians to adopt the essence of AMR stewardship. According to one study, 91% of veterinarians in the Indian state of Haryana were not familiar with the concept of antibiotic stewardship (Parkunan *et al.*, 2019). It is possible that tactics that have been proven effective in public health are also likely to be effective in animal health. Such implementation ought to be preceded by raising awareness, which would necessitate establishing a nationwide training programme that addresses the demands of the different stakeholder groups.

A restriction on antibiotic usage in food animals resulted in a 10–15% decrease in resistant microorganisms. The Theory of Change (ToC) method helps us better understand how change happens and lays out what has to be done to get the results we want. Identification and evaluation of strategies to prevent AMR can also be guided by the theory of change. The long-term objective of a task is laid out in a ToC method, together with all the prerequisites that must be met. The ToC method demonstrates how programme interventions relate to defined long-term objectives.

Interventions for AMR reduction can range from management to regulatory to educational, along with other measures. One goal of the Global Action Plan intervention is to raise awareness among all stakeholders. The Global Antibiotic Awareness Week (18–24 November) is celebrated every year to increase public understanding of antibiotic resistance and to promote actions that will slow its emergence and spread. Antibiotic usage standards would need to be revised and the changes may be impacted by a variety of policies.

6.11 Conclusions

When antimicrobials are used heavily to prevent disease and promote growth, it may favour the spread of organisms with elevated levels of resistance. Antibiotic prophylaxis at key junctures during the rearing period is frequently used to control bacterial diseases in animals. It would be ideal to determine each country's disease burden for each pathogen and, if necessary, implement prophylactic vaccination. Restricting access to antimicrobials in animal production, which are thought to be crucial for human medicine, would be a part of advisable practices. Future strategic planning for the animal sector and consumer expectations of the value and safeness of animal products remain as challenges. Recent years have seen an increase in research into the potential benefits of using botanicals to treat infections in animals. The development of new antibiotics is challenging but there is a need for consideration of alternatives for the antibiotics that are particularly effective against AMR and MDR strains. In order to increase biosecurity in the livestock industry and reduce the effects of AMR on human health, strategies like teaching excellent farming practices, limiting access to antibiotics and learning about the AMR profiles of livestock microbes can be adopted. Awareness programmes for the public should be designed and the policies regarding the purchase and accessibility of antibiotics should be revised as per the current scenario to avoid a post-antibiotic era. A multisectoral approach must be taken in unison to solve the complex problem of AMR. The One Health approach integrates different sectors and stakeholders involved in the layout and execution of projects, policies, legislation and research. This helps to improve public health outcomes for people and for both aquatic and terrestrial animal health as well as plant health, feed and food production and the environment.

References

Ahmed, M.O. and Baptiste, K.E. (2018) Vancomycin-resistant *Enterococci*: A review of antimicrobial resistance mechanisms and perspectives of human and animal health. *Microbial Drug Resistance* 24, 590–606. DOI: 10.1089/mdr.2017.0147.

Behera, B. and Mathur, P. (2011) High levels of antimicrobial resistance at a tertiary trauma care centre of India. *Indian Journal of Medical Research* 133(3), 343–345.

Behera, M., Parmanand, A., Roshan, M., Rajput, S., Gautam, D, *et al.* (2023) Novel aada5 and dfra17 variants of class 1 integron in multidrug-resistant *Escherichia coli* causing bovine mastitis. *Applied Microbiology and Biotechnology* 107, 433–446. DOI: 10.1007/s00253-022-12304-3.

CDC (2019) Antibiotic resistance threats in the United States, 2019. Centers for Disease Control and Prevention, US Department of Health and Human Services, Atlanta, Georgia.

Devasahayam, G., Scheld, W.M. and Hoffman, P.S. (2010) Newer antibacterial drugs for a new century. *Expert Opinion on Investigational Drugs* 19, 215–234. DOI: 10.1517/13543780903505092.

Elango, A., Dhanalakshmi, B., Pugazhenthi, T., Jayalalitha, V., Kumar, C. *et al.* (2009) RAPD-PCR characterization of *Campylobacter jejuni* isolates obtained from raw milk samples in Chennai. *Egyptian Journal of Dairy Science* 37, 175–181.

FDA (2019) 2018 Summary report on antimicrobials sold or distributed for use in food-producing animals. US Food and Drug Administration, White Oak, Maryland.

Jechalke, S., Heuer, H., Siemens, J., Amelung, W. and Smalla, K. (2014) Fate and effects of veterinary antibiotics in soil. *Trends in Microbiology* 22, 536–545.

Kaakoush, N.O., Castano-Rodriguez, N., Mitchell, H.M. and Man, S.M. (2015) Global epidemiology of *Campylobacter* infection. *Clinical Microbiology Reviews* 28, 687–720. DOI: 10.1128/CMR.00006-15.

Kanaan, H.F.M., Al-Isawi, A.J.O. and Mohamme, F.A. (2022) Antimicrobial resistance and antibiogram of thermotolerant *Campylobacter* recovered from poultry meat in Baghdad markets, Iraq. *Archives of Razi Institute* 77, 249–255. DOI: 10.22092/ARI.2021.356362.1828.

Khan, J.A., Rathore, R.S., Abulreesh, H.H., Qais, F.A. and Ahmad, I. (2018) Prevalence and antibiotic resistance profiles of *Campylobacter jejuni* isolated from poultry meat and related samples at retail shops in Northern India. *Foodborne Pathogens and Disease* 15, 218–225.

Laxminarayan, R. and Chaudhury, R.R. (2016) Antibiotic resistance in India: Drivers and opportunities for action. *PLoS Medicine* 13(3), e1001974. DOI: 10.1371/journal.pmed.1001974.

Loponte, R., Pagnini, U., Iovane, G. and Pisanelli, G. (2021) Phage therapy in veterinary medicine. *Antibiotics (Basel)* 10(4), 421. DOI: 10.3390/antibiotics10040421.

Ma, F., Xu, S., Tang, Z., Li, Z. and Zhang, L. (2021) Use of antimicrobials in food animals and impact of transmission of antimicrobial resistance on humans. *Biosafety and Health* 3, 32–38. DOI: 10.1016/j.bsheal.2020.09.004.

Martinez, J.L. (2009) Environmental pollution by antibiotics and by antibiotic resistance determinants. *Environmental Pollution* 157, 2893–2902.

Meade, E., Slattery, M.A. and Garvey, M. (2017) Antimicrobial resistance: An agent in zoonotic disease and increased morbidity. *Journal of Clinical and Experimental Toxicology* 1, 30–37.

Mutua, F., Sharma, G., Grace, D., Bandyopadhyay, A., Shome, B. *et al.* (2020) A review of animal health and drug use practices in India, and their possible link to antimicrobial resistance. *Antimicrobial Resistance and Infection Control* 9, 103. DOI: 10.1186/s13756-020-00760-3.

Nhung, N.T., Chansiripornchai, N. and Carrique-Mas, J.J. (2017) Antimicrobial resistance in bacterial poultry pathogens: A review. *Frontiers in Veterinary Science* 4, 126. DOI: 10.3389/fvets.2017.00126.

Parkunan, T., Ashutosh, M., Sukumar, B., Chera, J.S., Ramadas, S. *et al.* (2019) Antibiotic resistance: A cross-sectional study on knowledge, attitude and practices among veterinarians of Haryana State in India. *Veterinary World* 12(2), 258–265.

Roshan, M., Parmanand, A., Arora, D., Behera, M., Vats, A. *et al.* (2022) Virulence and enterotoxin gene profile of methicillin-resistant *Staphylococcus aureus* isolates from bovine mastitis. *Comparative Immunology, Microbiology and Infectious Diseases* 80, 101724. DOI: 10.1016/j.cimid.2021.101724.

Sachi, S., Ferdous, J., Sikder, M.H. and Hussani, S.A.K. (2019) Antibiotic residues in milk: Past, present, and future. *Journal of Advanced Veterinary and Animal Research* 6(3), 315.

Sharma, C., Rokana, N., Chandra, M., Singh, B.P., Gulhane, R.D. *et al.* (2018) Antimicrobial resistance: Its surveillance, impact and alternative management strategies in dairy animals. *Frontiers in Veterinary Science* 4, 237. DOI: 10.3389/fvets.2017.00237.

Sharma, G., Mutua, F., Deka, R.P., Shome, R., Bandyopadhyay, S. *et al.* (2022) Comparing the effectiveness of different approaches to raise awareness about antimicrobial resistance in farmers and veterinarians of India. *Frontiers in Public Health* 10, 837594. DOI: 10.3389/fpubh.2022.837594.

Smith, R. and Coast, J. (2013) The true cost of anti-microbial resistance. *British Medical Journal* 346, f1493. DOI: http://www.bmj.%20com/content/346/bmj.f1493.

van Boeckel, T.P., Gandra, S., Ashok, A., Caudron, Q., Grenfell, B.T. *et al.* (2014) Global antibiotic consumption 2000 to 2010: An analysis of national pharmaceutical sales data. *Lancet Infectious Diseases* 14(8), 742–750.

Vankerckhoven, V., Huys, G., Vancanneyt, M., Snauwaert, C., Swings, J. *et al.* (2008) Genotypic diversity, antimicrobial resistance and virulence factors of human isolates and probiotic cultures constituting two intraspecific groups of *Enterococcus faecium* isolates. *Applied and Environmental Microbiology* 74(14), 4247–4255.

Verma, A.K., Kumar, A., Singh, S.K., Rahal, A., Ahmed, I. *et al.* (2014) Prevalence and resistance to antimicrobial agents of *Campylobacter* sp. isolated from dogs in India. *Journal of Biological Sciences* 14, 142–148.

Vishnuraj, M.R., Kandeepan, G., Rao, H.K., Chand, S. and Kumbhar, V. (2016) Occurrence, public health hazards and detection methods of antibiotic residues in foods of animal origin: A comprehensive review. *Cogent Food and Agriculture* 2, 1235458.

Wang, L., Hu, C. and Shao, L. (2017) The antimicrobial activity of nanoparticles: Present situation and prospects for the future. *International Journal of Nanomedicine* 12, 1227–1249. DOI: 10.2147/IJN.S121956.

WHO (2021) Antimicrobial resistance. World Health Organization. Available at: https://www.who.int/news-room/fact-sheets/detail/antimicrobial-resistance

7 Safety Precautions in the Laboratory

Barkha Sharma* **and Meena Goswami**
U.P. Pandit Deen Dayal Upadhyay Veterinary University (DUVASU), Mathura, India

Abstract
In this ever-changing era of globalization and technological innovations, concerns are raised almost on a daily basis regarding the working conditions and safety protocols in the laboratories that serve as harbinger for these new ideas. Researchers have become more security conscious and aware about working in laboratories. Driven by the continuous and evolving need for developing safe and better laboratory equipment and ethical working conditions, new guidelines and approaches are being constantly evolved, standardized and enforced by legislation and regulation. Still, lack of better compliance and inability to follow standard protocols as well as lax judgement on the part of young researchers and the failure of authorities to make laboratory workers comply with the safety regulations have, every now and then, shown us that a lot still needs be done to attain safe laboratory practices, so that no mishap takes place anywhere in the world.

Keywords: zoonosis, goats, technology, diagnosis, legislation

7.1 Introduction

On 29 December 2018, a 23-year-old young Pakistani researcher, Seherbano Sangji, died as a result of severe second- and third-degree burns sustained while working in a laboratory headed by Patrick Herran, in the UCLA Molecular Sciences Building, USA. The researcher was alone in the laboratory at the time of the accident and working without her laboratory coat. What ensued was a long trial accusing Harran of criminal offences on four accounts. This was the first criminal procedure against an American academic for a laboratory accident. The incident startled the scientific community all over the world and prompted a debate over whose fault it really was (Allen, 2014). On 13 April 2011, in Yale University's chemistry laboratory, another young undergraduate student, Michele Dufault, lost her life working late alone (Van Noorden, 2011). In 2018, three students died in a blast at Beijing Jiaotong University while carrying out sewage treatment experiments (Pinghui, 2018; Kaufman, 2019). Online surveys at an Indian and an American university during 2020–2021 revealed that, even though almost all the students were aware and had received training regarding safety precautions and protocols, in real time poor compliance and negligence were rampant. Institutional policies and educators' attitudes seem to play a significant role in shaping students into following good lab practice (Sonawane *et al.*, 2023). Twenty-five years ago, in the aftermath of an accident in a UK laboratory involving the shooting of a metal piece into the abdomen of a student, steps were taken that led to improvements in adopted safety standards in Britain. Between January 2020 and December 2021, 56 unintended incidents involving exposure to harmful pathogens were reported from laboratories in England, Scotland and Wales.

*Corresponding author: barkha16vet@gmail.com

 The Handbook of Zoonotic Diseases of Goats (ed. T. Rana)
DOI: 10.1079/ 9781800622852.0007

In 2020, 42 unintended pathogen exposures were reported in Canada (Silver, 2022).

Now British researchers are required to write risk assessments before every experiment, something that is lacking in the USA and other parts of the world, but something that makes the experimenter responsible and aware of the risks involved (Van Noorden, 2011).

In 2008, in a Centres for Disease Control (CDC) laboratory, an unvaccinated repair worker was potentially exposed to an undisclosed pathogen because of a malfunctioning autoclave. In 2009, a dramatic series of cascading failures of safety systems inside one of the most advanced and secure laboratories in the world – the CDC biosafety level 4 (BSL-4) lab – caught the world by surprise. The CDC has been implicated in cover-ups of various such incidents occurring in its labs involving bioterror agents (Young, 2016).

More importantly, the alleged escape of the deadly SARS-COV2 virus from a virology research laboratory in Wuhan, China (Bloom *et al*., 2021) has already brought to the forefront the lax attitude of the research community towards compliance with laboratory biosafety procedures (Huising and Silbey, 2021). These accidents have raised serious concerns about the research practices, freedom and safe working conditions in academia (Huising and Silbey, 2011).

Carelessness in the laboratory may lead to simple injuries that include chemical burns, cuts from broken glass, inhalation of toxic fumes, absorption of chemicals through the skin and ingestion of toxic chemicals. Sometimes injuries may be so dangerous that they may lead to severe hazards to health and environment. There has been very little academic research into the prevalence and incidence of laboratory accidents. Ménard and Trant (2020) reported that many disastrous and hazardous accidents occurred in the past due to carelessness of professionals and workers. Upon reviewing media reports of lab accidents since 2001, the US Chemical Safety Board (CSB) concluded that safety practices at US universities leave a lot to be desired. After Sangji's debacle, UCLA revealed its latest safety initiative: a new centre for laboratory safety, the first in the USA to measure the effectiveness of safety policies and develop ways to improve scientists' approach to safety (Huising and Silbey, 2011). Likewise, the aftermath of these incidents is often followed by calls for reflection and re-examination of the academic discipline's approach to safety research and policy.

7.2 Laboratory Safety and Security: The Importance and Need

A scientific laboratory is a place where basic experimental skills are learnt by performing a set of prescribed experiments. These are the places where innovations and discovery take place for the progression of society and economics (Ejilemele, 2005). An efficient laboratory security system mitigates a number of risks and is complementary to existing laboratory security policies. In very broad terms, laboratory safety keeps people safe from chemicals, and laboratory security keeps chemicals safe from people. Safety procedure usually involves the Standard Operating Procedures (SOPs) regarding use, disposal and accidents associated with the specific type of research. Researchers should be well trained and aware of all the laboratory procedures and should abide by them at all times. They should maintain all the regulations and safety precautions while performing an experiment in the lab. Researchers should review information and procedures about safety issues, which includes an appropriate usage of protective equipment and clothing, safe handling of materials in laboratories, safe operation of equipment, safe disposal of materials, safety management and accountability, hazard assessment processes, safe transportation of materials between laboratories, safe design of facilities, emergency responses, etc. There are several safety aids available, which include posters, safety contracts, safety tests, safety citations, texts, handbooks on secondary science safety and a variety of safety equipment (Simmons *et al*., 2017).

7.3 Non-Compliance with Safety Protocols and Regulations in Laboratories: Probable Reasons

No one can possibly deny that research laboratories are hazardous (Ménard and Trant, 2020). There is always a risk of losing appendages or life or acquiring an infection if one is not careful enough. Even then, these accidents happen frequently all over the world. And one cannot help but think about the probable reasons. Commercialization of universities has forced the researchers to seek out external funding and most of the academics are engaged in enhancing their individual careers. In this process, they sometimes choose to neglect following safety protocols (Shore, 2008). Adoption of ethical regulations and constitution of institutional regulatory bodies (Stark, 2012) have generated a burden of compliance for researchers, making these policies a problem, instead of becoming a part of lab culture. Scientists often comply with these regulations by delegating the requirements to other staff members. Usually, compliance of any regulation in the absence of a credible regulatory enforcement is akin to giving a toddler the choice of taking a candy or bitter medicine. Everyone knows what that choice would be. Since the compliance is usually costly and not mandatory, it finally depends on the discretion of the researcher to follow it or simply let it go (Gunningham, 2005). In most universities, there are established power hierarchies where the Principal Investigator (PI) or the tenured faculty member is ranked higher than the untenured staff. Delegation of responsibilities by the higher-ranked person to other staff members renders the responsible person without any work and the actual workers without any real responsibility. Labs often become power domains, projecting unique cultures of their own, usually derived from personality and idiosyncrasies of the PI. Studies have shown that tenure and magnitude of funding available to a PI is an important predictor of non-compliance with regulatory safety procedures. A tenured scientist is more likely to ignore the safety regulations or delegate the responsibility to others, as compared with non-tenured peers (Basbug *et al.*, 2023).

7.4 Biosafety and Biosecurity Practices in the Laboratory

Generally, the terms biosafety and biosecurity are used interchangeably but there is a definite distinction. Biosafety includes all the measures taken to safeguard against the risk of being exposed to pathogens and their toxins while handling them in laboratory settings (Zaki, 2010). Biosecurity refers to the overall set of preventive strategies designed to protect the workers, the public and the environment against any exposure to potentially hazardous biological material. Academic laboratories are usually engaged in manipulation of highly pathogenic microorganisms and toxins for fundamental research purposes, diagnostics, drugs and vaccines development and are thus continually at risk of being exposed to these laboratory-acquired infections (LAIs). Anything can happen in a laboratory set-up that handles deadly microorganisms: accidental needle piercing of the skin, malfunctioning equipment, spilled beakers, a bite from an experimental animal. Life-threatening accidents can happen anywhere, at any time, even in the most secure BSL3 and BSL4 labs. Many surveys have indicated the widespread occurrence of LAIs in labs all over the world (Pike, 1979; Jacobson *et al.*, 1985; Walker and Campbell, 1999; Baron and Miller, 2008). The leading causes of LAIs seem to be *Brucella* spp., *Mycobacterium tuberculosis*, *Salmonella* spp., *Shigella* spp., *Rickettsia* spp., *Neisseria meningitides*, dimorphic fungi, or viruses like the human immunodeficiency virus (HIV), hepatitis B (HBV) and hepatitis C (HCV) (Peng *et al.*, 2018). The situation is even worse in developing countries where health and safety are still considered low-priority issues (Ejilemele and Ojule, 2004).

There have been many incidents when these bioterror agents have been intentionally or accidentally released and reported by media, causing fear and raising a sense of suspicion against biologists. Furthermore, the emergence and re-emergence of life-threatening diseases are of supreme concern and come under the biosafety and biosecurity agenda to circumvent LAIs. As a result, many countries have strengthened, or are in the process of strengthening, their biosecurity procedures and laws regulating the manufacture, transportation, import, export, possession, supply, transfer, acquisition and use of highly pathogenic microorganisms and toxins (Devaux, 2015).

7.5 Biohazard: Symbol, History and Meaning

A biological hazard, or biohazard, is any biological substance that poses a threat to living beings, especially humans, either directly through infection or indirectly through disruption of their surroundings. The biohazard symbol (Fig. 7.1) was created by Charles L. Baldwin of Dow Chemicals and Robert S. Runkle of the National Institutes of Health in 1966. It indicates the actual or probable presence of harmful viruses, toxins, or medical waste and warns people of potential exposure. The symbol is usually displayed prominently on the labels of chemicals, and can be of different colours (black, fluorescent orange, or orange-red), backgrounds, borders, etc. (Keith, 2014). The design and colour of the symbol were finalized after much deliberation. The fiery orange colour was adapted from Arctic exploration colours, due to its maximum visibility under most conditions. The design was three-sided and inspired by one of the oldest symbols of humanity: the Triskele (three intertwined human legs), which represents a threefold rotational symmetry so that the symbol remained recognizable even if it was put upside down. In Unicode, the biohazard symbol is U+2623.

7.5.1 UN/ISO Classification

The biohazard materials are put in different transportable categories with unique UN numbers, depending on their ability to cause harm.

1. Category A, UN 2814 – Infectious substance capable of causing permanent disability or life-threatening or fatal disease in otherwise healthy humans or animals upon exposure.
2. Category A, UN 2900 – Infectious substance affecting animals (only), not humans, when exposure occurs.
3. Category B, UN 3373 – Biological substance transported for diagnostic or investigative purposes.
4. Regulated Medical Waste, UN 3291 – Waste or reusable material derived from medical treatment of an animal or human, or from biomedical research, which includes the production and testing.

7.5.2 Biohazard levels

Various disease agents are also categorized in different biohazard levels by the United States CDC categories, Level one being minimum risk and Level four being extreme risk.

- **Biohazard Level 1:** Bacteria and viruses having minimal biohazard potential; requires gloves and facial protection. Examples include *Bacillus subtilis*, *Escherichia coli* and varicella (chickenpox), as well as some cell cultures and non-infectious bacteria.
- **Biohazard Level 2:** Bacteria and viruses that cause only mild disease to humans, or are difficult to contract via aerosol in a lab setting, such as hepatitis A, B and C, some influenza A strains, Human respiratory syncytial virus, Lyme disease, salmonella, mumps, measles, scrapie, dengue fever and

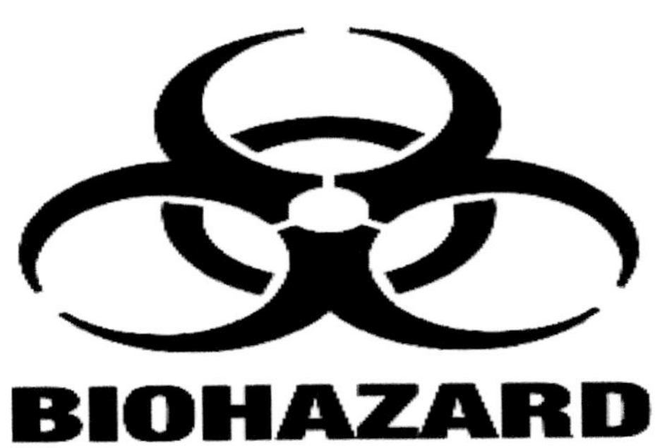

Fig. 7.1. The biohazard symbol. (Author's own image.)

HIV. These agents require Biosafety Level 2 practices and procedures.

- **Biohazard Level 3:** Bacteria and viruses that can cause severe to fatal disease in humans, but for which vaccines or other treatments exist, such as anthrax, West Nile virus, Venezuela equine encephalitis, SARS coronavirus, MERS coronavirus, SARS-CoV-2, Influenza A H5N1, hantaviruses, tuberculosis, typhus, Rift Valley fever (RVF), Rocky Mountain spotted fever, yellow fever and malaria. These require BSL-3 lab facilities.
- **Biohazard Level 4:** Viruses that cause severe to fatal disease in humans, and for which vaccines or other treatments are not available, such as Bolivian haemorrhagic fever, Marburg virus, Ebola virus, Lassa fever virus, Crimean–Congo haemorrhagic fever and other haemorrhagic diseases, as well as Nipah virus and Variola virus (smallpox). These require BSL-4 facilities. Currently there are no bacteria classified at this level.

7.6 Basic Safety Rules in Scientific Laboratories

People who work in scientific laboratories are exposed to a variety of possible hazards. Some of these hazards are not ordinarily encountered and need special precautions.

7.6.1 General safety and operational rules

- Running, jumping or talking loudly should not be permitted in working areas.
- Access to fire extinguishers, safety equipment and exits must be kept clear and unobstructed.
- Safety points like safety showers, eyewash stations and fire extinguishers should be located near the laboratory entrance and emergency exit routes should be well known to all working personnel.
- All the chemicals should be properly labelled with safety precautions.
- Unknown chemicals should be assumed as highly toxic and should not be tasted or intentionally sniffed.
- Mouth pipetting is not allowed. Skin and eye contact with chemicals should be avoided.
- Warning signs and biohazard signs must be posted at appropriate places.
- Any equipment should be used only for its designated purpose.
- All containers must have appropriate labels. Unlabelled chemicals should never be used.
- Eating, drinking, storing edibles and applying cosmetics should not be allowed in working or storage areas.
- Proper personal protection equipment (PPE) and laboratory safety glasses or goggles should be worn all the time while working in the lab and they should give protection against any accidental spill or splashes.
- No contact lenses should be worn around hazardous chemicals, even when wearing safety glasses.
- Closed-toe shoes must be worn at all times in the laboratory.
- Long hair and loose clothing must be pulled back and secured from entanglement or potential capture.
- Clothing made of synthetic fibres should not be worn while working with flammable liquids or when a hazard is present, as these materials tend to melt and stick to exposed skin.
- Laboratory coats should not be stored in offices or break-rooms, as this spreads contamination to other areas.
- Wash exposed areas of the skin prior to leaving the laboratory.
- Determine the potential hazards and appropriate safety precautions before beginning any work.
- Procedures should be developed that minimize the formation and dispersion of aerosols.
- Chemicals should not be poured down the drains. Proper protocols should be followed for their disposal.
- Keep all sink traps (including cup sink traps and floor drains) filled with water by running water down the drain at least monthly.

- Do not utilize fume hoods for evaporations and disposal of volatile solvents.
- Perform work with hazardous chemicals in a properly working fume hood to reduce potential exposures.
- Working alone in a laboratory should not be permitted if the procedures being conducted are hazardous.
- Laboratory employees should have access to a chemical inventory list, applicable safety data sheets (SDSs), departmental laboratory safety manual, and SOPs.
- Access to laboratories and support areas, such as stockrooms or specialized laboratories, should be limited to approved personnel only.
- All equipment should be regularly inspected for wear or deterioration.
- Equipment should be maintained according to the manufacturer's requirements and records of certification, maintenance, or repairs should be maintained for the life of the equipment.
- Designated and well-marked waste storage locations are necessary.
- No cell-phone or ear-bud usage is allowed in the active portion of the laboratories or during experimental operations.
- Computers and instrumentation should be labelled. Extension cords should not be used as a substitute for permanent wiring.
- Regular laboratory inspection and equipment maintenance is beneficial, to prevent laboratory accidents.

7.6.2 Responses in case of a laboratory emergency

The most common laboratory emergencies include chemical spills, fire or explosion, electric shock and personnel injuries. Most laboratory accidents occur due to poor planning or lack of attention.

General instructions

- Keep yourself safe first and remain calm.
- Call local emergency responders or a safety department, when possible, to report the emergency.
- Inform people nearby of what happened and pull the emergency alarm, when and if necessary.

Chemical spills

Chemical spills are the most common accidents when working in a chemical laboratory. Even a small-quantity spill of a hazardous chemical might threaten the lives of laboratory personnel. Therefore, caution needs to be taken when working with chemicals and PPE should always be worn to prevent bodily exposure in the case of a spill.

Chemical spilling onto surroundings

- Identify the area of the chemical spill, inform people around you and evacuate the area immediately.
- Identify the spilled chemical and ascertain it as major or minor, depending on the amount of chemical that has spilled. Refer to the chemical's SDS for hazard assessments.

For minor spills (spills of less than one gallon (4.5 litres) of low-hazard chemicals or less than 20 ml of hazardous chemicals):

- Wear proper PPE first before taking any action. Care should be taken to avoid bodily exposure to chemicals.
- If possible, modify the spill source to avoid further issues.
- If possible, turn off any nearby heat or ignition source if the chemical is flammable.
- Avoid breathing any vapours from spilled chemicals. This applies especially to chemicals that are toxic and volatile.
- Locate the spill kit and use appropriate kit tools to confine and contain the spill area.
- Use suitable adsorbent to cover the spill and neutralize the spill, if the chemicals are acidic or basic in nature.
- Collect the residues and place them into a suitable container.
- Report to EHS (Environment, Health & Safety) to dispose of any chemical spill waste.
- Refill the spill kit.

For major spills (spills of larger than one gallon (4.5 l) of low-hazard chemicals or larger than 20 ml of high-hazardous chemicals):

- Secure and evacuate the spilled area immediately and inform all nearby personnel about the major spill.
- Call emergency responders for help.
- Never attempt to clean up a major spill, even when wearing PPE.
- If possible, without exposure to the spill, shut down the power to any heat source if the spilled chemical is flammable.
- Help the emergency personnel identify the spilled area when they arrive.

Chemical spills onto the body

- Wash off all chemicals spilled on a body immediately, using a safety shower for at least 15 min. If clothes are saturated with spilled chemical, remove clothing immediately.
- If the spill splashed into eyes, use an eyewash right away for at least 15 min. Open the eyes to allow complete washing. Only attempt to remove contact lenses after eye washing has commenced.
- If the spilled chemical is a strong acid, wipe out the residues first before washing, to avoid excessive or painful burning.
- Call local responders for emergency assistance and alert people in the vicinity of the spill.

Fire or explosion

- Fire or explosion may occur from overheating, leakage, or spillage of flammable chemicals, or gases exposed to excessive heat, an open flame, or electric sparks in the laboratory. Be careful when working with flammable or explosive chemicals and avoid heat or electric sparks nearby. Safely operate electric equipment and any source of heat to prevent fire or explosion.
- In the case of a fire involving an individual's clothing, do not run, since it might accelerate the fire. Stop, drop onto the ground with hands covering the face, and roll to extinguish the fire. If possible, use the safety shower to extinguish the fire.
- In the case of a lab fire or explosion, ensure your safety first and call emergency responders immediately for help.
- Evacuate the building safely and pull fire alarms or notify nearby people, if possible.
- Do not use elevators. Use stairs and locate the nearest exit.
- If possible, shut down the electric power before evacuating.
- Use a wet towel to cover the mouth and nose, if there is heavy smoke.
- In the case of a small fire, use a proper fire extinguisher and make sure an easy exit is available if you fail to extinguish the fire.

Personal injuries

While working in a lab, a person may suffer personal injuries such as electric shock, heat burn, bleeding, or poisoning. Once this happens:

- Assess the situation before taking any actions.
- Ask the person what happened to them first, if they are conscious. Look for possible signs of injury if the person is unconscious and/or unresponsive.
- Call local emergency responders immediately if the person is in danger.
- Do not move the injured person unless imminent danger is present.
- Do not touch the person with bare hands. Use non-conductive material such as wood, glass, or rubber to pull the person away from the electric contact.
- If bleeding from minor cuts, flush with water to avoid contamination and treat with first aid supplies. If cuts are more serious, call for medical assistance.
- Initiate first aid to help, if possible.

Accidental exposure to a biohazard

The whole procedure to deal with accidental exposure to a biohazardous material through an accidental splash or splatter to facial mucous membranes, punctures with contaminated sharps and exposure to aerosols must be provided/listed in the SOPs, and must be available in the laboratory for continuous access. If an incident results in a bloodborne or other biohazard exposure (infectious agents, rDNA, biological toxins, etc.), by a needle-stick or other exposure (i.e. face and/or eye splash, cut or puncture with sharps, contact with non-intact skin, animal bites or scratches), proceed as follows.

1. **Clean it:** For skin exposure, immediately remove contaminated clothing and wash area with soap and water for 15 min; encourage needle sticks and cuts to bleed. For eye exposure, flush the eye with water for 15 min at an eyewash station or sink.
2. **Treat it:** For Risk Group (RG) 1 infectious agents it is necessary to seek medical attention within 1–2 hour so that treatment is instituted within a timeframe that increases effectiveness. If overtly exposed to recombinant or synthetic nucleic acid molecules or RG 2 infectious agents, seek immediate medical attention.
3. **Report it:** Report all exposures to the relevant authorities. Any accident involving recombinant DNA must be reported to the Institutional Biosafety Committee (IBC) office (or relevant environmental health authority) within 24 h.

7.7 Biosafety Level Requirements in Laboratory

Biosafety levels (BSLs) are individual safeguards designed to protect individuals as well as the surrounding environment and community from the high-risk agents on which various types of manipulations are done in these laboratories. There are four such biosafety levels that have increasingly complex and more stringent constraints and barriers put in place for the containment of these increasingly risky biological agents: BSL-1, BSL-2, BSL-3 and BSL-4 (Ma *et al.*, 2021).

7.7.1 Biosafety Level 1 (BSL-1)

The lowest level, BSL-1, needs no special containment equipment since it is used for working with minimum-threat, non-lethal agents that pose minimal potential hazard to the lab personnel as well as the environment. Examples of BSL-1 organisms are non-pathogenic strains of *E. coli*, *Aspergillus niger*, *Bacillus thuringiensis*, *Lactobacillus acidophilus*, *Neurospora crassa*, *Pseudomonas fluorescens*, *Serratia marcescens*, etc.

The work is done on open benches with no special containment or isolation required. The waste disposal should be after decontamination in an autoclave. Safety protocols for BSL-1 labs may include:

- mechanical pipetting (no mouth pipetting allowed)
- safe sharps handling
- avoidance of splashes or aerosols
- daily decontamination of all work surfaces when work is complete
- regular handwashing
- prohibition of food, drink and smoking materials
- use of PPE, such as goggles, gloves and a lab coat or gown
- biohazard signs.

7.7.2 Biosafety Level 2 (BSL-2)

BSL-2 laboratories are used to handle moderate-risk pathogenic agents capable of causing human diseases that are rarely serious and for which preventive and therapeutic interventions are available, if accidentally inhaled, swallowed or exposed to skin. Common examples of BSL-2 agents include bacteria like *Bacillus anthracis*, *Bordetella* spp., *Actinomyces* spp., *Actinobacillus* spp., *Borrelia* spp., *Mycobacterium* spp., *Brucella* spp., *Campylobacter*, *Chlamydia*, *Clostridium botulinum*, *Corynebacterium* spp., *Staphylococcus aureus*, *Enterobacter* spp., *Mycoplasma* pneumonia, *Yersinia* pseudotuberculosis, etc. and viruses like equine encephalitis viruses, IBR virus, herpes simplex virus (HSV), HIV, etc.

Personnel working in BSL-2 laboratories are expected to take greater care to prevent injuries, such as cuts and abrasions to the skin, ingestion and mucous membrane exposures. In addition to the safety protocols meant for BSL-1 labs, BSL-2 labs are required to have the following safety controls:

- use of PPE, including lab coats, gloves, eye protection and face shields
- biological safety cabinet in which to perform experiments causing infections with aerosols or splashes
- self-closing lockable doors.

7.7.3 Biosafety Level 3 (BSL-3)

BSL-3 is designed for handling indigenous or exotic agents that are associated with serious or lethal individual risk but low community risk and for which prophylactic or therapeutic interventions may be available. In this type of laboratory, appropriate protective clothing and equipment are mandatory for scientists working in a negative pressure facility. Common examples of microbes found in BSL-3 labs include yellow fever, West Nile virus and the bacterium that causes tuberculosis (*M. bovis*). The kind of work and the microbes handled in BSL-3 settings are strictly controlled and registered through the appropriate government agencies. Continuous medical surveillance and prophylactic immunization are often required for the personnel working in these laboratories. The access to a BSL-3 laboratory is restricted and controlled at all times. Common safety controls within a BSL-3 lab include:

- use of PPE, including goggles and gloves and respirators
- use of solid-front wraparound gowns, scrub suits and/or coveralls
- access to a hands-free sink and eyewash station near the exit
- sustained directional airflow to draw air into the laboratory from clean areas towards potentially contaminated areas (exhaust air cannot be recirculated)
- self-closing set of locking doors with access away from general building corridors.

7.7.4 Biosafety Level 4 (BSL-4)

BSL-4 is the highest, maximum-containment state-of-the-art facility constructed to handle dangerous and exotic biological agents that are likely to cause serious or lethal human disease with high individual and community risks, for which there are no preventive or therapeutic interventions usually available. This facility must be in complete isolation and the use of positive-pressure personnel suits is mandatory for its staff (WHO, 2004). In BSL-4 labs, highly dangerous and exotic microbes, such as the Ebola and Marburg viruses, are handled. These have a dedicated supply of exhaust air, as well as vacuum lines and decontamination systems. In addition to BSL-3 considerations, BSL-4 laboratories must follow these safety protocols:

- personnel must change clothing before entering the facility and shower upon exiting
- all materials must be decontaminated before leaving the facility
- personnel must wear the PPE from lower BSL levels, as well as a full-body, air-supplied, positive-pressure suit
- there must be access to a Class III biological safety cabinet.

7.8 Biosafety Regulatory Framework in India and Abroad

The countries that have biosecurity agencies are: Australia, Bulgaria, Canada, Chile, China, Cuba, Czech Republic, Denmark, Estonia, France, Georgia, Hungary, Indonesia, Ireland, Israel, Japan, Netherlands, New Zealand, Norway, Singapore, Slovakia, South Korea, Sweden, Thailand, Ukraine, United Kingdom and the United States.

In India, the rules regarding the Handling (Manufacture, Use, Import, Export and Storage) of the Hazardous Microorganisms/Genetically Engineered Organisms or Cells 1989 (known as 'Rules, 1989') come under the Environment (Protection) Act, 1986, promulgated by the Ministry of Environment and Forests (MoEF).

The Rules, 1989 are supported by Recombinant DNA Safety Guidelines, 1990 and 1994, Revised Guidelines for Research in Transgenic Plants and Guidelines for Toxicity and Allergenicity Evaluation, 1998 and Guidelines and SOPs for the conduct of Confined Field Trials of Transgenic Plant, 2008.

At present there are five competent authorities in India responsible for monitoring the research on rDNA or biohazardous materials. They are:

- Institutional Biosafety Committees (IBSCs): every institution engaged in research with biohazardous material is required to establish an IBSC to oversee and regulate such research. The IBSC has a nominee of the Department of Biotechnology (DBT) on its Committee.
- Review Committee of Genetic Manipulation (RCGM): established under the Department of Biotechnology (DBT), supervises research activities, including small-scale field trials.
- Genetic Engineering Approval Committee (GEAC): established under the MoEF, gives approvals for large-scale releases and commercialization of genetically modified organisms (GMOs).
- State Biotechnology Coordination Committee (SBCC)
- District Level Committee (DLC).

The SBCCs and DLCs have a major role in monitoring the research on biohazard materials at state and district levels.

Under the Rules 1989 of Environment (Protection) Act 1986, laboratory biosafety through appropriate containment has been identified as the fundamental part of any biological research. In this direction, the DBT had earlier published three guidelines, namely 'Recombinant DNA safety guidelines, 1990', 'Revised Guidelines for Safety in Biotechnology, 1994' and 'Revised guidelines for research in transgenic plants, 1998'. To regulate the recombinant DNA research, including storage and handling, import/export, manufacture, disposal, emergency procedure and facility certification of genetically engineered (GE) and non-GE hazardous microorganisms, DBT in consultation with RCGM promulgated the new guidelines 'Regulations and Guidelines for Recombinant DNA Research and Biocontainment 2017' under MoEF.

7.9 Occupational Safety and Health Administration (OSHA)

OSHA is a large regulatory agency of the US Department of Labor established in 1922 as the Bureau of Labor Standards and later, in 1970, was converted to OSHA. The Occupational Safety and Health Act grants OSHA the authority to issue workplace standards related to biosafety and health to promote a safe working environment, like The Bloodborne Pathogens Standard, The Hazard Communication Standard and The Personal Protective Equipment (PPE) Standard. It sets the permissible exposure limits (PELs) to protect workers against the ill effects of exposure to hazardous substances, including limits on the airborne concentrations of hazardous chemicals in the air. Under the OSHA law, employers are responsible for providing a safe and healthy workplace for their workers. OSHA's 'Laboratory Safety Guidance', issued on 13 October 2011, intends to minimize the risk of injuries or fatalities caused by chemical, biological and other hazards commonly found in research laboratories employing an estimated 500,000 individuals in the United States.

7.10 Conclusion

There is a marked absence of regulations concerning biosafety and biosecurity around the world. The goal of laboratory safety rules and regulations is to reduce the rate and severity of accidents in experimental laboratories and to ensure health and safety of lab personnel as well as to protect the expensive equipment, laboratory and buildings. Every person entering the lab should be well trained about the experiments, hazards and handling of hazards. PPE should always be used in combination with biological safety cabinets to ensure maximum containment of aerosols generated by many infectious procedures. A universal biohazard symbol must be posted with relevant information, including the laboratory's biosafety level. Regular pest control measures, biohazard waste management and use of biosafety cabinets are essential for a safe laboratory. Always make sure that all the policies for the safe handling of sharps, such as needles, scalpels, pipettes and broken glassware, are implemented. A laboratory-specific biosafety manual must be prepared and updated regularly as per the policy and guidelines from the WHO and made available to every person working in the lab. Everyone working in labs is responsible for their own safety and the safety of others. One should be cognizant of potential hazards by conducting all experiments and demonstrations prior to their implementation. Laboratory accidents are usually caused by carelessness of working personnel, defective equipment, slippery floors, rusty surfaces and equipment, failure of safe clothing, toxic chemicals, fumes, gas leaks, hazardous arrangement and improper ventilation and illumination. With so many newly emerging infectious diseases threatening the very existence of the human race, research in genetic engineering and biotechnology is necessary; however, there is a dilemma about the freedom or limitation of these investigations. Thus, gain-of-function (GOF) research or dual-use research (DUR) have arisen as an important concern, not only among the scientific community but also among the general population. We have a collective responsibility to make meaningful contributions to prevent synthetic biology from being misused. Increased public attention on these issues is important, which would ultimately put pressure on officials to take the necessary steps to ensure that safety rules and regulations are consistently followed and part of normal laboratory habitsKaufman, 2019.

References

Allen, K. (2014) A young lab worker, a professor and a deadly accident. *Toronto Star*. Available at: https://www.thestar.com/news/world/2014/03/30/a_young_lab_worker_a_professor_and_a_deadly_accident.html

Baron, E.J. and Miller, J.M. (2008) Bacterial and fungal infections among diagnostic laboratory workers: Evaluating the risks. *Diagnostic Microbiology and Infectious Disease* 60, 241–246. DOI: 10.1016/j.diagmicrobio.2007.09.016.

Basbug, G., Cavicchi, A. and Silbey, S.S. (2023) Rank has its privileges: Explaining why laboratory safety is a persistent challenge. *Journal of Business Ethics* 184, 571–587. DOI: 10.1007/s10551-022-05169-z.

Bloom, J.D., Chan, Y.A., Baric, R.S., Bjorkman, P.J., Cobey, S. *et al.* (2021) Investigate the origins of COVID-19. *Science* 372(6543), 694–694. DOI: 10.1126/science.abj0016.

Devaux, C.A. (2015) The hidden face of academic researches on classified highly pathogenic microorganisms. *Infection, Genetics and Evolution* 29, 26–34. DOI: 10.1016/j.meegid.2014.10.028.

Ejilemele, A.A. and Ojule, A.C. (2004) Health and safety in clinical laboratories in developing countries: Safety considerations. *Nigerian Journal of Medicine* 13(2), 182–188.

Ejilemele, A.A. and Ojule, A.C. (2005) Knowledge, attitude and practice of aspects of laboratory safety in pathology laboratories at the University of Port Harcourt Teaching Hospital, Nigeria. *Nigerian Journal of Clinical Practice* 8(2), 102–106.

Gunningham, N., Thornton, D. and Kagan, R.A. (2005) Motivating management: Corporate compliance with safety, health and environmental regulation. *Law and Policy* 27, 289–316. DOI: 10.1111/j.1467-9930.2005.00201.x.

Huising, R. and Silbey, S.S. (2011) Governing the gap: Forging safe science through relational regulation. *Regulation & Governance* 5(1), 14–42. DOI: 10.1111/j.1748-5991.2010.01100.x.

Huising, R. and Silbey, S.S. (2021) To protect from lab leaks, we need banal safety rules, not antiterrorism measures. *StatNews*. Available at: https://www.statnews.com/2021/08/13/banal-lab-safety-rules-keep-us-safe/

Jacobson, J.T., Orlob, R.B. and Clayton, J.L. (1985) Infections acquired in clinical laboratories in Utah. *Journal of Clinical Microbiology* 21, 486–489.

Kaufman, J.A. (2019) Killed in lab accidents: Memorial Wall. Available at: https://www.labsafety.org/memorial-wall

Keith, P. (2014) Safety Breaches at UK labs handling lethal viruses. *The Telegraph*. Available at: http://www.telegraph.co.uk/news/science/11274543/Safety-breaches

Ma, L., Ma, X., Zhang, J., Yang, Q. and Wei, K. (2021) A methodology for dynamic assessment of laboratory safety by SEM-SD. *International Journal of Environmental Research in Public Health* 18(12), 6545. DOI: 10.3390/ijerph18126545.

Ménard, A.D. and Trant, J.F. (2020) A review and critique of academic lab safety research. *Nature Chemistry* 12, 17–25. DOI: 10.1038/s41557-019-0375-x.

Peng, H., Bilal, M. and Iqbal, H.M.N. (2018) Improved biosafety and biosecurity measures and/or strategies to tackle laboratory-acquired infections and related risks. *International Journal of Environmental Research and Public Health* 15(12), 2697. DOI: 10.3390/ijerph15122697.

Pike, R.M. (1979) Laboratory-associated infections: Incidence, fatalities, causes, and prevention. *Annual Review of Microbiology* 33, 41–66. DOI: 10.1146/annurev.mi.33.100179.000353.

Pinghui, Z. (2018) Three students die in blast at Beijing University laboratory. *SCMP News*. Available at: https://www.scmp.com/news/china/society/article/2179543/three-students-die-blast-beijing-university-laboratory

Shore, C. (2008) Audit culture and illiberal governance: Universities and the politics of accountability. *Anthropological Theory* 8(3), 278–298. DOI: 10.1177/1463499608093815.

Silver, A. (2022) Why the world has no universal biosafety standards. *BMJ* 377, o954. DOI: 10.1136/bmj.o954.

Simmons, H.E., Matos, B. and Simpson, S.A. (2017) Analysis of injury data to improve safety and training. *Journal of Chemical and Health Safety* 24, 21–28.

Sonawane, S.L., Patil, V.J. and Tigaa, R.A. (2023) Evaluating and promoting chemical safety awareness in the chemical sciences. *Journal of Chemical Education* 100(2), 469–478.

Stark, L. (2012) *Behind Closed Doors: IRBs and the Making of Ethical Research*. University of Chicago Press, Chicago, Illinois.

Van Noorden, R. (2011) A death in lab. *Nature* 472, 270–271.

Walker, D. and Campbell, D. (1999) A survey of infections in United Kingdom laboratories, 1994–1995. *Journal of Clinical Pathology* 52, 415–418. DOI: 10.1136/jcp.52.6.415.

WHO (2004) *Laboratory Biosafety Manual*, 3rd edn. World Health Organization, Geneva.

Young, A. (2016) Newly disclosed CDC biolab failures, 'like a screenplay for a disaster movie'. *USA Today*. Available at: https://www.usatoday.com/story/news/2016/06/02

Zaki, A.N. (2010) Biosafety and biosecurity measures: Management of biosafety level 3 facilities. *International Journal of Antimicrobial Agents* 36, S70–S74. DOI: 10.1016/j.ijantimicag.2010.06.026.

8 One Health Approach to Zoonotic Diseases of Goats

Subir Singh*

Dept of Veterinary Medicine and Public Health, Faculty of Animal Science, Veterinary Science and Fisheries, Agriculture and Forestry University, Rampur, Chitwan, Nepal

Abstract

The One Health approach is a collaborative, multisectoral and transdisciplinary plan at local, regional, national and international levels with a goal to achieve optimal health outcomes recognizing the interconnection between people, animals, plants and their shared environment. Animals may carry harmful germs that can spread to people and cause illness, and vice versa. There is a close connection between people and animals regarding transmission of zoonotic diseases. There needs to be awareness of the common ways people can get infected with germs that can cause zoonotic diseases. The One Health approach prioritizes zoonotic diseases in goats that should be jointly addressed by human, animal and environmental health sectors in a country, region, or other area in a collaborative manner.

Keywords: One Health, zoonosis, goat, harmful agents, awareness

8.1 Introduction

The One Health concept emphasizes the interconnection between human, animal and environmental health (Fig. 8.1), recognizing that the health of each is interconnected and that disease emergence and transmission often occur at the interface of these domains. Zoonotic diseases (i.e. those transmissible between animals and humans) pose significant public health threats and may have devastating impacts on animal populations. Goats, as a commonly kept domesticated species, play a crucial role in the transmission of zoonotic diseases. This chapter explores the importance of adopting a One Health approach to address zoonotic diseases in goats, emphasizing the integration of veterinary, medical and environmental disciplines, with the focus on enhancing global health security and safeguarding the well-being of both animals and humans (Bond *et al.*, 2016).

8.1.1 The significance of zoonotic diseases in goats

Zoonotic diseases in goats hold significant importance due to their potential to pose serious threats to both human and animal health. As domesticated animals, goats serve as reservoirs for various zoonotic pathogens, facilitating the transmission of diseases to humans through direct contact, consumption of contaminated

*ssingh@afu.edu.np

DOI: 10.1079/ 9781800622852.0008

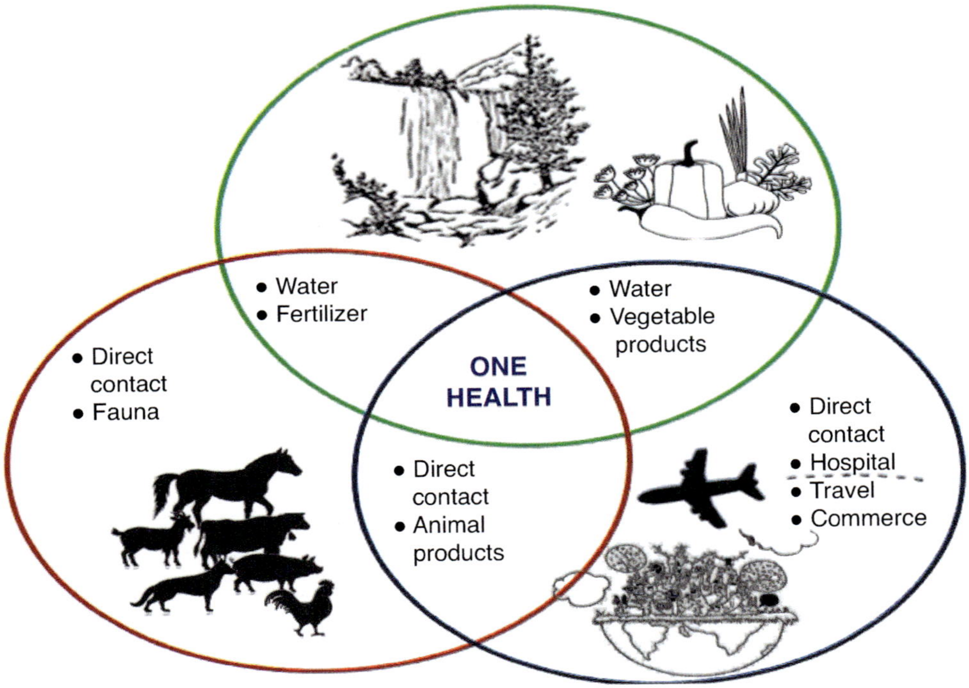

Fig. 8.1. Spreading processes of diseases at the human–animal–environment interface. (Author's own image.)

products, or exposure to environmental sources. These diseases can range from bacterial infections, such as brucellosis and Q fever, to parasitic diseases like cryptosporidiosis, causing a wide spectrum of clinical manifestations in both goats and humans. The implications of zoonotic diseases in goats extend beyond public health concerns, as they can also impact the livelihoods of communities relying on goat husbandry for food security and income. Addressing the significance of zoonotic diseases in goats necessitates a holistic One Health approach to develop effective prevention, surveillance and control strategies to safeguard the well-being of humans and animals.

8.1.2 The one health approach

The One Health approach in goat health represents a comprehensive and interconnected strategy that recognizes the intrinsic linkages between the health of goats, humans and the environment. As goats can serve as hosts for various zoonotic pathogens, understanding and managing their health becomes crucial in preventing disease transmission to humans and other animals. The One Health approach emphasizes interdisciplinary collaboration among veterinarians, medical professionals, epidemiologists, ecologists and public health experts. By integrating these diverse fields, the approach aims to enhance disease surveillance, early detection and response mechanisms. It also considers the broader environmental context, acknowledging the impact of ecological factors on disease transmission dynamics. Emphasizing preventive measures, such as vaccination programmes, biosecurity protocols and health monitoring, the One Health approach in goat health strives to create a more resilient and sustainable system that promotes the well-being of goats, humans and the ecosystem as a whole (Eibach *et al.*, 2012).

8.2 Zoonotic Diseases of Goats

Zoonotic diseases of goats represent a critical public health concern, due to their potential to cross the species barrier and infect humans. These diseases are caused by various pathogens, including bacteria, viruses, parasites and fungi, which can be transmitted from goats to humans through direct contact, ingestion of contaminated food or water, or exposure to infected animal products. Common zoonotic diseases of goats include brucellosis, Q fever, leptospirosis, campylobacteriosis and cryptosporidiosis, among others. These diseases can lead to a wide range of clinical symptoms in both goats and humans, ranging from mild to severe, and even fatal outcomes. Zoonotic diseases can have significant socioeconomic impacts, particularly in communities reliant on goat husbandry for sustenance and income. Effective control and prevention strategies are essential to reduce the risk of zoonotic disease transmission, necessitating a One Health approach. By addressing zoonotic diseases of goats holistically, we can protect human health, ensure the well-being of goat populations and minimize the potential for disease emergence and spread at the human–animal interface.

8.3 One Health Surveillance and Monitoring

One Health surveillance and monitoring in regard to goat health play a pivotal role in safeguarding both human and animal populations from zoonotic diseases and other health threats. By adopting an integrated approach that encompasses veterinary, medical and environmental perspectives, comprehensive surveillance systems can be established to detect potential disease outbreaks in goat populations and identify emerging zoonotic pathogens at the human–animal interface. Timely reporting of unusual health events in goats allows for early detection and rapid response, which is critical in containing and controlling the spread of diseases. Such surveillance efforts enable the identification of high-risk areas and populations, facilitating targeted interventions and preventive measures. Additionally, data sharing between relevant stakeholders enhances the effectiveness of surveillance programmes and fosters a deeper understanding of disease dynamics in goat populations. A proactive One Health surveillance and monitoring system is essential in mitigating the risks associated with zoonotic diseases in goats, ultimately contributing to global health security and reinforcing the interconnectedness between human, animal and environmental health.

8.3.1 Early detection and reporting

Early detection and reporting are critical components in safeguarding goat health and mitigating the risks associated with infectious diseases and zoonotic pathogens. Timely identification of health abnormalities, clinical signs, or unusual disease patterns in goat populations allows for swift intervention and implementation of appropriate control measures. Early detection is facilitated through regular and systematic health monitoring of goat herds, involving observation of clinical signs, routine veterinary examinations and diagnostic testing. Timely reporting of any suspicious or notifiable diseases to relevant authorities is essential to trigger a rapid response and prevent further disease spread. Effective communication channels between farmers, veterinarians and public health officials are crucial for facilitating early reporting and coordination of efforts. Early detection and reporting also contribute to the accumulation of valuable epidemiological data, enabling a better understanding of disease prevalence and dynamics. By prioritizing early detection and reporting in goat health, we can effectively protect both animal and human populations, enhance disease control measure and strengthen the foundation for a proactive One Health approach in addressing zoonotic diseases and other health challenges.

8.3.2 Integrated surveillance systems

Integrated surveillance systems in regard to goat health play a pivotal role in advancing One Health approaches to disease detection and control. These systems involve the harmonious integration of data from various sources, including veterinary clinics, diagnostic laboratories, public health agencies and environmental monitoring programmes. By collating and analysing information from multiple disciplines, integrated surveillance systems provide a comprehensive understanding of the health status of goat populations and their potential impact on human health. This approach facilitates the early detection of zoonotic diseases, emerging pathogens and other health threats in goats, allowing for timely and targeted responses to prevent disease spread. Moreover, integrated surveillance systems enable the identification of risk factors and high-risk areas, guiding the implementation of preventive measures and targeted interventions. Through efficient data sharing and real-time reporting mechanisms, these systems promote collaboration among stakeholders, fostering a proactive and synergistic response to goat health challenges. The establishment of robust integrated surveillance systems is essential for enhancing global health security, protecting the well-being of both animals and humans and bolstering the overall resilience of One Health initiatives (Jones *et al.*, 2013).

8.3.3 The role of data sharing and collaboration

The role of data sharing and collaboration in regard to goat health is paramount in fostering a comprehensive and proactive approach to disease management and prevention. Data sharing facilitates the integration of information from various sources, including veterinary clinics, research institutions, diagnostic laboratories and public health agencies. By consolidating diverse datasets, a more accurate and holistic understanding of goat health can be achieved, enabling early detection of disease outbreaks, surveillance of zoonotic pathogens and identification of emerging health threats. Collaboration among stakeholders, including veterinarians, researchers, farmers and public health officials, enhances the exchange of knowledge, expertise and resources. This synergy ensures a coordinated response to goat health challenges and enables the development of evidence-based strategies for disease control and prevention. Furthermore, data sharing and collaboration are essential for monitoring trends, evaluating intervention effectiveness and making informed policy decisions. Open communication and transparent data sharing not only strengthen goat health initiatives but also contribute to broader One Health efforts, recognizing the interconnections between human, animal and environmental health. Emphasizing the importance of data sharing and collaboration can lead to enhanced global health security, improved disease control measures and a more resilient approach to addressing zoonotic diseases and other health risks in goat populations.

8.4 The Role of Veterinary Medicine

The role of veterinary medicine in goat health is pivotal, encompassing both individual animal care and population-level health management. Veterinarians play a crucial role in disease prevention, diagnosis and treatment, as well as advising on animal husbandry practices that promote goat welfare and productivity. In the context of a One Health perspective, veterinarians are essential in recognizing the interconnectedness between human, animal and environmental health. By monitoring and controlling zoonotic diseases in goats, they contribute to the prevention of disease transmission to humans and other animals, thus safeguarding public health. Veterinary professionals also play a vital role in early detection and reporting of emerging diseases, which is critical for implementing timely and effective intervention measures. Collaboration between veterinarians, medical professionals, epidemiologists and environmental experts ensures a holistic approach to disease surveillance, research and control, considering the broader impact of goat health on overall ecosystem health. Additionally, veterinary education and capacity building are essential to empower communities with knowledge and skills for improved goat management practices, disease prevention and enhanced One Health awareness. The active involvement of veterinary medicine in goat health is integral to advancing One Health initiatives, creating a more resilient and sustainable future for both animal and human health.

8.4.1 Veterinary involvement in zoonotic disease prevention and control

Veterinary involvement in zoonotic disease prevention and control plays a crucial role in mitigating the risks posed by infectious diseases transmitted between animals and humans. Veterinarians are at the forefront of early detection, surveillance and diagnosis of zoonotic diseases in animal populations, including goats, which serve as significant reservoirs for these pathogens. Through regular health monitoring and diagnostic testing, veterinarians can identify zoonotic agents in animal hosts, thus providing early warning signals for potential human health threats. Veterinary professionals also play a key role in implementing preventive measures, such as vaccination programmes, biosecurity protocols and hygiene practices, to reduce the risk of zoonotic disease transmission from animals to humans. Their expertise in disease epidemiology and pathogenesis enables them to trace the source of outbreaks, identify high-risk areas and implement targeted control strategies. Moreover, veterinarians actively collaborate with public health officials and medical professionals in a One Health approach. By facilitating data sharing and communication among various stakeholders, veterinary involvement strengthens zoonotic disease surveillance, research and response efforts, fostering a holistic and proactive approach to protecting both animal and human populations from zoonotic diseases (Lee and Brumme, 2013).

8.4.2 Veterinarians as key players in one health initiatives

Veterinarians are indispensable key players in One Health initiatives, playing a critical role in bridging the gap between human, animal and environmental health. Their unique expertise in veterinary medicine enables them to understand and address health challenges that arise at the interface of these domains. As front-line professionals in animal health, veterinarians are instrumental in the early detection and surveillance of zoonotic diseases, such as those that may affect goats and pose a risk to human populations. By closely monitoring animal populations, veterinarians can identify potential disease outbreaks and emerging pathogens, contributing to timely intervention and prevention measures. Their understanding of disease transmission dynamics and control strategies is invaluable in designing comprehensive and integrated approaches to health management. Veterinarians also contribute to public health by advocating for responsible animal husbandry practices, promoting biosecurity and implementing vaccination programmes to reduce the risk of zoonotic disease transmission from animals to humans.

8.5 Case Studies

8.5.1 Successful one health interventions in zoonotic diseases of goats

The successful implementation of One Health interventions in zoonotic diseases of goats has demonstrated the potential of this integrated approach in mitigating health risks and protecting both human and animal populations. One notable case study involved the control of brucellosis, a zoonotic bacterial infection that poses a significant threat to goat herds and human health. In this intervention, veterinarians collaborated with medical professionals and public health officials to establish a comprehensive surveillance system for early detection of infected animals. Simultaneously, health education programmes were conducted to raise awareness among farmers about the importance of biosecurity measures and proper handling of goat products. Vaccination campaigns targeting both goats and high-risk human populations were implemented, effectively reducing the prevalence of brucellosis in both species. Another successful case study focused on the control of Q fever, a zoonotic disease caused by *Coxiella burnetii*. In this intervention, environmental experts collaborated with veterinarians to identify high-risk areas and develop control measures to reduce transmission from contaminated goat farms to neighboring communities. Concurrently, medical professionals improved the diagnosis and treatment of Q fever in humans, leading to earlier detection and better outcomes. These case studies illustrate the power of One Health collaborations, leveraging the expertise of multiple disciplines to develop effective and sustainable interventions for zoonotic diseases in goats. They highlight the importance of a coordinated and proactive approach to address health challenges at the human–animal–environment interface, promoting a safer and healthier future for both goat herds and human communities.

8.5.2 Lessons learned and best practices

The One Health approach regarding goat health has provided valuable lessons and best practices that can guide future efforts in disease prevention and control. First, the integration of veterinary, medical and environmental disciplines in the case study proved to be essential in addressing zoonotic diseases of goats comprehensively. Collaboration among experts from different fields allowed for a more holistic understanding of disease dynamics and the identification of shared risk factors. Secondly, early detection and reporting played a critical role in minimizing disease spread. Timely surveillance and reporting of unusual health events in goats enabled swift responses, preventing further transmission to humans and other animals. Thirdly, the case study emphasized the significance of data sharing and collaboration (Meurens *et al.*, 2021). Open communication among stakeholders facilitated the exchange of crucial information, improving decision making and resource allocation. Fourthly, the One Health approach highlighted the importance of health education and capacity building among communities. Empowering farmers and livestock keepers with knowledge about disease prevention and management practices proved effective in reducing disease incidence. Lastly, vaccination programmes targeting both goats and high-risk human populations were instrumental in preventing zoonotic disease transmission. This case study underscores the potential of the One Health approach to create a synergy among different disciplines, leading to better goat health outcomes, reduced zoonotic disease risks and enhanced global health security. By incorporating the lessons learned and best practices from this case study, stakeholders can strengthen their efforts in goat health management and contribute to a more resilient and interconnected approach to address health challenges at the human–animal–environment interface.

8.6 Importance and Challenges of One Health Regarding Zoonotic Goat Diseases

8.6.1 The importance of one health in tackling zoonotic diseases of goats

Goats, as common domesticated animals, can serve as reservoirs for various zoonotic pathogens, posing significant public health threats. The One Health approach facilitates a holistic understanding of disease transmission dynamics, enabling early detection, surveillance and control measures. By integrating veterinary, medical and environmental expertise, stakeholders can collaboratively identify high-risk areas, monitor disease trends and implement targeted interventions. This proactive approach not only prevents the transmission of zoonotic diseases from goats to humans but also safeguards the health and welfare of goat populations. The One Health perspective optimizes resources, promotes evidence-based decision making, enhances global health security, mitigates socio-economic impacts and safeguards the well-being of both human and animal populations. It lays the foundation for a more resilient and sustainable future, where proactive measures are taken to prevent, detect and control zoonotic disease threats at their source (Rahman *et al.*, 2020).

8.6.2 Future directions and challenges

Future directions and challenges in the context of One Health and zoonotic diseases of goats present exciting opportunities and complex tasks. As zoonotic diseases continue to emerge and evolve, the One Health approach must evolve in parallel to address new challenges. Integrating advanced technologies, such as genomics and big-data analytics, can enhance disease surveillance and facilitate the rapid identification of novel pathogens. Furthermore, strengthening international collaborations and data-sharing mechanisms is crucial for global disease monitoring and response. However, several challenges persist, including the need for increased awareness and education about zoonotic diseases among communities and healthcare professionals. Overcoming barriers to interdisciplinary cooperation and data sharing is critical to fully harness the potential of the One Health approach. Additionally, limited resources and infrastructure in certain regions may hinder effective disease surveillance and control. Addressing these challenges requires strategic investments in capacity building and infrastructural development. Moreover, the impact of climate change on disease dynamics underscores the need for a One Health approach that incorporates environmental considerations. By addressing these future directions and challenges, the One Health approach can pave the way for a more resilient and proactive response to zoonotic diseases of goats, safeguarding human and animal health while promoting the well-being of our shared ecosystems.

8.7 Conclusion

By adopting a One Health approach, we can effectively mitigate the risks associated with zoonotic diseases in goats and protect both human and animal populations. This chapter serves as a comprehensive resource for scientists, veterinarians, medical professionals, policy makers and other stakeholders involved in public health, animal health and environmental conservation, fostering collaboration and strengthening global efforts to combat zoonotic diseases.

References

Bond, K.A., Vincent, G., Wilks, C.R., Franklin, L., Sutton, B. *et al.* (2016) One health approach to controlling a Q fever outbreak on an Australian goat farm. *Epidemiology and Infection* 144(6), 1129–1141.

Eibach, R., Bothe, F., Runge, M., Fischer, S.F., Philipp, W. *et al.* (2012) Q fever: Baseline monitoring of a sheep and a goat flock associated with human infections. *Epidemiology and Infection* 140(11), 1939–1949.

Jones, B.A., Grace, D., Kock, R., Alonso, S., Rushton, J. *et al.* (2013) Zoonosis emergence linked to agricultural intensification and environmental change. *Proceedings of the National Academy of Sciences of the USA* 110(21), 8399–8404.

Lee, K. and Brumme, Z.L. (2013) Operationalizing the one health approach: The global governance challenges. *Health Policy Plan* 28, 778–785.

Meurens, F., Dunoyer, C., Fourichon, C., Gerdts, V., Haddad, N. *et al.* (2021) Animal board invited review: Risks of zoonotic disease emergence at the interface of wildlife and livestock systems. *Animal* 15(6), 100241.

Rahman, M.T., Sobur, M.A., Islam, M.S., Ievy, S., Hossain, M.J. *et al.* (2020) Zoonotic diseases: Etiology, impact, and control. *Microorganisms* 8(9), 1405.

9 Anthrax

Oluwawemimo Adebowale*
Department of Veterinary Public Health and Preventive Medicine, College of Veterinary Medicine, Federal University of Abeokuta, Abeokuta, Ogun State, Nigeria

Abstract
Anthrax is a neglected tropical zoonotic disease primarily of herbivores, such as goats, and which can be transmitted to humans. It is caused by a Gram-positive, aerobic, spore-forming and rod-shaped bacterium called *Bacillus anthracis*. Anthrax spores are naturally found in the soil and the disease occurs worldwide with varying occurrences in various geographical regions. It is a reportable disease that is endemic in some parts of Africa. Furthermore, anthrax is of huge concern because according to the Food and Drug Administration (FDA), anthrax is viewed as a possible biological weapon. Recent outbreaks were reported in 2023 in West Africa, including Nigeria, which affected several species of animals comprising cattle, sheep and goats. In Ghana, the disease and deaths were confirmed in both animals and humans. Fever, staggering, depression, incoordination, trembling and difficulty in breathing, followed by rapid collapse, terminal convulsions, bloody discharges from natural body orifices and death, are some typical clinical signs in goats. The transmission of disease to humans, depending on the route of exposure, may appear clinically in three distinct forms: cutaneous, gastrointestinal and pneumonic. The most effective strategy of disease prevention in humans is by vaccination of animal populations using the anthrax spore vaccine (Sterne attenuated spore vaccine). The human anthrax vaccine that is currently in use is not available to the general public. These vaccines are used only in high-risk groups. However, there is ongoing research to enhance the development of new third-generation vaccines, including recombinant sub-unit vaccines for use in humans. Also, multisectoral collaborations, efforts, initiatives, frameworks and integrated surveillance across the human, animal and environment sectors may be crucial for early warnings and mitigations.

Keywords: anthrax, goats, detection, control, prevention, biothreat

9.1 Introduction

Anthrax is a bacterial disease that primarily affects ruminant animals (such as cows, sheep and goats). It is caused by an aerobic spore-forming bacterium agent named *Bacillus anthracis* and becomes a serious zoonosis when it is transmitted from infected animals or animal products to humans via direct contact or through acts of bioterrorism. In addition, *B. anthracis* produces extremely potent toxins, that are lethal, and resistant spores that can contaminate and survive in the environment for many years, making the control or eradication of the disease very difficult once it becomes endemic, particularly in developing countries. Anthrax persistently threatens human and livestock health in developing countries (Les and Huwar, 2011). In recent times, Kenya (Munyua *et al.*, 2016), Uganda (Sekamatte *et al.*, 2018) and Nigeria (Ihekweazu *et al.*, 2021) have

*Corresponding author: adebowaleoluwawemimo1@gmail.com

DOI: 10.1079/ 9781800622852.0009

ranked the disease among the top five priority zoonoses using the 'One Health' approach and multisectoral collaborations to promote effective integrated surveillance, prevention and control strategies.

This chapter discusses goat anthrax in detail. Various sections in the chapter include: information on goat population and growth trends in Asia and Africa, which are major areas of high concentration of goats globally; the importance and benefits of goat keeping, especially for rural and smallholders in developing countries; the history of the disease; causative agent and ecology; host and pathogenicity; global disease epidemiology and distribution; clinical manifestations; detection/diagnostic methods; prevention and control strategies and the emerging bio-threat of anthrax.

9.2 Goat Population and the Benefits

The domestic goat, widely known as *Capra aegagrus hircus*, is distributed globally. Currently, there are over a billion goats worldwide, which has more than doubled in the past 40 years (Utaaker *et al.*, 2021). Over 90% of the global goat population are concentrated in developing countries, most especially Asia and Africa (Food and Agriculture Organization (FAO), 2021). This may be associated with the importance of goats to poor and smallholder farmers in these regions (Mahendra and Dilip, 2021). According to the Food and Agriculture Organization (FAO) (2021), India has the largest population of goats, estimated at 148,747,429, followed by China (133,443,170), Pakistan (80,326,000), Nigeria (76,292,153), Bangladesh (59,953,432), Ethiopia (47,309,695), Chad (43,735,657), Kenya (32,570,314), Sudan (32,420,404) and Mali (29,201,079). The goat population has increased with the growth in human population, which may be due to the higher demand for healthier red meat and milk products and it being an excellent source of protein (Kamer, 2022). Goat keeping or farming for meat and milk production is essentially a traditional practice, which may be a primary or secondary activity among the rural and semi-urban people living in many developing countries. For instance, in India, goats are kept mainly for milk production, both at commercial and household levels. In places like Nigeria, goats are traditionally kept in the household for meat consumption. Goats are resilient to many diseases, adapt to various environmental and climatic conditions, and have efficient conversion of feed into edible and high-quality meat, milk and hide, making it ideal for resource-limited/smallholder farmers to generate income (Mahendra and Dilip, 2021). Goat keeping or farming is making valuable contributions to livelihood, nutrition and poverty alleviation in many developing countries, especially rural and semi-urban areas.

9.3 History of Anthrax

Anthrax was one of the first zoonoses, described in 700 BC. It was postulated to be among the plagues in the Bible that struck ancient Egypt at the time of Moses and during the slavery era of the Israelites in Egypt. It was documented in the Book of Exodus as the fifth (death of livestock) and sixth (boils) plagues inflicted on Egypt (Sternbach, 2003). Anthrax was reported to persist, affecting humans and animals through the Middle Ages (Sternbach, 2003). In 1613, a disease ('Black Bane'), assumed to be most likely anthrax, swept through Europe, causing large numbers of human and animal deaths. It became an epidemic, which caused inhalation anthrax known as woolsorters' disease in the 18th century in England (Sternbach, 2003). This became the first occupational respiratory infectious disease to be described in history (Alam *et al.*, 2022). The clinical cutaneous form of anthrax was first described by Maret in 1752 and Fournier in 1769 (Alam *et al.*, 2022). In the 19th century (1877), Robert Koch experimentally injected mice with viable anthrax bacteria, leading to the development of the famous Koch postulates, which showed a causal relationship between the disease and the specific microorganisms – the germ theory of disease (Alam *et al.*, 2022). A few years later, in 1881, Louis Pasteur developed an effective live vaccine against the disease, making anthrax the first disease for which a vaccine was developed (Oncü *et al.*, 2003; Akula *et al.*, 2005). Several epidemics were later documented in the 20th century, with highest fatalities in domestic and wild animals. An outbreak of this disease was reported to have caused deaths in 30,000–60,000 animals in Rhodesia, Southern Africa, between 1978 and 1984 (Wilson *et al.*, 2016).

9.4 The Organism and Ecology

Anthrax is a deadly peracute, acute or subacute infectious disease of livestock and wildlife, and occasionally humans. It is caused by an aerobic, Gram-positive, non-motile, rod-shaped, 3–5 μm long and 1–1.2 μm wide, capsulated endospore-forming bacterium named *Bacillus anthracis*. *B. anthracis* belongs to the family Bacillaceae and is within the *Bacillus cereus* group. It is similar to *B. cereus* both genotypically and phenotypically and distinguishing *B. anthracis* and *B. cereus* can be difficult (Carroll *et al.*, 2020). However, a novel strategy using peptide mass fingerprints based on matrix-assisted laser desorption/ionization time-of-flight mass spectrometry (MALDI-TOF MS) has been shown to be reliable and safe for differentiating these species (Wei *et al.*, 2020).

B. anthracis was the first bacterium that was grown in pure culture and experimentally injected into animals to cause anthrax by Robert Koch in 1877. *B. anthracis* is a biosafety level 3 (BSL-3) bacterium that can be cultured on blood agar at 37°C where it produces non-haemolytic ground-glass-surface-like colonies and can be differentiated from *B. cereus*, which produces strongly beta-haemolytic colonies. Other characteristics of *B. anthracis* include absence of salicin fermentation, gelatin hydrolysis, and lack of growth on phenyl ethyl alcohol medium (Parry *et al.*, 1983).

The *B. anthracis* genome is tripartite and consists of a 5,227,419 bp circular chromosome and two large extrachromosomal DNA plasmids, namely pXO1 and pXO2, of 181,677 and 94,830 bp, respectively, which are responsible for its virulence. The pXO1 encodes a binary lethal factor (LF) and protective antigen (PA) or oedema (edema) factor (EF) and protective antigen (PA), which collectively (LF/PA and EF/PA) target multiple host functions, the immune responses and eventually cause death (NCBI, 2004; Keim *et al.*, 2009). There is less genomic variation in *B. anthracis* than in any other known bacterial species, hence making it genetically and phenotypically a highly homogeneous and stable species (Keim *et al.*, 2009). *B. anthracis* spores are primarily found in the soil. The bacteria spread by spores and contaminate soils where animals are kept, in animal products such as wool, hair, hides, skins, bones, bone meal and infected carcasses. The spores are resilient and may persist for many years in soil even under harsh dry and cold conditions, where it is metabolically dormant (Bergman, 2011). Exposure of the spores to oxygen will cause them to germinate, and vegetative spores multiply and become infectious in susceptible animals through uptake from the environment. The condition that appears most to favour long survival in the soil is dryness. Previous research evidence exists to show that anthrax spores could survive for many years in the environment. For instance, spores have been reported to have survived in dry soil for 60 years (Wilson and Russell, 1964). In South Africa's Kruger National Park, anthrax spores dated back to 200 ± 50 years old were recovered from bones retrieved during archaeological excavations (De Vos, 1990).

Also, past studies on the ecology of anthrax have documented an association between the disease and specific soil factors, such as alkaline pH, high moisture and high organic content. Specifically, soil with high levels of calcium (and limestone-rich) and a pH above 6.1 promotes and maintains spore vitality for prolonged periods, thereby increasing the chance of spores encountering and infecting a new host (Dragon and Rennie, 1995; Hugh-Jones and Blackburn, 2009). Another study, which investigated *Bacillus anthracis* spores in different soil types during a repeated anthrax outbreak in Bangladesh, showed that soil types, temperature, rainfall and a suitable pH range influenced the occurrence of anthrax spores (Ahsan *et al.*, 2013). Although *B. anthracis* spores can be long-lasting and highly resistant, they can be destroyed by several methods of sterilization, for example autoclaving at 121°C for 15 min (Todar, 2023).

Anthrax is a seasonal disease and various conditions such as temperature, heavy rainfall, flood, soil disturbance and/or drought, anthropogenic factors, or insect and animal population density may influence the disease occurrence and this may vary in different locations. However, the primary conditions affecting the seasonality of anthrax in any one place would appear to be temperature and rains (or drought) and humidity (Carlson *et al.*, 2018; Otieno *et al.*, 2021).

9.5 Epidemiology of Anthrax

Anthrax is a neglected and under-reported zoonosis that is distributed worldwide but endemic in continents such as Africa, Asia, North and South America and Australia (Dragon and Rennie, 1995). The World Organisation for Animal Health (WOAH) has shown that the disease is endemic in many countries, and that sporadic outbreaks are common (Ndiva Mongoh *et al.*, 2008). However, the global variation in anthrax endemism and outbreak intensity is still poorly characterized (Carlson *et al.*, 2019). A global ensemble distribution model conducted according to Carlson *et al.* (2019) showed well-established distribution of anthrax in Africa, China, Kazakhstan, North America, Turkey and Australia, and potential hotspots for human exposure. Another estimate of the global occurrence of anthrax based on studies of the prevalence of anthrax in cows, sheep, goats and buffalo species worldwide, using meta-analysis, reported a pooled prevalence of anthrax globally as 28% (Sushma *et al.*, 2021). The continent subgroup analysis using the random effects model revealed that the pooled prevalence of anthrax was highest in Africa, with a prevalence of 29%, and least in North America (21%). The prevalence rate of anthrax was also high in Asia and Europe (Sushma *et al.*, 2021). The high prevalence in Africa may be associated with the high livestock density, favourable climatic conditions, poor vaccination policy and low vaccination rates. Anthrax is probably eliminated in Austria, the Czech Republic, Denmark, Finland and Luxembourg (Schmid and Kaufmann, 2002).

Although anthrax outbreaks are commonly reported in bovines, several countries have estimated the disease prevalence in goats. A retrospective study conducted in a region in Northern Ethiopia among livestock from 2011 to 2020 reported two cases in goats (Seyoum *et al.*, 2022). In Mongolia, of the total number of animal cases of anthrax, 17% occurred in goats and sheep (Odontsetseg *et al.*, 2007). In 2012, an investigation into an outbreak of anthrax in Northern Tanzania showed that, out of 367 suspected animals studied, samples from goats (10%) were anthrax positive (Aminu *et al.*, 2020). In Kenya, a temporal and spatial patterns analysis of livestock anthrax from 1957 to 2017 reported occurred outbreaks involving goats, though lower compared with cattle (Nderitu *et al.*, 2021). Similarly, anthrax outbreak among goats in Ha Giang Province, Vietnam from 1999 to 2020 were documented (Luong *et al.*, 2023). Even though anthrax has been documented in Nigeria, past studies have reported 0% prevalence in goats (Okolo, 1985; Mawak *et al.*, 2006). This may be the reason why the live attenuated spore vaccine produced by the National Veterinary Research Institute, Vom, Nigeria (NVRI) is targeted for cattle only.

9.6 Host–Bacterial Interactions and the Pathogenic Mechanisms

Anthrax primarily affects herbivores such as goats, sheep and cattle since they are mostly raised in extensive grazing systems, which frequently infect them when sufficient concentrations of the anthrax spores in contaminated pastures are ingested or inhaled (von Terzi *et al.*, 2014).

The outcome of infection depends largely on the host susceptibility and infective dose. Animal exposure to the spores through inhalation, ingestion or wounds are first taken up by phagocytosis, and inflammatory signs are observed at the site of infection. The spores germinate, multiply and invade the animal tissues and then are carried to the lymph nodes and bloodstream, causing bacteraemia and necrosis, haemorrhages and oedema in the organs and tissues (WHO, 2008; Setlow, 2014).

Pathogenicity of *B. anthracis* is determined by two plasmids: pXO1 (toxin plasmid) and pXO2 (capsule plasmid) (Pilo and Frey, 2018). The toxin complex consists of three proteins, namely the protective antigen (PA), oedema factor (EF) and lethal factor (LF). The molecular basis for the pathogenicity of anthrax has been excellently explained by Pilo and Frey (2018) as follows:

> *B. anthracis* produces the four major virulence factors: the lethal toxin zinc metalloprotease (LF), the edema factor calmodulin-dependent adenylate cyclase (EF) and the adhesive subunit of the two toxins named 'protective antigen' (PA) all of which are encoded on plasmid pXO1, and the poly-D-glutamic acid polymer capsule (CAP) that allows survival of the bacterium in macrophages encoded on plasmid pXO2. PA binds to the receptors on the host cell, CMG2 and TEM8, and is subsequently cleaved by furin, allowing multimerization and binding of LF or EF. The PA-EF and PA-LF complexes are internalized by endocytosis in a dynamine-clathrin dependent way. In the acid environment of the endosomes, the PA-EF and PA-LF complexes change conformation in order to dissolve the complexes, transit to late endosomes and release the toxic subunits, which exert their activities by overproduction of cAMP by EF and apoptosis, release of proinflammatory cytokines, subsequent shock by proteolytic cleavage of MAPKK by LF.

The synergistic effects of the toxins severely impair the immune system, increase capillary endothelial permeability and delay blood clotting. The combined effect of three proteins causes more toxicity than each toxin effect individually (Abrami *et al.*, 2005).

9.7 Clinical Manifestations in Goats and Disease Exposure in Humans

The incubation period of anthrax is 1–20 days according to WOAH/OIE, for trade purposes. Under natural conditions this may be 1–14 days or more. The disease may present as peracute, acute, or subacute to chronic. In goats, the infection typically presents as peracute, while chronic or subacute cases are rare. In this section only the peracute and acute clinical manifestations will be discussed. For peracute, the animals are found dead without any premonition signs and usually in a few hours. The animal may be observed bloated, oedema may occur around the neck, thorax, abdomen and flank, with congestion and cyanosis of mucous membranes; staggering, convulsions, recumbency, spasms, dyspnoea and bloody discharges from natural body openings such as the nose, mouth, ears and anus are observed, followed by death within 48–72 hour (Ngetich, 2019). The acute form of the infection may manifest with fever, congestion and haemorrhagic mucous membranes, muscle spasms and laboured breathing, with terminal convulsions and death (Ngetich, 2019). This could also be preceded by a short phase of excitement followed by depression and listlessness. Animals that die of anthrax do not present rigor mortis.

The public health risk associated with anthrax is that humans may become exposed and infected by direct contact or by handling sick or dead animals. Also, contact with the hides, bones, blood, etc. from animals that died of the disease may expose humans to the infection (WHO, 2008). It is crucial to know that dead animals must not be opened, to avoid sporulation and the inhalation of spores by handlers. The spore inhalation may cause inhalational anthrax (wool sorter's disease), the most fatal form of anthrax in humans, associated with high fever, chest pain and high case fatality estimated at 90–100% regardless of treatment. Other routes of human exposure are through the cutaneous and intestinal transmissions resulting in cutaneous and gastrointestinal anthrax, respectively. Cutaneous anthrax is the most common pattern of the disease in humans and is acquired via wounds on the skin or mucous membranes and presented as vesicles, malignant pustule, necrotic ulcer and septicaemia (Pilo, 2011). The gastrointestinal form is rare and occurs through the ingestion of poorly cooked contaminated meat and meat products derived from infected animals.

To avoid spread and infection in humans, especially animal handlers, it is critical to notify a veterinarian immediately, as soon as these signs are observed, for guidance on handling, environmentally friendly disposal methods where dead animals are involved, and other precautions to ensure effective control of further dissemination into the environment, animals and humans (including handlers). Dead animals must be protected from scavengers, which may want to open the carcass, spill fluids and thereby aid sporulation and spread. Anthrax is a notifiable disease in many countries and any suspected case should be reported to the appropriate veterinary directorate and reporting channels for rapid government interventions.

9.8 Methods of Detection

Anthrax diagnosis can be made tentatively using the clinical manifestation of the disease. It is important to carry out necessary laboratory tests to confirm the pathogen. Specific diagnostic tests, which are microscopy, culture, serological and immunological (FAT, ELISA, lateral flow immunoassay) and molecular methods such as PCR-based techniques have been used successfully. A recent study used Active Anthrax Detect (AAD) Rapid Test lateral flow immunoassay to detect *B. anthracis* from animal tissues. AAD is used to detect the pathogen in human blood, serum and plasma but has been reported and described as a potentially effective tool for testing suspect animal cases (Kolton *et al.*, 2019). PCR-based methods and whole-genome sequencing (WGS) availability have enhanced rapid identification and genetic characterization of the bacteria from the animal tissues samples and environmental samples in several studies (Ellerbrok *et al.*, 2002; Levi *et al.*, 2003; Wielinga *et al.*, 2011; Be *et al.*, 2013; Aminu *et al.*, 2020; Galante *et al.*, 2021). The World Health Organization (WHO) recommended bacterial culture and PCR confirmatory tests (detection of genes specific to *B. anthracis*) – including phage and penicillin sensitivity – as being the gold standard approach for the diagnosis of animal anthrax (WHO, 2008; Aminu *et al.*, 2020).

Also several studies have used various molecular subtyping systems (single-nucleotide polymorphisms, variable-number tandem repeats and single-nucleotide repeats) to identify and describe the genetic characterization and diversity of *B. anthracis*. For instance, a study used the combination of variable-number tandem repeat (VNTR) and single-nucleotide repeat (SNR) typing systems to compare and describe the genetic diversity of *B anthracis* in Nigeria with Cameroon and Chad. The Nigerian multiple-locus VNTR analysis genotype was found to be genetically homologous to those in the neighbouring countries, further supporting that the strain belonged to the West African lineage (Blackburn *et al.*, 2015). VNTR genotyping in particular has been employed to describe the diversity of the pathogen in other countries, including the United States, France, Italy, Poland and Kazakhstan (Blackburn *et al.*, 2015).

It is important to note that strict biosecurity and biosafety measures must be ensured during sample collection, handling, transportation and microbial analysis. The pathogen, due to its associated high fatality, bioterrorism and trade risks, has been classified as a biosafety level 3 (BSL-3) pathogen requiring the use of a BSL-3 laboratory.

9.9 Prevention and Control in Goats

The most effective prevention strategies for anthrax in animals are surveillance and vaccination. Disease surveillance involves the systematic collection of field data on disease events, risk factors and other relevant parameters, which are then analysed with reference to temporal and spatial characteristics to enhance the development and implementation of necessary preventive measures (Chethan Kumar *et al.*, 2021). Surveillance, aside from being important in safeguarding animal health, protects international trade, food safety and human health. With efficient and robust surveillance data, trends and seasonality, pattern distributions and identification of hotspots, the magnitude of the disease, early detection and responses, informed policy making, targeted vaccination and education programme and implementations can be achieved and guided. Integrated systems (multisectoral and multidisciplinary) surveillance and responses for the disease from the One Health context are recommended, due to the inextricable linkage between animals, humans and the environment where anthrax is concerned. The impact should be measured at the human–animal–ecological interface. Furthermore, implementation of the One Health approach in the surveillance of anthrax for early detection, responses and control may be crucial due to the persistence of the disease in Africa, recent re-emerging outbreaks in countries such as Russia (2016), Sweden (2016) and other cold, high-latitude countries, and the potential to be used for future biowar and pandemic. The emerging bio threat of anthrax will be discussed in the last section of this chapter.

Vaccination helps animals develop active immunity to identify and neutralize anthrax antigens whenever introduced into the body system, and to control the disease. Anthrax spore vaccine (ASV, for veterinary use) has been successfully used to control anthrax in many developed countries. ASV is a non-pathogenic, non-encapsulated Sterne strain 34F2 variant of *B. anthracis* suspended in glycerol with saponin (adjuvants). Cold chain must be observed, usually stored in a refrigerator at 4°C and not frozen. ASV has been efficiently used to prevent anthrax not only in goats but also other ruminant animals. The recommended dose is 0.5–1.0 ml subcutaneously at the mid-thorax at the age of 6 months and given 2–4 weeks before the seasonal outbreak. Revaccination is recommended annually, especially in endemic areas. However, goats are known to react adversely to the vaccine, and one strategy in vaccinating goats is to pre-inoculate by giving the first dose as one-quarter of the standard recommended dose, and the second dose as the standard recommended dose, at a month's interval (WHO, 2008). The standard recommended dose is then given annually (WHO, 2008). The availability and implementation of mass vaccinations has been effective in many developed countries, with considerable reduction or complete eradication in animals and humans (D'Amelio *et al.*, 2015). However, the lack of vaccination programmes against anthrax has been a key risk for persistence of anthrax in developing countries. Vaccination against anthrax in sub-Saharan Africa is 0–6% (Carlson *et al.*, 2019). Livestock vaccination in most low-income countries is implemented as a reactive measure to major outbreaks, rather than preventive (Migisha *et al.*, 2021).

Containing anthrax outbreaks is essential to reducing spread, case morbidities and fatalities in animals and humans. During outbreaks of anthrax, according to FAO-EMPRESS (2016), control strategies can be implemented that include: (i) not opening up infected carcasses; (ii) isolation of sick animals; (iii) quarantine of affected farms and in-contact farms, animals and animal products; (iv) reactivated vaccination of the susceptible herds to promote immunity coverage and vaccination of humans at risk; (v) treatment of affected animals and, if necessary, in-contact or susceptible animals with antimicrobials such as treated with penicillin or oxytetracycline or other long-acting antibiotics; (vi) active outbreak investigations and surveillance to identify sources of infection and proffer mitigations; (vii) disposal of carcasses of infected animals by incineration and other alternative environmentally friendly and cost-effective methods; and (viii) disinfection of affected farms and environment with 10% formalin, 5% sodium hydroxide or 3% peracetic acid after disposal of the carcass. Implementation of annual vaccination campaigns is critical towards reducing the risk for future recurrence outbreaks

9.10 Anthrax and the Potential Biothreat

The deliberate use of viruses and bacteria as biological weapons and to harm or cause death in humans and animals is known as bioterrorism. Anthrax has been classified as one of the BSL-3 potential organisms of high biothreat and a biological weapon due to the highly resistant spores, virulence and lethality. Anthrax remains the most likely organism to be used in a bioterrorism attack. It can be easily produced, weaponized and released to induce deaths of thousands to millions of targeted populations (D'Amelio *et al.*, 2015), and there is a global concern that anthrax may be used as a bioweapon of war in the near future. Anthrax has been used as a biothreat since the First World War, when German scientists infected livestock and contaminated animal feed exported to Allied forces (Christopher *et al.*, 1997; Wallin *et al.*, 2007). In the Second World War, the spores were used in arsenals and as retaliation by Ishii on villages south of Shanghai for the assistance rendered to the USA during the attack on Tokyo in 1942 (D'Amelio *et al.*, 2015; Mondange *et al.*, 2022). Further bioterrorist attacks were reported in Tokyo in 1993 and in the USA in 2001 immediately after the '9/11' terrorist attack on 9 September, which involved dispatch of letters contaminated with anthrax spores to high-profile journalists and politicians (Mondange *et al.*, 2022). This incidence in the USA induced 11 cases with five deaths and prompted the US government to invest billions of dollars in biodefence, pathogen- and bioterrorism-related research, emergency preparedness and response to control the risk of attacks and potentially malicious use.

The deliberate use of anthrax as a potential emerging bioweapon for future human destruction must not be underestimated and lessons must be learnt from past experiences to protect future risks. It is important to note that every country is at risk, and multilateral coordination network and collaborative efforts are critical in preventing anthrax biothreats that may impact global health. Also, integrated (One Health) multisectoral monitoring and surveillance systems at local, national and global levels are crucial to promote effective emergency-response systems and mitigation.

9.11 Conclusion

The potential of anthrax as an emerging bioweapon is of immense global health concern. It has been prioritized as a One Health zoonosis requiring multisectoral and multidisciplinary collaborations and efforts for efficient prevention and control in many countries, especially in Africa. Improved surveillance and reporting systems and strengthened One Health coordination are crucial for monitoring the trend patterns and emergency responses. Improved capacity and resources for efficient integrated surveillance framework, laboratory infrastructure, anthrax research, risk assessment and communication, data analysis and reporting systems are critical to ensure early detection and response to outbreaks in humans and animals. In an anthrax endemic and hotspot countries, most especially for goats, it is recommended that vaccination and awareness campaign programmes should be implemented and enforced.

References

Abrami, L., Reig, N. and van der Goot, F.G. (2005) Anthrax toxin: The long and winding road that leads to the kill. *Trends in Microbiology* 13(2), 72–78. DOI: 10.1016/j.tim.2004.12.004.

Ahsan, M., Khan, M.F.R., Rahman, M.B., Hassan, J., Chowdhury, Z.H. *et al.* (2013) Investigation into *Bacillus anthracis* spore in soil and analysis of environmental parameters related to repeated anthrax outbreak in Sirajganj, Bangladesh. *Thailand Journal of Veterinary Medicine* 43(3), 449–454.

Akula, A., Gomedhikam, J.P., Kota, M.K., Bodhanapu, V.B., Kalagara, M. *et al.* (2005) Anthrax: An overview. *International Journal of Risk Assessment and Management* 5(1), 76–94. DOI: 10.1504/IJRAM.2005.006611.

Alam, M.E., Kamal, Md.M., Rahman, M., Kabir, A., Islan, Md.S. *et al.* (2022) Review of anthrax: A disease of farm animals. *Journal of Advanced Veterinary and Animal Research* 9(2), 323–334. DOI: 10.5455/javar.2022.i599.

Aminu, O.R., Lembo, T., Zadoks, R.N., Biek, R., Lewis, S. *et al.* (2020) Practical and effective diagnosis of animal anthrax in endemic low-resource settings. *PLoS Neglected Tropical Diseases* 14(9), e0008655. DOI: 10.1371/journal.pntd.0008655.

Be, N.A., Thissen, J.B., Gardner, S.N., McLoughlin, K.S., Fofanov, V.Y. *et al.* (2013) Detection of *Bacillus anthracis* DNA in complex soil and air samples using next-generation sequencing. *PloS ONE* 8(9), e73455. DOI: 10.1371/journal.pone.0073455.

Bergman, N.H. (2011) *Bacillus anthracis and Anthrax*. John Wiley & Sons, New Jersey.

Blackburn, J.K., Odugbo, M.O., Van Ert, M., O'Shea, B., Mullins, J. *et al.* (2015) *Bacillus anthracis* diversity and geographic potential across Nigeria, Cameroon and Chad: Further support of a novel West African lineage. *PLoS Neglected Tropical Diseases* 9(8), e0003931. DOI: 10.1371/journal.pntd.0003931.

Carlson, C.J., Getz, W.M., Kausrud, K.I., Cizauskas, C.A., Blackburn, J.K. *et al.* (2018) Spores and soil from six sides: Interdisciplinarity and the environmental biology of anthrax (*Bacillus anthracis*). *Biological Reviews* 93(4), 1813–1831. DOI: 10.1111/brv.12420.

Carlson, C.J., Kracalik, I.T., Ross, N., Alexander, K.A., Hugh-Jones, M.E. *et al*. (2019) The global distribution of *Bacillus anthracis* and associated anthrax risk to humans, livestock and wildlife. *Nature Microbiology* 4(8), 1337–1343. DOI: 10.1038/s41564-019-0435-4.

Carroll, L.M., Wiedmann, M. and Kovac, J. (2020) Proposal of a taxonomic nomenclature for the *Bacillus cereus* group which reconciles genomic definitions of bacterial species with clinical and industrial phenotypes. *mBio* 11(1), e00034–20. DOI: 10.1128/mBio.00034-20.

Chethan Kumar, H.B., Hiremath, J., Yogisharadhya, R., Balamurugan, V., Jacob, S.S. *et al*. (2021) Animal disease surveillance: Its importance & present status in India. *Indian Journal of Medical Research* 153(3), 299–310. DOI: 10.4103/ijmr.IJMR_740_21.

Christopher, G.W., Cieslak, T.J., Pavlin, J.A. and Eitzen, E.M. Jr. (1997) Biological warfare: A historical perspective. *Journal of American Medical Association* 278(5), 412–417. DOI: 10.1001/jama.1997.03550050074036.

D'Amelio, E., Gentile, B., Lista, F. and D'Amelio, R. (2015) Historical evolution of human anthrax from occupational disease to potentially global threat as bioweapon. *Environment International* 85, 133–146. DOI: 10.1016/j.envint.2015.09.009.

De Vos, V. (1990) The ecology of anthrax in the Kruger National Park, South Africa. *Salisbury Medical Bulletin* 68, 19–23.

Dragon, D.C. and Rennie, R.P. (1995) The ecology of anthrax spores: Tough but not invincible. *The Canadian Veterinary Journal* 36(5), 295–301.

Ellerbrok, H., Nattermann, H., Ozel, M., Beutin, L., Appel, B. *et al*. (2002) Rapid and sensitive identification of pathogenic and apathogenic *Bacillus anthracis* by real-time PCR. *FEMS Microbiology Letters* 214(1), 51–59. DOI: 10.1111/j.1574-6968.2002.tb11324.x.

Food and Agriculture Organization (FAO) (2021) Live Animals, Goats, World Total, Africa Total, America Total, Asia, Total, Europe Total, Oceania Total, Year 2021. Available at: http://www.fao.org/faostat/en/#data/QA (accessed 13 February 2021).

Galante, D., Manzulli, V., Serrecchia, L., Di Taranto, P., Hugh-Jones, M. *et al*. (2021) Investigation on anthrax in Bangladesh during the outbreaks of 2011 and definition of the epidemiological correlations. *Pathogens* 10(4), 481. DOI: 10.3390/pathogens10040481.

Hugh-Jones, M. and Blackburn, J. (2009) The ecology of *Bacillus anthracis*. *Molecular Aspects of Medicine* 30(6), 356–367. DOI: 10.1016/j.mam.2009.08.003.

Ihekweazu, C., Michael, C.A., Nguku, P.M., Waziri, E.E., Habib, A.G. *et al*. (2021) Prioritization of zoonotic diseases of public health significance in Nigeria using the one-health approach. *One Health* 13, 100257. DOI: 10.1016/j.onehlt.2021.100257.

Kamer, L. (2022) Goat population in Africa as of 2020 by country (in million heads). Available at: https://www.statista.com/statistics/1290087/goat-population-in-africa-by-country/ (accessed 13 February 2021).

Keim, P., Gruendike, J.M., Klevytska, A.M., Schupp, J.M., Challacombe, J. *et al*. (2009) The genome and variation of *Bacillus anthracis*. *Molecular Aspects of Medicine* 30(6), 397–405. DOI: 10.1016/j.mam.2009.08.005.

Kolton, C.B., Marston, C.K., Stoddard, R.A., Cossaboom, C., Salzeer, J.S. *et al*. (2019) Detection of *Bacillus anthracis* in animal tissues using InBios active anthrax detect rapid test lateral flow immunoassay. *Letters in Applied Microbiology* 68(6), 480–484. DOI: 10.1111/lam.13134.

Les, B. and Huwar, T. (2011) *Oxford Textbook of Zoonoses: Biology, Clinical Practice, and Public Health Control*, 2nd edn. Oxford University Press, London.

Levi, K., Higham, J.L., Coates, D. and Hamlyn, P.F. (2003) Molecular detection of anthrax spores on animal fibres. *Letters in Applied Microbiology* 36(6), 418–422. DOI: 10.1046/j.1472-765x.2003.01336.x.

Luong, T., Nguyen, T.T., Trinh, V.B., Walker, M.A., Hoang, T.T.H. *et al*. (2023) Informing one health anthrax surveillance and vaccination strategy from spatial analysis of anthrax in humans and livestock in Ha Giang Province, Vietnam (1999–2020). *American Journal of Tropical Medicine and Hygiene* 108(3), 492–502. DOI: 10.4269/ajtmh.22-0384.

Mahendra, L. and Dilip, B. (2021) The importance of goats in the world. *Professional Agricultural Workers Journal* 6(2), 9–21. Available at: https://tuspubs.tuskegee.edu/pawj/vol6/iss2/4

Mawak, J.D., Fayam, A.S., Lar, P.M., Zakari, H. and Ngbede, J. (2006) Seroprevalence of *Bacillus anthracis* in Jos and environs. *African Journal of Clinical and Experimental Microbiology* 7(3), 190–193. Available at: https://www.ajol.info/index.php/ajcem/article/view/7452

Migisha, R., Mbatidde, I., Agaba, D.C., Turyakira, E., Tumwine, G. *et al*. (2021) Risk factors for human anthrax outbreak in Kiruhura District, Southwestern Uganda: A population-based case control study.

PAMJ – One Health 5(13), 1–15. Available at: https://www.one-health.panafrican-med-journal.com/content/article/5/13/full/

Mondange, L., Tessier, É. and Tournier, J.N. (2022) Pathogenic bacilli as an emerging biothreat? *Pathogens* 11(10), 1186. DOI: 10.3390/pathogens11101186.

Munyua, P., Bitek, A., Osoro, E., Pieracci, E.G., Muema, J. *et al.* (2016) Prioritization of zoonotic diseases in Kenya, 2015. *PloS ONE* 11(8), e0161576. DOI: 10.1371/journal.pone.0161576.

NCBI Genomes (2004) *Bacillus anthracis* genomes. National Center for Biotechnology Information. Available at: https://www.ncbi.nlm.nih.gov/genomes/MICROBES/anthracis.html (accessed 28 February 2023).

Nderitu, L.M., Gachohi, J., Otieno, F., Mogoa, E.G., Muturi, M. *et al.* (2021) Spatial clustering of livestock anthrax events associated with agro-ecological zones in Kenya, 1957–2017. *BMC Infectious Diseases* 21, 191. DOI: 10.1186/s12879-021-05871-9.

Ndiva Mongoh, M., Dyer, N.W., Stoltenow, C.L., Hearne, R. and Khaitsa, M.L. (2008) A review of management practices for the control of anthrax in animals: The 2005 anthrax epizootic in north dakota – case study. *Zoonoses and Public Health* 55(6), 279–290. DOI: 10.1111/j.1863-2378.2008.01135.x.

Ngetich, W. (2019) Review of anthrax: A disease of animals and humans. *International Journal of Agriculture, Environment and Bioresearch* 4(1), 124–134.

Odontsetseg, N., Sh, T., Adiyasuren, Z., Uuganbayar, D. and Mweene, A.S. (2007) Anthrax in animals and humans in Mongolia. *Revue Scientifique et Technique de l'Office International Des Epizooties* 26(3), 701–710. DOI: 10.20506/rst.26.3.1777.

Okolo, M.I. (1985) Studies on anthrax in food animals and persons occupationally exposed to the zoonoses in Eastern Nigeria. *International Journal of Zoonoses* 12(4), 276–282.

Oncü, S., Oncü, S. and Sakarya, S. (2003) Anthrax – an overview. *Medical Science Monitor* 9(11), 276–283.

Otieno, F.T., Gachohi, J., Gikuma-Njuru, P., Kariuki, P., Oyas, H. *et al.* (2021) Modeling the potential future distribution of anthrax outbreaks under multiple climate change scenarios for Kenya. *International Journal of Environmental Research and Public Health* 18(8), 4176. DOI: 10.3390/ijerph18084176.

Parry, J.M., Turnbull, P.C.B. and Gibson, J.R. (1983) *A Color Atlas of Bacillus Species*. Wolfe Medical, London.

Pilo, P. and Frey, J. (2011) *Bacillus anthracis*: Molecular taxonomy, population genetics, phylogeny and patho-evolution. *Infection, Genetics and Evolution* 11(6), 1218–1224. DOI: 10.1016/j.meegid.2011.05.013.

Pilo, P. and Frey, J. (2018) Pathogenicity, population genetics and dissemination of *Bacillus anthracis*. *Infection, Genetics and Evolution* 64, 115–125. DOI: 10.1016/j.meegid.2018.06.024.

Schmid, G. and Kaufmann, A. (2002) Anthrax in Europe: Its epidemiology, clinical characteristics, and role in bioterrorism. *Clinical Microbiology and Infection* 8(8), 479–488. DOI: 10.1046/j.1469-0691.2002.00500.x.

Sekamatte, M., Krishnasamy, V., Bulage, L., Kihembo, C., Nantima, N. *et al.* (2018) Multisectoral prioritization of zoonotic diseases in Uganda, 2017: A one health perspective. *PloS ONE* 13(5), e0196799.

Setlow, P. (2014) Germination of spores of *Bacillus* species: What we know and do not know. *Journal of Bacteriology* 196(7), 1297–1305. DOI: 10.1128/JB.01455-13.

Seyoum, A.F., Bitew, A.B. and Negussie, H. (2022) A retrospective study on the epidemiology of anthrax among livestock from 2011 to 2020 in Awi Administrative Zone, Amhara region, Northwest Ethiopia. *Veterinary Medicine(Auckland, N.Z)* 13, 313–321. DOI: 10.2147/VMRR.S384794.

Sternbach, G. (2003) The history of anthrax. *The Journal of Emergency Medicine* 24(4), 463–467. DOI: 10.1016/s0736-4679(03)00079-9.

Sushma, B., Shedole, S., Suresh, K.P., Leena, G., Patil, S.S. *et al.* (2021) An estimate of global anthrax prevalence in livestock: A meta-analysis. *Veterinary World* 14(5), 1263–1271. DOI: 10.14202/vetworld.2021/1263-1271.

Todar, K. (2023) *Bacillus anthracis* and anthrax. In: *Todar's Online Textbook of Bacteriology. 'The Good, the Bad, and the Deadly*. Available at: https://www.textbookofbacteriology.net/Anthrax.html (accessed 25 February 2023).

Utaaker, K.S., Chaudhary, S., Kifleyohannes, T. and Robertson, L.J. (2021) Global Goat! Is the expanding goat population an important reservoir of *Cryptosporidium*? *Frontiers in Veterinary Science* 8, 648500. DOI: 10.3389/fvets.2021.648500.

von Terzi, B., Turnbull, P.C.B., Bellan, S.E. and Beyer, W. (2014) Failure of sterne- and pasteur-like strains of *Bacillus anthracis* to replicate and survive in the urban bluebottle blow fly *Calliphora vicina* under laboratory conditions. *PloS ONE* 9(1), e83860. DOI: 10.1371/journal.pone.0083860.

Wallin, A., Luksiene, Z., Zagminas, K. and Surkiene, G. (2007) Public health and bioterrorism: Renewed threat of anthrax and smallpox. *Medicina* 43(4), 278–284. DOI: 10.3390/medicina43040034.

Wei, J., Zhang, H.J., Zhang, H.F., Zhang, E., Zhang, B. *et al.* (2020) Novel strategy for rapidly and safely distinguishing *Bacillus anthracis* and *Bacillus cereus* by use of peptide mass fingerprints based on matrix-assisted laser desorption ionization–time of flight mass spectrometry. *Clinical Microbiology* 9(1), e02358–20. DOI: 10.1128/JCM.02358-20.

Wielinga, P.R., Hamidjaja, R.A., Ågren, J., Knutsson, R., Segerman, B. *et al.* (2011) A multiplex real-time PCR for identifying and differentiating *B. anthracis* virulent types. *International Journal of Food Microbiology* 145(1), 137–144. DOI: 10.1016/j.ijfoodmicro.2010.07.039.

Wilson, J.B. and Russell, K.E. (1964) Isolation of *Bacillus anthracis* from soil stored 60 years. *Journal of Bacteriology* 87, 237–238.

Wilson, J.B., Brediger, W., Albright, T.P. and Smith-Gagen, J. (2016) Reanalysis of the anthrax epidemic in Rhodesia, 1978–1984. *PeerJ* 4, e2686. DOI: 10.7717/peerj.2686.

World Health Organization (2008) *Anthrax in Humans and Animals*, 4. WHO Press, Geneva, Switzerland.

10 Brucellosis

Ranbir Singh Jatav[1]*, Aditya Pratap[1] and Tanmoy Rana[2]
[1]Department of Veterinary Medicine, College of Veterinary Science and Animal Husbandry, NDVSU, Jabalpur, M.P., India; [2]Department of Veterinary Clinical Complex, West Bengal University of Animal & Fishery Sciences, Kolkata, India

Abstract
Goats are considered very important domestic animals and can survive in harsh environments; as such, goat production plays a key role in livelihood security. Effective goat production is impaired by diseases such as brucellosis. Brucellosis is a serious disease with considerably lowered production of the goats, resulting in severe reproductive wastage and with declined economic implications, as well as being of zoonotic importance. *Brucella melitensis* and *Brucella ovis* are the common cause of brucellosis in both sheep and goats. *Brucella melitensis* infection also has major veterinary and human importance. Farmers and community animal health workers are the worst sufferers of infection caused by *B. melitensis* during handling of goats. Proper monitoring of disease prevalence with identification of the risk factors can reduce the veterinary and public health impacts of brucellosis in goats.

Keywords: brucellosis, goats, public health, production, zoonotic importance

10.1 Introduction

Brucellosis is one of the world's major zoonoses and is still of veterinary, public health and economic concern in many parts of the world. Caprine brucellosis is one of the most infectious zoonotic diseases, with potential reduction of economic status in society as well as having public health significance. The goat is considered as the 'poor man's cow' reared by marginal and small-household families. It is a source of basic animal protein needed by human beings. Chevon is the meat procured from a mature goat. Foodborne zoonotic significance and public health consequences are the most important key factors for rearing goats in the most hygienic way. Weak, debilitated, immunocompromised goats are the worst sufferers from brucellosis, as it is a highly infectious disease with a high morbidity rate. Symptoms include chills, weakness, anorexia, intermittent fever, sweats, endocarditis, myalgia, late-stage abortion, depression and osteo-articular complications. In addition, *Brucella melitensis* was considered to be a most powerful bioterrorist agent in the 20th century (Pappas *et al.*, 2006). The World Health Organization (WHO) considers brucellosis to be a neglected zoonosis because, despite its widespread distribution and effects on multiple species, it is not prioritized by national and international health systems (WHO, 2005).

10.2 History and Epidemiology

Because it was endemic in the Mediterranean island of Malta, brucellosis in humans was

*Corresponding author: hindoliya.ranbir@gmail.com

 The Handbook of Zoonotic Diseases of Goats (ed. T. Rana)
DOI: 10.1079/ 9781800622852.0010

widely known as Malta fever in the 19th century (Marston, 1863; Bruce, 1887; Wright and Smith, 1897; Vassallo, 1992; Wyatt, 2005). Another synonym is Mediterranean fever. D'Anastasio *et al.* (2009) reported that a possible brucellosis infection found in the skeleton of a hominin species from 2 million years ago might have been due to consumption of infected meat from wild animals. More widely, infection in humans has been attributed mainly to the consumption of unpasteurized milk from affected cows and goats. Goats are considered to have been the host of *B. melitensis* for centuries (Capasso, 2002; Foster *et al.*, 2009). Zeder and Hesse (2000) gave a comprehensive history of the domestication of goats some 10,000 years ago.

Brucellosis remains a major debilitating illness. It is more prevalent in western parts of Asia, India, the Middle East, Southern Europe and Latin American countries. Human brucellosis is found to have a significant presence in rural and nomadic communities where people live in close association with animals. Epidemiological investigation of brucellosis generally relies upon sero-prevalence studies. Animals with histories of reproductive failure and abortion are generally screened for brucellosis by the Rose Bengal plate test (RBPT), serum tube agglutination test (SAT) and enzyme-linked immunosorbent assay (ELISA) kits. There are ten host-specific *Brucella* species: *B. abortus* (cattle), *B. canis* (canids), *B. ceti* (cetaceans), *B. melitensis* (sheep and goats), *B. microti* (Microtusarvalis), *B. neotomae* (Neotomalepida), *B. ovis* (sheep), *B. pinipedialis* (pinnipeds), *B. suis* (pigs) and *B. inopinata* (isolated from a human patient who had undergone breast surgery).

Transmission of *Brucella* bacteria among animals mainly occurs through contact following an abortion. Contaminated pasture or animal houses are responsible for the spread of the organisms through ingestion, inhalation, conjunctival inoculation, skin contamination and udder inoculation from infected milking cups, among other modes. In calves, pooled colostrum for feeding newborn calves serves as a source. Artificial insemination procedures transmit the disease but sexual transmission plays a small role in bovines. The sharing of male breeding stock also promotes transfer of infection between farms. Sexual transmission probably plays a greater role in the transmission of *B. melitensis* in sheep and goats along with *B. suis* in swine and *B. canis* in dogs. Other risk factors involve mingling of different flocks and herds, entry of unscreened animal purchases into the farm, transhumance for summer grazing, mingling of animals at fairs and closed-space animal housing. As the disease is zoonotic in nature, transmission to humans takes place by eating or drinking unpasteurized or raw dairy products and by inhalation and can also enter wounds in the skin and mucous membranes directly from infected animals. Ingestion of raw milk and occupational exposure are the key modes. Person-to-person spread of brucellosis is extremely rare. Infected breast-feeding mothers may transmit the infection to their infants. Sexual transmission has rarely been reported and, while uncommon, transmission may also occur via tissue transplantation or blood transfusions (Singh *et al.*, 2015).

In India, brucellosis was first recognized in 1942 and is now endemic throughout the country. Rapid and easy travel and trade have the potential to increase the endemicity. The disease is reported in cattle, buffalo, sheep, goats, pigs, dogs and humans. Long-term serological studies have indicated that 5% of cattle and 3% of buffalo are infected with brucellosis (Renukaradhya *et al.*, 2002). Polding (1942) first reported the isolation of *B. melitensis* in goats. Thereafter, *B. abortus* was isolated from cases of abortion in Haryana (Mathur, 1967). *B. melitensis* biotype-1 was isolated in the states of Karnataka, Andhra Pradesh, Maharashtra and Gujarat, and *B. melitensis* biotype-1 and biotype-3 in Haryana (Sen and Sharma, 1975; Hemashettar *et al.*, 1987). After investigations of 50 isolates from goats and 38 from sheep, Mathur (1985) opined that *B. melitenses* and *B. abortus* infections were common in sheep and goats. The sheep isolates included 32 isolates of *B. melitensis* and six of *B. abortus* as compared with 39 isolates of *B. melitensis* and 11 *B. abortus* from goats. He concluded that *B. abortus* infections of these animals were much higher in India than compared with other countries. *B. abortus* biotype-4 has been observed as a predominant biotype in small ruminants of Tamil Nadu (Darshana *et al.*, 2016).

B. melitensis is the major cause of abortion in sheep and goats in many countries, including

India, where infection is widespread (Ghosh and Verma, 1985). Serological surveys of small-ruminant brucellosis have indicated varying levels of infection in different states: 4.9% of sheep and 7.6% of goats in Karnataka (Desai *et al.*, 1995), 11% of sheep and 18% of goats in the northern state of Delhi, 50% of sheep and 16% of goats in Punjab, 33% of sheep and 30% of goats in the western state of Rajasthan, 55% of goats in Andhra Pradesh (Mrunalini *et al.*, 2000) and 24% of goats and 4.7% of sheep in Uttar Pradesh (Singh *et al.*, 2000) have been recorded as suffering from the infection. It was observed that flocks with a history of abortions had high incidence of brucellosis (Mrunalini *et al.*, 2000).

10.3 Aetiology

Brucellosis is caused by members of the bacterial genus *Brucella*. These are facultative intracellular Gram-negative pathogens. The ability of *Brucella* bacteria to replicate and persist in host cells is directly linked with their capacity to cause persistent disease and to circumvent innate and adaptive immunity (Gorvel and Moreno, 2002).

The morphology of *Brucella* is fairly constant except in old cultures, where pleomorphic forms may be evident. *Brucella* species are non-motile. They do not form spores, flagella, or pili. True capsules are not produced. They are Gram-negative and usually do not show bipolar staining. They are not truly acid-fast but resist decoloration by weak acids, thus they are stained red by Stamp's modification of the Ziehl–Neelsen method, which is sometimes used for the microscopic diagnosis of brucellosis from smears of solid or liquid specimens (Alton *et al.*, 1988).

B. melitensis is present in and transmitted by goats and related animals and is most virulent for humans. *B. abortus* is the dominant species in cattle and *B. suis* is mainly confined to pigs. In India, different *B. abortus* biotypes (types 1, 2, 4, 6 and 9) have been isolated from cattle (Renukaradhya *et al.*, 2002). *B. abortus* was also isolated from buffalo and from goats and sheep. *B. melitensis* biotypes 1 and 3 have been isolated from goats, sheep and cattle. *B. suis* may also be present in cattle, buffalo and goats. Though *B. melitensis* is more infectious to humans than *B. abortus* and in general is the dominant causative agent of brucellosis, disease caused by infection with *B. abortus* is indistinguishable from that by *B. melitensis* and may be equally severe (Dokuzoğuz *et al.*, 2005).

The genomic sequences of *B. melitensis*, *B. abortus* and *B. suis* have been (partially) determined and this knowledge will help to improve our understanding of the biology and pathogenicity of these organisms and may be used to develop new acellular and safer vaccines (Sánchez *et al.*, 2001).

10.4 Pathogenesis

Brucellosis in small ruminants is mainly caused by *B. melitensis*, a pathogen that may also infect cattle and other ruminants (Verger *et al.*, 1995). This pathogen, which has three different biovars, is endemic in several parts of the world, particularly biovar-3 in Mediterranean and Middle Eastern countries. Some Latin American countries are also seriously affected by biovar-1, especially Mexico, Peru and Northern Argentina (Lucero *et al.*, 2008). *B. melitensis* infection of goats and sheep is characterized by abortion, reduced milk yield and orchitis. Although sexually mature animals of both genders are equally susceptible to the disease, the predominant sign of acute infection is reproductive failure, with abortion in the last trimester or birth of weak offspring. In small ruminants, transmission of the disease often occurs by contact of susceptible animals with contaminated secretions from the female genital tract. Approximately two-thirds of acute natural *B. melitensis* infections of goats during pregnancy lead to infection of the udder and excretion of the bacteria in milk during the subsequent lactation. Progressively, intermittent shedding of the agent in milk occurs in animals with persistent infection of the udder. *B. melitensis* may cause inflammation of the mammary tissue, which is the most probable cause of reduced milk production in infected animals. However, clinical signs of mastitis are usually not detectable in naturally infected goats.

Brucella spp. are capable of invading and surviving in both phagocytic and non-phagocytic host cells. Macrophages, dendritic cells (DCs) and trophoblasts represent the major target cells for *Brucella*, according to clinical manifestation of brucellosis in experimental and natural hosts, characterized by persistent infections in lymphoid tissues and inflammatory lesions in the reproductive tract of pregnant females. Bacterial entrance, survival and replication have been intensively investigated in phagocytes, but these mechanisms are poorly characterized in trophoblasts, which represents an important gap in our understanding of the disease and transmission in the natural host species (Pizarro-Cerdá *et al.*, 2000).

In order to reach their target cells, *Brucella* bacteria need to cross mucosal barriers of the respiratory, genitourinary or digestive tract, where they undergophagocytosis by resident macrophages and DCs, resulting in dissemination of the organism to lymphoid and reproductive organs (Anderson *et al.*, 1986). Invasion through the digestive tract is associated with epithelial transmigration of bacteria preferentially through microfold (M) cells. Intra-epithelial phagocytes may also transport *Brucella* from the intestinal lumen to the lamina propria.

Trophoblastic cells are the key target cell of *Brucella* infection during the late phase of gestation in ruminants (Meador and Deyoe, 1989). Growth of *Brucella* bacteria inside trophoblasts is apparently enhanced in the presence of high concentrations of steroid hormones and erythritol during the final third of gestation. The capacity to replicate rapidly and extensively in trophoblasts can compromise the integrity of the placenta and result in infection of the fetus, leading to abortion or the birth of weak offspring. In addition, hormonal changes in infected placentas may affect the occurrence of abortion, since an increase in prostaglandin 2α, oestrogen and cortisol and decrease in progesterone levels mimic what happens during parturition (Samartino *et al.*, 1994).

10.5 Clinical Signs

Although a variety of clinical signs has been described in artificially infected animals, the main clinical manifestations of brucellosis in sheep and goats are, as in all female ruminants, reproductive failure, i.e. abortion or birth of weak offspring. Abortion generally occurs during the last 2 months of pregnancy and is followed in some cases by retention of fetal membranes. In the male, localization in the testis, epididymis and accessory sex organs is common, and bacteria may be shed in the semen. This may result in acute orchitis and epididymitis and later in infertility. Arthritis is also observed occasionally in both sexes. There is no evidence that the clinical features of *B. melitensis* infection in sheep and goats vary according to the biovar involved (Fensterbank *et al.*, 1987).

Non-pregnant animals exposed to small numbers of organisms may develop self-limiting, immunizing infections, or they may become latent carriers. Persistent infection of the mammary glands and supra-mammary lymph nodes is common in goats, with constant or intermittent shedding of the organisms in the milk in succeeding lactations, while the self-limiting nature of the disease in sheep, which is seldom accompanied by prolonged excretion of the bacteria, has been observed (Alton *et al.*, 1988). The inflammatory changes in the infected mammary gland reduce milk production by an estimated minimum of 10%. Orchitis and epididymitis generally lead to a chronic infection.

The lesions, when present, are not pathognomonic. The following could be observed: necrotizing placentitis, palpable testicular alterations, necrotizing orchitis and epididymitis with subsequent granuloma, necrotizing seminal vesiculitis and prostatitis. Acute mastitis with palpable nodules and the production of clotted and watery milk may occur. Some aborted fetuses may have an excess of blood-stained fluids in the body cavities, with enlarged spleen and liver. Others appear normal. Infected fetal membranes show changes affecting part or all of the membrane.

10.6 Diagnosis

Brucellosis presents a great variety of clinical manifestations, making it difficult to diagnose clinically. Therefore, the diagnosis must be confirmed by laboratory tests. Accurate and fast diagnosis of brucellosis is very important, as delay or misdiagnosis usually results in treatment failure.

Diagnostic tools include isolation and identification of *Brucella* bacteria from clinical samples, with detection of antigen, genome and antibodies.

10.6.1 Isolation of bacteria

The only unequivocal method for the diagnosis of brucellosis in small ruminants is based on the isolation of *Brucella* bacteria (Alton *et al.*, 1988). The presumptive bacteriological diagnosis of *B. melitensis* can be made by means of the microscopic examination of smears from vaginal swabs, placentas or aborted fetuses stained with the Stamp modification of the Ziehl–Neelsen method. Vaginal swabs and milk samples are the best samples to isolate *B. melitensis* from sheep and goats. The spleen and lymph nodes (iliac, mammary and prefemoral) are the most reliable samples for isolation purposes in necropsied animals (Marin *et al.*, 1996).

Farrell's selective medium, developed for the isolation of *B. abortus* from milk (Farrell, 1974), is also recommended for the isolation of *B. melitensis* (Alton *et al.*, 1988).

10.6.2 Culture

Brucella members are aerobic, but some strains require an atmosphere containing 5–10% carbon dioxide (CO_2) added for growth, especially on primary isolation. The optimum pH for growth varies from 6.6 to 7.4, and culture media should be adequately buffered near pH 6.8 for optimum growth. The optimum growth temperature is 36–38°C, but most strains can grow between 20°C and 40°C.

Brucella bacteria require biotin, thiamine and nicotinamide. The growth is improved by serum or blood, but haemin (V-factor) and nicotinamide-adenine dinucleotide (X-factor) are not required. The growth of most *Brucella* strains is inhibited on media containing bile salts, tellurite or selenite.

Blood culture provides definite proof of brucellosis but may not provide a positive result for all patients. Lysis centrifugation and blood clot culture techniques have yielded encouraging results (Mantur *et al.*, 2007) in terms of sensitivity and rapidity. The modern automated blood culture systems have somewhat improved the speed of detection. Although bone marrow cultures are considered the gold standard in some studies (Gotuzzo *et al.*, 1986), results have not been universally reproducible. In such cases, bacteraemia might also be maintained from other sources of the reticulo-endothelial system. This could be the reason for the discrepancy in the results of blood and bone marrow cultures reported in the literature.

The time required for culturing field specimens can be long and tissues or fluids that are only contaminated with a low number of *Brucella* organisms may not be detected. Thus, in the case of tissues or fluids contaminated with non-viable or a low number of *Brucella*, PCR could be a potentially useful method for the diagnosis of brucellosis. Several authors reported a good sensitivity of PCR for detecting of *Brucella* DNA on pure cultures (Baily *et al.*, 1992).

Hence a preliminary bacteriological diagnosis can be made on smears from vaginal swabs, milk, placentas or aborted fetuses stained with Stamp's method. Confirmation on appropriate culture and selective media is recommended. Spleen and lymph nodes are most reliable from necropsy material. PCR is potentially a useful method in samples containing a low number of *Brucella* bacteria.

10.6.3 Serological tests

It is widely assumed that the serological tests used for *B. abortus* infection in cattle are also adequate for the diagnosis of *B. melitensis* infection in small ruminants. Accordingly, the Rose Bengal test and complement fixation test are the most widely used tests for the serological diagnosis of brucellosis in sheep and goats (Farina, 1985; Alton, 1990).

Rose Bengal test (RB test)

The Rose Bengal (RB) test was developed more than 20 years ago for the diagnosis of bovine brucellosis. Despite the scanty and sometimes conflicting information available, this test is internationally recommended for the screening of brucellosis in small ruminants.

Complement fixation test (CF test)

The Complement fixation (CF) test is the most widely used test for the serological confirmation of brucellosis in animals. As in cattle brucellosis, despite its complexity and the heterogeneity of the techniques used in different countries, there is agreement that this test is effective for the serological diagnosis of brucellosis in sheep and goats (Farina, 1985; Alton, 1990). When testing a limited number of sera obtained from *B. melitensis* culture-positive and *Brucella*-free goats, the CF test provided the same sensitivity as the RB and i-ELISA. However, under field conditions, the sensitivity of the CF test has been reported to be somewhat lower (88.6%) than those of the RB (92.1%) and i-ELISA (100%) for diagnosing *B. melitensis* infection in sheep (Blasco *et al.*, 1994).

10.6.4 Enzyme-immunoassay (EIA) Methods

The large majority of Enzyme-immunoassays (EIAs) in use in brucellosis diagnosis are indirect ELISAs (iELISAs). ELISAs are methods that involve the immobilization of one of the active components on a solid phase, and iELISAs are those in which the antigen is bound to a solid phase, usually a polystyrene micro-titre plate so that antibody, if present in a sample, binds to the immobilized antigen and may be detected by an appropriate anti-globulin–enzyme conjugate which, in combination with a chromogenic substrate, gives a coloured reaction indicative of the presence of antibody in the sample. It is this method that is now familiar to most diagnosticians.

Another method that is gaining prominence in publications on brucellosis diagnosis is the competitive ELISA (cELISA). In this test, *Brucella* antigen is immobilized on the plate as with the indirect ELISA. Following that, the serum under test and a monoclonal antibody directed against an epitope on the antigen are co-incubated. This anti-*Brucella* monoclonal antibody is conjugated to an enzyme, the presence of which is detected if it binds to the antigen. This will only occur if there is no antibody in the serum sample which is bound preferentially.

Relatively little information is available on the value of the ELISA for the diagnosis of *B. melitensis* in small ruminants. The indirect ELISA, using more or less purified S-LPS of *B. melitensis* as antigen and polyclonal conjugate (anti-IgG H + L), has been reported to be sensitive enough for the diagnosis of infection in sheep and goats (Blasco *et al.*, 1994).

While the use of ELISA for the diagnosis of bovine brucellosis is well developed, more extensive field trials are required to fully validate the test for use in sheep and goats. Further research is needed to develop serological tests of improved sensitivity for the diagnosis of brucellosis in sheep, especially assays that would be able to discriminate between infected and vaccinated animals.

10.6.5 Antiglobulin (Coombs') test

The antiglobulin test or Coombs' test (Coombs *et al.*, 1945) was developed to detect antibodies which, although they combine with cellular antigens of *Brucella*, do not give rise to agglutination. The presence of these so-called 'incomplete agglutinins' can be detected by using an antibody directed against the IgG fraction of the animal species being tested. Early in 1955, the test was described as the most effective immunological method for the detection of brucellosis in goats.

There is evidence (Unel *et al.*, 1969; Alton, 1990) suggesting that the antiglobulin test is effective in diagnosing brucellosis in sheep and goats, but because of the complexity of the technique its use may be restricted to special situations, for example for the detection of antibodies in anti-complementary sera. Its use is not recommended in bovines vaccinated with strain S19 or in small ruminants immunized with strain Rev. 1 vaccine (Farina, 1985), because of its low specificity as compared with the CF test.

10.6.6 Immunocapture test

The immunocapture test is a one-step technique, very easy to perform, able to detect antibodies of medium to high affinity against *Brucella*, and suitable for simple standardization and automation. The test is based on a blue-coloured cellular antigen of *Brucella melitensis* (strain 16M) and on anti-total species immunoglobulin-coated polystyrene microplates of 96 U-wells.

10.7 Preventive Cure and Management

The government of India has a centrally sponsored brucellosis control programme operating in all the states. The activities of this programme are generally restricted to investigation into abortion, infertility and serological surveys and have not contributed to any tangible approach towards disease control.

Vaccination is often the first step in the control of infectious diseases. There is agreement that vaccination of small ruminants is the only practical and effective procedure to reduce the incidence of brucellosis in many countries. In most developing countries and in some EU countries affected by *B. melitensis*, the vaccination of small ruminants continues to be applied in order to control the disease.

The live attenuated *B. melitensis* Rev. 1 strain is presently recognized as the best available vaccine for the prophylaxis of brucellosis in sheep and goats. Moreover, according to the WHO (1998) 'correctly standardized Elberg 101 strain Rev. 1 vaccine should continue to be considered as the basis of brucellosis control in small ruminants where vaccination is applied, until new safer and effective versions of *B. abortus* and *B. melitensis* vaccines, based on rough strains, are tested under controlled experimental and field conditions and shown to be at least equivalent to the Rev.1 vaccine'. The ability of the vaccine (Rev. 1 strain) to produce a high level of immunity against both artificial and natural challenges has been convincingly demonstrated for sheep and goats (Alton, 1990).

When Rev. 1 vaccine is administered in young replacement animals by the conjunctival route ($0.5–2 \times 10^9$ CFU contained in a small volume of 30–50 μl inoculated in the conjunctival sac), the protection conferred is similar to that induced by the classical subcutaneous method but the serological response evoked is significantly reduced. Thus, this route of vaccine administration is compatible with eradication programmes based on test-and-slaughter principles (Fensterbank *et al.*, 1987).

B. suis S2, a classically obtained *Brucella* attenuated strain with smooth LPS (lipopolysaccharide), was apparently successfully used in controlling brucellosis following oral administration to small ruminants in field conditions in China (Xin, 1986) and Libya (Mustafa and Abusowa, 1993). However, this vaccine showed no protective effect against *B. melitensis* in sheep in fully controlled experimental conditions (Verger *et al.*, 1995).

Other interesting approaches to develop new-generation vaccines, such as the construction of recombinant strains deleted in relevant diagnostic proteins, or DNA-based vaccines, are being currently investigated. It is probable that some of these vaccines will become candidates to replace the available classical vaccines in the near future. However, to date, none of these vaccines have been found to surpass the immunity conferred by the classical Rev. 1 vaccine.

Control of the disease in animals is a prerequisite to reduce its zoonotic spread. Control of infection in animal populations can be based on different strategies, the selection of which depends on numerous factors. Mass vaccination accompanied by a strict surveillance scheme is a first step to reduce the number of infected animals and hence the infection pressure. At a low level of infection, a test-and-slaughter programme can be applied in order to attain brucellosis-free flocks and zones. The creation of brucellosis-free flocks and zones is a second level, which requires that re-infection is prevented and that young replacement animals are available in a sufficient number. Application of a control and finally eradication programme can be negatively affected by traditional factors of husbandry of goats, in particular mixing of flocks in transhumance areas and movement of flocks to different places in the course of a year. Eradication programmes require constant surveillance and financial support from state authorities. Socioeconomic factors play an important role in eradication programmes.

10.8 Conclusion

Although infection by *B. melitensis* in sheep and goats resembles infection by *B. abortus* in cattle, differences exist. *Brucella* are facultative intracellular parasites of the reticulo-endothelial system. Virulence varies between species and strains. Infection occurs mainly through the mucous membranes of the oro-pharynx, upper respiratory tract, conjunctiva and genital tract. In pregnant animals the uterus is invaded, resulting in abortions. The udder is an important predilection site for *B. melitensis*. The predominant symptom of an acute *B. melitensis* infection is reproductive failure, with abortion and birth of weak offspring. Abortion occurs during the last 2 months of gestation. In males the reproductive organs are affected and bacteria may be shed with semen. Persistent infection of the udder is accompanied by intermittent discharge of the agent in milk. Inflammation of the mammary gland reduces milk production. Aborted fetuses may show increased amounts of bloody fluids in their body cavities and enlarged spleen and liver. Fetal membranes may be oedematous or necrotic. Elimination of the bacterium is possible, but a long-lasting persistent infection is the normal course of the disease, in particular in goats. There is agreement that vaccination of sheep and goats is the only practical and effective procedure to reduce the prevalence/occurrence of brucellosis in many countries. In most of the developing countries and in some EU Member States affected by *B. melitensis*, vaccination of sheep and goats continues to be indispensable to control the disease. The live attenuated *B. melitensis* Rev. 1 (Elberg 101) strain is the best classical vaccine available for prophylaxis of brucellosis in small ruminants. Its use is recommended by FAO (2010) and it has its own monograph in the EP.

References

Alton, G.G., Jones, L.M., Angus, R.D. and Verger, J.M. (1988) *Techniques for the Brucellosis Laboratory*. INRA, Paris.

Alton, G.G. (1990) Brucella melitensis. In: Nielsen, K. and Duncan, J.R. (eds) *Animal Brucellosis*. CRC Press, Boca Raton, Florida, pp. 383–409.

Anderson, T.D., Meador, V.P. and Cheville, N.F. (1986) Pathogenesis of placentitis in the goat inoculated with *Brucella abortus*. I. Gross and histologic lesions. *Veterinary Pathology* 23(3), 219–226.

Baily, G.G., Krahn, J.B., Drasar, B.S. and Stoker, N.G. (1992) Detection of *Brucella melitensis* and *Brucella abortus* by DNA amplification. *Journal of Tropical Medicine and Hygiene* 95(4), 271–275.

Blasco, J.M., Garin-Bastuji, B., Marin, C.M., Gerbier, G., Fanlo, J. *et al.* (1994) Efficacy of different Rose Bengal and complement fixation antigens for the diagnosis of *Brucella melitensis* infection in sheep and goats. *Veterinary Record* 134(16), 415–420.

Bruce, S.D. (1887) *Note on the discovery of a microorganism in Malta fever*. John Brigg.

Capasso, L. (2002) Bacteria in two-millennia-old cheese, and related epizoonoses in Roman populations. *Journal of Infection* 45(2), 122–127.

Coombs, R.R.A., Mourant, A.E. and Race, R.R. (1945) A new test for the detection of weak and 'incomplete' Rh agglutinins. *British Journal of Experimental Pathology* 26(4), 255.

D'Anastasio, R., Zipfel, B., Moggi-Cecchi, J., Stanyon, R. and Capasso, L. (2009) Possible brucellosis in an early hominin skeleton from sterkfontein, South Africa. *PLoS ONE* 4, e6439. DOI: 10.1371/journal.pone.0006439.

Darshana, U., Ganesan, P.I., Samuel, B.S.M., Vijayabharthi, M. and Rincy, T. (2016) Predominant prevalence of *Brucella abortus* biovar-4 in small ruminants in Tamilnadu. *International Journal of Advanced Veterinary Science and Technology* 5(2), 293–297.

Desai, T., Krishnappa, G. and Upadhye, A.S. (1995) Incidence of brucellosis in sheep, goats and some human risk groups. *Mysore Journal of Agricultural Sciences* 29, 348–351.

Dokuzoğuz, B., Ergönül, Ö., Baykam, N., Esener, H., Kılıç, S. *et al.* (2005) Characteristics of *B. melitensis* versus *B. abortus* bacteraemias. *Journal of Infection* 50(1), 41–45.

FAO (2010) *Brucella melitensis in Eurasia and the Middle East*. Food and Agriculture Organization, Rome.

Farina, R. (1985) Current serological methods in *Brucella melitensis* diagnosis. In: Plommet, M. and Verger, J.M. (eds) *Brucella Melitensis*. Martinus Nijhoff, Dordrecht, pp. 139–146.

Farrell, I.D. (1974) The development of a new selective medium for the isolation of *Brucella abortus* from contaminated sources. *Research in Veterinary Science* 16(3), 280–286.

Fensterbank, R., Verger, J.M. and Grayon, M. (1987) Conjunctival vaccination of young goats with *Brucella melitensis* strain Rev 1. *Annales de Recherches Vétérinaires* 18(4), 397–403.

Foster, J.T., Beckstrom-Sternberg, S.M., Pearson, T., Beckstrom-Sternberg, J.S., Chain, P.S. *et al.* (2009) Whole-genome-based phylogeny and divergence of the genus *Brucella*. *Journal of Bacteriology* 191(8), 2864–2870.

Ghosh, S.S. and Verma, P.C. (1985) Incidence of brucellosis in sheep and goat in Nagaland [India]. Short communication. *Indian Veterinary Journal* 62(4), 339–340.

Gorvel, J.P. and Moreno, E. (2002) Brucella intracellular life: From invasion to intracellular replication. *Veterinary Microbiology* 90(1–4), 281–297.

Gotuzzo, E., Carrillo, C., Guerra, J. and Llosa, L. (1986) An evaluation of diagnostic methods for brucellosis – the value of bone marrow culture. *Journal of Infectious Diseases* 153(1), 122–125.

Hemashettar, B.M., Patil, C.S., Jayakumar, K., Devaraj, M. and Nagalotimath, S.J. (1987) Isolation of *Brucella melitensis* biotype 1 from a cow and 2 of its attenders. *Indian Veterinary Journal* 64(10), 822–825.

Lucero, N.E., Ayala, S.M., Escobar, G.I. and Jacob, N.R. (2008) Brucella isolated in humans and animals in Latin America from 1968 to 2006. *Epidemiology & Infection* 136(4), 496–503.

Mantur, B.G., Amarnath, S.K. and Shinde, R.S. (2007) Review of clinical and laboratory features of human brucellosis. *Indian Journal of Medical Microbiology* 25(3), 188–202.

Marin, C.M., Alabart, J.L. and Blasco, J.M. (1996) Effect of antibiotics contained in two Brucella selective media on growth of *Brucella abortus*, *B. melitensis*, and *B. ovis*. *Journal of Clinical Microbiology* 34(2), 426–428.

Marston, J.A. (1863) *Report on Fever (Malta)*. Army Medical Department, London.

Mathur, T.N. (1967) Isolation of *Brucella abortus* from goats and sheep in the Punjab. *Indian Journal of Veterinary Science* 37, 277–286.

Mathur, T.N. (1985) The epidemiology of brucellosis. In: Proceedings of the Brucellosis symposium and annual sero-prevalence and molecular detection of *Brucella* species in pig producers of Punjab. *India Journal of Animal Research* 6(5), 9–10.

Meador, V.P. and Deyoe, B.L. (1989) Intracellular localization of *Brucella abortus* in bovine placenta. *Veterinary Pathology* 26(6), 513–515.

Mrunalini, N., Sastry, P.R., Pandarinadh, G.N. and Rao, M.R. (2000) Control of brucellosis epidemic in goats in a farm. *Indian Veterinary Journal* 77(11), 932–935.

Mustafa, A.A. and Abusowa, M. (1993) Field-oriented trial of the Chinese *Brucella suis* strain 2 vaccine on sheep and goats in Libya. *Veterinary Research* 24(5), 422–429.

Pappas, G., Panagopoulou, P., Christou, L. and Akritidis, N. (2006) Biological weapons: Brucella as a biological weapon. *Cellular and Molecular Life Sciences* 63, 2229–2236.

Pizarro-Cerdá, J., Moreno, E. and Gorvel, J.P. (2000) Invasion and intracellular trafficking of *Brucella abortus* in nonphagocytic cells. *Microbes and Infection* 2(7), 829–835.

Polding, J.B. (1942) Brucellosis in india. *Indian Journal of Veterinary Science* 13, 27–34.

Renukaradhya, G.J., Isloor, S. and Rajasekhar, M. (2002) Epidemiology, zoonotic aspects, vaccination and control/eradication of brucellosis in India. *Veterinary Microbiology* 90(1–4), 183–195.

Samartino, L.E., Truax, R.E. and Enright, F.M. (1994) Invasion and replication of *Brucella abortus* in three different trophoblastic cell lines. *Journal of Veterinary Medicine, Series B* 41(1-10), 229–236.

Sánchez, D.O., Zandomeni, R.O., Cravero, S., Verdún, R.E., Pierrou, E. *et al.* (2001) Gene discovery through genomic sequencing of *Brucella abortus*. *Infection and Immunity* 69(2), 865–868.

Sen, G.P. and Sharma, G.L. (1975) Speciation of seventy eight Indian strains of *Brucella*: An epidemiological study. *Indian Journal of Animal Sciences* 45, 537.

Singh, B.B., Dhand, N.K. and Gill, J.P.S. (2015) Economic losses occurring due to brucellosis in indian livestock populations. *Preventive Veterinary Medicine* 119(3–4), 211–215.

Singh, S.V., Gupta, V.K. and Singh, N. (2000) Comparative evaluation of a field-based dot-ELISA kit with three other serological tests for the detection of *Brucella* antibodies in goats. *Tropical Animal Health and Production* 32(3), 155–163.

Unel, S., Williams, C.F. and Stableforth, A.W. (1969) Relative value of the agglutination test complement fixation test and coombs (antiglobulin) test in the detection of *Brucella melitensis* infection in sheep. *Journal of Comparative Pathology* 79(2), 155–159.

Vassallo, D.J. (1992) The corps disease: Brucellosis and its historical association with the Royal Army Medical Corps. *BMJ Military Health* 138(3), 140–150.

Verger, J.M., Grayon, M., Zundel, E., Lechopier, P. and Olivier-Bernardin, V. (1995) Comparison of the efficacy of *Brucella suis* strain 2 and *Brucella melitensis* Rev. 1 live vaccines against a *Brucella melitensis* experimental infection in pregnant ewes. *Vaccine* 13(2), 191–196.

WHO (1998) *The Development of New/Improved Brucellosis Vaccines: Report of WHO Meeting, Geneva, Switzerland, 11-12 December 1997*. World Health Organization, Geneva.

WHO (2005) *The Control of Neglected Zoonotic Diseases*. Report of the first meeting on the control of neglected zoonotic diseases, WHO and Department for International Development-Animal Health Programme (DFID-AHP), with the participation of FAO and OIE 20-21, World Health Organization, Geneva.

Wright, A. and Smith, F. (1897) *On the application of the serum test to the differential diagnosis of typhoid and Malta fever: And on the further application of the method of serum diagnosis to the elucidation of certain problems in connexion with the duration of immunity and the geographical distribution of disease*.

Wyatt, H.V. (2005) How themistocles zammit found Malta fever (brucellosis) to be transmitted by the milk of goats. *Journal of the Royal Society of Medicine* 98(10), 451–454.

Xin, X. (1986) Orally administrable brucellosis vaccine: *Brucella suis* strain 2 vaccine. *Vaccine* 4(4), 212–216.

Zeder, M.A. and Hesse, B. (2000) The initial domestication of goats (*Capra hircus*) in the Zagros mountains 10,000 years ago. *Science* 287(5461), 2254–2257.

11 Campylobacteriosis

Ranbir Singh Jatav*, Nitin Vaishnav and Aditya Pratap
Department of Veterinary Medicine, College of Veterinary Science and Animal Husbandry, NDVSU, Jabalpur, M.P

Abstract
Campylobacter spp. in goats are generally transmitted via water, food, or the faecal–oral route. The most important ecological niche for *Campylobacter* spp. is the gastrointestinal tract of goats with zoonotic transmission to humans. *Campylobacter* contaminates the environment through grazing of animals. *Campylobacter* spp. can persist for prolonged periods in faeces, milk, water and urine, especially at temperatures close to 4°C. In adverse situations, this bacterium can convert to a viable non-culturable form that can be reactivated when ingested. Human foods can be contaminated with *Campylobacter* bacteria. People infected with campylobacteriosis show diarrhoea, nausea, fever, vomiting, abdominal pain, headache and muscle pain. Immunocompromised people are at higher risk for severe or recurrent infections.

Keywords: Campylobacteriosis, goats, contamination, grazing, food issues

11.1 Introduction

Goats are multipurpose animals, producing meat, milk, skin and hair, and they contribute greatly to food, rural employment and gross domestic product. Goats are affected by many diseases and campylobacteriosis is one of the important diseases among them. It is responsible for infertility and sterility and thus heavy economic losses to goat farmers. It is a highly contagious bacterial disease of farm animals and humans. *Campylobacter* bacteria cause enteric campylobacteriosis and genital campylobacteriosis and some species are zoonotic in nature. *Campylobacter* species were previously classified in the genus *Vibrio*, and the term 'vibriosis' has been retained for some of the disease conditions that they cause (Quinn *et al.*, 2011). One of the major concerns is contamination of meat products, milk and milk products by *Campylobacter*, the main bacterial cause of diarrhoea in humans. It is one of the most frequently isolated bacterial pathogens from the stools of infants with diarrhoea in several developing countries (Coker *et al.*, 2002; Padungton and Kaneene, 2003), particularly in poultry meat. *Campylobacter* spp. reside in the gut of domesticated animals and birds as part of the intestinal microflora (Salihu *et al.*, 2009). *Campylobacter jejuni* is now recognized as the leading bacterial cause of foodborne disease in both developed and developing countries (Oberhelman and Taylor, 2000; Han *et al.*, 2007; Calistri and Giovannini, 2008). Spiral *Campylobacter*-like organisms were first observed microscopically from the stools of children by the paediatrician Theodor Escherich in 1886. Between 1909 and 1944, there were a growing number of reports of

*Corresponding author: hindoliya.ranbir@gmail.com

DOI: 10.1079/ 9781800622852.0011

similar 'vibrio-like' organisms isolated from bovine and ovine sources, but they were not isolated from humans until 1938, in association with a milk-borne outbreak of gastroenteritis where blood cultures were positive for organisms resembling '*Vibrio jejuni*'. Goats can act as source of human infections as well as contamination of the environment (Uaboi-Egbenni *et al.*, 2011). The family Campylobacteraceae also contains the genetically misclassified species *Bacteroides ureolyticus* and strains originally described as *Sulfurospirillum* species. Species belonging to the genus *Sulfurospirillum* have no known pathogenicity for humans or animals, and are considered environmental organisms.

11.2 Aetiology

11.2.1 Aetiology for enteric campylobacteriosis

Campylobacter is a Gram-negative, non-spore-forming, spiral, flagellated bacterium. Daughter cells remain joined with parent cells and give a gull-winged appearance. It is microaerophilic (requiring 5–15% CO_2) and causes gastrointestinal tract infection in humans and animals. *Campylobacter jejuni* subsp. *jejuni* causes enteritis and abortion in sheep and goats. *Campylobacter fetus* subsp. *fetus* is also isolated from the gastrointestinal (GI) tract of goats. Some *Campylobacter* species are thermotolerant; for instance, *C. jejuni* and *Campylobacter coli*, which are of critical importance in food safety, grow optimally at 42°C. whereas *C. fetus* grows well at 25°C and 37°C and usually does not grow at 42°C (Penner, 1988; Goualié Gblossi *et al.*, 2012). A small number of *Campylobacter* cells may cause potent infection. There are two *C. fetus* subspecies: *C. fetus* subsp. *fetus*, which is associated with both ovine and bovine reproductive disorders as well as human infections; and *C. fetus* subsp. *venerealis*, which causes bovine-associated abortion and infertility. This species is most similar phenotypically and genetically to the two *Campylobacter hyointestinalis* subspecies: *C. hyointestinalis* subsp. *hyointestinalis* and *C. hyointestinalis* subsp. *lawsonni*.

11.2.2 Aetiology for genital campylobacteriosis

Campylobacter are spiral rod-shaped bacteria in the family Campylobacteriaceae. *Campylobacter fetus* subsp. *fetus* (also known as *Campylobacter fetus* subsp. *intestinalis* and *Vibrio fetus* var. *intestinalis*) cause infertility and enzootic abortion in goats. It is occasionally isolated from humans and has also been isolated from the intestines of healthy goats, sheep and cattle and from enteric lesions in cattle with enteritis. *C. fetus* subsp. *venerealis* is also responsible for disease in animals and humans.

11.3 Epidemiology and Transmission

Campylobacter species are found in several countries and are isolated from different animals like cattle, sheep, goats, birds, pets and the human population. *C. fetus* subsp. *fetus* is transmitted by ingestion of contaminated pastures or water in goats. Animals also get infection by direct contact with contaminated fomite, vaginal discharge, aborted material, etc. Humans get infection by ingestion of contaminated food, water and animal products. Raw goat's milk may transmit *C. jejuni* infection from animals to humans. *Campylobacter* species are primarily zoonotic, with a variety of animals implicated as reservoirs of infection, including a diverse range of domestic and wild animals and birds. In addition, water and the environment play a significant but poorly understood role in the epidemiology of campylobacteriosis. While sporadic *Campylobacter* infections are extremely common, campylobacteriosis outbreaks, defined as two or more persons epidemiologically linked by time and exposure, are relatively rare compared with other enteric pathogens. Outbreaks in the United States have been linked to a variety of foods, including poultry and other meats and fruit. However, the most common single food implicated in outbreaks of campylobacteriosis is unpasteurized milk.

11.4 Pathogenesis

After ingestion of contaminated feed and water, bacteria must cross the stomach barrier and reach the intestines, where they multiply in intestinal epithelium and cells of lamina propria. *Campylobacter* bacteria also lower the dissolved oxygen and reduce the oxygen supply and nutrients for embryo implantation, thus causing retarded implantation and development of the embryo. It has been shown that the expression of genes involved in motility (flaA and flhA) are essential for the mobility/passage of *Campylobacter* through the stomach and gut environment (Park, 2002). Colonization, epithelial cell invasion (cadF, docA, racR, virB11, ciaB, and iam genes), adherence and invasion of epithelial cells of the intestine (Konkel *et al.*, 1997; Carvalho *et al.*, 2001; Dasti *et al.*, 2010) and toxin production play an important role in the disease development (Humphrey *et al.*, 2007; Dasti *et al.*, 2010). *C. jejuni* is able to produce the superoxide dismutase (SOD) enzyme (encoded by the sodB marker), which catalyses the breakdown of superoxide radicals and hence plays a major role in defending *Campylobacter* species from oxidative damage (Pesci *et al.*, 1994). *Campylobacter* spp. possess a microcapsule or S layer, which consists of high-molecular-weight proteins arranged in a lattice formation. This S layer confers resistance to serum-mediated destruction and phagocytosis (Blaser and Pei, 1993).

11.5 Clinical Signs

Sheep and goats are natural reservoir hosts for *Campylobacter* spp. and mostly they are asymptomatic. Clinical signs depend upon the immune status of the affected animal. *Campylobacter* spp. cause infertility. Sporadic abortion has been reported in sheep and goats, although goats are known to be more resistant to *Campylobacter* infections, resulting in fewer abortions (Moeller, 2009), and enteritis has been reported in goats and kids. The animal will be depressed and may have fever and mucoid diarrhoea, which may contain blood. The bacteria may cause metritis, stillbirth and weak kids. Severe bacteraemia may occur in patients having low immunity levels. Infection of the udder by the organism is easy to establish, and the infection is persistent but subclinical for the most part. Infection of the udder is characterized by fine granular clots in the milk, very high cell counts and a transient episode of fever and swelling of the quarter (Constable *et al.*, 2017).

11.6 Necropsy Findings

On post-mortem examination, haemorrhagic enteritis is seen in the jejunum and ileum. The aborted fetus is usually autolysed. Round, necrotic lesions up to 2 cm in diameter with pale raised rims and dark depressed centres are evident on the liver (Quinn *et al.*, 2011) and the placenta becomes oedematous and leathery (necrotic placentitis).

11.7 Diagnosis

Faecal samples should be collected and transported at 4°C temperature (in transport media like Cary Blair, modified Cary Blair, modified Stuart medium, Campylobacter-thioglycollate (campy-thio) medium, alkaline peptone water) to the laboratory as early as possible for microscopic examination by dark field microscopy or phase contrast microscopy. On Gram staining, Gram-negative spiral bacteria are seen. The dilute carbol fuchsin staining procedure is also used, especially for recognizing *Campylobacter* species. Presumptive diagnosis can be given on the basis of demonstrating the organisms in fetal abomasal contents and birth fluids (Quinn *et al.*, 2011). In fresh wet preparations *Campylobacter* bacteria show rapid jerking motility and darting motility in dark-field microscopy (the sample should be placenta or fetal abomasum). Isolation of bacteria is done on selective media covered by defibrinated ox blood. *Campylobacter* bacteria show raised, round, translucent and sometime mucoid colonies on media (*C. fetus* shows small 'dew-drop' colonies after 2–3 days of incubation). Biochemical-test *Campylobacter* bacteria do not ferment carbohydrate. Immune diagnosis is based on ELISA and fluorescent antibody technique and the effective, sensitive and faster method of diagnosis of campylobacteriosis is PCR. Multilocus sequence typing (MLST) distinguishes between species within the *Campylobacter* genus (Quinn *et al.*, 2011).

11.7.1 Polymerase chain reaction (PCR)

Many PCR-based assays have been described to directly detect campylobacters in clinical and environmental specimens, although thus far they have been used only for research applications. Advantages of using a PCR approach include same-day detection and identification of campylobacters to the species level and identification of the less common *Campylobacter* species that are often missed by conventional culture. However, this approach is more expensive than culture and does not provide an isolate for further characterization.

11.7.2 Filtration method for isolation

A passive filtration technique that uses a non-selective medium developed by Steele and McDerrmott is an effective approach to isolate campylobacters, particularly *Campylobacter* species that are susceptible to the antibiotics in selective agar isolation procedures. The method is based on the principle that campylobacters can pass through membrane filters (0.45–0.65 µm) with relative ease (because of their small size and motility), while other stool flora are retained during the short processing time.

Nalidixic acid and cephalothin susceptibility testing have been used for species identification in the past. A presumptive *Campylobacter* strain that was hippurate-positive, sensitive to nalidixic acid and resistant to cephalothin was identified as *C. jejuni*. However, *Campylobacter* species that are fluoroquinolone-resistant and cross-resistant to nalidixic acid have become increasingly common, with rates reported to be as high as 80%. Therefore, antimicrobial susceptibility tests can no longer be relied upon for the phenotypic identification of *Campylobacter* isolates. Cellular fatty acid (CFA) analysis can be helpful in identifying *Campylobacter* and in differentiating some species; however, it cannot differentiate between *C. jejuni* and *C. coli*, the two most common species.

11.8 Treatment

It is a bacterial infection, so antibiotics should be administered along with supportive care. The preferred antibiotic is streptomycin at 25 mg/kg body weight by parental injection, sometimes combined with penicillin. Cephalosporin, clindamycin, gentamicin, chloramphenicol and tetracycline should be used for treatment.

11.8.1 Antimicrobial resistance

Antimicrobial-resistant strains in humans and animals are frequently isolated. This is a consequence of the massive use of antibiotics for therapy and prevention of diseases, as well as use of the same as growth promoters (Uaboi-Egbenni *et al.*, 2011). Antimicrobial resistance among *Campylobacter* species from faeces and carcasses of livestock have been reported (Karikari *et al.*, 2017). Increasing antibiotic resistance in campylobacters from animal sources is well reported globally (Saenz *et al.*, 2000; Abamecha *et al.*, 2015). Some species are showing resistance against fluoroquinolones, erythromycin, chloramphenicol and tetracycline. *C. jejuni* expresses a resistance-nodulation-division (RND)-type efflux pump (known as AcrAB-TolC in the former and cmeABC in the latter). In *Campylobacter*, the CmeABC efflux pump is responsible for high-level resistance to fluoroquinolones (Quinn *et al.*, 2011). Goats can act as a source of human infections as well as contamination of the wider environment (Uaboi-Egbenni *et al.*, 2011).

11.9 Zoonotic Implication

Zoonotic pathogens such as *Campylobacter* species cause disease and death, resulting in enormous social and economic losses (Asuming-Bediako *et al.*, 2019). Campylobacteriosis is a leading bacterial infection in humans who work on animal farms. Campylobacters are transmitted by a faecal–oral route; people can get infection by consumption of raw goat's milk, undercooked meat, contaminated food and water. Human populations are mostly affected by *C. jejuni*, *C. coli* and *C. fetus*. Untreated surface water has been implicated in *Campylobacter* outbreaks in New Zealand, Finland, England, Wales, Australia, the United States and Canada. The Walkerton, Ontario, waterborne outbreak of 2000 resulted from entry of *Escherichia coli* 0157:H7 and *Campylobacter* spp. from neighbouring cattle farms into the town water supply (Radostits *et al.*, 2007). *Campylobacter* bacteria cause enteritis and show clinical signs like fever, nausea, diarrhoea (sometimes containing blood), vomiting, abdominal pain. *Campylobacter* infection can also result in irritable bowel syndrome and Guillain-Barré syndrome. When humans are infected by opportunistic bacteria like *C. fetus*, systemic illness like fever, abdominal pain, splenomegaly and hepatomegaly occur. Subacute endocarditis and arthritis may occur. Diagnosis is based on clinical signs and laboratory tests.

11.10 Prevention and Control of Campylobacteriosis

A holistic, multiple-intervention One Health approach is required to better understand, prevent and control *Campylobacter* (Asuming-Bediako *et al.*, 2019). There is a chance of acquiring infection via consumption of raw and undercooked meat. Thus implementation of hygienic practices from the slaughterhouse to the retailers, proper handling and cooking of meat are very important in preventing *Campylobacter* infection (Hagos *et al.*, 2021)

11.10.1 Vaccination

Campylobacteriosis may be prevented by vaccination given shortly before breeding. Two inactivated vaccines are available in the United States. They contain both *C. fetus* and *C. jejuni*. A third vaccine is available in Australia and New Zealand. This may contain multiple *C. fetus* strains (DL42, 6/1, 132). Immunity develops in about 21 days (sheep and goat vaccine). Formalin-inactivated bivalent vaccine can increase the probability of live lambs by around 10%; there is variable efficacy depending on which strains are present (Constable *et al.*, 2017).

11.10.2 Disinfection

Chemical decontamination can also be an effective intervention for reducing Campylobacter load on food-animal carcasses. Chlorine, chlorine dioxide, acidified sodium chlorite, trisodium phosphate and peroxyacid are typically used in poultry processing (Butzler, 2004; WHO, 2015). Phenolic-based compounds, 70% ethyl alcohol, 1% sodium hypochlorite, 2% glutaraldehyde and formaldehyde are effective against *Campylobacter* bacteria. Autoclaving and dry heat and radiation also destroy the bacteria.

11.11 Control

To control the campylobacters, sanitation and hygiene in livestock farms should be very high and the effectiveness of biosecurity-related interventions in primary production should be based on a good understanding of the regional risk factors at the farm level (Asuming-Bediako *et al.*, 2019). The consumption of raw meat and milk should be avoided. Milk should be properly pasteurized and the core temperature of meat pieces should be up to 82°C. Isolation of affected goats and proper disposal of aborted material should be performed.

References

Abamecha, A., Assebe, G., Tafa, B. and Wondafrash, B. (2015) Prevalence of thermophilic Campylobacter and their antimicrobial resistance profile in food animals in Lare District, Nuer Zone, Gambella, Ethiopia. *Journal of Drug Research and Development* 1(2), 2470–1009.

Asuming-Bediako, N., Parry-Hanson Kunadu, A., Abraham, S. and Habib, I. (2019) Campylobacter at the human–food interface: The African perspective. *Pathogens* 8(2), 87.

Blaser, M.J. and Pei, Z. (1993) Pathogenesis of *Campylobacter fetus* infections: Critical role of high-molecular-weight S-layer proteins in virulence. *Journal of Infectious Diseases* 167(2), 372–377.

Butzler, J.P. (2004) Campylobacter, from obscurity to celebrity. *Clinical Microbiology and Infection* 10(10), 868–876.

Calistri, P. and Giovannini, A. (2008) Quantitative risk assessment of human campylobacteriosis related to the consumption of chicken meat in two italian regions. *International Journal of Food Microbiology* 128(2), 274–287.

Carvalho, A.C., Ruiz-Palacios, G.M., Ramos-Cervantes, P., Cervantes, L.E., Jiang, X. *et al.* (2001) Molecular characterization of invasive and noninvasive *Campylobacter jejuni* and *Campylobacter coli* isolates. *Journal of Clinical Microbiology* 39(4), 1353–1359.

Coker, A.O., Isokpehi, R.D., Thomas, B.N., Amisu, K.O. and Obi, C.L. (2002) Human campylobacteriosis in developing countries1. *Emerging Infectious Diseases* 8(3), 237.

Constable, P.D., Hinchcliff, K.W., Done, S.H. and Grunberg, W. (2017) *Veterinary Medicine: A text book of the diseases of cattle, horses, sheep, pigs and goats*, 11th edn. Saunders Elsevier, St Louis, Missouri, pp. 1904–1996.

Dasti, J.I., Tareen, A.M., Lugert, R., Zautner, A.E. and Gross, U. (2010) *Campylobacter jejuni*: A brief overview on pathogenicity-associated factors and disease-mediating mechanisms. *International Journal of Medical Microbiology* 300, 205–211.

Goualié Gblossi, B., Akpa, E.E., Kakou-N'Gazoa, E.S., Guessennd, N., Bakayoko, S. *et al.* (2012) Prevalence and antimicrobial resistance of thermophilic campylobacter isolated from chicken in cote d'Ivoire. *International Journal of Microbiology* 150612.

Hagos, Y., Gugsa, G., Awol, N., Ahmed, M., Tsegaya, Y. *et al.* (2021) Isolation, identification and antimicrobial susceptibility pattern of *Campylobacter jejuni* and *Campylobacter coli* from cattle, goat, and chicken meat in mekelle, Ethiopia. *PLoS ONE* 16(2), e0246755.

Han, K., Jang, S.S., Choo, E., Heu, S. and Ryu, S. (2007) Prevalence, genetic diversity, and antibiotic resistance patterns of *Campylobacter jejuni* from retail raw chickens in Korea. *International Journal of Food Microbiology* 114(1), 50–59.

Humphrey, T., O'Brien, S. and Madsen, M. (2007) Campylobacters as zoonotic pathogens: A food production perspective. *International Journal of Food Microbiology* 117(3), 237–257.

Karikari, A.B., Obiri-Danso, K., Frimpong, E.H. and Krogfelt, K.A. (2017) Antibiotic resistance of Campylobacter recovered from faeces and carcasses of healthy livestock. *Hindawi BioMed Research International* 2017(1), Article 4091856.

Konkel, M.E., Garvis, S.G., Tipton, S.L., Anderson, D.E. Jr. and Cieplak, W. Jr. (1997) Identification and molecular cloning of a gene encoding a fibronectin-binding protein (cadF) from *Campylobacter jejuni*. *Molecular Microbiology* 24(5), 953–963.

Moeller, R.B. (2009) Bacterial Abortions of Sheep and Goats. *Tri-County Goat News*, January 2009. University of California Agriculture and Natural Resources (UCANR), Hanford, California. Available at: http://cekings.ucanr.edu/newsletters/Tri-County_Goat_Newsletter16085.pdf

Oberhelman, R.A. and Taylor, D.N. (2000) Campylobacter infections in developing countries. In: Nachamkin, I. and Blaser, M.J. (eds) *Campylobacter*, 2nd edn. American Society for Microbiology, Washington, DC, pp. 139–153.

Padungton, P. and Kaneene, J.B. (2003) *Campylobacter* spp. in humans, chickens, pigs and their antimicrobial resistance. *Journal of Veterinary Medical Science* 65, 161–170.

Park, S.F. (2002) The physiology of *Campylobacter* species and its relevance to their role as foodborne pathogens. *International Journal of Food Microbiology* 74(3), 177–188.

Penner, J.L. (1988) The genus *Campylobacter*: A decade of progress. *Clinical Microbiology Reviews* 1, 157–172.

Pesci, E.C., Cottle, D.L. and Pickett, C.L. (1994) Genetic, enzymatic, and pathogenic studies of the iron superoxide dismutase of *Campylobacter jejuni*. *Infection and Immunity* 62, 2687–2694.

Quinn, P.J., Markey, B.K., Leonard, F.C., FitzPatrick, E.S., Fanning, S. *et al.* (2011) *Campylobacter* and *Helicobacter* species. In: Quinn, P.J. (ed.) *Veterinary Microbiology*, 2nd edn. Blackwell Publishing, Oxford, UK, pp. 342–350.

Radostits, O.M., Gay, C.C., Hinchcliff, K.W. and Constable, P.C. (2007) Diseases associated with bacteria – V. In: Radostits, O.M. (ed.) *Veterinary Medicine: A Textbook of the Diseases of Cattle, Horses, Sheep, Pigs and Goats*, 10th edn. Saunders Elsevier, St Louis, Missouri, p. 1086.

Saenz, Y., Zarazaga, M., Lantero, M., Gastánares, M.J., Baquero, F. *et al.* (2000) Antibiotic resistance in *Campylobacter* strains isolated from animals, foods, and humans in Spain in 1997–1998. *Antimicrobial Agents and Chemotherapy* 44(2), 267–271.

Salihu, M.D., Junaidu, A.U., Oboegbulem, S.I. and Egwu, G.O. (2009) Prevalence and biotypes of *Campylobacter* species isolated from sheep in Sokoto state, Nigeria. *International Journal of Animal Veterinary Advance* 1, 6–9.

Uaboi-Egbenni, P.O., Bessong, P.O., Samie, A. and Obi, C.L. (2011) Prevalence and antimicrobial susceptibility profiles of *Campylobacter jejuni* and *coli* isolated from diarrheic and non-diarrheic goat faeces in Venda region, South Africa. *African Journal of Biotechnology* 10(64), 14116–14124.

WHO (2015) *WHO Estimates of the Global Burden of Foodborne Diseases*. World Health Organization, Geneva.

12 Caseous Lymphadenitis

Kabita Roy* **and Saindla Rakesh**
Department of Veterinary Medicine, College of Veterinary Science & A.H, NDVSU, Jabalpur, Madhya Pradesh, India

Abstract
Caseous lymphadenitis (CLA) is a zoonotic bacterial infection that primarily affects sheep and goats and is caused by a Gram-positive intracellular bacterium, *Corynebacterium pseudotuberculosis* biovar *ovis* and is also known as 'thin ewe syndrome'. Although the illness is widespread worldwide, tropical and subtropical nations record the majority of cases. CLA is spread from one animal or person to another by the skin, ingestion, inhalation, or contact with contaminated objects. It multiplies within macrophages and survives the action of phagolysosomic enzymes, due to the external lipid layer of the cell wall. Abscessation of both internal (visceral) and exterior (superficial) lymph nodes is the most common symptom. A typical lesion is accompanied by suppurative bronchopneumonia. Diagnosis is routinely made based on bacteriological confirmation of clinical cases. Treatment includes drainage and lavage of the abscess along with antimicrobial therapy. A complete recovery might be quite challenging to achieve. No CLA vaccine offers complete protection against *C. pseudotuberculosis*.

Keywords: caseous lymphadenitis, sheep, goat, abscess, lymph nodes, bronchopneumonia

12.1 Introduction

Goats are one of the most economically important livestock in the world. A goat is often described as a poor man's cow (or mini-cow) because of its immense contribution to the poor man's economy. The main source of income for India's small, landless farmers is goat farming. The goat industry was given a lot of attention because of the increased demand for meat and skin in both domestic and international markets. But infections are a big problem for the goat industry, causing production losses since they reduce weight increase and milk output and increase mortality rates. Goats are susceptible to several infectious illnesses, which can cause morbidity and mortality as well as economic loss. Among these, corynebacterial infection is a significant issue that affects sheep and goats.

Caseous lymphadenitis (CLA) is a bacterial infection that affects sheep and goats; however, it has also been documented to afflict cattle, buffalo, camels and pigs (Fontaine and Baird, 2008). It has been categorized as an occupational zoonotic disease since *Corynebacterium pseudotuberculosis* biovar *ovis*, often known as *C. ovis*, the disease's causative agent, rarely affects humans. The illness primarily affects sheep and goats but can also infect cattle, horses and occasionally people (Williamson, 2001). It is also known as 'lympho' or 'cheesy gland' and is linked to 'thin ewe syndrome'. It occasionally makes irregular, enzootic appearances (Ivanovic *et al.*, 2009).

*Corresponding author: kabitaroy59@yahoo.in

DOI: 10.1079/9781800622852.0012

Localized inflammation at the site of bacterial entry and abscessation of both internal (visceral) and exterior (superficial) lymph nodes are the most common clinical symptoms (Glen, 2000). Sheep are more likely to get internal abscesses than goats, which develop external abscesses (Baird and Fontaine, 2007). The peripheral lymph nodes enlarge and develop abscesses in the superficial form, while systemic complications in the visceral form can lead to chronic debility in affected animals (Radostits *et al.*, 2007).

Diagnosis is routinely made based on bacteriological confirmation of clinical cases (Cetinkaya *et al.*, 2002). Strain variations have an impact on culture and biochemical testing and, as a result, molecular tests like the polymerase chain reaction (PCR) assay (Pacheco *et al.*, 2007), proteomics and sequencing are used as supplementary diagnostic tests (Silva *et al.*, 2017).

Due to decreased meat and milk production, loss of fertility, culling of affected animals, condemnation and downgrading of affected carcasses at the time of slaughter and meat inspection, caseous lymphadenitis poses a serious financial risk to the goat husbandry industry (Guimaraes *et al.*, 2011). Additionally, it may survive in the environment and responds poorly to several chemotherapeutic drugs. Consequently, it is particularly challenging to control once it is introduced into a flock (Williamson, 2001).

12.2 History

In 1888, an instance of lymphangitis in a cow led French bacteriologist Edward Nocard to isolate a unique bacterium (Nocard, 1896). Later, a similar bacterium was found in cultures from a ewe's renal abscess by the Bulgarian bacteriologist Hugo von Preisz (Preisz and Guinard, 1891). Due to these associated findings, the bacterium in question was given the name 'Preisz Nocard bacillus'. The bacterium was named *Bacillus pseudotuberculosis* as a result of numerous findings linked to it. The second designation, which persisted until the end of the 19th century, was given under the presumption that there was a clinical similarity of lesions between caseous nodules and *Mycobacterium pseudotuberculosis*. The organism was placed in the genus of *Corynebacterium* and at the same time renamed to become recognized as *Corynebacterium ovis*. The species name had to be changed because the later term indicated specialization and completely ignored the generic ability that may infer for other mammalian species that may also be a host for the same agent (Baird and Fontaine, 2007).

12.3 Aetiology

Corynebacterium pseudotuberculosis, a microaerophilic intracellular bacterium that multiplies inside the macrophage, is a Gram-positive, small, or pleomorphic coccobacillus that causes CLA. It is a member of the Actinobacteria class and family Corynebacteriaceae (Baird and Fontaine, 2007). This bacterial species can be found in the goat's faeces, intestines and abscesses (Muthukumar *et al.*, 2020). *C. pseudotuberculosis* is classified into two biovars (Biberstein *et al.*, 1971). The biovar *ovis*, which primarily affects sheep and goats and causes superficial and visceral abscesses, and the biovar *equi*, which primarily affects horses, are the most common (Connor *et al.*, 2000, 2007). The organism has also been isolated from laboratory animals, llamas, camels, deer, pigs, buffalo and other species (Williamson, 2001; Dorella *et al.*, 2006). Overcrowding and unsanitary environments might contribute to the disease's onset (Kumar and Kumar, 2010).

12.4 Epidemiology

Although the illness is spread throughout the world, tropical and subtropical nations record the majority of cases. Numerous western nations have recorded cases of CLA (Kuria and Ngatia, 1990; Paton *et al.*, 2003; Osman *et al.*, 2015; Akgul *et al.*, 2018).

12.5 Transmission

CLA is spread from one animal or person to another by the skin, ingestion, inhalation, or contact with contaminated objects, places, pastures and watering troughs. The *C. pseudotuberculosis* bacteria are resilient and can endure up to 2 years in the soil, even in dry environments with a lot of sun exposure. Animals that are infected, with or without showing clinical symptoms, can contaminate the soil, water, feed, pastures and facilities with their nasal secretions, faeces and pus from spontaneously draining abscesses. Infected animals that do not present clinical symptoms can eliminate the bacteria through their respiratory tract (Guimaraes *et al.*, 2011). Routine management procedures like shearing, dipping, vaccination, etc. as well as environmental pollution from soil and termites, make it simple for *C. pseudotuberculosis* to spread throughout the herd (Brown and Olander, 1987).

Since *C. pseudotuberculosis* has been isolated from the bodies of domestic flies (a mechanical vector) as well as from fly intestines and faeces, it is important to take into account the role of insects (namely, flies) in the disease's transmission (biological vector) (Braverman *et al.*, 1999).

12.6 Pathogenesis

The microorganisms may stay on the skin as pollutants and could enter the tissues through cuts and other wounds. Being a facultative intracellular bacterium, *C. pseudotuberculosis* multiplies within macrophages after entering the host, which typically happens through the oral, nasal and ocular mucosae, or through skin wounds, surviving the action of phagolysosomic enzymes due to the external lipid layer of the cell wall, and disseminates freely or within macrophages to regional lymph nodes and internal organs (Dorella *et al.*, 2006).

Although other virulence factors have been hypothesized, the exotoxin phospholipase D (PLD) and a mycolic acid surface lipid are what make *C. pseudotuberculosis* pathogenic. PLD results in dermal necrosis, which is characterized by inflammation, necrosis and increased vascular permeability. This promotes the invasiveness of the organism and its transport by phagocytes to the local lymph nodes, where it is ultimately destroyed. However, in most challenged animals, local lymphadenitis ensues, followed by suppuration and destruction of the lymph node; recovery from this stage is infrequent. The inflammatory response may stop the infection from spreading beyond the cutaneous lesion (Windsor, 2011). The bacterium's lipid cell layer is pyogenic but not immunogenic, which increases its virulence (cytotoxicity), survival inside macrophages and ability to create abscesses by the release of lysosomal enzymes. Because of virulence factors including phospholipase D and mycolic acid, the development of chronic lesions in CLA with many abscesses is thought to be caused by bacterium's capacity to evade the host immune system and move to different organs (Baird and Fontaine, 2007). Besides participating in pathogenicity, mycolic acid appears to be important for the survival of this bacterium in the environment (West *et al.*, 2002).

12.7 Clinical Signs

In sheep and goats, CLA can manifest both internally and externally. Sheep are more likely to get internal abscesses than goats, which develop exterior abscesses (Baird and Fontaine, 2007). An abscess in superficial lymph nodes, such as the pre-scapular, pre-femoral, inguinal, mediastinal and mesenteric lymph nodes, as well as in subcutaneous tissues, characterizes CLA in its external form. In contrast, CLA's internal form manifests as an abscess in internal organs and lymph nodes, particularly the lungs, liver, kidneys and mediastinal, bronchial and lumber lymph nodes (Gowda *et al.*, 2012). These two forms can coexist and other less common sites can also be affected, such as the mammary gland, scrotum, central nervous system and joints. In rare situations, CLA cases can also result in orchitis, cellulitis, mastitis, or even death (Baird and Fontaine, 2007). Internal abscesses are typically accompanied by weakness and weight loss, a condition known as the thin ewe syndrome in sheep. The mature abscesses easily leak through fistulas, releasing purulent whitish-green discharges into the environment or the affected organ. Only a necropsy can reveal internal abscesses. External abscesses typically cause disease transmission but internal abscesses are the lethal ones (Ivanovic *et al.*, 2009).

It has been noted that the locations of the abscesses differ between sheep and goats, with the visceral form occurring more frequently in sheep and the superficial form in goats (Brown and Olander, 1987). Goats are more likely to develop external abscesses in their head and neck lymph nodes, whereas sheep are more likely to get these infections in their sub-iliac and pre-scapular lymph nodes (Brown and Olander, 1987; Smith and Sherman, 1994). There have also been reports of differences between the appearance of abscess contents in sheep and goats. In sheep, the contents have a laminar structure when cut, resembling the layers of an onion. This is due to the formation of layers of fibrous tissue and thick caseous material, while abscesses in goats have a thin and pasty exudate (Brown and Olander, 1987).

Hussain *et al.* (2013) reported that symptoms in goats exposed to CLA include a sharp increase in body temperature, inappetence, gradual emaciation, lethargy and enlargement of pre-scapular and submandibular lymph nodes. However, Gururaj *et al.* (2018) reported that the most affected lymph nodes in goats with CLA were 63.09% pre-scapular and post-scapular followed by 29.53% pre-femoral and 6.04% mandibular, and 1.34% of goats had an internal abscess. They stated that the abscess was covered by a thick fibrous layer and that thick, caseous and greenish-tinged pus oozed out on the incision.

12.8 Post-Mortem Findings

The most typical sign of caseous lymphadenitis in sheep is abscessation of internal organs, particularly the lungs, whereas the condition is more frequently seen in goats as abscessation of superficial lymph nodes. Necropsy revealed that the most prevalent lesions in *C. pseudotuberculosis* infection were in the subcutaneous lymph nodes and extended to the lungs, where caseous multiple abscesses were filled with yellow, thick creamy pus. A typical lesion of CLA is accompanied by suppurative bronchopneumonia. Lung parenchyma may grossly show numerous abscesses that range in size from a pea to a walnut (discrete nodules). The damaged lungs are solid, pale and red to grey in colour. Additionally, various lobes of the lungs and even the chest wall may show caseo-calcified nodules of varying sizes. Sectioning of affected lobes may reveal suppurative exudates (greenish pus).

Mediastinal and trachea-bronchial lymph nodes are diffusely enlarged and replaced by abscesses having calcified granules. The mediastinal lymph node's cut surfaces reveal a thick, semi-solid fluid with greenish-yellow inspissated pus, concentrically lamellated layers of fibrous connective tissue and alternating zones of caseous and friable material, giving it a look similar to the skin of an onion (pathognomonic signs of CLA) (Sonawane *et al.*, 2016; Singh *et al.*, 2018).

A granulomatous lesion with caseous necrosis in the lesion's centre and surrounded by inflammatory cells, including neutrophils, lymphocytes and macrophages, may be seen during histopathological examination of CLA-affected tissues. The accumulation of living and dead neutrophils, macrophages, lymphocytes, multinucleated giant cells, bacteria and tissue cells around caseous necrosis in the centre comprises a granuloma with concentric layers separated by inspissated caseous liquefied material (Gururaj *et al.*, 2018).

12.9 Diagnosis

Diagnosis is routinely made based on bacteriological confirmation of clinical cases (Cetinkaya *et al.*, 2002). Strain variations have an impact on culture and biochemical testing and, as a result, molecular tests like the PCR assay (Pacheco *et al.*, 2007), sequencing and proteomics are employed as additional diagnostic procedures (Silva *et al.*, 2017). Decreased time consumptions in DNA isolation (Nassar *et al.*, 2015) and reduced cost are the driving factors behind the use of such molecular tests for the diagnosis of CLA.

12.9.1 Bacteriological diagnosis

For bacteriological identification of *C. pseudotuberculosis*, lesion contents and pus should be collected aseptically after sterilization by ethanol. Isolation is mostly performed under aerobic conditions, occasionally under anaerobic conditions. The organism is grown on a highly enriched medium at 37°C for 48–72 hour in a pH of 7.0–7.2 with the addition of blood or serum for enhancing the growth (Baird and Fontaine, 2007). For bacterial isolation, nutrient agar, 5% sheep blood agar and MacConkey agar were incubated aerobically at 37°C for 48–72 hour and for identification of *C. pseudotuberculosis* the isolates were further inoculated on cystine tellurite blood agar (cystine tellurite agar base added with 5% defibrinated sheep blood and 5% v/v of 1% potassium tellurite) and incubated at 37°C for 48 hour. The colony morphology, Gram's stain and biochemical characteristics were used to identify the isolates.

The bacterial culture examination reveals the presence of bacterial growth forming cream-white, dry, waxy colonies with a narrow zone of β-haemolysis. Gram's staining could show pleomorphic, Gram-positive coccobacilli organized in a 'Chinese pattern' or standard palisade pattern (Singh *et al.*, 2018). *C. pseudotuberculosis* on cystine tellurite blood agar produces black colonies (Tripathi *et al.*, 2016).

12.9.2 Biochemical characteristics

Differential biochemical tests, such as those for nitrate reduction, catalase, urease, synergistic haemolysis with *Rhodococcus equi* and antagonistic haemolysis with *Staphylococcus aureus* for the production of phospholipase D (PLD), are the basis for the definitive identification of *C. pseudotuberculosis* (Guimaraes *et al.*, 2011). Catalase, urease and PLD were all positive while nitrate reduction was negative in *C. pseudotuberculosis* (Tripathi *et al.*, 2016).

12.9.3 CAMP (Christie-Atkins-Munch-Peterson) test

CAMP assays can be used as rapid presumptive tests for *C. pseudotuberculosis*, *R. equi* and *Corynebacterium renale*, interacting with the beta-haemolysin of *Staphylococcus aureus*. The staphylococcal beta-haemolysin is inhibited by *C. pseudotuberculosis* (reverse CAMP test), whereas its activity is enhanced by *R. equi* and *C. renale*. On sheep blood agar, *R. equi* (also known as '*R. equi* factors') and *C. pseudotuberculosis* had a synergistic haemolytic effect (Quinn *et al.*, 2013).

12.9.4 Polymerase chain reaction

The adoption of molecular diagnostics for the diagnosis of CLA is motivated by the reduced time requirements for DNA isolation (Nassar *et al.*, 2015) and lower cost and speed of analysis. When validating the diagnosis of CLA, the sensitivities of PCR and bacterial culture are relatively close. However, PCR has advantages over bacterial culture in terms of rapidity, simplicity and its ability to also detect non-viable or fewer germs in pus samples. Tripathi *et al.* (2016) performed PCR assays targeting putative oligopeptide/dipeptide ABC transporter, nicotinamide adenine dinucleotide phosphate oxidoreductase coenzyme F420-dependent and proline aminopeptidase genes of *C. pseudotuberculosis* carried out directly on the DNA extracted from pus and reported that the selection of these three specific genes as target confers specificity to the assay.

12.9.5 Serological tests

For caseous lymphadenitis in goats and sheep, several diagnostic methods have been developed, including complement fixation, immunodiffusion in agar gel, indirect haemagglutination and hypersensitivity tests (Baird and Fontaine, 2007). With a sensitivity of 91% and a specificity of 98%, INF-γ detection by ELISA has been utilized to diagnose infection by *C. pseudotuberculosis*, suggesting its potential for application in caseous lymphadenitis eradication campaigns (Sunil *et al.*, 2008).

12.10 Differential Diagnosis

1. Actinobacillosis
2. Tuberculosis

3. Superficial abscesses caused by *Staphylococcus aureus* and *Actinomyces pyogenes*
4. Pulmonary adenomatosis
5. Scrapie
6. Pneumonias caused by *Mycobacterium bovis*, *Pasteurella haemolytica*, *Pasteurella multocida*, or ovine progressive pneumonia (Guimaraes *et al.*, 2011).

12.11 Treatment

Treatment for the external form entails locating the sick animals before the abscess ruptures and isolating them from the main flock or herd. If the disease is uncommon in the flock or herd, treatment may involve the culling of sick animals. To prevent the infected material from contaminating the farm environment, lance the abscess, flush the abscess cavity with an antiseptic solution and pack the cavity with gauze or other bandage material (Dorella *et al.*, 2006). Treatment of abscesses caused by *C. pseudotuberculosis* involve drainage and lavage of the abscess in combination with antimicrobial therapy that includes penicillin, doxycycline, trimethoprim–sulfonamide, or a combination of these. A promising treatment is the injection of a specific antibiotic right into the diseased lymph node. Long-term antibiotic therapy is necessary for the treatment of caseous lymphadenitis of the internal organs. Complete recovery might be quite challenging to achieve (Schreuder *et al.*, 1986). Antibiotic therapy is another option for treatment, although it is not particularly effective even though *C. pseudotuberculosis* is responsive to practically all studied drugs *in vitro*. The treatment is not usually attempted, because the abscess is encapsulated, and because the intracellular location of the bacteria and the development of biofilm in spontaneous infections decrease drug efficiency, making antimicrobials ineffective under these circumstances (Olson *et al.*, 2002; Radostits *et al.*, 2007). Antibiotic therapy is an unviable alternative for herd-level disease management, due to its ineffectiveness and high cost.

Even after the abscess has been removed, the disease is likely to reoccur. Additionally, the existence of internal abscesses is a significant barrier to effective therapy (Dorella *et al.*, 2006). It is preferable to cull all affected animals from the intensive farm or entirely depopulate the current herd. After taking the appropriate biocontrol measures, replace with newer livestock.

12.12 Prevention: Vaccination

Although vaccination has been demonstrated to reduce infection spread and cause a progressive drop in prevalence, none of the CLA vaccines that are now available offer complete protection against *C. pseudotuberculosis* (Baird and Fontaine, 2007). PLD is the main *C. pseudotuberculosis* component used in the formulation of vaccines. The rationale behind its application is the high level of immunity that results from giving goats this toxin as an immunization. The majority of commercial *C. pseudotuberculosis* vaccines use inactivated PLD linked to antigens of other pathogens, including *Clostridium tetani*, *Clostridium perfringens* type D, *Clostridium novyi* and *Clostridium chauvoei* (de Pinho *et al.*, 2021).

The Glanvac® six vaccine (Zoetis, Australia) is a multivalent vaccine that has been approved for use in goat flocks in numerous countries to manage clostridial infections as well as control CLA (de Pinho *et al.*, 2021). In 1984, it was the first commercial vaccination to hit the market. Field trial results for the formalin-inactivated exotoxin vaccine for PLD showed rates of protection ranging from 25% to 90%. According to the procedure, 1 ml of vaccine must be administered beneath the skin close to the neck. Four weeks later, a second vaccination completes the initial course. To prevent CLA, it is advised to administer annual booster doses at least one month before lambing or shearing (Gascoigne *et al.*, 2020).

Brazil has granted permission for the use of the Pfizer vaccine Biodectin® in goats. Caseous D-T®, another commercial vaccine that has been examined (Colorado Serum Co., Canada), consists of two formulations, one of which contains clostridial toxoids and the other of which contains *C. pseudotuberculosis* and clostridial toxoids together (Paton *et al.*, 2003). According to preliminary findings, the second formulation offers superior infection resistance to the first, resulting in fewer interior and exterior lesions (Piontkowski and Shivvers, 1998).

The effectiveness of these vaccinations in preventing exposure to CLA has been questioned because using PLD toxoids for the immunization of adult goats can have some side effects, such as decreased milk supply, fever, ventral oedema and ataxia, but not in young animals. Therefore, farm practitioners should be aware of the vaccination's limits and alert owners to the vaccine's potential negative effects before providing the vaccine for goats (Williamson, 2001).

12.13 Zoonotic Importance

Even though infections in humans are rather uncommon, *C. pseudotuberculosis* is regarded as an occupational zoonosis. The majority of documented occurrences of human lymphadenitis in Australia involve workers who frequently come into touch with diseased sheep (Schlicher *et al.*, 2021)

The consumption of raw goat's meat and cow's milk was implicated in the 1988 diagnosis of the first case of zoonotic *C. pseudotuberculosis*. By 2005 there had been about 25 documented examples of this bacterium infecting humans (Liu *et al.*, 2005). Peel *et al.* (1997) studied 22 cases, wherein infected people typically displayed constitutional symptoms, lymphadenitis and abscesses. Mills *et al.* (1997) documented the case of a boy's suppurative granulomatous lymphadenitis brought on by contact with tainted farm animals. Most of the patients underwent surgical lymph node removal and antibiotic therapy. A 12-year-old girl in France was diagnosed with *C. pseudotuberculosis* necrotizing lymphadenitis, according to a report (Join-Lambert *et al.*, 2006), believed to be the earliest known incidence of the disease in childhood.

12.14 Control and Eradication

Eradication is a very challenging process that starts with the culling of all animals displaying clinical symptoms and is followed by the culling of those animals that still test positive after being tested using an enzyme-linked immunosorbent assay (ELISA).

1. Isolation of all infected animals before abscesses get ruptured.
2. Immunization of animals against *Corynebacterium*.
3. Periodical serological monitoring of outbreak.
4. In recurrent cases, culling will be the advisable option.
5. Purchase of flock from CLA-free flocks or herds.
6. Removal of lambs and kids born to infected animals immediately after birth.
7. Infected animals should be sheared last.
8. Shear from youngest to oldest, since older animals are more likely to be infected.
9. Immediately disinfect any equipment or any areas that get contaminated with pus.
10. Decrease stock density in holding pens after shearing.
11. Dip the healthy animals first, followed by the suspected animals and then positive animals last (Muthukumar *et al.*, 2020).

12.15 Conclusion

Corynebacterium pseudotuberculosis biovar *ovis*, also known as *C. ovis*, is the cause of the chronic bacterial infection known as caseous lymphadenitis (CLA), which primarily affects sheep and goats but can also infect cattle, horses and, in rare cases, humans. For this reason, the illness has been dubbed an occupational zoonotic disease (Williamson, 2001). It is also known as 'lympho' or 'cheesy gland' and is linked to thin ewe syndrome. It occasionally makes irregular, enzootic appearances (Ivanovic *et al.*, 2009). In sheep and goats, CLA can manifest both internally and externally. Sheep are more likely to get internal abscesses than goats, which develop exterior abscesses (Baird and Fontaine, 2007). The peripheral lymph nodes enlarge and develop abscesses in the superficial form, while in the visceral form, systemic complications can lead to chronic debility in affected animals (Radostits *et al.*, 2007).

On bacteriological confirmation of clinical cases, a definitive diagnosis is typically made (Cetinkaya *et al.*, 2002). Strain variations have an impact on culture and biochemical testing and, as a result, molecular tests like the PCR assay (Pacheco *et al.*, 2007) are used for the diagnosis of CLA. Caseous lymphadenitis poses a serious financial risk to the goat industry. Additionally, the therapy is typically avoided due to the abscess encapsulation, the intracellular location of the bacteria and the development of biofilm in naturally occurring infections, which render antimicrobials ineffective under these circumstances (Olson *et al.*, 2002; Radostits *et al.*, 2007). Antibiotic therapy is an unviable alternative for herd-level disease management, due to its ineffectiveness and high cost. Even after the abscess has been removed, the disease is likely to recur. Therefore, for efficient prevention and control of CLA on a farm, it is preferable to slaughter all the infected animals or entirely depopulate the current stock from an intensive farm and replace it with newer livestock after following proper biocontrol measures.

References

Akgul, G., Demirbilek, S.K., Celik, O.Y., Irak, K., Akgul, B.S. *et al.* (2018) *Corynebacterium pseudotuberculosis* case in a Boer Goat X Turkish Hair Goat crossbred. *Erciyes Universitesi Veteriner Fakultesi Dergisi* 15(1), 82–85.

Baird, G.J. and Fontaine, M.C. (2007) *Corynebacterium pseudotuberculosis* and its role in ovine caseous lymphadenitis. *Journal of Comparative Pathology* 137(4), 179–210.

Biberstein, E.L., Knight, H.D. and Jang, S. (1971) Two biotypes of *Corynebacterium pseudotuberculosis*. *The Veterinary Record* 89(26), 691–692.

Braverman, Y., Chizov-Ginzburg, A., Saran, A. and Winkler, M. (1999) The role of houseflies (*Musca domestica*) in harbouring *Corynebacterium pseudotuberculosis* in dairy herds in Israel. *Revue Scientifique et Technique (International Office of Epizootics)* 18(3), 681–690.

Brown, C.C. and Olander, H.J. (1987) Caseous lymphadenitis of goats and sheep: A review. *Veterinary Bulletin* 57, 1–12.

Cetinkaya, B., Karahan, M., Atil, E., Kalin, R., De Baere, T. *et al.* (2002) Identification of *Corynebacterium pseudotuberculosis* isolates from sheep and goats by PCR. *Veterinary Microbiology* 88(1), 75–83.

Connor, K., Fontaine, M., Rudge, K., Baird, G. and Donachie, W. (2007) Molecular genotyping of multinational ovine and caprine *Corynebacterium pseudotuberculosis* isolates using pulsed-field gel electrophoresis. *Veterinary Research* 38(4), 613–623.

Connor, K.M., Quirie, M.M., Baird, G. and Donachie, W. (2000) Characterization of United Kingdom isolates of *Corynebacterium pseudotuberculosis* using pulsed-field gel electrophoresis. *Journal of Clinical Microbiology* 38(7), 2633–2637.

de Pinho, R.B., de Oliveira Silva, M.T., Bezerra, F.S.B. and Borsuk, S. (2021) Vaccines for caseous lymphadenitis: Up-to-date and forward-looking strategies. *Applied Microbiology and Biotechnology* 105, 2287–2296.

Dorella, F., Pacheco, L.G.C., Oliveira, S., Miyoshi, A. and Azevedo, V. (2006) *Corynebacterium pseudotuberculosis*: Microbiology, biochemical properties, pathogenesis and molecular studies of virulence. *Veterinary Research* 37(2), 201–218.

Fontaine, M.C. and Baird, G.J. (2008) Caseous lymphadenitis. *Small Ruminant Research* 76, 46–48.

Gascoigne, E., Ogden, N., Lovatt, F. and Davies, P. (2020) Update on caseous lymphadenitis in sheep. *In Practice* 42(2), 105–114.

Glen, J.S. (2000) Caseous lymphadenitis in goat. Available at: http://www.saanedoah.com/GlennCL2000. html

Gowda, K.H., Baddi, S.Y. and Nagesh, A.M. (2012) Caseous lymphadenitis and its management in a goat. *Intas Polivet* 13(1), 81–82.

Guimaraes, A., do Carmo, F.B., Pauletti, R.B., Seyffert, N., Ribeiro, D. *et al.* (2011) Caseous lymphadenitis: Epidemiology, diagnosis, and control. *IIOAB Journal* 2, 11.

Gururaj, K., Singh, D.D., Pawaiya, R.V.S., Andani, D., Gangwar, N.K. *et al.* (2018) Investigation of an outbreak of caseous lymphadenitis in goats. *Indian Journal of Small Ruminants* 24(1), 95–100.

Hussain, S.A., Ali, M., Turkar, S., Hassan, N., Rais-ul-Islam, M. *et al.* (2013) Caseous lymphadenitis in goats: First report of two clinical cases from Punjab (India). *Applied Biological Research* 15(1), 83–84.

Ivanovic, S., Zutic, M., Pavlovic, I. and Zujovic, M. (2009) Caseous lymphadenitis in goats. *Biotechnology in Animal Husbandry* 25, 999–1007.
Join-Lambert, O.F., Ouache, M., Canioni, D., Beretti, J.L., Blanche, S. *et al.* (2006) *Corynebacterium pseudotuberculosis* necrotizing lymphadenitis in a twelve-year-old patient. *The Pediatric Infectious Disease Journal* 25(9), 848–851.
Kumar, S.P. and Kumar, M. (2010) Bacterial diseases. In: Sharma, R.D., Kumar, M. and Sharma, M.C. (eds) *Textbook of Preventive Veterinary Medicine and Epidemiology*, 1st edn. Directorate of Information and Publications of Agriculture, ICAR, New Delhi, pp. 211–212.
Kuria, J.K.N. and Ngatia, T.A. (1990) Caseous lymphadenitis of sheep and goats in Kenya. *Bulletin of Animal Health and Production in Africa* 38(1), 15–18.
Liu, D.T.L., Chan, W.M., Fan, D.S.P. and Lam, D.S.C. (2005) An infected hydrogel buckle with *Corynebacterium pseudotuberculosis*. *British Journal of Ophthalmology* 89(2), 245–246.
Mills, A.E., Mitchell, R.D. and Lim, E.K. (1997) *Corynebacterium pseudotuberculosis* is a cause of human necrotising granulomatous lymphadenitis. *Pathology* 29(2), 231–233.
Muthukumar, S., Ronald, B.S.M., Hemalatha, S. and Sughanthi, S.M.S. (2020) Outbreak of caseous lymphadenitis in an organized goat farm. *Journal of Entomology and Zoology Studies* 8(3), 9–11.
Nassar, A.F.D.C., Daniel, G.T., Ruiz, R., Miyashiro, S., Scannapieco, E.M. *et al.* (2015) Diagnostic comparison of *Corynebacterium pseudotuberculosis* through microbiological culture and PCR in sheep samples. *Arquivos do Instituto Biológico* 82, 1–6.
Nocard, E. (1896) On ulcerous lymphangitis simulating farcin snot in the horse. *Annales de l'Institut Pasteur* 10, 609–609.
Olson, M.E., Ceri, H., Morck, D.W., Buret, A.G. and Read, R.R. (2002) Biofilm bacteria: Formation and comparative susceptibility to antibiotics. *Canadian Journal of Veterinary Research* 66(2), 86.
Osman, A.Y., Abdullah, F.F.J., Chung, E.L.T., Abba, Y., Sadiq, M.A. *et al.* (2015) Caseous lymphadenitis in a goat: A case report. *International Journal of Livestock Research* 5(3), 128–132.
Pacheco, L.G., Pena, R.R., Castro, T.L., Dorella, F.A., Bahia, R.C. *et al.* (2007) Multiplex PCR assay for identification of *Corynebacterium pseudotuberculosis* from pure cultures and for rapid detection of this pathogen in clinical samples. *Journal of Medical Microbiology* 56(4), 480–486.
Paton, M.W., Walker, S.B., Rose, I.R. and Watt, G.F. (2003) Prevalence of caseous lymphadenitis and usage of caseous lymphadenitis vaccines in sheep flocks. *Australian Veterinary Journal* 81(1-2), 91–95.
Peel, M.M., Palmer, G.G., Stacpoole, A.M. and Kerr, T.G. (1997) Human lymphadenitis due to *Corynebacterium pseudotuberculosis*: Report of ten cases from Australia and review. *Clinical Infectious Diseases* 24(2), 185–191.
Piontkowski, M.D. and Shivvers, D.W. (1998) Evaluation of a commercially available vaccine against *Corynebacterium pseudotuberculosis* for use in sheep. *Journal of the American Veterinary Medical Association* 212(11), 1765–1768.
Preisz, H. and Guinard, L. (1891) *Journal Medicine Veterinaire* 16, 563.
Quinn, P., Markey, B., Carter, M. and Carter, G.R. (2013) *Clinical Veterinary Microbiology*, 2nd edn. Mosby, St Louis, Missouri, p. 141.
Radostits, O.M., Gay, C.C., Hinchcliff, K. and Constable, P.D. (2007) *Veterinary Medicine: A Textbook of the Diseases of Cattle, Horses, Sheep, Pigs, and Goats*, 10th edn. Saunders Elsevier, Philadelphia, Pennsylvania.
Schlicher, J., Schmitt, S., Stevens, M.J., Stephan, R. and Ghielmetti, G. (2021) Molecular characterization of *Corynebacterium pseudotuberculosis* isolated over a 15-year period in Switzerland. *Veterinary Sciences* 8(8), 151.
Schreuder, B.E.C., Ter Laak, E.A. and Griesen, H.W. (1986) An outbreak of caseous lymphadenitis in dairy goats: First report of the disease in the Netherlands. *Veterinary Quarterly* 8(1), 61–67.
Silva, W.M., Folador, E.L., Soares, S.C., Souza, G.H., Santos, A.V. *et al.* (2017) Label-free quantitative proteomics of *Corynebacterium pseudotuberculosis* isolates reveals differences between Biovars *ovis* and *equi* strains. *BMC Genomics* 18(1), Article no.451.
Singh, R., Singh, R., Kamdi, B., Kamari, S., Singh, S. *et al.* (2018) Pathology of caseous lymphadenitis in slaughtered goats associated infection with *Corynebacterium pseudotuberculosis*. *Journal of Animal Research* 8(3), 497–500.
Smith, M.C. and Sherman, D. (1994) *Goat Medicine*, 1st edn. Lea and Febiger, Philadelphia, Pennsylvania.
Sonawane, G.G., Kumar, J. and Sisodia, S.L. (2016) Etio-pathological study of multiple hepatic abscesses in a goat. *Indian Journal of Veterinary Pathology* 40, 257–260.

Sunil, V., Menzies, P.I., Shewen, P.E. and Prescott, J.F. (2008) Performance of a whole blood interferon-gamma assay for detection and eradication of caseous lymphadenitis in sheep. *Veterinary Microbiology* 128(3–4), 288–297.

Tripathi, B.N., Kumar, J., Sonawane, G.G., Kumar, R. and Dixit, S.K. (2016) Microbiological and molecular investigation of clinically suspected caseous lymphadenitis cases in goats. *Agricultural Research* 5, 413–419.

West, D.M., Bruere, A.N. and Ridler, A.L. (2002) Caseous lymphadenitis. In: *The Sheep: Health, Disease and Production*, 2nd edn. Foundation for Veterinary Continuing Education, Massey University, Palmerston North, New Zealand, pp. 274–279.

Williamson, L.H. (2001) Caseous lymphadenitis in small ruminants. *Veterinary Clinics of North America: Food Animal Practice* 17(2), 359–371.

Windsor, P.A. (2011) Control of caseous lymphadenitis. *Veterinary Clinics: Food Animal Practice* 27(1), 193–202.

13 Chlamydiosis (Enzootic Abortion)

Subir Singh*
Dept of Veterinary Medicine and Public Health, Faculty of Animal Science, Veterinary Science and Fisheries, Agriculture and Forestry University, Rampur, Chitwan, Nepal

Abstract
Chlamydiosis, a bacterial zoonotic disease in goats, is caused by *Chlamydia abortus*. Pregnant goats can shed large volumes of *C. abortus* in the placenta as well as uterine discharges when they abort or give birth. Goats are generally affected mainly with abortion in the later phase of gestation. In human beings, chlamydiosis can cause flu-like signs including fever, body aches, headache, reddened eyes and pneumonia. Pregnant women should avoid all contact with ewes when the flock is highly infected with *C. abortus*.

Keywords: chlamydiosis, ewes, placenta, zoonosis

13.1 Introduction

Caprine chlamydiosis, known as enzootic abortion, is a pivotal reproductive affliction causing abortion in goats. Attributed to the Gram-negative intracellular bacterium and zoonotic agent *Chlamydia abortus*, this ailment has been acknowledged since 1950 as the catalyst for enzootic abortion, typically manifesting in the final 2–3 weeks of gestation, characterized by stillborn offspring and inflamed placentas. The economic strain inflicted upon the goat industry is noteworthy, stemming from compromised reproductive efficacy and elevated mortality rates. This chapter endeavours to comprehensively explore multiple facets of caprine chlamydiosis, encompassing its origins, spread, clinical attributes, diagnostic modalities, prevention, control mechanism and implications for zoonosis (Iraninezhad *et al.*, 2020).

13.2 Aetiology

The Chlamydiaceae family comprises a solitary genus, named *Chlamydia*, encompassing 11 distinct member species. Within this group, *Chlamydia abortus* (*C. abortus*) holds notable significance due to its capacity to trigger abortion in sheep and goats, raising concerns about potential zoonotic transmission. Operating as an obligate intracellular bacterium of the Gram-negative nature, *C. abortus* stands as the causal agent behind chlamydiosis in goats. In the past, *C. abortus* was denoted as *Chlamydia psittaci*, specifically immunotype 1. It is worth noting that the term chlamydiosis retains its pertinence, given that *Chlamydia* is a bacterial genus within the family Chlamydiaceae and order Chlamydiales (Nietfeld, 2001). Predominantly affecting placental and fetal tissues, *C. abortus* precipitates abortion, stillbirths and weakened offspring. This bacterium's distinct biphasic life

*Corresponding author: ssingh@afu.edu.np

DOI: 10.1079/ 9781800622852.0013

cycle involves infectious elementary bodies (EB) and reticulate bodies (RB), a strategic adaptation aiding in evading host immune responses. Notably, the elementary bodies produced by *C. abortus* exhibit resilience against various chemical and physical factors, affording them the ability to endure prolonged periods of extracellular exposure. *C. abortus* is a leading cause of infectious abortion in sheep and goats across North America and the United Kingdom, concurrently triggering persistent subclinical infections in non-pregnant and multiparous caprines and ovines (Marsilio *et al.*, 2005).

13.3 Epidemiology

Chlamydiosis is a zoonotic disease with a global distribution. Goats become infected through inhalation of contaminated aerosols, ingestion of contaminated feed and water, or contact with infected birth fluids and tissues. Vertical transmission from dam to offspring can also occur. The disease is more prevalent in intensively managed herds, where close contact facilitates its spread.

13.4 Transmission and Pathogenesis

The primary route of *C. abortus* transmission is through oronasal contact with contaminated materials like aborted tissues, vaginal discharge, or infected neonates. Certain birds, including pigeons and sparrows, might serve as carriers of the bacterium, while ticks and insects could potentially contribute to its spread. The extent of infection from environmental and wildlife sources remains uncertain. Once introduced through the tonsils, these intracellular bacteria remain dormant within an unidentified cell population. While the exact immunological mechanisms driving pathogenesis are not fully elucidated, disease progression follows a consistent pattern. Following experimental subcutaneous inoculation around day 70 of gestation, *C. abortus* is detectable in cotyledonary trophoblasts by day 85 and undergoes significant replication around day 115, mirroring observations in naturally occurring cases. At this stage, extensive intracellular organism proliferation leads to cotyledon necrosis, hindering nutrient transfer across the placentome and resulting in fetal demise (Giannitti *et al.*, 2016).

In post-abortion scenarios, infected female goats (does) shed substantial quantities of the bacterium in uterine discharge and placental tissues for approximately 3 weeks. In cases of primiparous abortions caused by *C. abortus*, subsequent pregnancies may be normal, yet the organism continues to be shed in low quantities in vaginal secretions. Although *Chlamydia* has been isolated from experimentally infected ram semen for up to 29 days post-inoculation, this mode of transmission is not regarded as primary. Additionally, instances of abortion outbreaks in goats due to dual infections involving both *C. abortus* and *Coxiella burnetii* have been documented (Essig and Longbottom, 2015).

13.5 Clinical Manifestations

Infections can lead to the birth of stillborn kids or weak offspring that do not survive beyond 48 hour. However, it is noteworthy that infected does can also give birth to healthy offspring. The occurrence of impending abortion is seldom predictable, although observable changes in behaviour and vulval discharge might manifest within the final 48 hour of pregnancy. Comparable to its impact in goats, chlamydial abortion holds significance in sheep and, to a lesser extent, cattle, pigs, horses and even wild ruminants may experience its effects.

On farms where *C. abortus* is established, abortions primarily affect first-time mothers (primiparous females). Following an initial bout of transient fever and general discomfort during the initial infection, persistently infected ewes and does may remain asymptomatic until the abortion occurs. Affected does and ewes may experience a brief and mild episode of pneumonia and hepatitis, accompanied by loss of appetite, fever and a bloody vaginal discharge a couple of days before abortion. Although typically delivered in a fresh state, the fetus can occasionally be retained within the uterus for a day or two, leading to autolysis. Some weak newborns might survive, while a small number of females could experience retained placentas.

Additionally, instances of pneumonia in young animals might be observed during periods of increased abortion rates (Selim, 2016).

13.6 Lesions

Chlamydiosis in goats is characterized by enzootic abortion, usually occurring late in pregnancy. Infected does may exhibit vaginal discharge, fever and generalized weakness. Aborted fetuses may have hepatic necrosis, splenomegaly and fibrinous placentitis.

Examination of the placenta will reveal regional to generalized thickening, brownish exudate, opacity of the inter-cotyledonary space, and white-grey foci on the chorionic surface of cotyledons. Severity of lesions will vary between animals and between placentomes of the same placenta, and necrotizing vasculitis of placental vessels is observed microscopically.

Goat fetuses may occasionally show white spots on the liver, identifiable in gross specimens, but on histopathological examination, most fetuses are found to have some combination of hepatitis, splenitis, bronchopneumonia, or encephalitis (Barati *et al.*, 2017).

13.7 Diagnosis

Accurate diagnosis plays a pivotal role in the effective management and control of the condition. Several diagnostic techniques are employed, including polymerase chain reaction (PCR), enzyme-linked immunosorbent assay (ELISA), and immunohistochemistry. These methods can identify the presence of *Chlamydia* DNA, antibodies, or antigen in clinical specimens such as vaginal swabs, placental tissues, and blood.

In goats, the occurrence of abortion in late pregnancy, accompanied by the expulsion of necrotic fetal membranes, serves as a diagnostic indicator. Swift diagnosis can be achieved through the visualization of elementary bodies in trophoblast impression smears extracted from cotyledons or uterine discharge. The application of specialized stains like Gimenez or modified Ziehl–Neelsen enhances cytological detection. Fluorescent antibody techniques can be employed to scrutinize impression smears of cotyledons (Essig and Longbottom, 2015). A conclusive diagnosis is established through positive culture or PCR analysis of fresh placenta, stomach contents, or fetal tissue. Notably, PCR assays conducted on vaginal swabs exhibit elevated specificity and sensitivity. Given that *C. abortus* primarily affects the placenta, traditional histopathological examination, culture and PCR analysis of fetal tissue might yield limited results. A more effective diagnostic approach involves scrutinizing the placenta using special stains like Giemsa or modified Ziehl–Neelsen. Immunohistochemistry studies or PCR assays performed on formalin-fixed paraffin-embedded placental tissue can be considered a less sensitive alternative if fresh tissue is unavailable. It is important to note that PCR assay sensitivity diminishes as tissues are stored for longer durations in formalin.

Ewes and does demonstrate significant antibody increase against *C. abortus* post-abortion. Diagnosis can be aided by analysing paired serum samples from the aborting female, collected 2–3 weeks apart, or by detecting antibodies in fetal serum. While complement fixation testing and various ELISA methods prove useful in evaluating sera for *C. abortus* antibodies, they may yield false-negative outcomes due to cross-reactivity with *Chlamydia pecorum* antigen. In contrast, recently developed ELISA tests targeting outer membrane protein fragments exhibit heightened sensitivity and are devoid of cross-reactivity with *C. pecorum* (Marsilio *et al.*, 2005).

13.8 Treatment

Controlling outbreaks in fibre-producing animals has shown success through a strategy involving the administration of tetracycline to all females in the flock during the last 4–6 weeks of gestation. Incorporating tetracycline (400–500 mg/head/day) into their feed for a duration of 2 weeks has been demonstrated to prevent the disease. In dairy herds, a common practice involves individually treating non-lactating does with injections of long-acting oxytetracycline (20 mg/kg SC) at intervals of 10–14 days. A viable approach may encompass an initial injection of long-acting oxytetracycline 6–8 weeks prior to parturition, followed by a second injection 3 weeks after parturition. Whenever feasible, we prefer incorporating tetracycline into the feed or energy-protein supplements. Irrespective of the administration method chosen, the use of antibiotics to suppress the organism can curtail further placental damage and minimize the shedding of *C. abortus* (Nietfeld, 2001).

Another potential treatment involves Tylosin administration (20 mg/kg IM, once or twice daily), which has demonstrated effectiveness. Additionally, *C. abortus* infection has exhibited responsiveness to Rifamicin and Chloramphenicol, although it is important to note that the use of these drugs is subject to restrictions in certain countries.

13.9 Prevention and Control

The prevention and control of chlamydiosis demand a comprehensive approach. In order to control the disease, the culling of ewes and does that have previously experienced abortions due to *C. abortus* infection should be considered. Avoiding the introduction of replacement females from endemic herds into naive populations is also crucial. Implementing embryo transfer (ET) from endemic farms to disease-free recipients has been suggested as a means to uphold a farm's disease-free status or curtail the spread within and between farms.

Vaccination proves effective in reducing abortion rates among susceptible animals. Both inactivated and attenuated vaccines are available, offering reported success in preventing abortions and decreasing excretion. However, while these vaccines contribute to disease control, complete eradication is not guaranteed. Some countries have initiated compulsory vaccination programmes due to the serious economic implications of enzootic abortion. While killed vaccines for sheep are accessible in specific regions and live vaccines are available in Europe, their use in goats may lead to localized and systemic reactions, potentially resulting in fetal wastage if administered during the initial month of pregnancy (Iraninezhad *et al.*, 2020). If employed, the vaccine should be administered through intramuscular or subcutaneous injection, 8 weeks before breeding, followed by a booster 4 weeks later. Despite sheep trials demonstrating protection against abortion for about 3 years, annual revaccination is advised. It is important to note that while vaccination aids in preventing abortion, it might not completely eliminate infection and should not be regarded as fully foolproof.

Biosecurity measures are instrumental in curtailing disease transmission. Isolating sick animals, maintaining proper sanitation and thorough premises disinfection are vital components. Aborting females must be isolated from the herd for a minimum of 3 weeks, and fetuses and placentas not submitted for diagnostics should be safely disposed of through burning or burial. Stringent precautions should be taken to prevent feed and water contamination, including avoiding direct offering of supplemental feedstuffs on the ground and designing feeders to prevent animal intrusion and feed contamination. Timely identification and culling of carriers also contribute significantly to disease control endeavors (Giannitti *et al.*, 2016).

13.10 Zoonosis of Chlamydiosis

Zoonosis constitutes a significant facet of chlamydiosis (enzootic abortion) in goats, underscoring the potential transmission of the culpable agent, *C. abortus*, from goats to humans. Human infection can arise from handling products of abortion or parturition or from inadequate management of laboratory cultures of the organism. This spectrum of infection may encompass inconspicuous subclinical instances to pronounced flu-like symptoms. Therefore, meticulous bio-risk measures should be implemented when dealing with cultures and potential exposure. Particularly vulnerable are women engaged in the handling of livestock, especially aborted animals, putting them at heightened risk of contracting the infection. Aside from provoking systemic septicaemia, the bacterium can instigate stillbirths or abortions in pregnant women.

Although chlamydiosis primarily targets goats' reproductive systems, it poses a potential threat to individual humans in close contact with infected animals or their byproducts, including veterinarians, farmers and slaughterhouse staff. Direct transmission may occur through contact with birth fluids, placental tissues, or contaminated equipment. A significant proportion (approximately 94%) of animal-acquired chlamydiosis cases result in fetal loss, while 6.3% lead to maternal mortality. Clinical manifestations in humans range from acute febrile conditions, respiratory distress, fatigue, and malaise, to liver and kidney dysfunction, shock, disseminated intravascular coagulopathy and eventual fatality. The chlamydial organism targets the placenta, proliferating within trophoblast epithelial cells, causing detrimental effects on placental vitality. Infected females display elevated C-reactive protein levels and reduced platelet counts. In non-pregnant females, the infection can manifest as 'pelvic inflammatory disease'. Recent research highlighted that out of 23 cases of gestational chlamydiosis, 20 were traced back to exposure to sheep and goats. Notably, a veterinary researcher's case featured atypical pneumonia attributed to *C. abortus* (Essig and Longbottom, 2015).

Cases demonstrating human placentitis and abortion stemming from *C. abortus* of ovine/caprine origin underscore the heightened vulnerability of pregnant women, necessitating stringent precautionary measures. To mitigate the zoonotic risk associated with chlamydiosis in goats and safeguard both animal handlers and the broader community, adherence to proper hygiene protocols, utilization of personal protective equipment and implementation of biosecurity measures are imperative.

13.11 Economic Impact

Chlamydiosis-induced abortion incurs economic losses, attributed to diminished milk production, escalated veterinary expenses and compromised reproductive efficiency. Notably, reduced kidding rates and heightened neonatal mortality further exacerbate the economic repercussions. This impact is felt across various scales, affecting both large-scale commercial farms and smallholders, thereby impinging on the overall sustainability of the goat industry.

13.12 Path Forward

Continued research is pivotal to deepening our understanding of chlamydiosis in goats, encompassing its epidemiology, pathogenesis and the intricate interplay of host immune responses. Progressing towards more efficacious vaccines and enhanced diagnostic tools will significantly contribute to disease prevention and management. Moreover, investigations centred around the zoonotic potential of *C. abortus* will augment awareness of public health concerns and facilitate effective surveillance efforts.

13.13 Conclusion

Chlamydiosis (enzootic abortion) stands as a substantial reproductive ailment exerting considerable influence on goats, imparting extensive economic ramifications. A profound comprehension of its aetiological underpinnings, epidemiological dynamics, clinical manifestations, diagnostic intricacies and robust control measures is imperative for the efficacious governance of this malady. The strategic deployment of comprehensive preventive paradigms, accompanied by the propulsion of research endeavours, emerges as paramount in mitigating the deleterious imprint of chlamydiosis on the goat industry. This concerted approach not only facilitates the amelioration of chlamydiosis-induced adversity but also bolsters the prospect of fostering enduring sustainability within goat production paradigms.

References

Barati, S., Moori-Bakhtiari, N., Najafabadi, M.G., Momtaz, H. and Shokuhizadeh, L. (2017) The role of zoonotic chlamydial agents in ruminants abortion. *Iran Journal of Microbiology* 9(5), 288–294.

Essig, A. and Longbottom, D. (2015) *Chlamydia abortus*: New aspects of infectious abortion in sheep and potential risk for pregnant women. *Current Clinical Microbiology Reports* 2, 22–34.
Giannitti, F., Anderson, M., Miller, M, *et al*. (2016) *Chlamydia pecorum*: Fetal and placental lesions in sporadic caprine abortion. *Journal of Veterinary Diagnostic Investigation* 28(2), 184–189.
Iraninezhad, Z., Azizzadeh, M., Taghavi Razavizadeh, A., Mehrzad, J. and Rashtibaf, M. (2020) Seroepidemiological feature of *Chlamydia abortus* in sheep and goat population located in Northeastern Iran. *Veterinary Research Forum* 11(4), 423–426.
Marsilio, F., Martino, B., Francesco, C.E, *et al*. (2005) Diagnosis of ovine chlamydial abortions by PCR-RFLP performed on vaginal swabs. *Veterinary Research Communications* 29(Suppl. 1), 99–106.
Nietfeld, J.C. (2001) Chlamydial infections in small ruminants. *Veterinary Clinics of North America: Food Animal Practice* 17(2), 301–314.
Selim, A. (2016) *Chlamydophila abortus* infection in small ruminants: A review. *Asian Journal of Animal and Veterinary Advances* 11, 587–593.

14 Colibacillosis

Gaurav Charaya[1]*, Jasleen Kaur[2] and Yudhbir Rana[1]
[1]Department of Veterinary Medicine, Lala Lajpat Rai University of Veterinary and Animal Sciences, Hisar, India; [2]Department of Veterinary Microbiology, Lala Lajpat Rai University of Veterinary and Animal Sciences, Hisar, India

Abstract
Colibacillosis is a significant disease affecting goat kids, leading to severe economic losses due to high morbidity and mortality rates. The disease is caused by *Escherichia coli*, which is a normal inhabitant of the intestinal tract, but certain strains can cause disease, especially in young animals, characterized by diarrhoea. Goat kids born in litters, particularly triplets, are more susceptible. Disease incidence decreases with age, due to the development of resistance in intestinal cells. Transmission occurs through the faecal–oral route, exacerbated in crowded conditions. Serotyping distinguishes *E. coli* strains based on surface antigens. Different pathotypes, including enteropathogenic and uropathogenic, cause varying types of diarrhoeal illnesses. Diagnosis and distinguishing various serotypes can be done by serological and molecular assays. Treatment typically involves antibiotics, but alternative approaches like herbal remedies, probiotics and homeopathy are explored to mitigate antibiotic resistance. Prevention focuses on sanitation, hygiene, vaccination and passive immunization through colostrum intake.

Keywords: colibacillosis, diarrhoea, goat kids, passive immunization, serotyping

14.1 Introduction

Colibacillosis is an acute to peracute disease mainly affecting kids and leading to diarrhoea. It causes huge economic losses due to its severity in terms of high morbidity and high mortality. Disease is caused by a bacterium named *Escherichia coli*. The majority of strains are commensals inhabiting the intestinal tract of humans and warm-blooded animals and rarely cause diseases. Intestinal pathogenic *E. coli* is one of the leading causes of diarrhoea in young animals and represents a global health problem for mammals, including humans.

14.2 Epidemiology

Goat kids are especially susceptible to colibacillosis during the first 2 weeks of life. Colibacillosis is the single major cause of death in neonatal goat kids, with a reported morbidity rate of 60%, mortality rate of 15–30% and case fatality rate of 24% in kids. The mortality rate has been reported to increase with increase in litter size and to be higher in kids born as triplets, followed by twins and singles. This can be attributed to direct negative correlation of litter size with that of body weight at birth, which is an important factor in determining the survival of kids. There is no significant effect of parity on disease attributes, but the disease is more often seen in first

*Corresponding author: gcharaya9@luvas.edu.in

DOI: 10.1079/ 9781800622852.0014

parity because of poor letdown of milk and low milk production, which fail to provide sufficient passive immunization. It increases in fourth and fifth parities where chances of multiple birth increase, leading to the birth of low-weight kids. Passive transfer of immunity plays important role in the outcome of disease: kids with poor immune status may succumb to death within 0–7 days of life, whereas those with stronger immune systems survive. Disease incidence is seen to be correlated with age: as age advances, disease incidence becomes lower. This can be attributed to the development of resistance of intestinal cells to pilus attachment or replacement of cells by new cells that lack pilus attachment receptors as age progresses. No sex predilections have been reported in the disease, although males have higher survival rates owing to their higher body weight.

Disease transmission occurs by the faecal–oral route. Goats suffering from disease shed the bacteria in their faeces and the situation becomes worse in intensive farming, with overcrowding resulting in high morbidity. The disease can be seen in extensive systems where kidding seasons coincide with periods of extreme weather conditions, like heat stress, excessive cold or during heavy rains. In semi-intensive rearing systems, outbreaks have been limited to the season coinciding with kidding.

14.3 Aetiology

Historically, *E. coli* was first identified by the German paediatrician Theodor Escherich in 1885. He discovered the bacterium in the faeces of healthy infants and named it after himself. Since its discovery, *E. coli* has been extensively studied and has become a model organism for scientific research.

Escherichia coli is a Gram-negative, rod-shaped bacterium that belongs to the family Enterobacteriaceae. It is a normal inhabitant of the intestinal tract of humans and animals and is commonly found in the environment. While most strains of *E. coli* are harmless, some can cause serious illness, including diarrhoea, urinary tract infections and even death.

Morphologically, *E. coli* has a thin peptidoglycan cell wall surrounded by an outer membrane. The bacterium is approximately 1–2 µm in length and 0.5–1 µm in width. *E. coli* cells are motile, with the help of flagella that are distributed all over the cell surface. Under a microscope, *E. coli* has a distinct, pinkish-red colour.

Bacteriologically, *E. coli* can be cultured on a variety of media, including MacConkey agar, eosin methylene blue (EMB) agar and Levine's EMB agar. These media contain specific nutrients that allow *E. coli* to grow and form colonies. *E. coli* colonies on these media appear as small, round and pink-coloured with a metallic sheen (Fig. 14.1).

14.3.1 Serotypes of *E. coli*

Serotyping is a technique used to identify and classify different strains of bacteria based on the specific antigens present on their cell surface. In *E. coli*, serotyping is commonly used to differentiate between different strains of the bacterium based on the presence or absence of specific surface antigens (Fig. 14.2), known as O, H and K antigens. The O antigen is a component of the outer membrane of the bacterial cell wall and is used to identify different serotypes of *E. coli*. The H antigen is a component of the bacterial flagellum, which is a long, whip-like structure used for motility. The K antigen is a component of the bacterial capsule, a protective layer that surrounds the bacterial cell. There are over 170 different O antigens, more than 50 hour antigens, and a smaller number of K antigens that have been identified in *E. coli*. By combining the results of tests for the presence or absence of these different antigens, it is possible to assign a specific serotype to a given strain of *E. coli*. Serotyping is an important tool for public health officials and researchers studying outbreaks of *E. coli* infections, as it can help to identify the specific strain of the bacterium responsible for the outbreak and track its spread.

14.3.2 Pathotypes of *E. coli*

Pathogenic *E. coli* bacteria are divided into two types: enteropathogenic *E. coli* and uropathogenic *E. coli*. Enteropathogenic *E. coli* is further

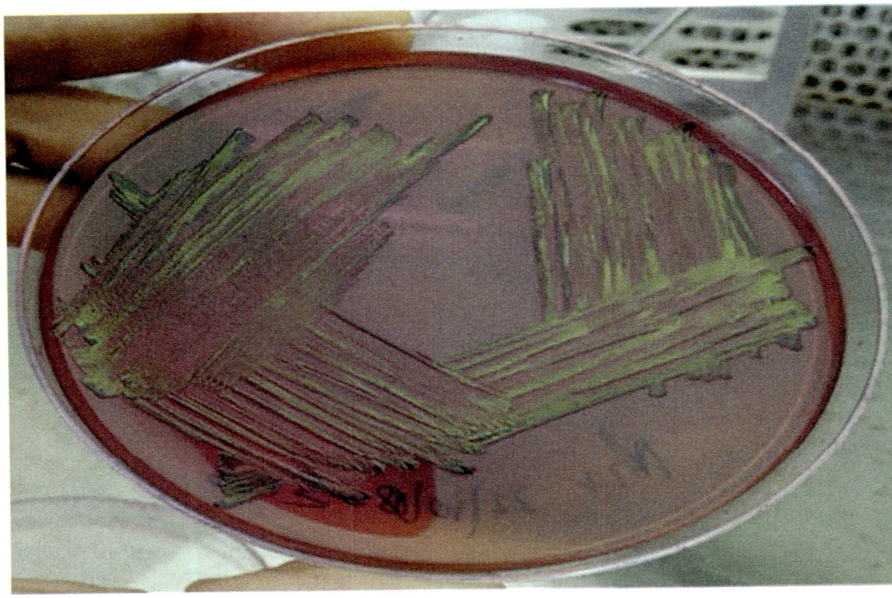

Fig. 14.1. *E. coli* colonies on EMB showing typical metallic sheen. (Author's own image.)

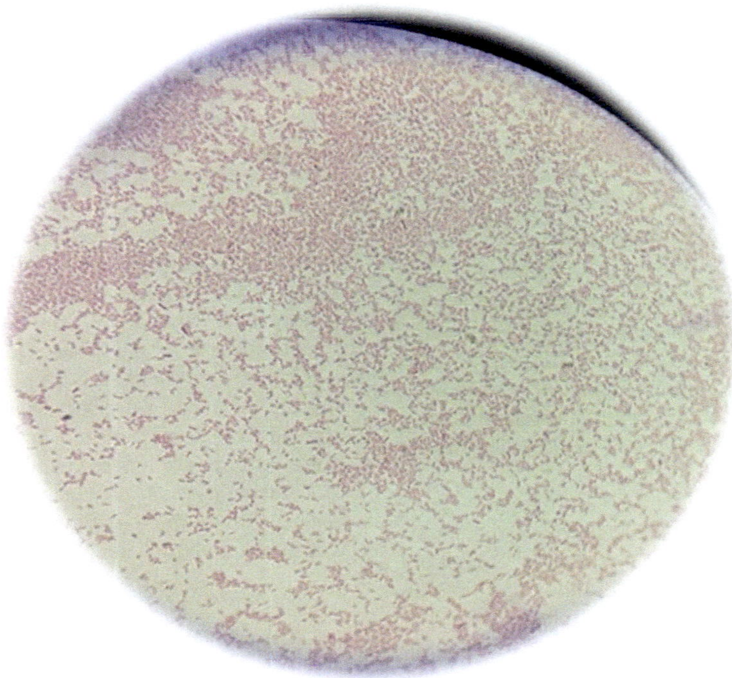

Fig. 14.2. Gram-staining reaction of colonies from *E. coli* culture depicting Gram-negative rod-shaped bacteria. (Author's own image.)

grouped into enterotoxigenic *E. coli* (ETEC), enteropathogenic *E. coli* (EPEC), enteroinvasive *E. coli* (EIEC), enteroaggregative *E. coli* (EAggEC or EAEC) and enterohaemorrhagic *E. coli* (EHEC), which are responsible for causing diarrhoea or related illness.

Diarrhoeagenic *E. coli* bacteria can be categorized into seven major categories: enteropathogenic *E. coli* (EPEC), atypical EPEC (ATEC), locus of enterocyte effacement (LEE)-positive and LEE-negative Shiga toxin (Stx)-producing *E. coli* (STEC), enterotoxigenic *E. coli* (ETEC), enteroinvasive *E. coli* (EIEC) and enteroaggregative *E. coli* (EAEC).

- EPEC is a major aetiological agent of infant diarrhoea predominantly in developing countries. EPEC colonizes the small intestine and causes typical attaching-and-effacing lesions characterized by the degeneration of microvilli and intimate adherence of bacteria to epithelial membranes. EPEC form microcolonies on hist intestinal cells.
- ATEC causes very little damage to the body.
- Stx-producing *E. coli* (STEC) can result in a spectrum of outcomes ranging from asymptomatic carriage to uncomplicated diarrhoea but also to bloody diarrhoea and the haemolytic-uraemic syndrome (HUS). Shiga toxins have been further categorized on the basis of toxin neutralization assay.
- ETEC, a cause of traveller's diarrhoea in humans, is another pathotype and is further classified as heat labile and heat stable ETEC, depending on their ability to produce particular toxins.
- EIEC is associated with watery diarrhoea and fever. After invading intestinal cells, EIEC induces polarized actin comets, propelling the bacteria through the cytoplasm of host cells, also allowing cell-to-cell spread.
- EAEC bacteria are responsible for sporadic and persistent diarrhoea. All these pathotypes differ from each other in terms of presence of different virulence factors and their mode of action.

14.3.3 Determination of pathotypes of *E. coli*

Bacterial genomes are extremely dynamic, and the ability of the organisms to acquire genetic elements, such as pathogenicity islands and virulence factors, from one another in the environment makes it difficult to identify the pathogens (Ochman *et al.*, 2000). Diagnostic assays have been employed for diagnosis of pathotypes. Different methodologies have different principles; some of them target single factors/indicators and others use multiple factors for screening of pathotypes.

Simplex PCR assay

The simplex method uses specific gene targets for identification of different pathotypes. However, it has the limitation of identifying a single gene in a single reaction. Therefore, for identification of multiple pathotypes, multiple genes need to be targeted in different reactions, which makes the method cumbersome, time consuming and uneconomical.

Multiplex PCR assay

In this methodology, multiple genes can be targeted and amplified at the same time in one reaction. This protocol has an added advantage of using a single reaction to generate multiple amplicons and distinguish them on the basis of product size. This strategy can be used for simultaneous identification of five major different diarrhoeagenic *E. coli* pathotypes. Ohmura-Hoshino *et al.* (2022) developed one such single-step multiplex PCR assay for simultaneous diagnosis of different pathotypes (Fig. 14.3). They used ten different primer pairs to amplify ten virulence genes specific to the different pathotypes (i.e. stx1 and stx2 for EHEC, elt and sth for ETEC, eaeA and bfpA for EPEC, aggR and astA for EAEC, and ipaH and invE for EIEC) and to generate DNA fragments of sufficiently different sizes to be unequivocally resolved. This method has a limitation of being an end-point Polymerase chain reaction (PCR) assay where gel electrophoresis needs to

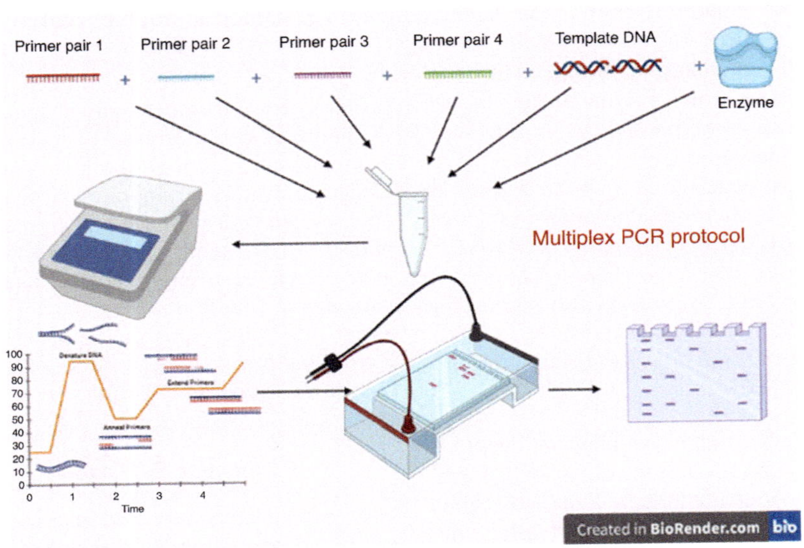

Fig. 14.3. Flowchart of protocol of multiplex PCR assay. (Created in BioRender.com.)

be undertaken each time for visualization of the results.

Real-time PCR assay

Barbau-Piednoir *et al.* (2018) developed a real-time PCR system based on a combination of 13 SYBR Green qPCR which is able to detect, differentiate and discriminate *E. coli* pathotypes. Shigatoxigenic (STEC) (including enterohaemorrhagic (EHEC)), enteropathogenic (EPEC), enteroaggregative (EAggEC), enteroaggregative shigatoxigenic (EAggSTEC), and enteroinvasive (EIEC) *E. coli* were the different pathotypes identified using this system. qPCR assays target the uidA, ipaH, eae, aggR, aaiC, stx1 and stx2 genes. They used two primer pairs for each gene to ensure sufficient detection even in the case of polymorphism or deletion.

DNA microarrays

This method explores the genome at molecular level and screens multiple markers. It is unable to determine the genetic and virulence markers which helps to differentiate between strains. This method can also predict the emergence of new pathotypes. Using oligonucleotide probes as compared with cDNA probes is a cost-effective methodology. Palaniappan *et al.* (2006) developed an oligonucleotide spotted array (70-mers) representing the known *E. coli* pathotype virulence genes (those of EHEC, EPEC, UPEC, ETEC, EAEC and EIEC), specific genes (those of *E. coli* O157 EDL933, *E. coli* K-12 MG1655 and *E. coli* CFT073), common genes (those of *E. coli* O157 EDL933, *E. coli* K-12 MG1655 and *E. coli* CFT073) and negative controls (core genes of *Salmonella* and dimethyl sulfoxide buffer without oligonucleotides).

Whole-genome sequencing

This is a comprehensive method for analysing the entire genome order of nucleotides and can be used for determination of variations. The *E. coli* genome varies in size from 4.5 to 5.5 Mb

14.4 Clinical Signs

Clinical signs of colibacillosis in goats can vary depending on the severity of the infection. In mild cases, goats may exhibit decreased appetite, depression and diarrhoea. In severe cases, goats may develop dehydration, fever, abdominal pain and systemic infection. In newborn kids, colibacillosis can cause septicaemia, which can lead to sudden death.

Animals suffering from disease have severe colitis characterized by abdominal pain and pasty white to watery brown faeces. In severe cases diarrhoea, dehydration, loss of appetite, depression, weakness and severe enteritis are seen. Death usually occurs due to severe dehydration. Typical symptoms may include watery and frequently bloody diarrhoea, abdominal cramping and a low-grade fever.

14.5 Zoonotic Importance

Goat's meat or milk may serve as a reservoir for foodborne transmission of the organism. Some strains of *E. coli* that infect goats can also cause illness in humans. These strains can cause gastrointestinal illness, including bloody diarrhoea and abdominal pain. Shiga toxin-producing *E. coli* (STEC) is one of the significant foodborne pathogens. The clinical manifestations of STEC infection range from asymptomatic carriage, diarrhoea, or haemorrhagic colitis (HC) to the potentially life-threatening complication, haemolytic uraemic syndrome (HUS), which can lead to acute renal failure (Majowicz *et al.*, 2014). Recent studies have suggested that goats and sheep are also significant sources of human STEC infection (Álvarez-Suárez *et al.*, 2016). Transmission from animals to humans can occur by different means, for example animal slaughter processes or exposure to faecal-matter-contaminated water, soils, animal-derived food and agricultural products. The importance of the existence of STEC lies with the fact that Stx-converting prophages act as horizontal gene transfer elements leading to conversion of normal intestinal commensal microbes to pathogenic ones.

Haemorrhagic colitis (HC) and haemolytic uraemic syndrome (HUS) caused by Shiga toxin (Stx)-producing *E. coli* (STEC) are the two important diseases in human beings spread through the faeces. Yang *et al.* (2022) used whole-genome sequencing to identify the STEC and showed that goat-derived Stx2k-STEC strains share similar genetic backbones with human patient-derived strains. The high prevalence of Stx2k-STEC in goats suggests that there is a risk of cross-species spread and that these strains may pose pathogenetic potential to humans.

14.6 Diagnosis

14.6.1 Clinical signs and history

Kids are more affected than adults. In young kids, the disease can cause diarrhoea, dehydration, fever, loss of appetite, weakness and lethargy. In adult goats, the disease can cause mastitis, metritis, septicaemia, or urinary tract infections, which can lead to decreased milk production, weight loss and even death.

14.6.2 Identification of bacteria in faeces (bacteriological examination)

Identification of *E. coli* is based on a combination of morphological, biochemical and genetic characteristics. Biochemical tests such as the oxidase test, catalase test and Gram staining are used to identify the bacterium. *E. coli* is negative for the oxidase test and positive for the catalase test. It is also Gram-negative, which means it stains pinkish-red under a microscope. IMViC (indole, methyl red, Voges-Proskauer, citrate) tests can be used to differentiate *E. coli* from other Enterobactericae family members.

14.6.3 ELISA

Enzyme-linked immunosorbent assay (ELISA) is a serological test that detects antibodies to *E. coli* in the blood or milk of the infected goat. This test is useful for detecting chronic or subclinical infections, as well as for monitoring the efficacy of treatment. Different ELISAs have been developed in the past and in 2016 a competitive ELISA was developed by Shan *et al.* (2016) with a detection sensitivity of the *E. coli* serotype O157:H7 that was 20 cfu/ml with the cascade signal amplification in ELISA, which was 1000-fold higher than that of traditional

ELISA. Furthermore, the novel method can be used to detect *E. coli* O157:H7 in milk (2 cfu/g).

14.6.4 DNA-based diagnostics

This test is based on detection of DNA and further sequencing/downstream processing to determine the pathotypes. PCR allows rapid and sensitive detection of the bacterium in clinical samples. This test is particularly useful for detecting low levels of the bacterium in faeces or milk.

14.7 Therapeutic Measures

Treatment of colibacillosis in goats typically involves the use of antibiotics, such as penicillin, ampicillin, or tetracycline. Supportive care, such as fluid therapy, electrolyte supplementation and nutritional support, is given to manage the clinical signs of the disease.

With the inadvertent and indiscriminate use of antibiotics, the world is facing the huge problem of antibiotic resistance and antibiotic residue. Therefore, alternative medicinal approaches for treatment of colibacillosis in goats can be used, which include herbal remedies, probiotics, homeopathy and aromatherapy.

14.7.1 Herbal remedies

Herbal remedies have been used for centuries to treat various diseases in both humans and animals. When it comes to colibacillosis in goats, several herbs have been found to be effective in managing the symptoms of the disease. These include echinacea, garlic, goldenseal and chamomile.

- Echinacea is a natural immune booster that can help goats fight off the bacterial infection. It can be given to goats in the form of capsules or tinctures.
- Garlic has natural antibacterial properties that can help kill the *E. coli* bacteria in goats. It can be added to their feed or given in the form of capsules.
- Goldenseal is a natural antimicrobial herb that can help kill the *E. coli* bacteria in goats. It can be given to goats in the form of capsules or tinctures.
- Chamomile has natural anti-inflammatory properties that can help soothe the digestive system and reduce diarrhoea in goats. It can be given to goats in the form of tea or tinctures.

14.7.2 Probiotics

Probiotics are live microorganisms that can be beneficial to the digestive system of goats. They can help restore the balance of bacteria in the gut and improve the overall health of the animal. Probiotics can be given to goats in the form of supplements or fermented foods such as yogurt.

14.7.3 Homeopathy

Homeopathy is a form of alternative medicine that uses highly diluted substances to stimulate the body's natural healing process. When it comes to colibacillosis in goats, several homeopathic remedies have been found to be effective in managing the symptoms of the disease. These include arsenicum album, nux vomica and veratrum album.

- Arsenicum album can be used to treat diarrhoea in goats caused by colibacillosis. It can be given in the form of pellets or liquid.
- Nux vomica can be used to treat goats with diarrhoea and abdominal pain caused by colibacillosis. It can be given in the form of pellets or liquid.
- Veratrum album can be used to treat goats with diarrhoea and dehydration caused by colibacillosis. It can be given in the form of pellets or liquid.

14.7.4 Aromatherapy

Aromatherapy is a form of alternative medicine that uses essential oils to promote healing and relaxation. When it comes to colibacillosis in goats, essential oils such as lavender and peppermint can be used to soothe the digestive system and reduce stress in the animal.

14.8 Prevention and Control

Prevention of colibacillosis in goats involves good management practices, including proper sanitation and hygiene. Goats should be housed in clean, dry and well-ventilated facilities, and their living areas should be cleaned and disinfected regularly. Kids should receive colostrum from healthy does to help protect them from infection. Vaccines are available for some strains of *E. coli* in goats, but their efficacy can vary.

14.8.1 Role of passive immunization

In ruminants, placental immunoglobulin transfer does not take place and consequently the neonate is born agammaglobulinaemic (without immunoglobulin), having neither received maternal immunoglobulin nor initiated their own production of immunoglobulins. Instead, these species are born with an 'open gut' allowing Fc-receptor-mediated immunoglobulin transfer from the gut to the circulation for approximately the first 24 hour after birth, assuring the very quick establishment of the necessary circulating levels of maternal immunoglobulins through ingestion of colostrum, which in these species contains high concentrations of IgG (Cervenak and Kacskovics, 2009).

Immunization by administration of immunoglobulins has been known for a long time as a very efficient means of obtaining immediate, short-lived protection against infection and/or against the disease-causing effects of toxins from microbial pathogens and from other sources. This plays a crucial role in the modern animal production sector as a means of controlling infectious diseases, even more importantly in the era of antimicrobial resistance where they can be used as an alternative to antibiotics. Administration of immunoglobulin establishes instant immunity and provides short-term protection with no induction of immunological memory. Maternal antibodies also do not interfere with the passive immunity provided by the immunoglobulins.

14.8.2 Vaccination for protection

It has been proven that vaccination reduces the incidence of disease and its outcome. Vaccination of pregnant goats can be used as a means of restricting the incidence of cases of neonatal colibacillosis in goats. In an experimental study, pregnant goats of the Barbari and Jamnapari breeds were vaccinated with two doses of vaccine subcutaneously 40–50 and 15–20 days before parturition against the natural form of enteric colibacillosis. Kids born from non-vaccinated does had 54.2% and 58.8% diarrhoea and 31.2% and 17.6% succumbed to colibacillosis in the Barbari and Jamnapari breeds, respectively. No deaths have been reported by the researchers. Administering immunomodulator along with the vaccine results in an increase in further immunity and decreases the incidence.

14.8.3 Sanitation and hygiene

The disease can be controlled following the maintenance of strict hygienic and sanitary measures in addition to antibiotic therapy.

References

Álvarez-Suárez, M.E., Otero, A., García-López, M.L., Dahbi, G., Blanco, M. *et al.* (2016) Genetic characterization of Shiga Toxin-producing *Escherichia Coli* (STEC) and atypical Enteropathogenic *Escherichia Coli* (EPEC) isolates from goat's milk and goat farm environment. *International Journal of Food Microbiology* 236, 148–154. DOI: 10.1016/j.ijfoodmicro.2016.07.035.

Barbau-Piednoir, E., Denayer, S., Botteldoorn, N., Dierick, K., De Keersmaecker, S.C.J. *et al.* (2018) Detection and discrimination of five *E. coli* pathotypes using a combinatory SYBR® green qPCR screening system. *Applied Microbiology and Biotechnology* 102(7), 3267–3285. DOI: 10.1007/s00253-018-8820-0.

Cervenak, J. and Kacskovics, I. (2009) The neonatal Fc receptor plays a crucial role in the meatbolism of igG in livestock animals. *Veterinary Immunology and Immunopathology* 128(1–3), 171–177. DOI: 10.1016/j.vetimm.2008.10.300.

Majowicz, S.E., Scallan, E., Jones-Bitton, A., Sargeant, J.M., Stapleton, J. *et al.* (2014) Global incidence of human Shiga toxin-producing *Escherichia coli* infections and deaths: A systematic review and knowledge synthesis. *Foodborne Pathogens and Disease* 11, 447–455. DOI: 10.1089/fpd.2013.1704.

Ochman, H., Lawrence, J.G. and Groisman, E.A. (2000) Lateral gene transfer and the nature of bacterial innovation. *Nature* 405, 299–304.

Ohmura-Hoshino, M., Miyaki, Y. and Yashima, S. (2022) A one-step multiplex PCR-based assay for simultaneous detection and classification of virulence factors to identify five diarrheagenic *E. coli* pathotypes. *Heliyon* 8(8), e10231. DOI: 10.1016/j.heliyon.2022.e10231.

Palaniappan, R.U.M., Zhang, Y., Chiu, D., Torres, A., DebRoy, C. *et al.* (2006) Differentiation of *Escherichia coli* pathotypes by oligonucleotide spotted array. *Journal of Clinical Microbiology* 44(4), 1495–1501.

Shan, S., Liu, D., Guo, Q., Wu, S., Chen, R. *et al.* (2016) Sensitive detection of *Escherichia coli* O157:H7 based on cascade signal amplification in ELISA. *Journal of Dairy Science* 99(9), 7025–7032. DOI: 10.3168/jds.2016-11320.

Yang, X., Liu, Q., Bai, X., Hu, B., Jiang, D. *et al.* (2022) High prevalence and persistence of *Escherichia coli* strains producing Shiga toxin subtype 2k in goat herds. *Microbiology Spectrum* 10(4), e0157122. DOI: 10.1128/spectrum.01571-22.

15 Bovine Tuberculosis

J.B. Kathiriya*

Department of Veterinary Public Health & Epidemiology, College of Veterinary Science & AH, Kamdhenu University, Junagadh, Gujarat, India

Abstract

This chapter provides a quick summary of the data accessible in the literature from the early 20th century onwards to evaluate the current state of bovine tuberculosis (bTB) in India. The epidemiology, transmission and diagnosis of bTB are examined in depth. In addition, the chapter discusses prevention and control techniques, emphasizes the relationship between human and animal health, and suggests immunizing cattle to stop the spread of infection to humans and other animals. The literature on investigations of risk factors at the herd level is reviewed here. India will be better able to combat tuberculosis (TB) if it adopts the One Health concept, which acknowledges the connection of human and animal health.

Keywords: Bovine tuberculosis, zoonosis, cattle, contamination, immunity

15.1 Introduction

Bovine tuberculosis (bTB) is a chronic sickness that mostly affects cattle. It is a significant public health risk and causes productivity loss in animals. In many nations, including India, where national control programmes have not yet been implemented, accurate estimates of tuberculosis prevalence are lacking, despite the disease's substantial economic implications and zoonotic hazard (Cousins, 2005). Because most underdeveloped countries do not regularly collect surveillance data, the full burden of the disease is unknown. Although India is making good progress towards the 'end TB' target, bTB is still mostly unknown. Furthermore, the lack of research on bTB in India could cause undue complacency, therefore it must be carefully monitored to avoid creating any misconceptions. To stop the spread of bTB to humans, to improve food safety and to protect people's livelihoods, it is essential to prevent and control the disease at the animal–human interface. Implementing multisectoral techniques and tactics based on international norms will enable improved animal illness detection and diagnosis, hence lowering the danger to people, in order to achieve this goal. This chapter also provides a quick summary of the data accessible in the literature from the early 20th century onwards to evaluate the current state of bTB in India.

Clinical evidence of TB in cattle is uncommon in nations with tuberculosis eradication initiatives, because the intradermal tuberculin test allows for presumptive diagnosis and removal of diseased animals before symptoms manifest. However, clinical indications of TB were often seen prior to the national initiatives to eradicate the disease (Cousins, 2001).

Bovine TB is one of the most difficult endemic illnesses that the governments, the

*Corresponding author: jbkathiriya@gmail.com

 The Handbook of Zoonotic Diseases of Goats (ed. T. Rana)
DOI: 10.1079/ 9781800622852.0015

veterinary profession and the farming sector in some countries are now dealing with. The epidemiology of the disease is infamously complicated, and the scientific literature supports both cattle-to-cattle and wildlife-to-cattle transmission pathways (De Lisle, 2001). In order to develop more efficient methods of minimizing this kind of transmission, it is critical to comprehend the risk variables that affect whether bovine TB is present in cattle herds or not. The purchase of cattle, the presence of bovine TB in contiguous herds and the surrounding area, as well as herd size, are among the risk factors linked to bovine TB herd breakdowns. These risk factors have been identified by epidemiological studies. Several studies have discovered additional characteristics, such as herd and farm management techniques including the spreading slurry, utilizing specific types of housing, having numerous farms and using silage clamps. In general, the most consistently identified risk factors are biologically plausible and consistent with known transmission routes involving cattle–cattle and wildlife–cattle pathways.

15.1.1 Aetiology

Bovine TB is usually described as a chronic, crippling illness, but it can sometimes proceed more quickly. As well as cattle, other domesticated animals, and some free or captive wildlife species, are susceptible to bTB, which is caused by acid-fast bacilli. The causative agent of bTB is *Mycobacterium bovis*. Being a zoonotic organism, *M. bovis* needs to be handled like a risk/hazard group III organism and proper care needs to be taken to avoid infecting humans. The disease is often marked by the development of tubercles, which are nodular granulomas. While lesions can occur in any area of the body, they are most commonly seen in the lymph nodes (especially those of the head and thorax), lungs, intestines, liver, spleen, pleura and peritoneum.

Even in more severe instances when numerous organs may be affected, the infection often has a chronic course and no symptoms at all. Clinical indications can vary when they occur; for example, a cough indicative of lung involvement may be brought on by temperature changes or physical pressure applied to the trachea. Additional indications of lung involvement include dyspnoea and other symptoms of low-grade pneumonia.

Advanced instances frequently have significantly swollen lymph nodes, which might block blood arteries, the alimentary tract, or airways. Visibly afflicted head and neck lymph nodes may occasionally burst and drain. Constipation and sporadic diarrhoea are signs of digestive tract involvement in certain cases. In the later stages of TB, extreme emaciation and severe respiratory distress are possible outcomes. There might be lesions on the female genitalia. Male genitalia are seldom involved.

Tubercles may be the sole tissue damaged during necropsy, and they are most commonly observed in the bronchial, mediastinal, retropharyngeal and portal lymph nodes. The surfaces of bodily cavities as well as the liver, spleen and lung are frequently impacted. Palpation is a common method for detecting early nodular pulmonary lesions. The lesions often do not smell. It is important to look into any other affected anatomical areas.

A tuberculous granuloma is typically caseous, caseo-calcareous, or calcified in consistency, and it typically has a yellowish appearance under the microscope. It can occasionally have a purulent look. Cervids and camelids may have a more purulent appearance. Certain non-tuberculous granulomas could be macroscopically identical to tuberculous granulomas.

Usually dry and hard, the caseous core is encased in a fibrous connective capsule that varies in thickness. Lesions can range in size from tiny enough to be invisible to the unassisted eye to involving a large portion of an organ. It could be necessary to slice organs and tissues in sequence in order to find the little lesions that are present inside the tissue. Histologically speaking, *M. bovis* lesions are frequently paucibacillary (meaning that they contain few organisms), and TB can still be present in lymphadenitis with an unclear aetiology even in the absence of acid-fast organisms. Thin-walled purulent abscesses without a clear aetiology should raise the possibility of TB in cervids and certain non-native species.

In the majority of countries where mycobacteria isolates from patient samples have been thoroughly characterized, *M. bovis* has been found in humans. Urban residents have a lower incidence of pulmonary TB caused by *M. bovis* than do agricultural and abattoir workers. The pasteurization of milk eliminates the possibility of *M. bovis* infection in humans from milk and its by-products. Reductions in sickness and mortality from bovine TB in the human population are among the outcomes of initiatives to eradicate the disease.

15.1.2 Bovine TB in wildlife

Several domesticated and wild species have been documented as afflicted with *M. bovis*, but cattle are thought to be the actual hosts of the illness. Animals that have been isolated include buffalo, bison, sheep, goats, pigs, wild boar, camels, equines, dogs, cats, foxes, mink, badgers, ferrets, rats, primates and South American camelids. A few predatory felines that have been isolated include lions, tigers, leopards and lynx.

Bovine tuberculosis in wildlife was first reported in 1929 in greater kudu (*Tragelaphus strepsiceros*) and common duiker (*Sylvicapra grimmi*) in South Africa, and by the 1940s the disease was found to be endemic in greater kudu. In 1982 in Uganda, a prevalence of 10% in African buffalo and 9% in warthog (*Phacochoerus aethiopicus*) was found, and in Zambia, *M. bovis* infection has been reported in Kafue lechwe (*Kobus leche* subsp. *kafuensis*) and in a single eland (*Traurotragus oryx*). An outbreak of tuberculosis in wild olive baboons (*Papio cynocephalus anubis*) was reported in Kenya. *M. bovis* infection has also been diagnosed in African buffalo in the Kruger National Park in South Africa (Bengis *et al.*, 1996), and more recently spilling over to other species such as chacma baboon (*Papio ursinus*), lion (*Panthera leo*) and cheetah (*Acynonyx jubatus*).

In several places, the elimination of *M. bovis* infection from farmed bovine herds has been achieved via the strict implementation of tuberculin testing and reactor animal culling, but this approach has not proven to be effective elsewhere. Numerous studies on the infrequent recurrence of *M. bovis* have demonstrated the existence of wildlife reservoirs in some countries, which can serve as a source of infection for deer, cattle and other animals. Depending on the unique epidemiological circumstances for the species and the surrounding environment, the risk that these reservoirs of infection provide to both domestic animals and people varies greatly (Morris *et al.*, 1994; Corner, 2006). In order to identify infection in a population of animals, epidemiological data analysis must be combined with bacteriological inquiry or the use of a reliable testing technique specific to the species in question (not all species respond well to the tuberculin test). It has been demonstrated that a number of wild-living species in Africa, the brush-tail possum (*Trichosurus vulpecula*) in New Zealand (Animal Health Division, 1986), wild boar (*Sus scrofa*) in Spain (Naranjo *et al.*, 2008), and the badger (*Meles meles*) in the United Kingdom (Wilesmith, 1991) and the Republic of Ireland (O'Reilly and Daborn, 1995) are all capable of sustaining *M. bovis* infection. Reducing or eliminating the contaminated wildlife population has been the main strategy used to control the complicated process of transmission from the wild population to farmed animals.

It has proved possible to isolate *M. bovis* from both farmed and wild cervids. The illness may proceed at a different rate and be either chronic or subacute. Some animals may have severe symptoms within months after infection, while others may take years to show clinical symptoms associated with lesions in the animal. The resulting lesions (caseating granulomatous inflammation that is often mineralized) may mimic those observed in cattle. The lesions may resemble purulent material-filled, thin-walled abscesses with little calcification.

Llamas have also been reported to have thin-walled abscesses. When abscess-like lesions without a recognized cause are seen in cervids, TB should be taken into consideration. Usually, the head and thoracic lymph nodes are the afflicted ones. There might be a big abscess at the location of the afflicted mesenteric lymph nodes. The incubation period prior to examination, the method of infection and the infectious dosage will all affect the distribution of lesions.

Deer raised on farms can be tested for tuberculin. The side of the neck is where the test has to be performed. Valid findings can only be obtained by accurately injecting tuberculin intradermally, trimming hair around the injection site, and using callipers to measure the thickness of the skin both before and after the injection (Clifton-Hadley and Wilesmith, 1991).

Further research is being done on the use of vaccination to manage the illness in some animals.

15.1.3 Mycobacterium tuberculosis complex

Notably, despite having identical 16s RNA sequences and over 99.9% genome sequence similarity, additional members of the *Mycobacterium tuberculosis* (Mtb) complex previously thought to be *M. bovis* have been recognized as novel species. These include *M. pinnipedii* (Cousins *et al.*, 2003), a pathogen of fur seals and sea lions, and *M. caprae* (Aranaz *et al.*, 2003), which is thought to be a main pathogen of goats in various areas. It is established that these two new species are zoonotic. *M. caprae* has been found to be a prevalent cause of TB in cows in central Europe (Prodinger *et al.*, 2005). The disease produced by *M. caprae* may be diagnosed using the same assays as for that caused by *M. bovis*, and it is not thought to differ much from that disease.

15.2 Diagnostic Techniques

Clinical signs of TB in cattle typically do not appear until extremely large lesions have formed. This made it impossible to diagnose the disease in individual animals and to launch an eradication campaign before Koch discovered tuberculin in 1890. The illness can be identified using tuberculin, a concentrated sterile culture filtrate of tubercle bacilli produced on glycerinated beef broth and, more recently, on synthetic medium.

15.2.1 Skin testing

The most common method for diagnosing bovine TB is skin testing with tuberculin based on delayed-type hypersensitivity, in which an infected animal is given an intradermal injection of at least 2000 IU of bovine pure protein derivative (PPD) antigen in the middle third of its neck skin. Because pathogenic and non-pathogenic environmental mycobacteria share mycobacterial antigen, leading to false-positive findings, the specificity of tuberculin skin testing is poor. The interferon gamma (IFN-γ) test and the lymphocyte proliferation test have a better sensitivity for detecting cell-mediated immunity (CMI) and can identify infection at an early stage of the illness. Although serologically based assays are less specific and sensitive for diagnosing TB in cows, they are nevertheless a good option to CMI-based tests because to their ease of use, low cost and capacity to create additional side diagnostic tests. The specificity of diagnostic tests can be enhanced by employing refined and more specific antigens, including MPB-70, CFP-10 and ESAT-6. Bovine TB diagnosis has entered a new age thanks to molecular diagnostic tests. These tests use expensive molecular reagents and complex equipment, yet they are fast, accurate and have excellent sensitivity and specificity.

15.2.2 Other identification techniques

Although skin testing can have practical difficulties, immunological responses to *M. bovis* infections in cattle are still being investigated in an effort to create better or alternative diagnostic techniques. The commercially available interferon gamma test is being used more often as a diagnostic blood test for TB in cattle and other animals (such as goats and buffalo). In farmed red deer, both the lymphocyte proliferation test and the immunoglobulin G1 (IgG1) enzyme-linked immunosorbent assay (ELISA) have shown promise as supplemental serial (for improving specificity) and parallel (for improving sensitivity) testing.

Examination of tissue slices or stained smears can reveal the presence of *M. bovis* in clinical and post-mortem specimens. The organism can then be cultivated on primary isolation medium to confirm the presence of *M. bovis*. When possible, single-use plastic disposable containers with a 50 ml capacity can be used for a variety of specimen types. Collection containers should be clean and preferably sterile (using sample containers contaminated by environmental mycobacteria may result in the failure to identify *M. bovis* infection, due to the rapid growth of the environmental mycobacteria).

The likelihood of *M. bovis* being recovered culturally is significantly increased by timely specimen transmission to the laboratory. Specimens to be delivered to the laboratory need to be packaged carefully to avoid breaking or crushing during travel, and they need to be cushioned and sealed to prevent leaks. When exporting specimens from a suspected zoonotic illness, adherence to the International Air Transport Association's (IATA) Dangerous Goods Regulations (DGR) is mandatory. Specimens should be frozen or chilled if delivery delays are expected, in order to protect the mycobacteria and slow the development of contaminants. Boric acid (0.5% (w/v) final concentration) may be applied as a bacteriostatic agent under warm ambient settings when refrigeration is not practicable, but only for brief periods of time – no more than 1 week. It is important to take precautions against laboratory staff contracting infections. A biological safety cabinet should be used for any process requiring culture.

15.2.3 Microscopic examination

M. bovis can be demonstrated microscopically on direct smears from clinical samples and on prepared tissue materials. The acid fastness of *M. bovis* is normally demonstrated with the classic Ziehl–Nielsen stain (Fig. 15.1), but a fluorescent acid-fast stain may also be used. Immunoperoxidase techniques may also give satisfactory results. The presumptive diagnosis of mycobacteriosis can be made if the tissue has characteristic histological lesions (caseous necrosis, mineralization, epithelioid cells, multinucleated giant cells and macrophages). As lesions are often paucibacillary, the presence of acid-fast organisms in histological sections may not be detected, although *M. bovis* can be isolated in culture. However, large numbers of acid-fast organisms are seen in lesions in primates, felids, mustelids (badgers) and marsupials (brush-tailed possums).

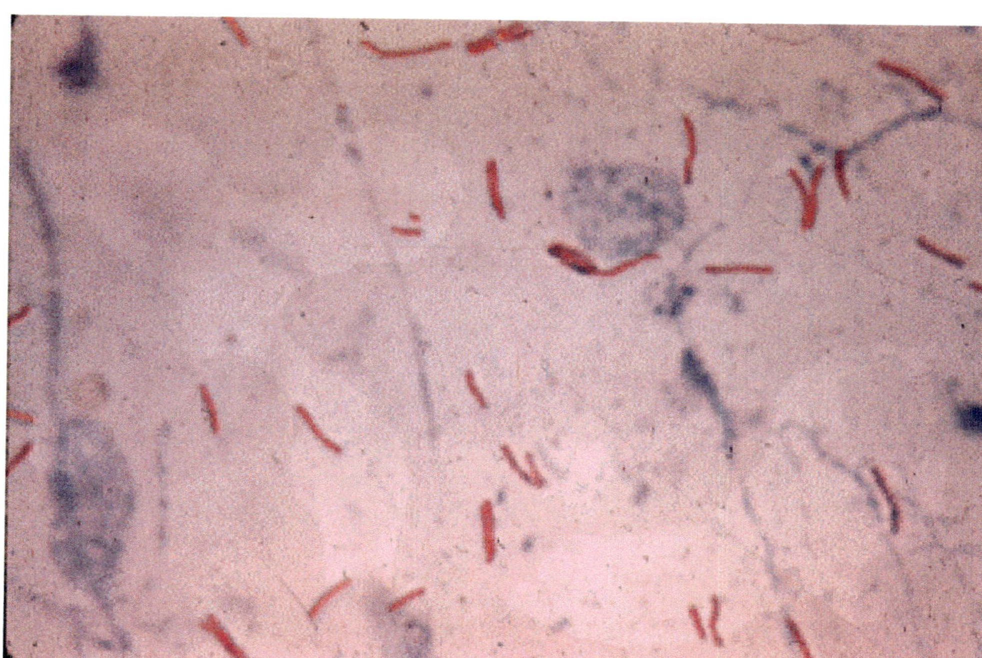

Fig. 15.1. Acid-fast bacilliin Ziehl–Nielsen staining. (Author's own image.)

15.2.4 Culture

In order to prepare specimens for culture, the tissue must first be homogenized using a stomacher, blender, or mortar and pestle. Next, the tissue must be decontaminated using an acid (5% oxalic acid), an alkali (2–4% sodium hydroxide), or a detergent (such as 0.375–0.75% hexadecylpyridinium chloride (HPC)). After shaking the alkali or acid combination at room temperature for 10–15 min, it is neutralized. Utilizing HPC does not necessitate neutralization. The sediment is utilized for culture and microscopic analysis after the suspension is centrifuged and the supernatant is disposed of. In cases where animals tested positive for tuberculin or interferon during post-mortem inspection do not have obvious lesions, it is advised that, at the very least, pooled lymph node samples from the head and thorax be cultured.

A set of solid egg-based media, such as Lowenstein-Jensen, Coletsos base, or Stonebrinks, are often injected with the sediment for primary isolation; these media should include either pyruvate or pyruvate plus glycerol (Fig. 15.2). It is also possible to utilize a blood-based agar medium (Cousins *et al.*, 1989) or an agar-based media like Middlebrook 7H10 or 7H11.

Cultures are cultured at 37°C with or without CO_2 for a minimum of 8 weeks (and ideally for 10–12 weeks). To prevent desiccation, the medium must be kept in tubes that are securely closed. Slopes are periodically checked during the incubation period for macroscopic growth. Smears are made and stained using the Ziehl–Neelsen method once growth is apparent. Depending on the medium, *M. bovis* typically grows 3–6 weeks after incubation.

Certain hospital and veterinary laboratories often employ liquid culture systems, where growth is evaluated using fluorometric or radiometric techniques.

The culture procedure should be redone using the retained inocula and a different decontaminating agent if there is significant contamination of the culture media. The low quality of the samples supplied is frequently the limiting factor in isolation, hence every effort should be made to ensure that the laboratory obtains high-quality samples.

Though each isolate must be verified, distinctive growth patterns and colony morphology might lead to a preliminary diagnosis of *M.*

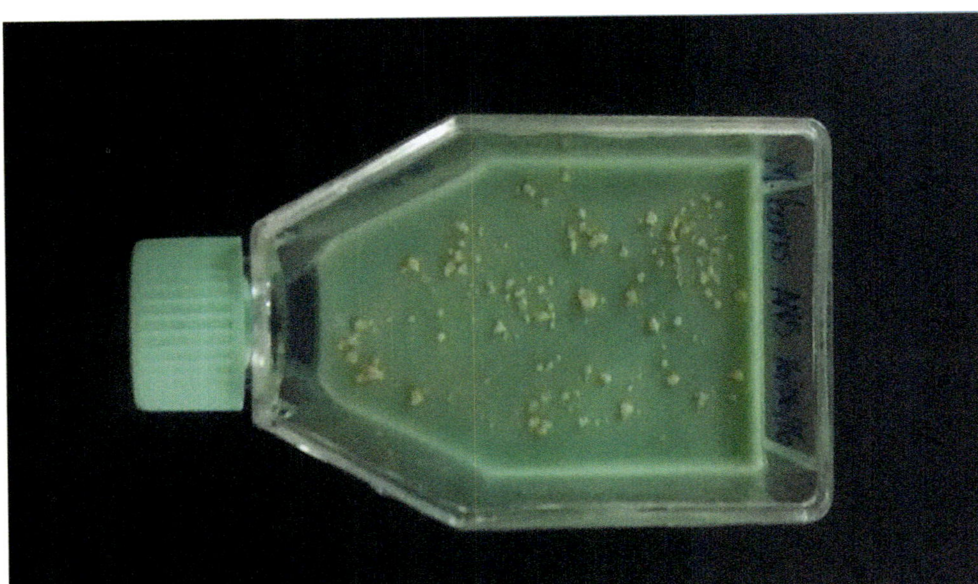

Fig. 15.2. Colonies of *M. bovis* on Stonebrink media. (Author's own image.)

bovis. *M. bovis* must be distinguished from the other members of the *Mycobacterium tuberculosis* complex, which include *M. pinnipedii* (fur seals and sealions, as noted earlier), *M. caprae*, *M. microti* (the 'vole bacillus', an uncommon organism), *M. africanum* (which occupies a phenotypic position intermediate between *M. tuberculosis* and *M. bovis*) and *M. tuberculosis* (the primary cause of tuberculosis in humans).

Without producing the usual symptoms, *M. tuberculosis* can infect cattle and make them more susceptible to bovine tuberculin. Sometimes lesions in cattle that resemble TB can be used to isolate *M. avium* or other environmental mycobacteria. In these situations, a thorough diagnosis is required, and a mixed *M. bovis* infection has to be ruled out.

By identifying conventional cultural and biological features, isolates can be recognized. The smooth, off-white (buff) colonies of *M. bovis* are grown on an appropriate pyruvate-based solid medium. At 37°C, the organism develops slowly; at 22°C or 45°C, it does not grow. Isonicotinic acid hydrazide (INH) and thiophen-2-carboxylic acid hydrazide (TCH) are both effective against *M. bovis*. Growth on 7H10/7H11 Middlebrook agar medium or on media containing eggs can be used to test for this. Pyruvate is known to block INH, and as it may have a similar impact on TCH (an analogue of INH), it is best to avoid using it in the preparation of the egg medium. This will prevent false-positive (resistant) findings. Certain strains of *M. bovis* are also susceptible to streptomycin and para-amino salicylic acid. The optimal medication concentrations for agar- and egg-based media vary. In *M. bovis*, the results for nitrate reduction and niacin generation are negative. *M. bovis* tests negative for nicotinamidase and pyrazinamidase but positive for urease in the amidase test. It is a non-chromogenic, microaerophillic bacterium.

15.2.5 Nucleic acid recognition methods

The Gen Probe TB complex DNA probe, polymerase chain reaction (PCR) targeting 16S–23S rRNA, the insertion sequences IS6110 and IS1081, and genes coding for *M. tuberculosis* complex-specific proteins, such as MPB70 and the 38 kDa antigen b, have all been used to quickly identify isolates to the level of *M. tuberculosis* complex. A specific mutation at nucleotide positions 285 in the oxyR gene, 169 in the pncA gene, 675/756/1311/1410 and 1450 of the gyrB gene, and the presence or absence of regions of difference (RDs) can be targeted by PCR to specifically identify an isolate as *M. bovis* (Espinos de los Monteros *et al.*, 1998; Niemann *et al.*, 2000; Parsons *et al.*, 2002; Huard *et al.*, 2003). As an alternative, *M. bovis* isolates can be identified using molecular-typing techniques like spacer oligotyping (spoligotyping), which also yields some molecular-typing information on the isolate that is useful for epidemiology (Kamerbeek *et al.*, 1997).

PCR has recently been used to diagnose TB in animals. It has been extensively tested for the identification of the *M. tuberculosis* complex in clinical samples (mostly sputum) in human patients. Several in-house techniques and commercial kits have been tested for identifying the *M. tuberculosis* complex in both fresh and preserved tissues. As previously mentioned, several primers have been employed. Amplification results have been examined using gel electrophoresis or hybridization using probes. In interlaboratory comparisons, commercial kits and in-house techniques using fresh, frozen, or boric acid-preserved tissues have shown inconsistent and subpar findings (Noredhoek *et al.*, 1996). The test's reliability has been lowered by false-positive and false-negative findings, especially in specimens with low bacilli counts. Low numbers of bacilli and a low copy number of the target sequence per bacillus have been linked to variability in the findings. Additional factors that have been linked to variability include decontamination processes, DNA extraction protocols, polymerase enzyme inhibitor removal methods, internal and external controls, and cross-contamination avoidance protocols. Development of standardized and reliable techniques is necessary to increase the PCR test's accuracy in identifying the *M. tuberculosis* complex in fresh clinical specimens. The biggest issue with this kind of application is cross-contamination, which is why appropriate controls need to be established before every amplification. However, several laboratories now routinely utilize PCR to identify the *M. tuberculosis* group in tissues fixed in paraffin (Miller *et al.*, 1997, 2002). To confirm a live

M. bovis infection, culture should be employed in tandem with direct PCR, even if it can yield a result quickly.

For epidemiological objectives, a range of DNA fingerprinting methods have been developed to differentiate the isolates of the *M. tuberculosis* complex. These techniques allow for the differentiation of *M. bovis* strains and will make it possible to characterize the patterns of origin, transmission and dissemination of *M. bovis* (Durr *et al.*, 2000a, b). Spoligotyping, also known as 'spacer oligotyping', is the most often employed technique. It permits strain differentiation within each species of the *M. tuberculosis* complex, including *M. bovis*, and also has the ability to differentiate *M. bovis* from *M. tuberculosis* (Kamerbeek *et al.*, 1997; Heifets and Jenkins, 1998). To enable cross-border profile comparison, the adoption of a uniform nomenclature for the spoligotypes based on the database Mbovis.org (http://www.mbovis.org) is suggested.

Other methods include restriction endonuclease analysis (REA), restriction fragment length polymorphism (RFLP), the direct repeat (DR) region probe, the PGRS (polymorphic GC repeat sequence) probe (Skuce *et al.*, 1996), and the pUCD probes (O'Brian *et al.*, 2000) using the IS6110 (Fig. 15.3) probe (especially where there are >3–4 copies of IS6110 in the isolate). To improve the differentiation of the *M. tuberculosis* complex species, the variable number tandem repeat (VNTR)–mycobacterial interspersed repetitive units (MIRU) typing method has also been developed (Frothingham and Meeker-O'Connell, 1998; Supply *et al.*, 2000). To achieve the greatest degree of strain discrimination, a variety of methods are frequently employed (Cousins *et al.*, 1998).

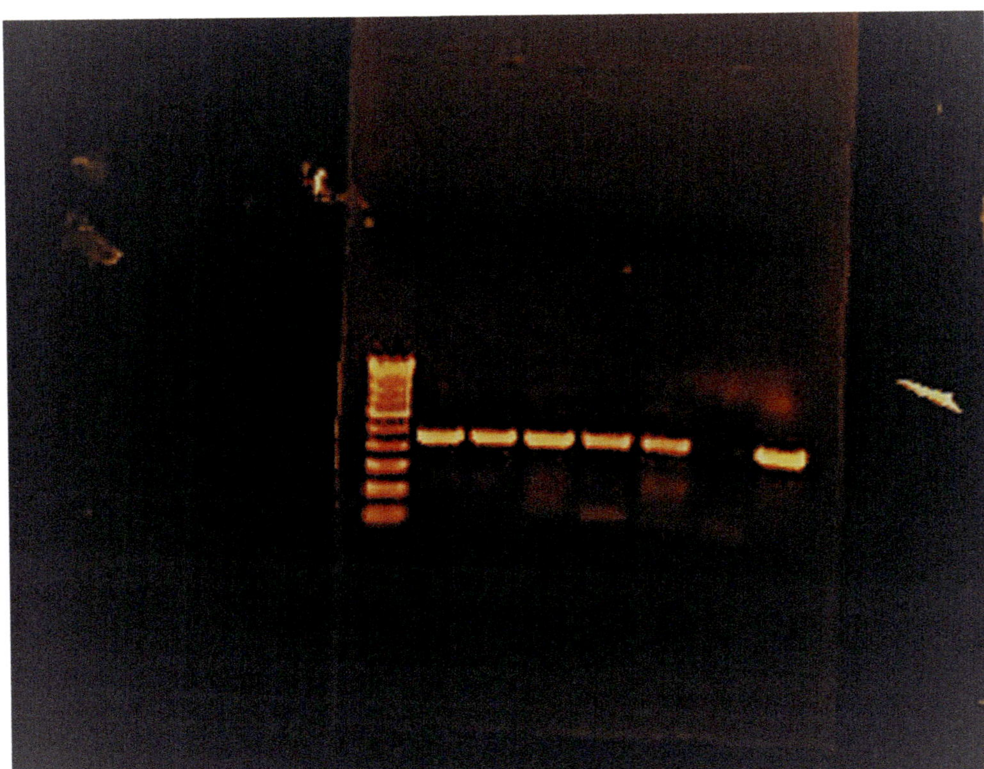

Fig. 15.3. PCR targeting MTB complex specific insertion sequence IS6110 producing 445 bp amplicon in all MTB complex *Mycobacterium*. (Author's own image.)

The genome of *M. bovis* has been sequenced (Garnier *et al.*, 2003), and this knowledge has helped to create PCR tests that distinguish the several subspecies of the *M. tuberculosis* complex and to enhance genetic fingerprinting techniques.

15.3 Delayed Hypersensitivity Test

15.3.1 The tuberculin test

The prescribed test for international trade is the tuberculin test, which involves injecting bovine tuberculin PPD subcutaneously and monitoring for swelling (delayed hypersensitivity) at the injection site for 72 hour, is the usual procedure for diagnosing tuberculosis in cows (Fig. 15.4). This may be done either as a comparison test between avian and bovine tuberculins, or using bovine tuberculin alone. The tuberculin test is typically conducted on the mid-neck but the caudal fold of the tail can also be used. Compared with the skin of the caudal fold, the skin of the neck is more susceptible to tuberculin. In the caudal fold, larger dosages of tuberculin may be administered to make up for this discrepancy.

After infection, delayed hypersensitivity cannot appear for 3–6 weeks. Delaying testing should thus be taken into consideration in order to lower the likelihood of false-negative results if a herd or animal is suspected of having had recent contact with sick animals. It is improbable that a single tuberculin test will be sufficient to eradicate tuberculosis from a herd, due to the test's less than 100% sensitivity. It should be acknowledged that the tuberculin test may not work when administered to animals with severe pathology and chronic infection. In the majority of non-cervid and non-bovid species, the validity of the tuberculin test has been questioned.

Animals reacting to bovine tuberculin as a consequence of exposure to other mycobacteria and those infected with *M. bovis* are distinguished from one another using the comparative

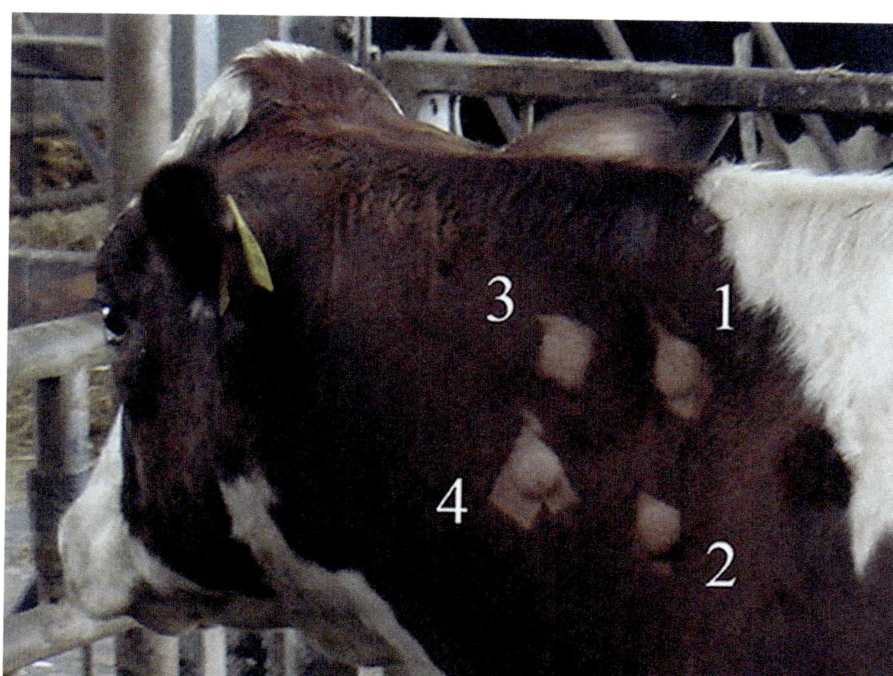

Fig. 15.4. Detection of swelling in delayed hypersensitivity test at the site of injection for 72 hours. (Author's own image.)

intradermal tuberculin test. The antigenic cross-reactivity between mycobacterial species and related taxa is responsible for this sensitization. Bovine and avian tuberculin are intradermally injected into separate locations, often on the same side of the neck, and the reaction is measured 3 days later.

Potency of tuberculins is measured in International Units (IU) and must be determined biologically by comparing them with standard tuberculins. If the estimated potency of bovine tuberculin ensures that each bovine dosage in cattle is at least 2000 IU (± 25%), then it is deemed appropriate in various countries. Doses of up to 5000 IU of bovine tuberculin are advised in national eradication efforts, and greater doses are required in calves with reduced allergic sensitivity. Every injectable dose's volume cannot be more than 0.2 millilitres.

15.3.2 Test procedure

Injection method

Using the right injection method is crucial. It is necessary to clean and trim the injection sites. Before injecting, the location is indicated and a skin fold within each clipped region is measured using callipers (Fig. 15.5). An obliquely inserted short needle with a bevel edge outwards and a graded syringe connected and charged with tuberculin is introduced into the deeper layers of the skin. After that, the tuberculin dosage is administered. It is acceptable to use a multiple injection gun or multiple dosage syringe as long as safety and volume delivery are guaranteed. An injection of tuberculin must include a minimum of 2000 IU of either bovine or avian tuberculin. At each injection location, feel for a little, pea-sized swelling to check that the injection was done correctly. The two injections should be spaced apart by around 12–15 cm. One injection must be administered on either side of the neck at the same locations in the middle third of the neck for young animals if there is not enough space to adequately divide the sites on one side of the neck. Seventy-two hours following injection, each injection site's skin-fold thickness is assessed again. The skin should be measured by the same person both before and after the test is read.

Evaluation

Several alternative approaches to evaluating the results of the skin test have been implemented

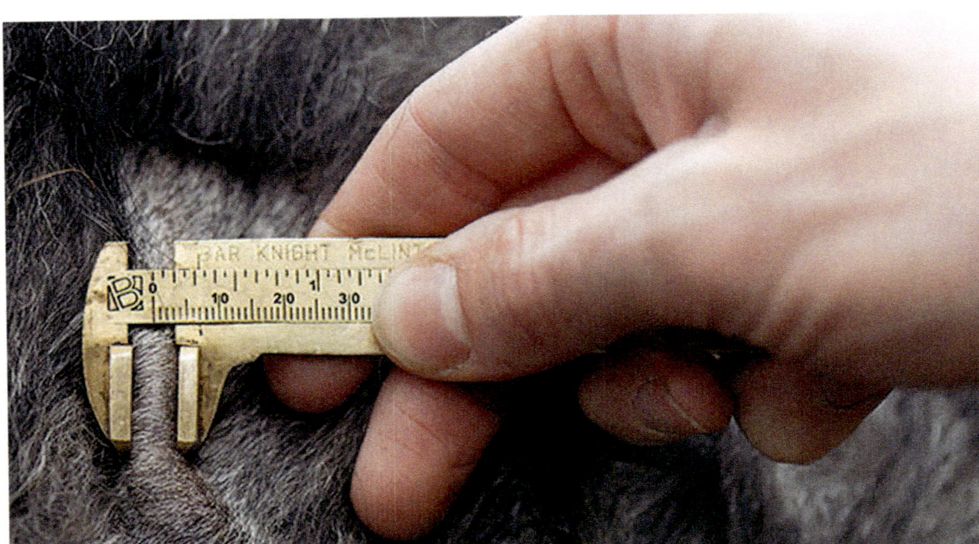

Fig. 15.5. Skin fold measurement with callipers. (Author's own image.)

in recognition of the possibility that local inflammation and other mycobacteria-induced sensitization might result in false-positive findings. It is critical to understand that sensitivity and specificity must coexist in balance, and that reaching high concurrent values might not be achievable. Policies should be implemented in accordance with risk and disease prevalence (e.g. when a wildlife reservoir is present). Based on observation and the observed increases in skin-fold thickness, an interpretation has been made. When a single injection of bovine tuberculin is required for the single intradermal test, the reaction is typically regarded as negative if there is only mild swelling that increases by no more than 2 mm and no clinical signs, such as diffuse or extensive oedema, exudation, necrosis, pain, or inflammation of the lymphatic ducts or lymph nodes in that area. If the increase in skin-fold thickness is greater than 2 mm but less than 4 mm, and none of these clinical indications are seen, the reaction is deemed inconclusive. If the above-mentioned clinical indications are seen, or if the skin-fold thickness increases by 4 mm or more, the reaction is deemed positive. Furthermore, any visible or palpable swelling in cattle infected with *M. bovis* should be interpreted as positive. A stricter interpretation is occasionally applied, especially when dealing with in-contact animals or populations at high danger. After 42 days, animals who test negative for a single intradermal test should undergo another test to enable desensitization to wear off (in certain places, 60 days are used for cattle and 120 days for deer). Animals should be considered positive for the test if they do not test negative for the second time. A blood test or a comparative intradermal test may be administered to animals that test positive for the single intradermal test. Every re-test ought to be conducted in compliance with the guidelines established by regional or national control programmes.

Interpretation

A reaction is often interpreted as positive in the intradermal comparative test if the rise in skin thickness at the injection location in the bovine is more than 4 mm larger than the reaction at the injection site in the avian. If there is a difference of less than 4 mm between the avian and bovine sites of injection in terms of skin thickness growth, the reaction is deemed inconclusive. If the rise in skin response at the avian injection site is equal to or less than the increase in skin thickness at the bovine injection site, the reaction is deemed negative. This interpretation scheme is based on Council Directive 64/432/EEC (EU, 1980) and is implemented in Member States of the European Union (EU). Occasionally, a stricter interpretation is used.

Caudal fold test

To perform the caudal fold test, a small needle with a bevel edge outwards is inserted obliquely into the skin's deeper layers on the fold's lateral aspect, halfway along it and halfway between the fold's ventral aspect and hairline. Any discernible or tangible change is generally understood to constitute a response. There is also a modified interpretation in use: any felt or visible swelling at the injection site with a 4 mm difference in caudal fold thickness from the opposite caudal fold is considered a positive test. If an animal has only one caudal fold, it is considered to be test-positive if the caudal fold thickness is 8 mm or more (Fig. 15.4).

15.4 Identification of the Agent

15.4.1 Blood-based laboratory test

Numerous blood tests have been employed in addition to the traditional intradermal tuberculin test (Haagsma, 1993). Laboratory-based assays are typically employed as additional tests to increase the identification of infected animals (parallel testing) or to validate or refute the results of an intradermal skin test (serial testing), due to their higher cost and more sophisticated nature. Additionally, there is evidence that an improved blood test can take place the week after an infected animal is skin tested. This improves the ability to distinguish between *in vitro* blood test answers, increasing test accuracy. Cellular immunity is measured by the interferon gamma test and

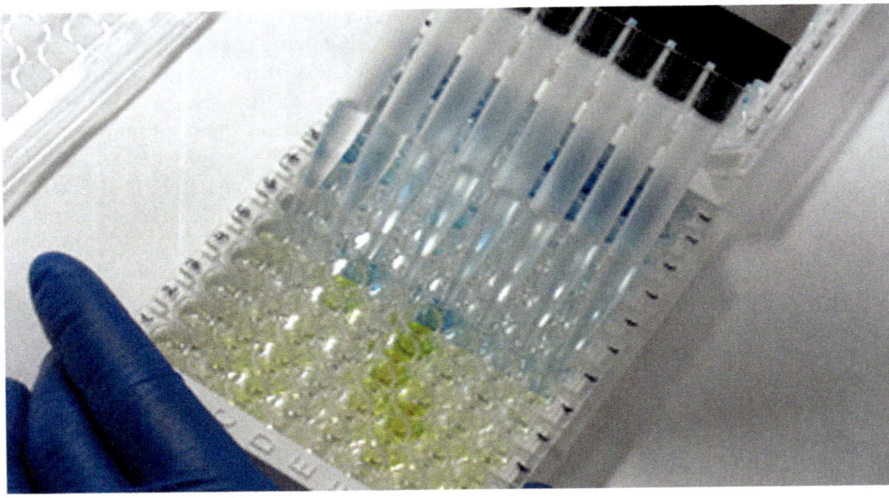

Fig. 15.6. IFN-gamma-bovine-tuberculosis. (Author's own image)

the lymphocyte proliferation assay; humoral immunity is measured by ELISA.

15.4.2 Interferon gamma assay

This test measures the release of interferon gamma (IFN-γ) from a lymphokine in a whole-blood culture system. The test relies on sensitized lymphocytes releasing IFN-γ after 16–24 hours of incubation with a particular antigen (PPD-tuberculin) (Wood *et al.*, 1990). The assay compares the production of IFN-γ from birds and cows after stimulation with PPD. Using two monoclonal antibodies to bovine interferon gamma, a sandwich ELISA is used to detect bovine IFN-γ (Fig. 15.6). As soon as feasible, but no later than the day following blood collection, the blood samples should be brought to the laboratory and the test set up (Ryan *et al.*, 2000; Coad *et al.*, 2007). Certain regions, particularly those where 'non-specificity' is common, have raised questions over the accuracy. However, the use of both tests in parallel allows for the detection of a larger number of infected animals before they become a source of infection for other animals or a source of environmental contamination, due to the early infection detection capability of the IFN-γ test (Gormley *et al.*, 2006). According to Buddle *et al.* (2001), the use of specified mycobacterial antigens like CFP-10 and ESAT six has promise for increased specificity. These antigens are used for serial testing in several nations, including the UK and New Zealand. Such antigens may also make it possible to distinguish between animals that have received the BCG (bacillus Calmette–Guérin) vaccination and those that have not. The IFN-γ test has an advantage over the skin test in situations when the animals are difficult or dangerous to handle, such as agitated cattle or other bovids, because only one catch is required. Several national programmes in the UK, Australia, New Zealand, the EU and the United States have authorized the use of the IFN-γ test. For example, the IFN-γ test is utilized for both parallel and serial testing in the UK and New Zealand to improve sensitivity and specificity, respectively. The test is offered as commercial kits for use on primates and bovine animals, but it has only been validated for a small number of these taxa.

15.4.3 Lymphocyte proliferation assay

The reactivity of peripheral blood cells to tuberculin PPD (PPD-B) and a PPD from *Mycobacterium avium* (PPD-A) is compared in this kind of *in vitro* experiment. The test may be run on isolated lymphocytes from peripheral blood samples (Griffin *et al.*, 1994) or whole blood (Buddle *et al.*, 2001). By eliminating the immune system's reaction to 'non-specific' or cross-reactive antigens linked to non-pathogenic mycobacteria species that the animal may have been exposed to, these techniques aim to improve the assay's specificity. The value acquired in reaction to PPD-B minus the value obtained in response to PPD-A is often used to evaluate the results. The B–A score therefore has to be higher than a variable cut-off point to enhance the sensitivity or specificity of the diagnosis. The assay has scientific merit, but it is rarely utilized for routine diagnosis since it takes a long time and needs difficult logistics and laboratory execution (it uses radioactive nucleotides and extended incubation durations). The lymphocyte proliferation assay should be carried out very soon after blood is drawn, much as the IFN-γ test. The examination could be helpful for zoo and wild animals. It has been found that a blood test combining ELISA and lymphocyte transformation assays has a high sensitivity and specificity for identifying *M. bovis* infection in deer (Griffin *et al.*, 1994). The test has not yet undergone interlaboratory comparisons and is somewhat costly.

15.4.4 Enzyme-linked immunosorbent assay

Several failed attempts have been made to create clinically relevant sero-diagnostic tests for TB. Of all the antibody-detection tests, the ELISA seems to be the most appropriate. It may be used in conjunction with cellular immunity tests rather than as a substitute for them. It could aid deer and livestock who are agitated. The ease of use of the ELISA is one of its benefits; nevertheless, its sensitivity is restricted mostly to cattle because of irregular and delayed humoral immune response development during the illness. When complex antigens like tuberculin or *M. bovis* culture filtrates are utilized on cattle, specificity is likewise low. Nonetheless, it has been demonstrated that comparing antibody levels to PPD-B and PPD-A might help to improve ELISA specificity (Griffin *et al.*, 1993). However, the antibody response in deer appears to develop more reliably and sooner, with reports of up to 85% sensitivity in a comparative ELISA (Griffin *et al.*, 1993). Combining several antigens, such as proteins (e.g. MPB70 and MPB83, which are specific yet insensitive), may improve the situation. Furthermore, it has been shown that an anamnestic increase occurs in *M. bovis*-infected animals, leading to improved ELISA findings 2–4 weeks following a standard tuberculin skin test (Lyashchenko *et al.*, 2004). The detection of *M. bovis* infections in wildlife may potentially benefit from the use of ELISA. For farmed deer in New Zealand, the ELISA test can be performed as an auxiliary parallel test 13–33 days following the mid-cervical skin test (Griffin *et al.*, 1994). Different forms for serum tests have also been created. For instance, it has been demonstrated that the lateral flow-based rapid test (TB StatPak) is effective in identifying tuberculous animals, especially in certain domestic animals, wildlife (Lyashchenko *et al.*, 2008), and zoo animals like South American camelids, badgers (Greenwald *et al.*, 2003), non-human primates, or elephants (Greenwald *et al.*, 2009), in which skin testing has been shown to be unreliable and where cellular immunity tests like the interferon gamma tests are unavailable. In cattle, nevertheless, its sensitivity is comparatively modest. This test is now licensed in the USA by the USDA for species such as elephants and non-human primates and is approved for use in the UK for badgers.

15.5 Requirements for Vaccine

Originally known as human and bovine tuberculins, respectively, tuberculin preparations were prepared from the heat-treated byproducts of the growth and lysis of *M. tuberculosis* or *M. bovis* cultured in glycerol broth. The 'old' tuberculins were superseded in the 1940s by 'heat-concentrated synthetic medium tuberculins', or HCSM tuberculins, which were made from cultures in a synthetic liquid medium. The old and HSCM tuberculins have been replaced, almost worldwide, by the purified protein derivatives or PPDs. Bovine PPDs prepared with the *M. bovis* production strain AN5 are more specific for detecting bovine tuberculosis than human PPDs prepared with *M. tuberculosis*.

Currently, the sole vaccination that can prevent *M. bovis* infections is the live, attenuated strain of *M. bovis* known as bacillus Calmette–Guérin, or BCG. According to Skinner *et al.* (2001), there have been inconsistent results with this vaccine's effectiveness in cow trials. This might be due to a number of factors, such as the vaccine's composition, the method of administration, and the degree of exposure to environmental mycobacteria. Many additional vaccines have been tested, but none have been shown to provide better protection against BCG. It has been demonstrated that BCG's effectiveness varies in a way that is comparable to human reports. Numerous novel vaccination candidates are presently being tested. The full genome sequences of *M. tuberculosis*, *M. bovis* and BCG (Pasteur) have been released, and in-depth studies of the genetic make-up of the tuberculosis organism are underway (Cole *et al.*, 1998; Brosch *et al.*, 2002; Garnier *et al.*, 2003). This might be especially helpful in finding virulence-associated genes and moving towards a subunit vaccination. BCG vaccination may be used to stop the spread of the virus in cattle in afflicted nations without testing or slaughter control programmes, but there is no conclusive evidence of a long-term decrease in prevalence or environmental and human safety. It is necessary to optimize the vaccination schedule for the local environment prior to starting a vaccination plan. A standard dosage would be subcutaneous delivery of 104–106 colony-forming units (CFUs). According to the WHO/FAO/OIE (1994), the vaccine should be based on the standard reference strain, either Danish or BCG Pasteur. It is critical to understand that using vaccines can affect immunological tests that rely on tuberculin as a diagnostic antigen, such as skin testing. Vaccinating cattle should thus not be done in countries that have trade or control policies based on these kinds of test. But a lot of work has gone into creating so-called Differentiating Infected from Vaccinated Animals (DIVA) antigens that enable BCG-vaccinated animals to be distinguished from *M. bovis*-infected animals, especially when the interferon gamma test is employed (Buddle *et al.*, 1999; Vordermeier *et al.*, 2001; Cockle *et al.*, 2006; Sidders *et al.*, 2008). These antigens are derived from *M. bovis* gene regions that are either not secreted by BCG (like Rv3615c) (Sidders *et al.*, 2008), under-expressed in some BCG strains (like MPB83), or deleted in BCG (like ESAT-6 and CFP-10) (Buddle *et al.*, 1999; Vordermeier *et al.*, 2001). It is also possible that, when these reagents have undergone complete validation and the relevant regulatory framework has been modified, BCG vaccination may be used in conjunction with such DIVA tests. Moreover, BCG vaccinations can stop *M. bovis* from spreading among wildlife reservoirs of infection. Validating the vaccine's delivery strategy for the specific animal species is crucial before utilizing it. It is also necessary to take into account how the vaccination may affect other animal species in the area.

15.6 Production of Tuberculin

15.6.1 Seed management

Characteristics of the seed

Strains of *M. bovis* used to prepare seed cultures must be identified to species level by appropriate tests. A record must be kept of their origins and subsequent history. Seed cultures must not be passaged more than five times. The production strains *M. bovis* AN5 or Vallee are the most commonly used.

Method of culture

The organism must be modified to develop as a floating culture if the original culture was grown on solid material (for example, by adding a sterile potato slice to the culture flasks containing liquid media, such Watson Reid's medium). The culture can be used to create the master seed lot, which is freeze-dried and conserved, once it has been converted to a liquid medium. This serves as the inoculation medium for the secondary seed lots, which can only be produced using a maximum of four culture passes from the master seed. Production cultures are inoculated with the secondary seed (Angus, 1978; Haagsma and Angus, 1994).

International standards

It must be demonstrated that the production culture substrate can provide a product that complies with internationally acknowledged standards (the WHO, European Pharmacopoeia, or other recognized control agencies). It has to be devoid of substances that are known to trigger allergic or harmful responses.

Validation

The strains of *M. bovis* used as seed cultures must be shown to be free from contaminating organisms. Seed lots must be shown to be efficacious in producing tuberculin with sufficient potency.

15.6.2 Method of manufacture

The organism is cultivated in a synthetic medium, after which the protein in the filtrate is chemically precipitated (TCA or ammonium sulfate are employed), washed and resuspended. Since PPD tuberculin may be more accurately standardized, it is advised.

An antimicrobial preservative (no more than 0.5% [w/v]) such as phenol may be added, which does not cause false-positive results. As a stabilizer, add 2.2% [w/v] of glucose or up to 10% [w/v] of glycerol. Utilizing mercurial derivatives is not advised. Additionally, the substance is aseptically distributed into sterile, neutral glass containers that are sealed to prevent contamination. The item might be dried in the freezer.

15.6.3 In-process control

After being inoculated from adequate seed cultures, the production flasks are given the proper amount of time to incubate. After autoclaving, any flasks exhibiting contamination or noticeably aberrant growth should be thrown away. The surface growth of many cultures becomes wet during incubation and has the potential to sink into the medium or to the flask's bottom. The so-called concentrated tuberculin, which is the dissolved precipitate in PPD tuberculins, should have a pH of 6.6–6.7.

Kjeldahl or another appropriate technique is used to determine the protein content of the PPD concentrate. It is common practice to compare total nitrogen and TCA precipitable nitrogen. The final product should be bioassayed in guinea pigs. Potency and specificity assays are carried out in comparison with a reference tuberculin (PPD). Further dilutions are made with a buffer according to the protein content and the required final concentration, usually 1.0mg/ml (Angus, 1978; Haagsma and Angus, 1994).

15.7 Tuberculin Batch Control

Samples should comply with the officially recognized standards for the production of tuberculin as set out in the European Pharmacopoeia or equivalent regulatory standards.

15.7.1 Sterility

Sterility testing is generally performed according to international guidelines.

15.7.2 Safety

Into two guinea pigs that weigh no less than 250g and have not had any prior treatment that might affect the test, 0.5 cc of the tuberculin under test is subcutaneously administered. Within 7 days, no unusual effects should manifest.

Testing for live mycobacteria in tuberculin can be done on samples extracted from the final containers or on the tuberculin itself right before it is distributed into those containers. At least two guinea pigs must receive an intraperitoneal injection of a minimum of 10 ml, with the dosage being divided between them. It is preferable to use a bigger sample – say, 50 ml – and concentrate any leftover mycobacteria using membrane filtering or centrifugation. Following at least 42 days of observation, the guinea pigs are inspected macroscopically at the post-mortem. Any lesions discovered are analysed both by culture and under a microscope.

15.7.3 Sensitizing effect

In order to assess the sensitizing effect, 500IU of the preparation under test in a 0.1 ml volume is intradermally injected three times into guinea pigs that have not previously received any treatment that would interfere with the test. Each guinea pig receives an intradermal injection of the same dosage of tuberculin 15–21 days following the third injection, along with three control guinea pigs that have not received an injection before. When tested 24–28 hour later, there should not be a substantial difference in reactions between the two groups of guinea pigs.

15.7.4 Potency

In guinea pigs sensitized to *M. bovis*, potency is assessed by comparison with a reference preparation of bovine tuberculin.

The European Economic Community acknowledged an EEC standard for bovine PPD in the 1960s. The drug was supplied in lyophilized form and had a strength of 50,000 provisional EEC tuberculin units per mg of PPD. Regretfully, there were not enough freeze-dried ampoules to meet WHO guidelines, thus a new preparation of bovine PPD was created so that it could be approved by the WHO as the new global standard for bovine PPD tuberculins.

It was necessary to calibrate the new bovine PPD standard against the current EEC standard. According to worldwide collaborative testing conducted on cattle and guinea pigs, the new bovine standard was shown to have a relative potency of 65% in comparison with the EEC standard. As a result, the WHO formally established 32,500 IU/mg as the worldwide standard for bovine PPD tuberculins in 1986. This indicates that the IUs and the temporary EEC tuberculin units are equipotent. The European Pharmacopoeia is acknowledged as the international standard for bovine PPD by the WHO.

It is desired that the countries where bovine PPD tuberculin is manufactured develop their own national reference preparations for bovine PPD as working standards in order to preserve the stock of the genuine international standard. It is imperative that these national reference preparations, for both guinea pigs and cattle, have been calibrated against the approved worldwide standard for bovine PPD (Maxild *et al.*, 1976; Schneider *et al.*, 1979; WHO, 1987).

15.7.5 Standardization of bovine tuberculin in guinea pigs

Five to seven weeks before the test, the guinea pigs are sensitized to a low dosage (e.g. 0.001 or 0.0001 mg wet weight) of live bacilli of a virulent strain of *M. bovis*. One millilitre is deeply injected intramuscularly into the medial side of the thigh after the bacilli are suspended in physiological saline. The low dose of *M. bovis* infection should have left the guinea pigs healthy at the time of the assay, and multiple post-mortem examinations performed soon after the standardization assays should demonstrate that the guinea pigs do not have open tuberculosis and are therefore not excreting tubercle bacilli.

For laboratories lacking isolation spaces for the safe housing of diseased guinea pigs, a different potency test that does not need live pathogenic mycobacteria can be employed. Regarding the welfare of the animals used in experiments, this alternative is also more practical. The procedure for this tuberculin potency test is as follows. Using an eight-point assay that consists of four dilutions that equate to roughly 20, 10, 5, or 2.5 IU, the PPD tuberculin is bio-assessed in homologous sensitized guinea pigs against the standard for bovine PPD tuberculin. There is 0.1 ml of injection volume. This assay uses a Latin square design, eight intradermal injections per animal, and compares two test tuberculins with standard tuberculin in eight guinea pigs. Inactivated *M. bovis* bacilli are used to sensitize the guinea pigs 5–7 weeks before the test. Freund's incomplete adjuvant is used to create an emulsion from the suspended bacilli in buffer. A 0.5 ml dosage is administered deeply intramuscularly on the medial side of the thigh.

The following is an appropriate potency assay. A six-point test consisting of three dilutions of each tuberculin at fivefold intervals is used to bioassay the generated PPD tuberculins in homologous sensitized guinea pigs against the standard for bovine PPD tuberculin. In an isotonic buffer solution containing 0.0005% (w/v) polysorbate 80 (Tween 80), the tuberculin preparations are diluted. The worldwide standard for PPD is 32, 6.4 and 1.28 IU, respectively. Volumes of 0.001, 0.0002 and 0.00004 mg tuberculoprotein, which correspond to these values, are selected because they produce well-readable skin responses within acceptable bounds. There is a 0.2 ml injection volume. Using a balanced incomplete Latin square design and eight intradermal injections per animal, two test tuberculins are compared with the standard tuberculin in a single experiment on nine guinea pigs (Finney, 1964).

Although a second reading can be carried out after 48 hour, the tests are normally examined 24 hour after the tuberculin injection. Using callipers, the various erythema diameters are measured in millimetres and noted on assay sheets. Finney (1964) stated that the data are statistically assessed using conventional statistical techniques for parallel-line tests. The slopes of the log dose–response curves for each preparation (increase in mean reaction per unit increase in log dose) and the F ratios for deviations from parallelism are used to compute the relative potencies of the two test tuberculins along with their 95% confidence limits.

The estimated strength of bovine tuberculins must be at least 66% and not more than 150% of the potency specified on the label, according to the European Pharmacopoeia.

15.7.6 Standardization of bovine tuberculin in cattle

Potency testing should be carried out in the animal species and in the circumstances in which the tuberculins will be used in practice, according to WHO Technical Report Series No. 384 (WHO, 1987). This implies that in naturally tuberculous cattle, bovine tuberculins should be tested. Since meeting this criterion is challenging, potency testing in guinea pigs is routinely carried out. However, standard preparations always need to be calibrated in cattle, and recurrent testing is required in tuberculous animals. If it is known that the standard preparations are indicative of the common problem tuberculins and that the production techniques provide consistency, then testing cattle less often is necessary.

The following is an appropriate potency assay for bovine tuberculins in cattle. Using two dilutions of each tuberculin spaced five times apart, the test tuberculins are tested using a four-point assay against a standard for bovine PPD tuberculin. Since these quantities correspond to around 3250 and 650IU if the international standard for bovine PPD turberculin is employed, 0.1 and 0.02 mg of tuberculoprotein are injected as part of the standard. The test tuberculins are diluted such that the same protein weights are used. The middle cervical region injection sites are spaced 15–20 cm apart, and the injection volume is 0.1 ml. Using a balanced full Latin square design and eight intradermal injections on both sides of the neck per animal, eight tuberculous cattle are used in one experiment to compare three test tuberculins with the standard tuberculin. As precisely as feasible, the thickness of the skin at the injection site is measured using callipers in tenths of a millimetre both before and 72 hour after the injection (Haagsma *et al.*, 1984).

The same industry-standard procedures for parallel-line assays used in the guinea-pig potency testing are used to statistically assess the results.

15.7.7 Specificity

An appropriate assay for determining specificity would be as follows. In heterologously sensitized guinea pigs, four-point assay consisting of two dilutions at 25-fold intervals of each tuberculin is used to assay three bovine test tuberculins against the standard for avian PPD tuberculin (or three avian test tuberculins against the standard for bovine PPD tuberculin). Test tuberculoprotein dosages of 0.03 mg and 0.0012 mg, or around 975 and 39 IU, were selected because they produce easily interpreted skin responses. The normal injectable dosages are 0.001 mg and 0.00004 mg, which are lower. Using a balanced full Latin square design and eight intradermal injections per animal, three test tuberculins are compared with the reference tuberculin in a single experiment. With the potency test, the interpretation of the findings and the statistical analysis are the same.

15.7.8 Stability

The tuberculins may be used until the expiration date indicated in the licence for tuberculin manufacturing, provided that they meet the legal requirements needed for production, are stored at a temperature of between 2°C and 8°C, and are shielded from light. It is advised to store PPD in a concentrated form rather than a diluted form for extended periods of time, and to store the concentrate in a dark, dry place.

15.7.9 pH control

The pH should be between pH 6.5 and 7.5.

15.7.10 Storage

Liquid bovine tuberculin should be kept at 5 ± 3°C and shielded from light throughout storage. The quality of the liquid product might be harmed by freezing. On the other hand, freeze-dried preparations can be made and kept at temperatures greater than 25°C as long as they are kept out of direct sunlight. Avoid spending too much time in the sun or at temperatures that are higher than normal.

15.7.11 Preservatives

Any additional ingredients or antimicrobial preservatives that could be added to a tuberculin product need to be demonstrated not to compromise the product's efficacy and safety.

The highest amount of phenol (0.5% w/v) and glycerol (10% v/v) that can be present is allowed.

15.7.12 Precautions (hazards)

It was discovered through experience with both people and animals that injecting intradermally with suitably diluted tuberculin causes a confined response at the injection site without causing widespread symptoms. Severe, widespread responses are exceedingly rare and restricted, even in highly sensitive individuals. However, past experiences have demonstrated that a hypersensitive operator may get severe, all-encompassing symptoms following inadvertent intradermal (needle stab) wound exposure to bovine tuberculin. It is advisable to caution these people against performing the skin test for tuberculin with a high dosage of 2000–5000 IU tuberculin, which is about 1000 times the human dose of 5 IU.

15.7.13 Test on the final product

A test for the absence of toxic or irritant properties must be carried out.

Biological techniques must be used to determine the potency of tuberculins. These procedures, which are based on comparing the tuberculins to be tested with a standard reference preparation of the same kind, are required for HCSM and PPD tuberculins.

15.8 Prevention and Control

In India, where tuberculosis is common and a sizeable percentage of animals are affected, test-and-kill policies are an efficient way to reduce the disease in cattle. It is possible to use test-and-segregation techniques to distinguish sick animals from healthy ones. Personnel handling and managing affected animals should be kept apart from those handling healthy, non-infected animals. Periodically re-testing affected herds is necessary to weed out livestock that could shed the bacterium.

Management practices, such as requiring animal handlers to be in good health and free of tuberculosis, refraining from nursing calves on tuberculous dams, disinfecting contaminated surfaces, feeding animals a balanced diet, etc. can stop the transmission of illness from infected animals to other vulnerable animals. The agent's ability to spread across the herd may be inhibited by sanitation and disinfection. *M. bovis* needs extended contact periods to become inactivated, since it is comparatively resistant to disinfectants. Disinfectants that work well include glutaraldehyde, formaldehyde, 5% phenol, and iodine solutions with high accessible iodine concentrations. 1% sodium hypochlorite applied over an extended period of time is also effective in situations containing modest amounts of organic waste. Furthermore, biosecurity protocols on farms reduce wildlife–domesticated animal encounters. The only vaccination against TB that is now available is the BCG vaccine, but in India we are unable to utilize this vaccine in our cattle due to the fact that it does not provide complete protection against tuberculosis sickness, and that vaccination will prevent skin tests for tuberculin from being conducted on animals. In the near future, we will need to create new, more effective vaccines in addition to developing new DIVAs, or diagnostic tests, that will allow us to distinguish between animals who are infected and those that have received vaccinations.

References

Angus, R.D. (1978) Production of reference PPD tuberculins for veterinary use in the United States. *Journal of Biological Standardization* 6, 221.

Animal Health Division (New Zealand) (1986) Possum research and cattle tuberculosis. *Surveillance* 13, 18–38.

Aranaz, A., Cousins, D., Mateos, A. and Dominiguez, L. (2003) Elevation of *Mycobacterium tuberculosis* subsp. caprae to species rank as *Mycobacterium caprae* comb. nov., sp. nov. *International Journal of Systematic and Evolutionary Microbiology* 53, 1785–1789.

Bengis, R.G., Kriek, N.P.J., Keet, D.F., Rath, J.P., De Vos, V. *et al.* (1996) An outbreak of tuberculosis in A free-living african buffalo (*Syncerus caffer*, sparrman) population in the Kruger National Park: A preliminary report. *Onderstepoort Journal of Veterinary Research* 63, 15.

Brosch, R., Godon, S.V., Marmiesse, M., Brodin, P., Buchrieser, C. *et al.* (2002) A new evolutionary scenario for the *Mycobacterium tuberculosis* complex. *Proceedings of the National Academy of Sciences USA* 99, 3684–3689.

Buddle, B.M., Parlane, N.A., Keen, D.L., Aldwell, F.E., Pollock, J.M. *et al.* (1999) Differentiation between *Mycobacterium bovis* BCG-vaccinated and *M. bovis*-infected cattle by using recombinant mycobacterial antigens. *Clinical and Diagnostic Laboratory Immunology* 6, 1–5.

Buddle, B.M., Ryan, T.J., Pollock, J.M., Anderson, P. and De Lisle, G.W. (2001) Use of ESAT-6 in the interferon- gamma test for diagnosis of bovine tuberculosis following skin testing. *Veterinary Microbiology* 80, 37–46.

Clifton-Hadley, R.S. and Wilesmith, J.W. (1991) Tuberculosis in deer: A review. *Veterinary Record* 129, 5–12.

Coad, M., Hewinson, R.G., Clifford, D., Vordermeier, H.M. and Whelan, A.O. (2007) Influence of skin testing and blood storage on interferon-gamma production in cattle affected naturally with *Mycobacterium bovis*. *Veterinary Record* 160, 660–662.

Cockle, P.J., Gordon, S.V., Hewinson, R.G. and Vordermeier, H.M. (2006) Field evaluation of a novel differential diagnostic reagent for detection of *Mycobacterium bovis* in cattle. *Clinical and Vaccine Immunology* 13, 1119–1124.

Cole, S.T., Brosch, R., Parkhill, J., Garnier, T., Churcher, C. *et al.* (1998) Deciphering the biology of *Mycobacterium tuberculosis* from the complete genome sequence. *Nature* 393, 537–544.

Corner, L.A.L. (2006) The role of wild animal populations in the epidemiology of tuberculosis in domestic animals: How to assess the risk. *Veterinary Microbiology* 112, 303–312.

Cousins, D.V. (2001) *Mycobacterium bovis* infection and control in domestic livestock. *Revue Scientifique et technique. Office international des épizooties* 20, 71–85.

Cousins, D.V. and Florisson, N. (2005) A review of tests available for use in the diagnosis of tuberculosis in non-bovine species. *Revue scientifique et technique. Office international des épizooties* 24, 1039–1059.

Cousins, D.V., Bastida, R., Cataldi, A., Quse, V., Redrobe, S. *et al.* (2003) Tuberculosis in seals caused by a novel member of the *Mycobacterium tuberculosis* complex: *Mycobacterium pinnipedii* sp. nov. *International Journal of Systematic and Evolutionary Microbiology* 53, 1305–1314.

Cousins, D.V., Francis, B.R. and Gow, B.L. (1989) Advantages of a new agar medium in the primary isolation of *Mycobacterium bovis*. *Veterinary Microbiology* 20, 89–95.

Cousins, D.V., Skuce, R.A., Kazwala, R.R. and Van Embden, J.D.A. (1998) Towards a standardized approach to DNA fingerprinting of *Mycobacterium bovis*. *International Journal of Tuberculosis and Lung Disease* 2, 471–478.

De Lisle, G.W., Mackintosh, C.G. and Bengis, R.G. (2001) *Mycobacterium bovis* in free-living and captive wildlife, including farmed deer. *Revue scientifique et technique. Office international des épizooties* 20, 86–111.

Durr, P.A., Clifton-Hadley, R.S. and Hewinson, R.G. (2000a) Molecular epidemiology of bovine tuberculosis II. Applications of genotyping. *Revue scientifique et technique. Office international des épizooties* 19, 689–701.

Durr, P.A., Hewinson, R.G. and Clifton-Hadley, R.S. (2000b) Molecular epidemiology of bovine tuberculosis. I. *Mycobacterium bovis* genotyping. *Revue scientifique et technique. Office international des épizooties* 19, 675–688.

Espinos de los Monteros, L.E., Galan, J.C., Gutierrez, M., Samper, S., Garcia Marin, J.F. *et al.* (1998) Allele-specific PCR method based on *pncA* and *oxyR* sequences for distinguishing *Mycobacterium bovis* from *M. tuberculosis: Intraspecific M. bovis pncA sequence polymorphism*. *Journal of Clinical Microbiology* 36, 239–242.

European Union (1980) Council Directive 80/219, amending Directive 64/432, Annex B.

Finney, D.J. (1964) *Statistical Methods in Biological Assays*, 2nd edn. Charles Griffin, London.

Frothingham, R. and Meeker-O'Connell, W.A. (1998) Genetic diversity in the *Mycobacterium tuberculosis* complex based on variable numbers of tandem DNA repeats. *Microbiology* 144, 1189–1196.

Garnier, T., Eiglmeier, K., Camus, J.C., Medina, N., Mansoor, H. *et al.* (2003) The complete genome sequence of *Mycobacterium bovis*. *Proceedings of the National Academy of Sciences USA* 100, 7877–7882.

Gormley, E., Doyle, M.B., Fitzsimons, T., McGill, K. and Collins, J.D. (2006) Diagnosis of *Mycobacterium bovis* infection in cattle by use of the gamma-interferon (Bovigam) assay. *Veterinary Microbiology* 112, 171–179.

Greenwald, R., Esfandiari, J., Lesellier, S., Houghton, R., Pollock, J. *et al.* (2003) Improved serodetection of *Mycobacterium bovis* infection in badgers (*Meles meles*) using multiantigen test formats. *Diagnostic Microbiology and Infectious Disease* 46, 197–203.

Greenwald, R., Lyashchenko, O., Esfandiari, J., Miller, M., Mikota, S. *et al.* (2009) Highly accurate antibody assays for early and rapid detection of tuberculosis in African and Asian elephants. *Clinical and Vaccine Immunology* 16, 605–612.

Griffin, J.F.T., Hesketh, J.B., Mackintosh, C.G., Shi, Y.E. and Buchan, G.S. (1993) BCG vaccination in deer: Distinctions between delayed type hypersensitivity and laboratory parameters of immunity. *Immunology & Cell Biology* 71, 559–570.

Griffin, J.F.T., Cross, J.P., Chinn, D.N., Rogers, C.R. and Buchan, G.S. (1994) Diagnosis of tuberculosis due to *Mycobacterium bovis* in New Zealand red deer (*Cervus elaphus*) using a composite blood test (BTB) and antibody (ELISA) assays. *New Zealand Veterinary Journal* 42, 173–179.

Haagsma, J. (1993) *Working Paper on Recent Advances in the Field of Tuberculosis Control and Research*. World Health Organization Meeting on Zoonotic Tuberculosis with Particular Reference to *Mycobacterium bovis*, 15 November 1993, Geneva, Switzerland.

Haagsma, J. and Angus, R.D. (1994) Tuberculin production. In: Steele, J.H. and Thoen, C.O. (eds) *Mycobacterium bovis Infections in Humans and Animals*. Iowa State University Press, Ames, Iowa, USA.

Haagsma, J., O'Reilly, L.M., Dobbelaar, R. and Murphy, T.M. (1984) A comparison of the relative potencies of various bovine PPD tuberculins in naturally infected tuberculous cattle. *Journal of Biological Standardization* 10, 273.

Heifets, L.B. and Jenkins, P.A. (1998) Speciation of *Mycobacterium* in clinical laboratories. In: Gangadharam, P.R. and Jenkins, P.A. (eds) *Mycobacteria I. Basic Aspects*. Chapman and Hall, New York, USA, pp. 308–350.

Huard, R.C., De Oliveira Lazzarini, L.C., Butler, W.R., Van Soolingen, D. and Ho, J.L. (2003) PCR-based method to differentiate the subspecies of the *Mycobacterium tuberculosis* complex on the basis of genomic deletions. *Journal of Clinical Microbiology* 41, 1637–1650.

Kamerbeek, J., Schouls, L., Kolk, A., Van Agterveld, M., Van Soolingen, D. *et al.* (1997) Simultaneous detection and strain differentiation of *Mycobacterium tuberculosis* for diagnosis and epidemiology. *Journal of Clinical Microbiology* 35, 907–914.

Lyashchenko, K., Whelan, A.O., Greenwald, R., Pollock, J.M., Andersen, P. *et al.* (2004) Association of tuberculin-boosted antibody responses with pathology and cell-mediated immunity in cattle vaccinated with *Mycobacterium bovis* BCG and infected with *M. bovis*. *Infection and Immunity* 72, 2462–2467.

Lyashchenko, K.P., Greenwald, R., Esfandiari, J., Chambers, M.A., Vicente, J. *et al.* (2008) Animal-side serologic assay for rapid detection of *Mycobacterium bovis* infection in multiple species of free-ranging wildlife. *Veterinary Microbiology* 132, 283–292.

Maxild, J., Bentzon, M.W., Moller, S. and Zachariassen, P. (1976) Assays of different tuberculin products performed in guinea pigs. *Journal of Biological Standardization* 4, 171.

Miller, J., Jenny, A., Rhgyan, J., Saari, D. and Saurez, D. (1997) Detection of *Mycobacterium bovis* in formalin-fixed, paraffin-embedded tissues of cattle and elk by PCR amplification of an IS6110 sequence specific for *M. tuberculosis* complex organisms. *Journal of Veterinary Diagnostic Investigation* 9, 244–249.

Miller, J.M., Jenny, A.L. and Payeur, J.B. (2002) Polymerase chain reaction detection of *Mycobacterium tuberculosis* complex and *Mycobacterium avium* organisms in formalin-fixed tissues from culture-negative organisms. *Veterinary Microbiology* 87, 15–23.

Morris, R.S., Pfeiffer, D.U. and Jackson, R. (1994) The epidemiology of *Mycobacterium bovis* infections. *Veterinary Microbiology* 40, 153–157.

Naranjo, V., Gortazar, C., Vicente, J. and De La Fuente, J. (2008) Evidence of the role of European wild boar as a reservoir of *Mycobacterium tuberculosis* complex. *Veterinary Microbiology* 127, 1–9.

Niemann, S., Harmsen, D., Rusch-Gerdes, S. and Richter, E. (2000) Differentiation of clinical *Mycobacterium tuberculosis* complex isolates by gyrB DNA sequence polymorphism analysis. *Journal of Clinical Microbiology* 38, 3231–3234.

Noredhoek, G.T., Van Embden, J.D.A. and Kolk, A.H.J. (1996) Reliability of nucleic acid amplification for detection of *Mycobacterium tuberculosis*: An international collaborative quality control study among 30 laboratories. *Journal of Clinical Microbiology* 34, 2522–2525.

O'Brian, R., Danilowicz, B.S., Bailey, L., Flynn, O., Costello, E. *et al.* (2000) Characterisation of the *Mycobacterium bovis* restriction fragment length polymorphism DNA probe pUCD and performance comparison with standard methods. *Journal of Clinical Microbiology* 38, 3362–3369.

O'Reilly, L.M. and Daborn, C.J. (1995) The epidemiology of *Mycobacterium bovis* infections in animals and man: A review. *Tubercle and Lung Disease* 76(Suppl. 1), 1–46.

Parsons, L.M., Brosch, R., Cole, S.T., Somoskovi, A., Loder, A. *et al.* (2002) Rapid and simple approach for identification of *Mycobacterium tuberculosis* complex isolates by PCR-based genomic deletion analysis. *Journal of Clinical Microbiology* 40, 2339–2345.

Prodinger, W.M., Brandstatter, A., Naumann, L., Pacciarini, M., Kubica, T. *et al.* (2005) Characterization of *Mycobacterium caprae* isolates from Europe by mycobacterial interspersed repetitive unit genotyping. *Journal of Clinical Microbiology* 43, 4984–4992.

Ryan, T.J., Buddle, B.M. and De Lisle, G.W. (2000) An evaluation of the gamma interferon test for detecting bovine tuberculosis in cattle 8 to 28 days after tuberculin skin testing. *Research in Veterinary Science* 69, 57–61.

Schneider, W., Dobbelaer, R., Dam, A., Jorgensen, J.B., Gayot, G. *et al.* (1979) Collaborative assay of EEC standards for bovine tuberculins. *Journal of Biological Standardization* 7, 53.

Sidders, B., Pirson, C., Hogarth, P.J., Hewinson, R.G., Stoker, N.G. *et al.* (2008) Screening of highly expressed mycobacterial genes identifies Rv3615c as a useful differential diagnostic antigen for the *Mycobacterium tuberculosis* complex. *Infection and Immunity* 76, 3932–3939.

Skinner, M.A., Wedlock, D.N. and Buddle, B.M. (2001) Vaccination of animals against *Mycobacterium bovis*. *Revue scientifique et techniques. Office international des épizooties* 20, 112–132.

Skuce, R.A., Brittain, D., Hughes, M.S. and Neill, S.D. (1996) Differentiation of *Mycobacterium bovis* isolates from animals by DNA typing. *Journal of Clinical Microbiology* 38, 2469–2474.

Supply, P., Mazars, E., Lesjean, S., Vincent, V., Gicquel, B. *et al.* (2000) Variable human minisatellite-like regions in the *Mycobacterium tuberculosis* genome. *Molecular Microbiology* 36, 762–771.

Vordermeier, H.M., Whelan, A., Cockle, P.J., Farrant, L., Palmer, N. *et al.* (2001) Use of synthetic peptides derived from the antigens ESAT-6 and CFP-10 for differential diagnosis of bovine tuberculosis in cattle. *Clinical and Diagnostic Laboratory Immunology* 8, 571–578.

WHO (1987) Requirements for Biological Substances no.16, Annex 1: Requirements for Tuberculins. Technical Report Series no.745. World Health Organization, Geneva, Switzerland, 31-59.

WHO/FAO/OIE (World Health Organization/Food and Agriculture Organization of the United Nations/ Office International Des Epizooties (1994) *Report on Consultation on Animal Tuberculosis Vaccines*. WHO/CDS/VPH/94.138. Geneva: WHO Veterinary Public Health Unit.

Wilesmith, J.W. (1991) Epidemiological methods for investigating wild animal reservoirs of animal disease. *Revue scientifique et techniques. Office international des épizooties* 10, 205–214.

Wood, P.R., Corner, L.A. and Plackett, P. (1990) Development of a simple, rapid *in vitro* cellular assay for bovine tuberculosis based on the production of gamma interferon. *Research in Veterinary Science* 49, 46–49.

16 Methicillin-resistant *Staphylococcus aureus*

Aliyu Mohammad Bashir*
Department of Veterinary Public Health and Preventive Medicine, Faculty of Veterinary Medicine, Ahmadu Bello University, Zaria, Nigeria

Abstract
Methicillin-resistant *Staphylococcus aureus* (MRSA) is an opportunistic human pathogen, basically associated with invasive as well as life-threatening infections. The bacteria threaten both human and animal health, due to development of resistance to various antibiotics. MRSA can transmit across host-species barriers through direct contact, the environment, or the food chain. Goats are generally considered as agricultural animals and are used as an important source of milk and meat. Goat mastitis can cause significant economic losses due to the reduced quality, as well as quantity, of milk, and a source of infection from slaughter of the animal to food consumption. The economic loss in relation to mastitis in goats is further exacerbated by antibiotic resistance, making it harder to treat the goats. MRSA isolates were generally transmitted to goats from the farm environment or vice versa. The emergence of livestock-associated MRSA is a global threat to human health due to antibiotic resistance. Livestock workers may transmit the disease to their household members. The appropriate preventive measures should be taken to counteract the antibiotic resistance as well as infection of MRSA.

Keywords: methicillin-resistant *Staphylococcus aureus*, global threat, immunocompromised, antibiotic resistance, zoonosis

16.1 Introduction

Staphylococcus aureus is a round-shaped, Gram-positive, non-motile bacterium that does not form spores. The organism can function as a commensal bacterium, sometimes as a facultative pathogen that can survive different antimicrobials (Fig. 16.1).

There are certain variants of *S. aureus* that are methicillin-resistant and have been shown to have a global occurrence, especially at livestock farms, within communities and in health facilities (Crespo-Piazuelo and Lawlor, 2021).

Methicillin resistance of *S. aureus* is mostly associated with the mecA gene, which usually results in resistance to all beta-lactam antibiotics. It has been established that the mecA gene originated from staphylococcal species found in animals and has moved to other staphylococci species through the SCCmec mobile genetic element (Turner *et al.*, 2019).

Contact with infected animals has been shown to be a major risk factor for the emergence, dissemination, and colonization of MRSA in humans. MRSA has the ability to colonize several animal species, hence resistance to antimicrobials can move from one species to

*Corresponding author: mailaliyu@gmail.com

DOI: 10.1079/ 9781800622852.0016

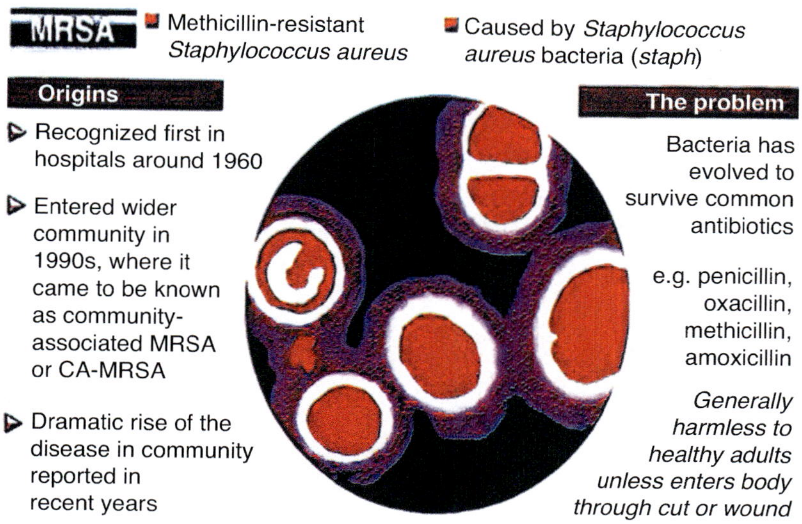

Fig. 16.1. A summary of methicillin-resistant *Staphylococcus aureus*. (Author's own image.)

another. Pets and livestock animals are of most concern due to the high usage of antimicrobials among these animals and their high frequency of contact with humans, so there is a risk to the animals of acquiring MRSA from colonized humans.

MRSA has been categorized into three major groups based on the origins: livestock-associated MRSA (LA-MRSA), healthcare-associated MRSA (HA-MRSA) and community-associated MRSA (CA-MRSA) (Dweba *et al.*, 2018).

In humans, MRSA causes infectious diseases such as otitis media, pyogenic endocarditis, osteomyelitis, food poisoning, suppurative pneumonia, etc. MRSA could cause a localized purulent infection and botryomycosis in horses; localized pyogenic infection and severe acute mastitis, caseous lymphadenitis in ruminants; pustular dermatitis and food poisoning in cats and dogs; exudative epidermatitis in pigs; and bumble-foot in birds (Algammal *et al.*, 2020).

16.2 MRSA in Goats

Generally, *S. aureus* causes diseases ranging from mild skin infection to invasive systemic infection. MRSA was initially referred to as a disease of humans until udder infection in cows caused by MRSA was reported in the late 1990s (Udoh *et al.*, 2019). Over the years, there has been a consistent increase in MRSA infection in small ruminants and cattle. Hence, LA-MRSA is an emerging zoonosis that causes infection among farm animals, farm personnel and also consumers of farm produce along the food chain and distribution (Papadopoulos *et al.*, 2018). LA-MRSA in goats has been reported to be mostly associated with dairy goats, hence the primary cause of mastitis in these dairy farms (Fig. 16.2). The presence of MRSA in these dairy farms usually results in the colonization of farm personnel and contamination of the environment. The colonization is due to the ability of cross-transmission of LA-MRSA to occur between the goat, the environment and humans (El-Deeb *et al.*, 2022).

16.3 Epidemiology/Prevalence

There is a global distribution of MRSA, and world surveillance has reported it as a major concern, hence the urgent need for a global molecular epidemiological study (Kumar *et al.*, 2021). LA-MRSA includes major *S. aureus* and other staphylococci species found in livestock and has been reported in virtually every country of the world (Butaye *et al.*, 2016).

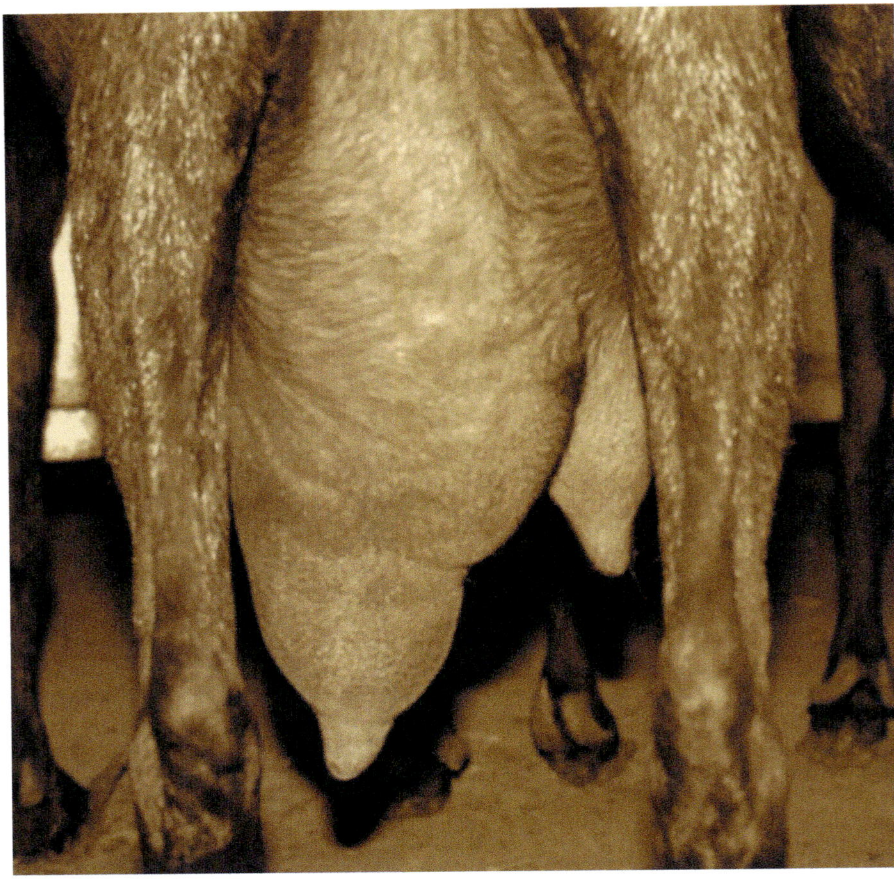

Fig. 16.2. A case of mastitis in a Kano brown goat. (Author's own image.)

However, there were reports of not detecting MRSA in goat farms in Sweden, despite earlier reports of MRSA in both animals and humans, thus indicating the absence of dissemination of MRSA in the Swedish dairy goat herds (Persson *et al.*, 2021).

The occurrence of LA-MRSA among apparently healthy goats and goats with subclinical mastitis plays a vital role in the epidemiology of the disease, making them serve as reservoirs for human infection. Previous studies have indicated genetic similarities among MRSA isolated from goats and the farm environment. Analysis of molecular genotypes and plasmids suggested that the isolates originated from humans where they also manifest multiple drug resistance (El-Deeb *et al.*, 2022).

16.4 Transmission

MRSA in goats can be transmitted from one animal to another, involving interspecies and intraspecies transmission. The transmission also occurs between the animal and the environment, because a study established MRSA isolates in goats that were identical to isolates from the environment.

Asymptomatic colonization with MRSA, including both nasal and rectal carriage, has been reported in animals and the organism can colonize more than one site. Carrier animals may serve as a reservoir for disease in themselves and may transmit MRSA to other animals or people.

The spread of MRSA among farm animals and humans is aided by the presence of some apparently healthy animals which can serve as a reservoir for the distribution of the MRSA (Abdel-Moein and Zaher, 2019).

To better understand the transmission and spread of MRSA between goats, humans and the environment, there is a need for more DNA sequence studies using a One Health approach (Venkatvasan *et al.*, 2020).

16.5 Risk Factors

A major risk factor for MRSA is individuals who are in close contact with animals, especially animals that are positive for MRSA. This usually leads to the individuals being colonized by LA-MRSA (Sergelidis and Angelidis, 2017).

Another important risk factor is the ability of goats to serve as reservoirs of MRSA, and the bacterium can be transmitted to humans in close contact with MRSA-colonized goats. People in direct contact with MRSA-positive animals have a high probability of becoming MRSA-positive. Such risks have also been established for individuals working with companion animals, or in equine clinics and livestock production environments.

16.6 Public Health and Economic Significance

MRSA in goats usually occurs as mastitis, rendering a great loss, especially for dairy goats. *S. aureus* has been established as a major cause of mastitis in goats (McDougall *et al.*, 2014). Mastitis in dairy goats (Fig. 16.3) causes great economic losses resulting from low milk yield and poor-quality milk (Novac and Andrei, 2020). Another aspect of the economic losses is antibiotic resistance, because most farmers usually make efforts to exhaust all available antibiotics to treat mastitis.

LA-MRSA has created public health concerns due to its role as a source of antimicrobial-resistant bacteria, which can be transmitted to humans.

S. aureus is not only a mastitis-causing organism, but also its role in the possible transmission of MRSA from goats to humans contributes to significant public health importance (Udoh *et al.*, 2019).

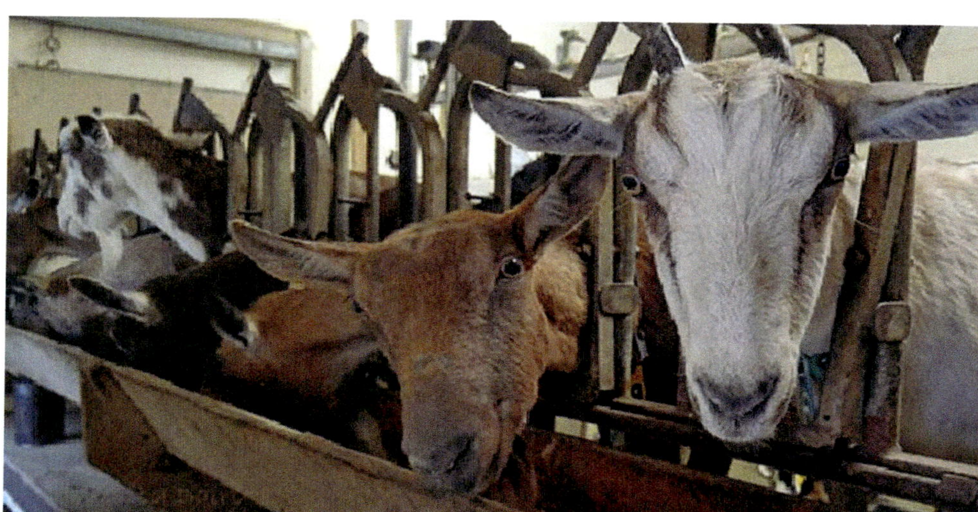

Fig. 16.3. A section of a dairy goat farm. (Author's own image.)

MRSA isolated from goats has shown phenotypic resistance to multiple antibiotics such as trimethoprim-sulfamethoxazole, which is used for decolonization patients with MRSA, leading to a reduction of treatment options for humans and animals (El-Deeb *et al*., 2022).

The increasing resistance of *S. aureus* to multiple antibiotics and the burden of MRSA significantly impact the economy, public health and livestock farming.

16.7 Prevention and Control

The high prevalence of MRSA among small ruminants calls for concern regarding their roles as reservoirs and the need for control and prevention (Ali *et al*., 2017). The occurrence in apparently healthy animals makes them serve as the linkage to humans. Hence, there is a need to implement a holistic approach to whole-genome sequencing surveillance in livestock and farm environments, so as to better establish the transmission of methicillin-resistant staphylococci and to design hygienic and control measures that can adequately break the transmission cycle (El-Deeb *et al*., 2022). It is also recommended that unnecessary contact with MRSA-positive goats should be avoided.

Because MRSA is transmitted from goats to humans via contact and consumption of undercooked meat, there is a need for frequent microbiological surveillance in goat farms and abattoirs, so as to determine the virulent and drug-resistant *S. aureus* and to implement preventive measures (Mechesso *et al*., 2021).

References

Abdel-Moein, K.A. and Zaher, H.M. (2019) Occurrence of multidrug-resistant methicillin-resistant *Staphylococcus aureus* among healthy farm animals: A public health concern. *International Journal of Veterinary Science and Medicine* 7(1), 55–60. DOI: 10.1080/23144599.2019.1689630.

Algammal, A., Hetta, H.F., Elkelish, A., Alkhalifah, D., Hozzein, W. *et al*. (2020) Methicillin-resistant *Staphylococcus aureus* (MRSA): One health perspective approach to the bacterium epidemiology, virulence factors, antibiotic-resistance, and zoonotic impact. *Infection and Drug Resistance* 13, 3255–3265. DOI: 10.2147/IDR.S272733.

Ali, A.A., Basha, O.A. and Ibrahim, M.S. (2017) Incidence of methicillin-resistant *Staphylococcus aureus* isolation from sheep and goat. *Alexandria Journal of Veterinary Sciences* 54, 142–148. DOI: 10.5455/ajvs.244291.

Butaye, P., Argudín, M.A. and Smith, T.C. (2016) Livestock-associated MRSA and its current evolution. *Current Clinical Microbiology Reports* 3(1), 19–31. DOI: 10.1007/S40588-016-0031-9.

Crespo-Piazuelo, D. and Lawlor, P.G. (2021) Livestock-associated methicillin-resistant *Staphylococcus aureus* (LA-MRSA) prevalence in humans in close contact with animals and measures to reduce on-farm colonisation. *Irish Veterinary Journal* 74(1), 1–12. DOI: 10.1186/S13620-021-00200-7.

Dweba, C.C., Zishiri, O.T. and El Zowalaty, M.E. (2018) Methicillin-resistant *Staphylococcus aureus*: Livestock-associated, antimicrobial, and heavy metal resistance. *Infection and Drug Resistance* 11, 2497–2509. DOI: 10.2147/IDR.S175967.

El-Deeb, W., Cave, R., Fayez, M., Alhumam, N., Quadri, S. *et al*. (2022) Methicillin resistant staphylococci isolated from goats and their farm environments in Saudi Arabia genotypically linked to known human clinical isolates: A pilot study. *Microbiology Spectrum* 10(4), e0038722. DOI: 10.1128/spectrum.00387-22.

Kumar, S., Anwer, R., Yadav, M., Sehrawat, N., Singh, M. *et al*. (2021) Molecular typing and global epidemiology of *Staphylococcus aureus*. *Current Pharmacology Reports* 7(5), 179–186. DOI: 10.1007/s40495-021-00264-7.

McDougall, S., Malcolm, D. and Prosser, C.G. (2014) Prevalence and incidence of intramammary infections in lactating dairy goats. *New Zealand Veterinary Journal* 62(3), 136–145. DOI: 10.1080/00480169.2013.865294.

Mechesso, A.F., Moon, D.C., Ryoo, G.S., Song, H.J., Chung, H.Y. *et al*. (2021) Resistance profiling and molecular characterization of *Staphylococcus aureus* isolated from goats in Korea. *International Journal of Food Microbiology* 336, 108901. DOI: 10.1016/j.ijfoodmicro.2020.108901.

Novac, C.S. and Andrei, S. (2020) The impact of mastitis on the biochemical parameters, oxidative and nitrosative stress markers in goat's milk: A review. *Pathogens* 9(11), 772. DOI: 10.3390/pathogens91110882.

Papadopoulos, P., Papadopoulos, T., Angelidis, A.S., Boukouvala, E., Zdragas, A. *et al.* (2018) Prevalence of *Staphylococcus aureus* and of methicillin-resistant *S. aureus* (MRSA) along the production chain of dairy products in North-Western Greece. *Food Microbiology* 69, 43–50. DOI: 10.1016/j.fm.2017.07.016.

Persson, Y., Börjesson, S., Myrenås, M. and Pedersen, K. (2021) No detection of methicillin-resistant *Staphylococcus aureus* in dairy goats. *Dairy* 2(1), 65–70. DOI: 10.3390/dairy2010005.

Sergelidis, D. and Angelidis, A.S. (2017) Methicillin-resistant *Staphylococcus aureus*: A controversial food-borne pathogen. *Letters in Applied Microbiology* 64(6), 409–418. DOI: 10.1111/LAM.12735.

Turner, N.A., Sharma-Kuinkel, B.K., Maskrinec, S.A., Eichenberger, E.M., Shah, P.P. *et al.* (2019) Methicillin-resistant *Staphylococcus aureus*: An overview of basic and clinical research. *Nature Reviews Microbiology* 17(4), 203–218. DOI: 10.1038/s41579-018-0147-4.

Udoh, E.K., Kwaga, J., Umoh, J. and Abiola, R.M. (2019) Occurrence of mastitis and methicillin resistant *Staphylococcus aureus* in goats in Zaria, Kaduna state, Nigeria. *Nigerian Veterinary Journal* 40(2), 164–177. DOI: 10.4314/nvj.v40i2.8.

Venkatvasan, R., Antony, P.X., Mukhopadhyay, H.K., Jayalakshmi, V., Srinivas, V.M.V. *et al.* (2020) Characterization of methicillin-resistant *Staphylococcus aureus* from goats and their relationship to goat handlers using Multi-Locus Sequence Typing (MLST). *Small Ruminant Research* 186, 106097. DOI: 10.1016/J.SMALLRUMRES.2020.106097.

17 Salmonellosis

Md. Saiful Islam and Md. Tanvir Rahman*
Department of Microbiology and Hygiene, Faculty of Veterinary Science, Bangladesh Agricultural University, Mymensingh, Bangladesh

Abstract
Salmonellosis is a bacterial infection caused by *Salmonella* species and is one of the most common causes of diarrhoea in small ruminants, including goats. This chapter focuses on the issue of salmonellosis in goats and its impact on both animal and human health. The chapter provides an overview of the epidemiology of salmonellosis in goats, including the risk factors and modes of transmission of the bacteria. The impact of salmonellosis on goat health is also discussed, including the symptoms and treatment options for infected goats. The zoonotic significance of goat salmonellosis, which refers to the potential for the bacteria to be transmitted from infected animals to humans, is also explored. The chapter concludes by highlighting the importance of implementing effective measures to prevent and control salmonellosis in goats, including proper hygiene practices and the use of vaccines, as well as the need for ongoing surveillance and research to better understand this important issue.

Keywords: salmonellosis, goat, zoonoses, public health, epidemiology, risk factors, prevention and control

17.1 Introduction

Multiple infectious diseases arise and spread due to the interplay between humans, animals and their environments (Rahman *et al.*, 2020). Animals are the source of newly emerging diseases in humans, and consuming goods from animals is directly linked to the spread of these diseases. Most of the emerging zoonotic diseases originated from animals. A zoonosis is a disease or infection that can spread from animals to humans or vice versa. Salmonellosis, caused by *Salmonella* species, is widely recognized as one of the deadliest zoonotic illnesses. About 1.5 billion individuals are infected with *Salmonella* bacteria every year, making it a major public health concern worldwide (Talukder *et al.*, 2021). This disease can affect both humans and animals, including goats. The disease is characterized by inflammation of the intestinal tract and can result in severe symptoms, including fever, diarrhoea and vomiting (Tawyabur *et al.*, 2020). Goats are susceptible to a variety of *Salmonella* species and the disease can have a significant impact on goat health and production. The symptoms of salmonellosis in goats can range from mild to severe and may lead to significant economic losses for farmers and producers (Bedaso *et al.*, 2015). Understanding the causes, transmission, diagnosis and prevention of salmonellosis in goats is important for the health and welfare of the animals and the protection of public health. The disease can be easily transmitted to humans, making it essential to take appropriate measures to control its spread. This chapter provides a comprehensive overview

*Corresponding author: tanvirahman@bau.edu.bd

DOI: 10.1079/ 9781800622852.0017

of salmonellosis in goats, including the latest research findings and practical information for goat farmers and veterinarians.

17.2 Classification of *Salmonella* Species

Salmonella is a genus of Gram-negative, facultative anaerobic, rod-shaped bacteria that are widely distributed in the animal kingdom, including humans. The genus was named after Daniel Elmer Salmon (1850–1914), an American veterinarian and pathologist (Monte and Sellera, 2020). *Salmonella* is one of the most important genera of foodborne pathogens, causing a wide range of diseases, ranging from gastroenteritis to invasive infections such as sepsis and meningitis. The genus *Salmonella* is a member of the family *Enterobacteriaceae*, which includes many other medically important genera such as *Escherichia*, *Shigella*, *Klebsiella* and *Yersinia* (Dekker and Frank, 2015).

The classification of *Salmonella* species is based on a combination of phenotypic and genotypic criteria, including morphological, cultural, biochemical and serological properties, as well as molecular biology techniques such as DNA–DNA hybridization, ribotyping, pulsed-field gel electrophoresis and whole-genome sequencing. The genus *Salmonella* currently includes over 2500 serovars (subtypes) grouped into two species: *Salmonella enterica* and *Salmonella bongori* (Dekker and Frank, 2015).

Salmonella enterica is the most commonly isolated species and is responsible for the majority of human salmonellosis cases. This species is further divided into six subspecies: *S. enterica* subsp. *enterica*, *S. enterica* subsp. *salamae*, *S. enterica* subsp. *arizonae*, *S. enterica* subsp. *diarizonae*, *S. enterica* subsp. *houtenae* and *S. enterica* subsp. *indica*. *S. enterica* subsp. *enterica* is the most clinically relevant and includes more than 1500 serovars, many of which are associated with different types of human disease. *Salmonella bongori* is a recently recognized species that was previously classified as a subspecies of *S. enterica*. *S. bongori* is less clinically relevant than *S. enterica* and is mainly associated with animal infections (Monte and Sellera, 2020).

17.3 Typhoidal and Non-Typhoidal Salmonellosis

The two main forms of salmonellosis are typhoidal and non-typhoidal salmonellosis, which differ in their clinical presentation, epidemiology and pathogenesis (Dekker and Frank, 2015). Understanding the differences between these two forms of salmonellosis is important for the diagnosis, treatment and control of salmonellosis.

Typhoidal salmonellosis is a systemic disease that is caused by specific serovars of *S. enterica*, such as *S. enterica* serovar Typhi and *S. enterica* serovar Paratyphi. This form of salmonellosis is characterized by fever, headache, muscle aches, abdominal pain and a rash and can progress to more severe symptoms such as hepatitis, meningitis and sepsis. Typhoidal salmonellosis is primarily a human disease and is transmitted from person to person via the faecal–oral route or through contaminated food or water. The disease is more common in developing countries with poor sanitation and hygiene, and it is estimated to cause about 11 million cases and 128,000 deaths per year worldwide (Dekker and Frank, 2015).

Non-typhoidal salmonellosis is a less severe form of salmonellosis caused by a wide variety of *Salmonella* serovars, including *S. enterica* serovar Enteritidis, *S. enterica* serovar Newport and *S. enterica* serovar Thompson. This form of salmonellosis is characterized by gastroenteritis, which is an inflammation of the stomach and intestines that results in symptoms such as diarrhoea, abdominal cramps, vomiting and fever. Non-typhoidal salmonellosis is usually transmitted through the consumption of contaminated food, such as undercooked meats, raw eggs and dairy products (Dekker and Frank, 2015). The disease is more common in industrialized countries and is estimated to cause about 1.35 million cases and 450 deaths per year in the United States alone (CDC, 2022a).

The pathogenesis of typhoidal and non-typhoidal salmonellosis is also different. In typhoidal salmonellosis, the bacteria invade the host's bloodstream and cause systemic infections; while in non-typhoidal salmonellosis, the bacteria primarily colonize the gastrointestinal tract and cause local infections. The virulence factors and mechanisms of invasion and colonization vary between different *Salmonella* serovars, and some serovars are more virulent and invasive than others. For example, *S. enterica* serovar Typhi has a specialized mechanism for invading the host's bloodstream and avoiding the host's immune system, while *S. enterica* serovar Enteritidis primarily colonizes the host's intestines and causes local infections (Dekker and Frank, 2015).

17.4 Salmonella Pathogenicity Islands

Salmonella pathogenicity islands (SPIs) are specific genomic regions found in the bacterium *Salmonella enterica* that play a crucial role in its virulence and pathogenesis. They are responsible for the ability of the bacterium to cause disease in humans and animals. SPIs are composed of clusters of genes involved in various functions, including host invasion, intracellular survival and modulation of the host immune response. They are distinct from the rest of the *Salmonella* genome, in terms of both sequence and gene content, and are thought to have been acquired through horizontal gene transfer. SPI-1, for example, is involved in the bacterium's ability to invade and replicate within host cells, while SPI-2 is responsible for the formation of a specialized organelle called the *Salmonella*-containing vacuole (SCV), where the bacterium can persist and evade the host's immune response. The presence and number of SPIs can vary among different strains of *Salmonella*, and some strains can even have additional SPIs not found in others. This variation can have a significant impact on the virulence and disease-causing potential of the bacterium (Marcus *et al.*, 2000).

17.5 Interaction of *Salmonella* with Animal Host

The interaction between *Salmonella* and its animal host is a complex process that involves multiple stages and can be influenced by various factors, including the virulence of the bacterium and the host's immune response. The first stage of interaction is the bacterium's entry into the host. This can occur through ingestion of contaminated food or water, inhalation of contaminated air, or direct contact with contaminated surfaces. Once inside the host, *Salmonella* must overcome the host's physical and chemical barriers, such as the acidity of the stomach and the antimicrobial properties of mucus, to reach the intestinal epithelium. Once in contact with the intestinal epithelium, *Salmonella* can invade the host cells and establish itself within a specialized vacuole called the SCV. The bacterium can persist within the SCV and replicate, leading to a systemic infection. The host's immune response is another crucial factor in the interaction between *Salmonella* and its animal host. The bacterium has evolved various mechanisms to modulate the host's immune response, such as secreting proteins that interfere with signalling pathways and impairing the function of immune cells (Wiedemann *et al.*, 2015).

17.6 Salmonellosis in Goats

17.6.1 Possible causal agents

Salmonella is a genus of bacteria that consists of over 2500 different serovars (strains). Goats can be infected with a variety of *Salmonella* serovars, but the most common are *Salmonella* Dublin, *Salmonella* Typhimurium and *Salmonella* Newport (Dekker and Frank, 2015).

17.6.2 Modes of transmission

The transmission of salmonellosis in goats can occur through several different routes, including faecal–oral transmission, horizontal transmission and vertical transmission. Understanding the mode of transmission is important for controlling and preventing the spread of salmonellosis in goat populations (Grünberg, 2022; Nesser *et al.*, 2023). The mode of transmission of *Salmonella* (Fig. 17.1) in goats includes the following.

- **Faecal–oral transmission** is the most common mode of transmission of

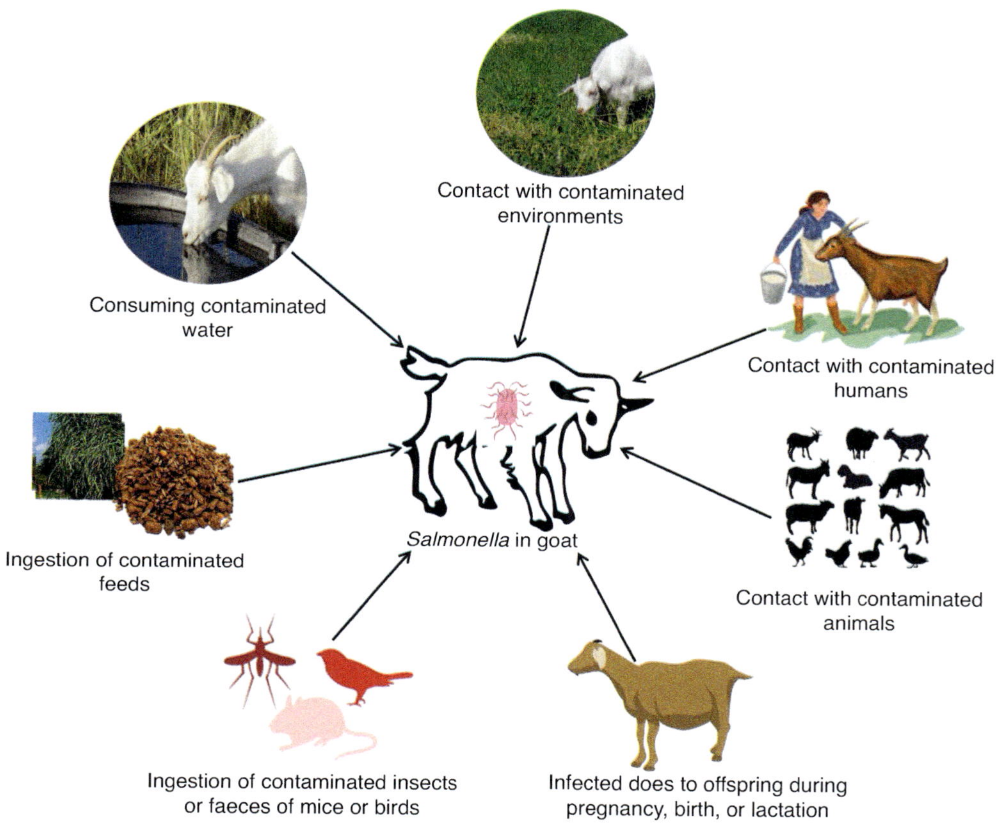

Fig. 17.1. The possible transmission pathways of *Salmonella* to goats. (Author's own image.)

salmonellosis in goats and other livestock. This occurs when contaminated faeces from infected animals are accidentally ingested by other animals, either directly or through contaminated feed, water, or the environment. Faecal–oral transmission can occur rapidly in crowded and unsanitary conditions, and it is particularly important in the spread of salmonellosis in feedlot operations and intensive goat farming systems.

- **Horizontal transmission** occurs when infected animals come into direct contact with healthy animals and spread the bacteria through their saliva, nasal secretions, or wounds. This mode of transmission is particularly important in outbreaks of salmonellosis in captive and wild animal populations, where close contact between animals is common.
- **Vertical transmission** occurs when infected does pass the bacteria to their offspring during pregnancy, birth, or lactation. This mode of transmission can result in the rapid spread of salmonellosis in goat populations and is particularly important in dairy goat farming operations, where close contact between does and their offspring is common.

17.6.3 Risk factors and predisposing conditions

The risk of salmonellosis in goats is influenced by a variety of factors, including the age and health of the animals, the environment in which they live and the management practices used. Young goats are particularly susceptible to the disease, as their immune systems are still developing. Goats that are housed in crowded or unsanitary conditions, or those that are under stress or have other underlying health problems, are also at an increased risk of contracting the disease (Cummings *et al.*, 2012; Nesser *et al.*, 2023).

- Poor nutrition and weakened immune systems are also significant risk factors for salmonellosis in goats. Malnutrition can lead to a weakened immune system, making goats more susceptible to infection. In addition, stress, such as from transportation, changes in management practices, or disease, can also weaken the immune system and increase the risk of salmonellosis.
- Poor hygiene practices, such as failing to wash hands after handling infected animals or contaminated materials, can also increase the risk of transmission. In addition, the use of contaminated equipment, such as feed buckets, water troughs, or milking machines, can spread the bacteria from one animal to another.
- Certain breeds of goats may be more susceptible to salmonellosis, while individual animals may have differences in their immune responses to *Salmonella* bacteria. Additionally, young and elderly goats are often more susceptible to salmonellosis, as they may have weaker immune systems.
- In addition to these general risk factors, certain predisposing conditions can also increase the risk of salmonellosis in goats. These conditions can include parasites, such as coccidia or worms, which can weaken the immune system and make goats more susceptible to infection. In addition, other diseases, such as pneumonia, can also increase the risk of salmonellosis.

17.6.4 Clinical signs and symptoms of salmonellosis in goats

Salmonellosis in goats is a bacterial infection caused by the *Salmonella* species that results in a range of symptoms, including gastrointestinal, respiratory and systemic manifestations. The clinical signs of salmonellosis in goats can vary, depending on the strain of *Salmonella* involved, the age, breed and health status of the goat, and the duration and severity of the infection (Goatlink, 2009; Nesser *et al.*, 2023).

- One of the most common clinical signs of salmonellosis in goats is diarrhoea, which is often severe and watery. Diarrhoea may contain mucus, blood, or other abnormal substances and may be accompanied by abdominal pain and discomfort. Vomiting is also a common symptom, which can be caused by the infection's effect on the goat's digestive system.
- Fever is another common clinical sign of salmonellosis in goats, which is caused by the body's immune response to the infection. Goats with salmonellosis may also display lethargy, lack of appetite and a decrease in feed and water intake. These symptoms can lead to dehydration, which can further exacerbate the symptoms and progress of the infection.
- In severe cases of salmonellosis in goats, respiratory symptoms, such as coughing, nasal discharge and difficulty in breathing, may also occur. This is likely due to the infection's spread to the goat's respiratory system, which can result in pneumonia or other respiratory infections.
- Systemic symptoms, such as joint pain, muscle stiffness and lameness, may also occur in some cases of salmonellosis in goats. This is likely due to the bacterium's ability to spread throughout the body and affect other organs and systems, such as the musculoskeletal system.
- In severe cases, salmonellosis can lead to septicaemia, which is a life-threatening infection that spreads throughout the body. Septicaemia can cause organ failure and death in severe cases.
- Pregnant goats are especially susceptible to *Salmonella* infection, as the bacteria can cross the placenta and infect the fetus. Clinical signs of *Salmonella* infection in pregnant goats may include abortion, premature delivery, stillbirth, or neonatal death.

It is important to note that not all goats with salmonellosis will display all of these symptoms and some may not display any symptoms at all. Additionally, the symptoms of salmonellosis in goats can be similar to those of other bacterial or viral infections, making it important to obtain a definitive diagnosis.

17.6.5 Examples of studies on salmonellosis in goats

In a study of goat operations in the United States from September 2019 to March 2020, Hempstead *et al.* (2022) found a low occurrence (0.7%, n = 35/4917) of *Salmonella* in goat faeces. They identified a wide range of serotypes, including S. Bareilly (35%). They also reported that *Salmonella* isolates were biofilm formers (14/35) and resistant to tetracycline (1/35).

A study conducted in Egypt (Hawwas *et al.*, 2022) examined the occurrence of *Salmonella* in goats and characterized the bacteria using molecular methods. The study found that *Salmonella* was present in 7% of the goat herds tested and identified the presence of other infected animals, as well as poor sanitation practices, as the main risk factors for contamination.

Another study conducted in Egypt (Farouk *et al.*, 2021) investigated the prevalence of *Salmonella* in goat farms and identified the risk factors associated with contamination. The study found that *Salmonella* was present in 3.63% of the goat farms tested and identified poor hygiene practices, overcrowding and the presence of other infected animals as the main risk factors for contamination.

A study conducted in Australia (Al-Habsi *et al.*, 2018) investigated goat samples and detected *Salmonella* in 26.5% (106/400) of the samples. They also determined the antimicrobial resistance of *Salmonella* isolated from goats and identified the prevalence of resistance to different antibiotics. The study found that *Salmonella* isolates were resistant to azithromycin, tetracycline, ampicillin, cefoxitin, amoxiclav, trimethoprim/sulfamethoxazole, gentamicin and streptomycin.

These studies highlight the importance of identifying the risk factors for *Salmonella* infection in goats, as well as the need for effective measures to prevent and control salmonellosis in this species.

17.7 Diagnosis of Salmonellosis in Goats

The diagnosis of salmonellosis in goats involves identifying the presence of the *Salmonella* bacteria in the goat's body and determining the specific strain involved. This is important for determining the appropriate treatment and controlling the spread of the infection. There are several diagnostic methods used to diagnose salmonellosis in goats (Grünberg, 2022).

17.7.1 Clinical examination

A thorough clinical examination of the goat can provide important information about its overall health and the presence of any signs or symptoms of salmonellosis. This may include a physical examination, blood tests and other diagnostic tests as indicated by the veterinarian.

17.7.2 Bacterial culture

A bacterial culture of a sample of the goat's faeces or other body fluids, such as blood or saliva, can be used to identify the presence of *Salmonella* bacteria. This test involves growing the bacterium in a laboratory and analysing its characteristics to determine the specific strain involved.

17.7.3 Polymerase chain reaction (PCR) test

This test is a molecular diagnostic technique that can detect the presence of *Salmonella* bacteria in a sample of the goat's faeces or other body fluids. This test is highly sensitive and specific and can provide results within a few hours.

17.7.4 Serological tests

Serological tests can be used to detect antibodies against *Salmonella* in the goat's blood, which indicates a previous or current infection. These tests are often used in combination with other diagnostic methods to confirm a diagnosis of salmonellosis.

17.7.5 Differential diagnoses

The clinical signs of salmonellosis in goats can be similar to those of other bacterial and viral infections, such as *Escherichia coli* and rotavirus infections. To differentiate between these conditions, a comprehensive diagnostic evaluation, including laboratory testing, is necessary.

17.8 Treatment of Salmonellosis in Goats

Salmonellosis in goats is a bacterial infection that requires prompt and appropriate treatment to prevent the spread of the infection and minimize its impact on the health and well-being of the goat. The treatment of salmonellosis in goats depends on several factors, including the specific strain of *Salmonella* involved, the severity of the infection and the overall health and well-being of the goat. The following are some of the most common treatments for salmonellosis in goats (Goat-link, 2009).

17.8.1 Antibiotic therapy

Antibiotics are the mainstay of treatment for salmonellosis in goats and are used to kill the *Salmonella* bacteria. The specific type and duration of antibiotics used will depend on the specific strain of *Salmonella* involved, the severity of the infection and the overall health and well-being of the goat. Antibiotics such as potentiated sulfonamides, ampicillin, amoxicillin and tetracycline are among the medications that have been suggested for treating salmonellosis in goats. However, it is important to use these agents judiciously, as overuse can contribute to the development of antimicrobial-resistant strains of *Salmonella*. In addition, the use of antibiotics in food-producing animals is regulated and may have implications for human health.

17.8.2 Supportive care

In addition to antibiotics, supportive care is important in the treatment of salmonellosis in goats. This may include fluid therapy to prevent dehydration, proper nutrition to support the goat's immune system, and other measures to support its overall health and well-being. Treatment includes rehydrating the patient and restoring electrolyte balance, focusing on potassium levels; an electrolyte solution can be fortified with sodium bicarbonate and potassium. The addition of glucose supplements is also quite useful. Non-steroidal anti-inflammatory medicines, such as Banamine, can be used to treat shock and reduce discomfort.

17.8.3 Isolation and disinfection

To prevent the spread of the infection, it is important to isolate the infected goat and thoroughly disinfect its rearing area. This can help prevent the spread of the *Salmonella* bacteria to other goats and prevent re-infection of the affected goat.

17.9 Prevention and Control of Salmonellosis in Goats

Salmonellosis is a bacterial infection that affects goats and can have serious consequences for the health and well-being of the affected animals and humans who come into contact with them. The prevention and control of salmonellosis in goats is an important aspect of maintaining the health and productivity of the herd. The following are some of the most effective strategies for preventing and controlling salmonellosis in goats (Fig. 17.2) (Pezzanite *et al.*, 2009; Karthik and Prabhu, 2021; CDC, 2022b; Veterinary Handbook, 2023).

17.9.1 Biosecurity

Maintaining good biosecurity practices is one of the most effective ways to prevent the spread of salmonellosis in goats. This includes separating sick goats from healthy goats, practising proper hygiene and sanitation and regularly disinfecting living areas, feed and water containers and equipment.

17.9.2 Vaccination

Vaccination is an effective way to prevent salmonellosis in goats. There are vaccines available that protect against certain strains of *Salmonella*, and it is important to discuss the appropriate vaccine with a veterinarian to determine which is best for the herd. Currently, there are several *Salmonella* vaccines available for goats, including live and inactivated vaccines. The type and frequency of vaccination should be determined based on the specific *Salmonella* serovars present in the area and the risk of infection.

17.9.3 Good nutrition

Providing goats with a balanced and nutritious diet is important for maintaining their overall health and well-being and can help prevent salmonellosis by supporting their immune system.

17.9.4 Proper management practices

Proper management practices, such as proper feeding and watering, good ventilation and

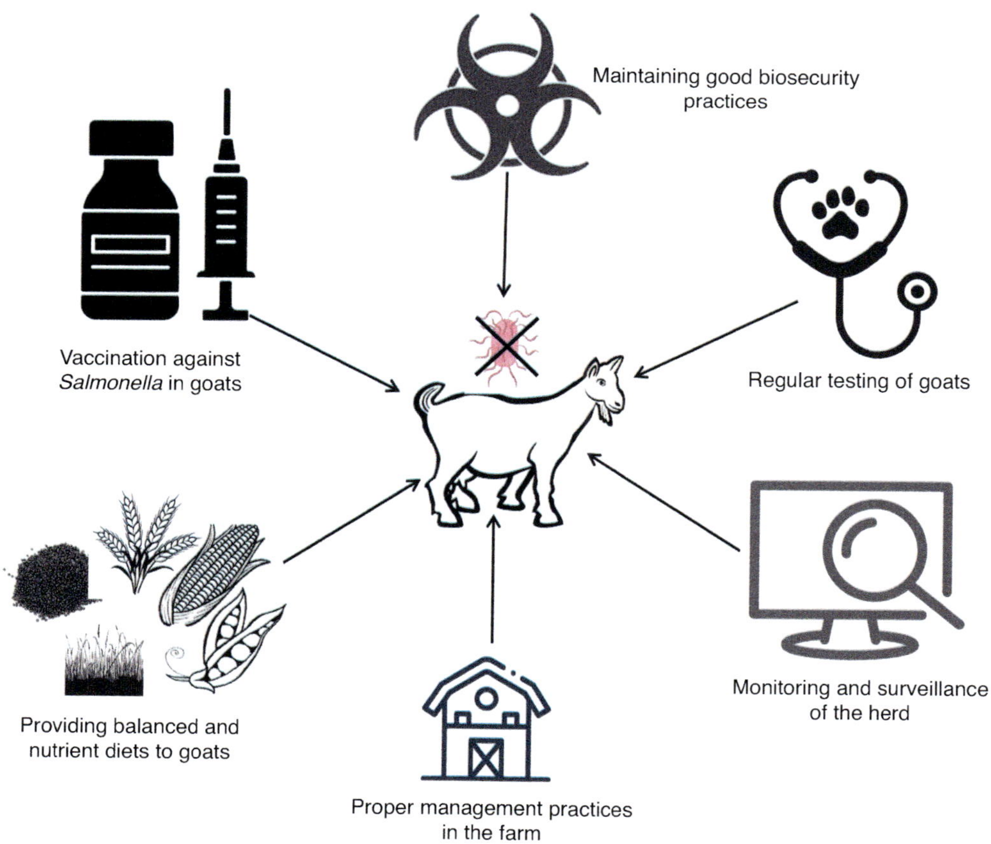

Fig. 17.2. Prevention and control strategies of salmonellosis in goat. (Author's own image.)

reducing overcrowding, can help reduce the risk of salmonellosis in goats.

17.9.5 Monitoring and surveillance

Regular monitoring and surveillance of the herd for signs of salmonellosis are important for early detection and prompt treatment. This includes monitoring for changes in behaviour, feeding habits and the presence of any clinical signs or symptoms.

17.9.6 Testing

Regular testing of goats for salmonellosis can help determine the presence of the bacteria in the herd and provide information about the specific strain involved. This information can be used to develop a management plan to prevent the spread of the infection and minimize its impact on the herd.

17.10 Human Health Aspect of Goat Salmonellosis

Goat salmonellosis is a bacterial infection caused by *Salmonella* species that can affect both humans and goats. While goats can serve as a source of infection for humans, the disease can also have a significant impact on human health. Understanding the human health aspect of goat salmonellosis is crucial in order to prevent and control outbreaks and minimize the harm caused by this disease. A possible mode of transmission of *Salmonella* from goats to humans is illustrated in Fig. 17.3.

Salmonellosis is a foodborne illness that affects millions of people worldwide each year. The infection is usually acquired by consuming contaminated food or water, and the symptoms can range from mild to severe. Common symptoms include fever, headache, abdominal pain, diarrhoea, nausea and vomiting. In severe cases, the infection can lead to complications such as dehydration, septicaemia and meningitis, which can be fatal in some cases (Hawwas *et al.*, 2022).

Goats can serve as a source of salmonellosis infection for humans through the consumption

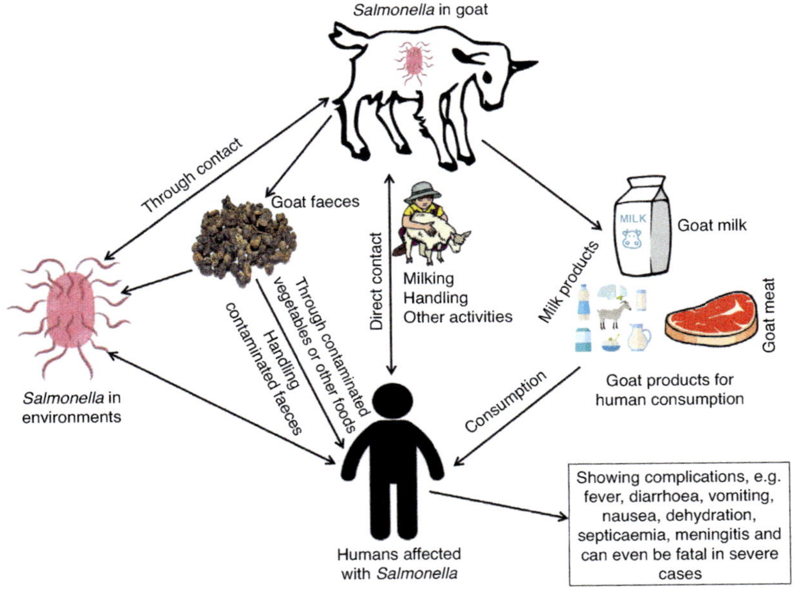

Fig. 17.3. Possible transmission pathways of *Salmonella* from goats to humans. (Author's own image.)

of contaminated food or water. This can occur when goat's milk, cheese, or other milk products are contaminated with *Salmonella* or when humans consume vegetables or other foods that have been contaminated by goat faeces (Fig. 17.3). In addition to foodborne transmission, salmonellosis can also be transmitted from goats to humans through direct contact with infected animals. This can occur when humans handle contaminated goat faeces or when they have direct contact with infected goats, such as during milking or other husbandry activities (Fig. 17.3) (CVM, 2023).

The human health impact of goat salmonellosis can be significant and it is important to take steps to minimize the risk of infection. Children are especially susceptible to infection from goats, as they are more likely to have direct contact with the animals and may not have fully developed immunity. In addition, individuals with weakened immune systems, such as the elderly, pregnant women and people with chronic health conditions, are also at increased risk of infection and are more likely to experience severe symptoms (CDC, 2022b).

Antibiotic resistance is a growing concern in public health, as it can lead to the spread of infections that are difficult to treat (Islam *et al.*, 2021). This problem is particularly relevant in the case of goat *Salmonella* serovars, which can cause serious illness in both humans and animals. The development of antibiotic resistance in goat *Salmonella* serovars poses a significant threat to public health. Goat *Salmonella* serovars are particularly prone to the development of antibiotic resistance, as these bacteria can be found in a variety of environments, including in the intestines of infected animals and in contaminated food and water. Additionally, the use of antibiotics in livestock production can contribute to the development of resistance in goat *Salmonella* serovars, as these drugs are often used to prevent and treat infections in animals. The problem of antibiotic resistance in goat *Salmonella* serovars is particularly relevant in the context of public health, as these bacteria can be transmitted from infected animals to humans through the consumption of contaminated food and water, as well as through direct contact with infected animals (Argudín *et al.*, 2017). When antibiotics are used excessively in livestock production, the development of resistance in goat *Salmonella* serovars can make it more difficult to treat infections in humans, as these bacteria may no longer respond to commonly used antibiotics (Umeh and Enwuru, 2014; Economou and Gousia, 2015).

In order to address the problem of antibiotic resistance in goat *Salmonella* serovars, it is important to implement measures that can reduce the overuse and misuse of antibiotics. This includes implementing good agricultural practices, such as reducing the use of antibiotics in livestock production and ensuring that these drugs are used only when necessary, as well as following food safety guidelines to minimize the risk of contamination of food and water with *Salmonella*. It is also important to invest in research and development to find new treatments and strategies to combat antibiotic resistance. This includes the development of new antibiotics, as well as the use of alternative treatments, such as probiotics and other natural remedies, which can help to reduce the need for antibiotics (Economou and Gousia, 2015).

To minimize the risk of goat salmonellosis, it is important to implement appropriate biosecurity measures to reduce the risk of infection. This includes proper sanitation practices, such as regularly cleaning and disinfecting goat housing and feeding areas, as well as implementing measures to minimize the spread of faeces and other contaminated materials. Additionally, good hygiene practices, such as washing hands thoroughly after handling goats or coming into contact with their faeces, can help to reduce the risk of infection.

Goat farmers and dairy producers should also take steps to minimize the risk of *Salmonella* contamination of their products. This includes implementing good agricultural practices, such as regularly testing goat's milk and dairy products for *Salmonella* and implementing measures to prevent cross-contamination between contaminated and non-contaminated products. In addition, goat farmers and dairy producers should follow food safety guidelines and ensure that their products are properly stored, handled and prepared, to reduce the risk of contamination.

It is also important to raise awareness of the zoonotic significance of goat salmonellosis among the public, especially in communities where goat farming and dairy production are common. This can be done through public health education campaigns and the distribution of informational materials, such as brochures and posters, which can help to educate people about the risks associated with goat salmonellosis and the measures that can be taken to prevent infection.

17.11 Conclusion

Salmonellosis is a significant health concern for goat farmers and requires a comprehensive approach to prevent and control its spread. This chapter has provided an overview of the causes and transmission, clinical signs and diagnosis, and prevention and control measures for the disease. It is important to understand the impacts of salmonellosis on goat health, production and human health and to implement effective biosecurity measures, such as controlling the movement of animals and people, regular cleaning and disinfection, and monitoring and surveillance. Additionally, the judicious use of vaccines and antimicrobial agents can help to reduce the spread of the disease. Research is needed to improve the understanding of the epidemiology of salmonellosis in goats and to develop more effective control strategies.

References

Al-Habsi, K., Jordan, D., Harb, A., Laird, T., Yang, R. *et al*. (2018) *Salmonella enterica* isolates from western Australian rangeland goats remain susceptible to critically important antimicrobials. *Scientific Reports* 8(1), 1–8.

Argudín, M.A., Deplano, A., Meghraoui, A., Dodémont, M., Heinrichs, A. *et al*. (2017) Bacteria from animals as a pool of antimicrobial resistance genes. *Antibiotics* 6(2), 12.

Bedaso, K.K., Dinsefa, J.H., Kifle, A.L. and Biniam, T. (2015) Study on prevalence and distribution of *Salmonella* isolates from apparently healthy sheep and goats slaughtered at Addis Ababa Abattoir enterprise, Ethiopia. *Journal of Veterinary Science and Technology* 6(6).

CDC (2022a) Salmonella. Available at: https://www.cdc.gov/salmonella/index.html

CDC (2022b) Salmonella Infection. Available at: https://www.cdc.gov/healthypets/diseases/salmonella.html

Cummings, K.J., Warnick, L.D., Davis, M.A., Eckmann, K., Gröhn, Y.T. *et al*. (2012) Farm animal contact as risk factor for transmission of bovine-associated *Salmonella* subtypes. *Emerging Infectious Diseases* 18(12), 1929.

CVM (2023) Zoonotic Diseases from Sheep/Goats. Available at: https://www.vet.cornell.edu/animal-health-diagnostic-center/programs/nyschap/modules-documents/zoonotic-diseases-sheepgoats

Dekker, J.P. and Frank, K.M. (2015) Salmonella, Shigella, and Yersinia. *Clinics in Laboratory Medicine* 35(2), 225–246.

Economou, V. and Gousia, P. (2015) Agriculture and food animals as a source of antimicrobial-resistant bacteria. *Infection and Drug Resistance* 8, 49–61.

Farouk, M.M., El-Molla, A., Salib, F.A. and Soliman, Y.A. (2021) Epidemiology of *Salmonella* species in diarrheic sheep and goats. *Pakistan Journal of Zoology* 54, 1–9.

Goat-link (2009) Salmonellosis. Available at: https://goat-link.com/content/view/185/183/90

Grünberg, W. (2022) Salmonellosis in Animals. Available at: https://www.msdvetmanual.com/digestive-system/salmonellosis/salmonellosis-in-animals

Hawwas, H.A.E.H., Aboueisha, A.K.M., Fadel, H.M. and El-Mahallawy, H.S. (2022) *Salmonella* serovars in sheep and goats and their probable zoonotic potential to humans in Suez Canal Area, Egypt. *Acta Veterinaria Scandinavica* 64(1), 17.

Hempstead, S.C., Gensler, C.A., Keelara, S., Brennan, M., Urie, N.J. *et al*. (2022) Detection and molecular characterization of *Salmonella* species on US goat operations. *Preventive Veterinary Medicine* 208, 105766.

Islam, M.S., Nayeem, M.M.H., Sobur, M.A., Ievy, S., Islam, M.A. *et al*. (2021) Virulence determinants and multidrug resistance of *Escherichia coli* isolated from migratory birds. *Antibiotics* 10(2), 190.

Karthik, K. and Prabhu, M. (2021) Bacterial diseases of goat and its preventive measures. In: Kukovics, S. (ed.) *Goat Science*, 17th edn. IntechOpen, London.

Marcus, S.L., Brumell, J.H., Pfeifer, C.G. and Finlay, B.B. (2000) *Salmonella* pathogenicity islands: Big virulence in small packages. *Microbes and Infection* 2(2), 145–156.

Monte, D.F. and Sellera, F.P. (2020) Salmonella. *Emerging Infectious Diseases* 26(12), 2955–2955.

Nesser, J.A., Henton, M.M. and Fenwink, S.G. (2023) Ovine and caprine salmonellosis. Available at: https://www.anipedia.org/resources/ovine-and-caprine-salmonellosis/943

Pezzanite, L., Neary, M., Hutchens, T. and Scharko, P. (2009) Common diseases and health problems in sheep and goats. *Animal Sciences* AS-595-W. Purdue University Cooperative Extension Service, West Lafayette, Indiana. Available at: https://www.extension.purdue.edu/extmedia/as/as-595-commondiseases.pdf

Rahman, M.T., Sobur, M.A., Islam, M.S., Ievy, S., Hossain, M.J. *et al.* (2020) Zoonotic diseases: Etiology, impact, and control. *Microorganisms* 8(9), 1405.

Talukder, M., Islam, M.S., Ievy, S., Sobur, M.A., Ballah, F.M. *et al.* (2021) Detection of multidrug resistant *Salmonella* spp. from healthy and diseased broilers having potential public health significance. *Journal of Advanced Biotechnology and Experimental Therapeutics* 4(2), 248–255.

Tawyabur, M., Islam, M.S., Sobur, M.A., Hossain, M.J., Mahmud, M.M. *et al.* (2020) Isolation and characterization of multidrug-resistant *Escherichia coli* and *Salmonella* spp. from healthy and diseased turkeys. *Antibiotics* 9(11), 770.

Umeh, S.I. and Enwuru, C.P. (2014) Antimicrobial resistance profile of *Salmonella* isolates from livestock. *Open Journal of Medical Microbiology* 4(4), 242.

Veterinary Handbook (2023) Salmonellosis. In: *Veterinary Handbook for the Livestock Export Industry*. Australian Livestock Export Corporation (LiveCorp) and Meat & Livestock Australia (MLA). Available at: http://www.veterinaryhandbook.com.au/Diseases.aspx?diseasenameid=247

Wiedemann, A., Virlogeux-Payant, I., Chaussé, A.M., Schikora, A. and Velge, P. (2015) Interactions of *Salmonella* with animals and plants. *Frontiers in Microbiology* 5, 791.

18 Johne's Disease (Paratuberculosis)

Shivangi Udainiya[1]*, Amita Tiwari[2], Brejesh Singh[2], Apoorva Mishra[3] and Tanmoy Rana[4]

[1]Veterinary Polytechnic College, Bhopal, Madhya Pradesh, NDVSU, Jabalpur, India; [2]Department of Veterinary Medicine, College of Veterinary Science and Animal Husbandry, NDVSU, Jabalpur, Madhya Pradesh, India; [3]Department of Veterinary Surgery and Radiology, College of Veterinary Science and Animal Husbandry, NDVSU, Jabalpur, Madhya Pradesh, India; [4]Department of Veterinary Clinical Complex, West Bengal University of Animal & Fishery Sciences, Kolkata, India

Abstract

Johne's disease, also known as paratuberculosis, is worldwide in distribution and many countries have national control programmes for this disease. It has a global distribution. The infective organism of the disease is resistant to heat, cold and drying, and can survive for extended periods in soil and even longer in water. This disease also has zoonotic importance and can be defined as a chronic infectious enteric disease that affects domestic and wild ruminants. It is characterized by a slowly progressive wasting of the animal and increasingly severe diarrhoea. It is caused by *Mycobacterium avium* subsp. *paratuberculosis* (MAP), which is common in the environment but does not multiply outside a living host. Infection is mainly spread by the faecal–oral route. Generally the age of onset of faecal shedding and clinical disease varies with dose, age of infection, host susceptibility to infection and herd management factors. Faecal shedding can be intermittent and usually precedes clinical signs. In goats, the main clinical signs are cachexia, production loss, a dull and crustaceous hair coat, exercise intolerance, selective food intake (leaving the concentrate) and sometimes intermittent diarrhoea. Diagnosis is generally performed on the basis of clinical signs, histopathology evaluation, post-mortem lesions and diagnostic tests.

Johne's disease has zoonotic importance, as *M. paratuberculosis* has been found occasionally in patients with Crohn's disease. Every country in different regions of the world adopts different control strategies for Johne's disease, depending upon the epidemiology. The strategies include management modification, testing, culling and vaccination.

Keywords: chronic, goat, Johne's disease, paratuberculosis, zoonotic

18.1 Introduction

Johne's disease, also known as paratuberculosis, is an economically important bacterial disease seen primarily in ruminants. including cattle, sheep and goats. It has zoonotic importance and has also been reported in captive and free-ranging wild ruminants, as well as omnivores and carnivores such as wild rabbits, foxes, weasels, pigs and non-human primates. Johne's disease is worldwide in distribution and many countries have national control programmes for this disease.

Paratuberculosis be defined as a chronic infectious enteric disease that affects domestic and wild ruminants and is characterized by a slowly progressive wasting of the animal

*Corresponding author: shivangiud15@gmail.com

DOI: 10.1079/ 9781800622852.0018

and increasingly severe diarrhoea. It is a listed disease by the OIE World Organisation for Animal Health (WOAH), meaning it is a priority disease for international trade. It is caused by a bacterium, *Mycobacterium avium* subsp. *paratuberculosis* (MAP), which affects several animal species, predominantly ruminants (cattle, sheep, goats, deer, etc.) (Verdugo *et al.*, 2014). MAP is resistant to heat, cold and drying and can survive for extended periods in soil (more than a year) and even longer in water. Goats have a less efficient humoral immunity reaction to MAP (Kostoulas *et al.*, 2013) and clinical illness develops at an earlier stage in the pathogenesis. The economic importance of Johne's disease, especially in goats, has been difficult to establish because infection with MAP does not always produce clinical illness. The disease has an endemic distribution globally, reducing production of food in developed as well as developing countries (Quinn *et al.*, 2013). In most instances it is restricted to subclinical infection, but there is rapid loss in condition leading to quick death because of nutritional deficiency as a result of absorption loss from the gut (Collins *et al.*, 2010).

18.2 Aetiology

Johne's disease is caused by a slow-growing, non-motile, aerobic, Gram-positive and acid-fast bacillus named *Mycobacterium avium* subsp. *paratuberculosis* (MAP). The bacilli do not possess an external cell membrane and the cell wall is very thick, waxy and hydrophobic (due to the high content of mycolic acid). This cell wall is one of the main reasons for the difficulty in eliminating infections caused by MAP. It is not susceptible to exposure to many antibiotics, disinfectants and environmental degradation. MAP is a subspecies requiring a host to replicate and it can survive for an extended period of time (3–24 months) in soil or water. It is a facultative intracellular pathogen preferentially replicating within macrophages. Residing intracellularly is one of the qualities that make MAP infection generally untreatable, as it is inaccessible to many antimycobacterial drugs (Cocito *et al.*, 1994). There are mainly two types, or strains, on the basis of phenotypic characteristics (growth rate as well as pigmentation): Type I/III and Type II, or MAP-S (sheep type) and MAP-C (cattle type), respectively (CFSPH, 2007; Ghosh *et al.*, 2012; Bryant *et al.*, 2016).

18.3 Epidemiology

Generally the age of onset of faecal shedding and clinical disease varies with dose, age of infection, host susceptibility to infection and herd management factors. Faecal shedding can be intermittent and usually precedes clinical signs. Investigations into prevalence in goats have been reported from Europe (including Iceland and Britain), South Africa, Australia and New Zealand, where goat industries are relatively more important than in North America. Few large prevalence studies have been done; however, paratuberculosis can be an important infection in small ruminants in certain regions. Prevalence of Johne's disease in goats has been reported from all over the world, with prevalence of 7.9% in the Republic of Cyprus (Liapi *et al.*, 2011), 76.9% in the USA (Manning *et al.*, 2002), 74.3% in Chile (Salgado *et al.*, 2007), 62.9% in France (Mercier *et al.*, 2010), 79.4% in India (Singh *et al.*, 2013) and 44.1% in Argentina (Fiorentino *et al.*, 2012).

Clinical paratuberculosis can be a significant cause of culling within individual herds. In Norway the infection rate in heavily infected goat herds approached 50%; annual slaughter surveys detected paratuberculosis in 4.7–9% of goats tested during a 15 year period (Saxegaard and Fodstad, 1985). Few studies have examined herd or individual animal prevalence in goat herds in North America. The age of infected animals ranged from 1 to 5 years, with the highest infection rates detected in older animals. In another investigation, poor weight gain and lesions at slaughter were a common finding in yearling bucks (Fawcett *et al.*, 1995). Due to a high local prevalence of infected goats, the practice of supplementing young crias (i.e. young lamoids) with goat colostrum was cited as a potential source of infection; however, the use of goat colostrum was not confirmed in the reported cases. The typical range for appearance of clinical disease is 2–7 years of age; however, the author has observed animals in heavily infected goat and deer herds with faecal shedding and with clinical infection at 1 year of age or younger. Risk factors in a severely infected deer herd included overcrowding, build-up of faecal material on overgrazed pastures and faecal contamination of water sources. Identified risk factors in the goat herd included the abundant presence of a number of does in late stages of infection. During Year 1, kids were reared on these does, rather than being segregated and fed with milk replacer. This practice resulted in infection with faecal shedding in more than 60% of Year 1's kid crop when these kids became yearlings.

18.4 Zoonotic Importance

Johne's disease has a zoonotic importance, as the organism that causes Johne's disease (*M. avium subsp. paratuberculosis*) has been found occasionally in patients with Crohn's disease. Crohn's disease is a chronic, painful, diarrhoeal inflammatory disease of the intestinal tract in humans that resembles Johne's disease. There is widespread exposure of MAP to the human population and Crohn's disease has been associated with this exposure. These bacteria are generally found in the intestinal tract of some healthy people (Fig. 18.1). Some investigators have also suggested that MAP might play a role in the onset or progression of a variety of other diseases (such as sarcoidosis, diabetes mellitus types 1 and 2, multiple sclerosis, HIV infection and Hashimoto's thyroiditis), based mainly on the presence of antibodies to this organism. One review described weak but consistent evidence for a possible association with diabetes mellitus type one in some studies, but not all. For the other diseases, any role appears to be speculative at this time. Humans are exposed to MAP from various sources that could be contaminated from infected animals, such as drinking water contaminated with faeces, milk, etc. (McNees *et al.*, 2015). Susceptible individuals with a compromised immune system, due to other illness or genetic factors, may be at higher risk for infection and disease. In these individuals, MAP may survive and multiply inside gut

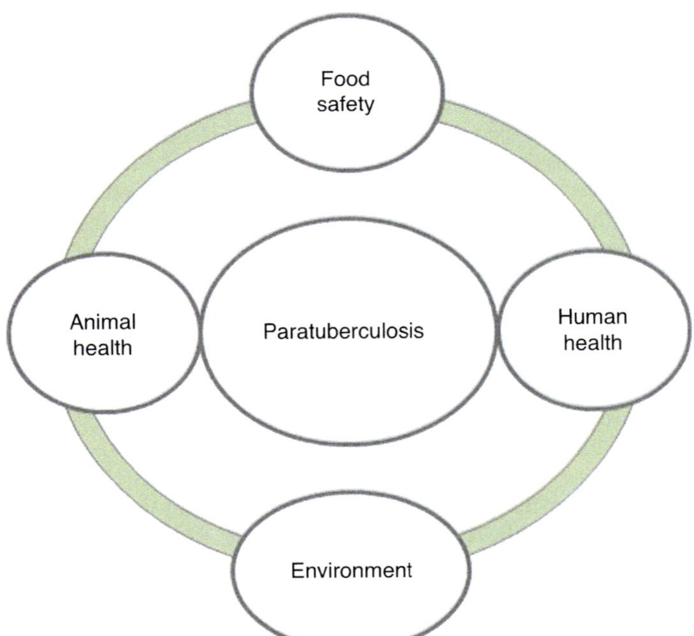

Fig. 18.1. The zoonotic impact of paratuberculosis (Johne's disease) on food safety, animal health, human health and environment. (Author's own image.)

macrophages, leading to immune dysregulation and inflammation of the intestinal wall, resulting in a 'leaky gut'. Microbes and food materials penetrate the leaky gut, causing massive wall inflammation leading to chronic inflammatory bowel disease. Initially, only anti-tuberculosis drugs were used for treatment of MAP infections in humans, but the results were not promising. Later macrolides (e.g. azithromycin and erythromycin), rifabutin and clofazimine have been used with limited success, but the treatment regimen is very lengthy. For treatment of this infection currently combinations of anti-inflammatory, anti-mycobacterial and immunosuppressant drugs are used or in trials. More studies are needed to identify novel drugs and targets for the development of better therapeutics against MAP to shorten and simplify the treatment. Several species of mammals and birds have been listed as susceptible species, including Bovidae, Cervidae and Leporidae, but there was no consensus on the zoonotic risk of MAP in the context of human diseases, such as Crohn's disease (Rathnaiah *et al.*, 2017).

18.5 Transmission

Paratuberculosis is a contagious infection which is spread mainly by the faecal-oral route. MAP is common in the environment, especially on contaminated farms; however, it does not multiply outside a living host. According to some researchers, data suggest that it could become dormant for a limited time in the environment. It can survive for a year or more on some pastures, although infectivity is reported to decrease significantly within a few months. In young animals, transmission occurs mainly through ingestion of contaminated colostrum and milk of infected dams. Infection enters by ingesting faecal contamination on the teats of their mother or other goats. If the mother is in advanced stages of infection, the kid can also be infected from drinking her milk or, less often, a kid can become infected before birth. MAP is capable of being transmitted from the infected pregnant dam to its her fetus through the placenta (Park *et al.*, 2017). Male animals may carry MAP in accessory reproductive organs and to some extent in semen. Embryos from infected animals may carry infection and will transmit it when transplanted in other animals. The infected animals shed large numbers of organisms in the faeces. Others may shed bacteria intermittently, transiently or not at all during the subclinical stage.

18.6 Pathogenesis

Pathogenesis of Johne's disease is found to be same in all animals and it starts when the organism gets entry into the body through the faecal–oral route. The bacterium infects the intestinal mucosa mediated by M-cells overlying Peyer's patches. After entry, the organism specifically invades the sub-epithelial macrophages with accelerated cell-mediated immune (CMI) response–initial T-cell response (Milner *et al.*, 1990; Clarke and Little, 1996; Corpa *et al.*, 2000; Henderson *et al.*, 2000).

18.7 Clinical Signs and Symptoms

Paratuberculosis can affect the animal at any age, with an accelerated tendency to infect more during the first week of life. The incubation period of paratuberculosis is long and highly variable (Robbe-Austerman, 2011). In goats, the main clinical signs are cachexia, production loss, a dull and crustaceous hair coat, exercise intolerance (Windsor and Whittington, 2010), selective food intake (leaving the concentrate) and sometimes intermittent diarrhoea (Figs. 18.2 and 18.3). In a study of 54 goats with paratuberculosis, 54% had normal faeces, 24% had pasty faeces, 15% had intermittent diarrhoea and only 7% suffered from chronic diarrhoea. Dairy goats generally do not reach the 'diarrhoea stage', possibly because they are removed earlier due to declining production. In contrast, pygmy goats do get to the diarrhoea stage. The only systematic clinical sign is cachexia without anorexia (Fernandez-Silva *et al.*, 2014). Therefore, it is impossible to diagnose paratuberculosis only by clinical observation and examination. In the case of goats, the clinical signs are mostly seen at the ages of 2–4 years. The clinical manifestations associated with

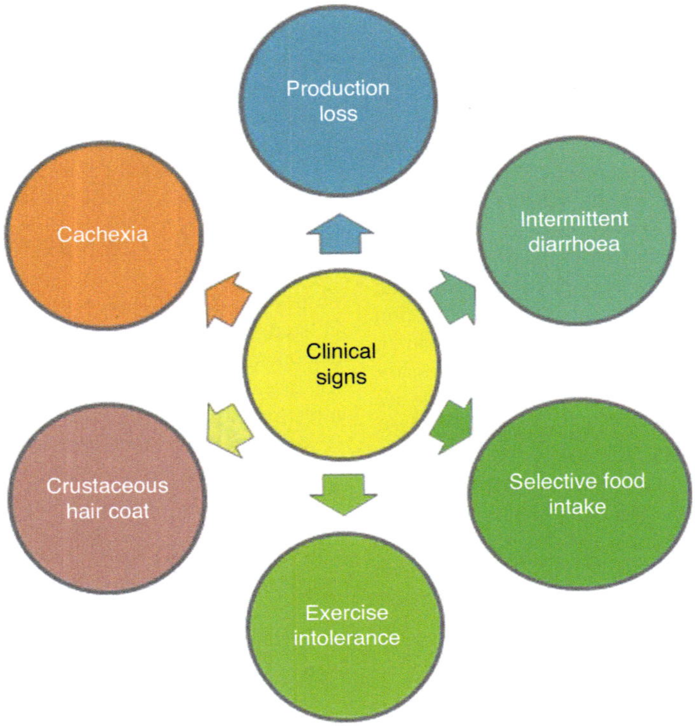

Fig. 18.2. Various clinical signs in a goat affected with paratuberculosis (Johne's disease). (Author's own image.)

the disease include poor hair coat, dullness, progressive weight loss, depression, anaemia, submandibular oedema, fragile skin, emaciation and dehydration. Stress can cause onset of diseases (Whittington and Sergeant, 2001). Reduced ruminal motility and decreases in haematocrit, haemoglobin and albumin levels in affected goats is also reported (Lybeck *et al.*, 2011). Paratuberculosis must be differentiated from other causes of chronic weight loss, including parasitism, internal abscesses due to *Corynebacterium pseudotuberculosis*, caprine arthritis–encephalitis (CAE) or ovine progressive pneumonia (OPP) virus infections in goats, and malnutrition (inadequate macronutrients, energy and protein and/or micronutrients, such as cobalt or copper).

18.8 Pathology

In cases of paratuberculosis, lesions may not be evident in the early stages but in clinical cases they can be seen. Lybeck *et al.* (2011) reported lesions in goats affected with MAP; enlargement of lymph nodes in the jejunum was evident, with yellowish necrotic foci on the cortex. Enteritis is usually seen with ulcerated intestinal mucosae and MAP can be isolated from lesions in the intestine and draining lymph nodes of clinically affected animals. Oedema can be found in the body cavity. Histopathological examinations exhibit diffused granulomatous enteritis, accumulation of epithelioid giant cells and macrophage in intestinal submucosa and mucosa (Almujalli and Al-Ghamdi, 2012).

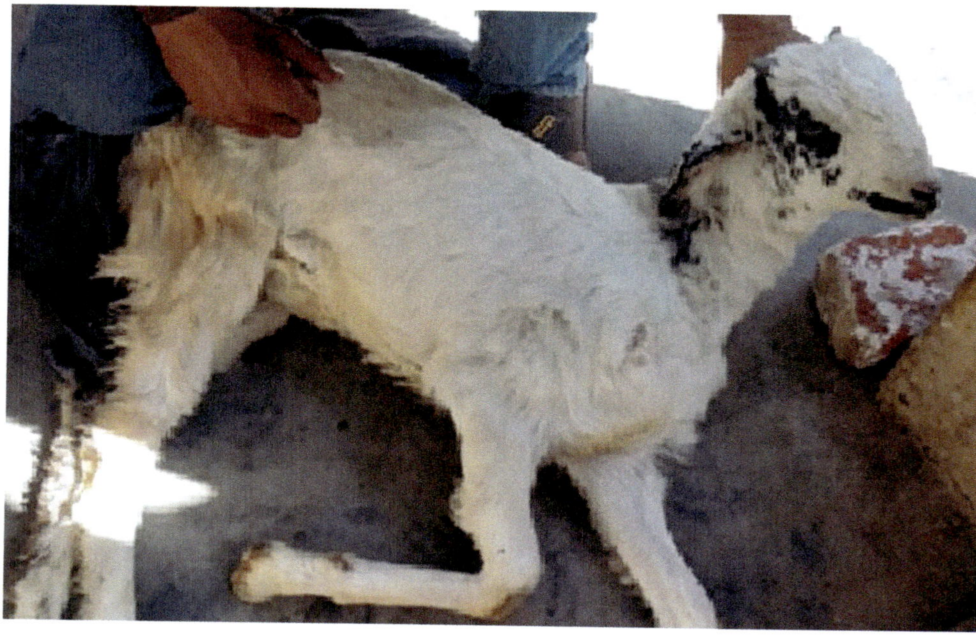

Fig. 18.3. Cachectic condition of a goat affected with paratuberculosis (Johne's disease). (Author's own image.)

18.9 Diagnosis

Animals with chronic, non-responsive diarrhoea and progressive emaciation, coupled with a normal appetite, should be viewed with suspicion. Johne's disease is confirmed by a postmortem examination where increased thickness and transverse folds in the intestinal lining are observed. It may be difficult to detect infected animals that do not exhibit clinical signs. Culture of faeces for MAP is expensive because of the long time required to grow the organism. Cultures must be incubated for up to 4 months before they can be called negative. Intermittent shedding also makes a negative faecal culture difficult to interpret. Several blood tests are available but the number of false positives and negatives makes these tests unreliable.

Diagnosis of MAP is difficult for its long incubation period (4 months to 15 years) and is performed on the basis of clinical signs with postmortem lesions, histopathology and diagnostic tests, including direct tests (e.g. faecal smears, faecal culture and polymerase chain reaction (PCR)) and indirect tests (e.g. interferon assay, delayed-type hypersensitivity (DTH), enzyme-linked immunosorbent assay (ELISA), complement fixation test (CFT) and agar gel immunodiffusion (AGID)). Differential diagnosis includes kidney failure, gastrointestinal parasitism, renal amyloidosis, peritonitis, chronic salmonellosis, lymphosarcoma and other chronic infectious diseases, copper deficiency and starvation.

18.9.1 Direct tests

Faecal smears

Examination of faecal smears is the simple and easy method for detection of aetiological agents. Acid-fast stain (Ziehl–Neelson or Wright's stain) is used to highlight the pathogen in the smear and observations under oil immersion (×1000) are positive when clumps of three to four acid-fast MAP are seen (Manning and Collins, 2001). The sensitivity of the particular test is very low if used in the preclinical stages of paratuberculosis but it is helpful when the clinical phase starts (Ansari *et al.*, 2013).

Faecal culturing

Many authorities consider faecal culturing as the most specific and sensitive method of MAP detection. Initially MAP was grown on an egg-based medium (Twort and Ingram, 1912), then egg yolk was used instead of whole egg because egg white retarded microbial growth (Herrold, 1931), but later antiformin and malachite green were used for decontamination.

Polymerase chain reaction (PCR)

PCR is a better and advanced technique that is able to detect MAP and distinguish it from other species and subspecies of *Mycobacteria*. The IS900 and IS901 insertion elements are considered unique to MAP and can be used in a PCR gene amplification technique for diagnosis (Slana *et al.*, 2009). The detection limit of PCR in MAP cases is 104 organisms per gram; it is also a limitation of its use. Addition of pretreatment of faecal samples using silica membrane mini-columns and magnetic particles can enhance the detection rate of MAP by PCR (Sting *et al.*, 2014).

18.9.2 Indirect tests

Detection of antibodies

This method is generally used for screening at mass but antibodies against paratuberculosis are late in forming because it is a chronic disease and they have a long incubation period; also they are difficult to detect in the preclinical stage, and sometimes even at clinical stages an animal fails to develop its antibodies against MAP. Cross-reactivity of MAP with other organisms can make antibody interpretation difficult.

Enzyme-linked immunosorbent assay (ELISA)

The sensitivity of ELISA in present condition changes from low (where minor shedding is present) to high (clinical stage is reached); so it can be said that sensitivity of ELISA in MAP cases will increase with disease progression (Donat *et al.*, 2014). This method can also detect antibodies in milk and blood (Gupta *et al.*, 2012).

Agar gel immunodiffusion (AGID) test

This test is economical and mostly reliable in small ruminants. The AGID test is unsatisfactory for subclinical cases, due to low specificity and sensitivity (Ferreira *et al.*, 2002), but it gives reliable results in clinical cases.

Complement fixation test (CFT)

This test can be applied for mass screening of infected animals but interpretation is reliable only at the clinical stage (Slana *et al.*, 2009).

Flow cytometry method (FCM)

This method is capable of distinguishing MAP-infected from MAP-non-infected cattle as well as MAP from *M. avium* subsp. *avium* and *M. scrofulaceum*. The FCM assay is rapid (completed in less than 4 hour) and technically easy and can be automated for handling large numbers of samples (Eda *et al.*, 2005).

Interferon-γ assay

This method is successfully used for detection of cytokines for the indication of CMI to check exposure of an animal to MAP (Nielsen and Toft, 2008). The test shows low sensitivity when used to detect infection in a herd with mixed infection of tuberculosis and paratuberculosis.

Delayed-type hypersensitivity (DTH) reaction

Delayed-type hypersensitivity is measured by injecting intradermal antigens (Johnin or avian purified protein derivative) into the skin to detect cell-mediated immunity (CMI). The reaction is allowed to occur and after 72h a thickness of 2 mm will indicate a positive result (Robbe-Austerman *et al.*, 2006). This is not reliable, because MAP antigens are already present in the environment (Whittington *et al.*, 2003).

18.10 Treatment

For Johne's disease there is no specific treatment or cure that provides better or satisfactory results. Generally a combination of various drugs has been used, mostly with isoniazid, clofazimine and rifampin (Borody *et al.*, 2007). The use of probiotics has also been explored. More recently, lactic acid bacteria (LABATCC 334) have been used as probiotics for treatment of experimentally induced Johne's disease in mice. Treatment may result in clinical improvement and prolong the animal's life, but lifelong treatment is thought to be necessary, and some animals nevertheless relapse. Milk or meat from treated animals should not be used for human consumption.

18.11 Control

Every country in different regions of world adopts different control strategies for Johne's disease depending upon the epidemiology. It includes management modification, tests, culling and vaccination (Al-Ghamdi, 2013) (Fig. 18.4).

18.11.1 Good managemental practices

Healthy managemental as well as controlling strategies are the good practices that are the basic integral approach for combating caprine paratuberculosis in small or marginal herds. The good and effective management practices include:

- feeding of uncontaminated and clean colostrum as well as milk replacement products;
- rearing of young stock apart from the adults;
- separation of offspring from their dams;
- lowering the chances of any contact between infected adult goats with other animals; and
- avoiding any exposure of healthy goats to highly infected adult animals, or with their manure, as well as contaminated

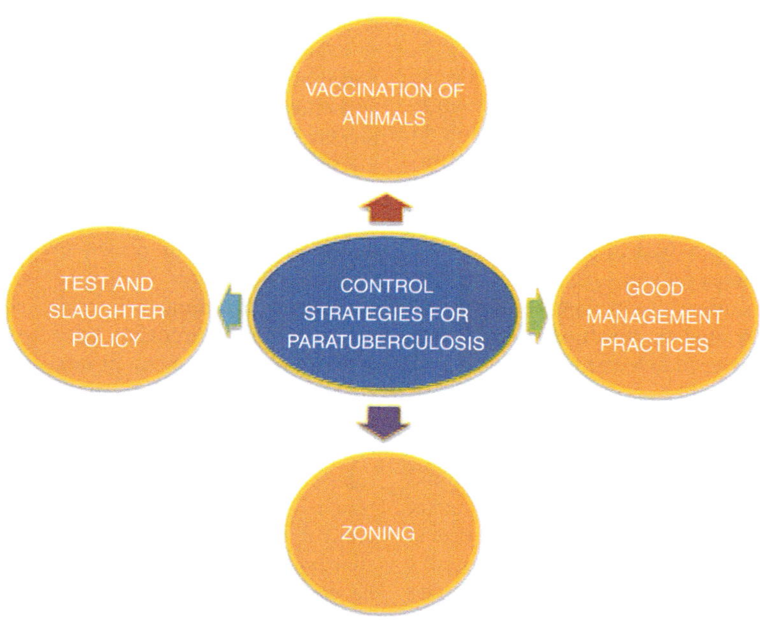

Fig. 18.4. Various control strategies for paratuberculosis in goats. (Author's own image.)

environments within farms (Bauman *et al.*, 2016).

Johne's disease infests animals at a younger age so they should be kept under proper management practices. Parturition should be in a clean and manure-free area to avoid early contact with MAP for newborn kids. Semen may contain MAP having potential to transmit and cause disease to inseminated animals and newborns, so breeding bulls should be tested for MAP and semen samples must undergo laboratory examination. Management of the periparturient period is also an important task to be considered, to avoid transmission of MAP from dams to young ones. MAP can survive exposure to many disinfectants, but 5% formalin, 2% calcium hypo-chloride and 2.5% phenol can kill the pathogen. The presence of organic matter may reduce effectiveness of disinfectants but detergents can be used on faeces to allow penetration by disinfectants.

Good manure management and disposal techniques are also important, as the manure may harbour the infection. Manure build-up should be prevented and surfaces should be kept clean. Grewal *et al.* (2006) observed that thermophilic composting is more effective than pack storage in reducing MAP in dairy manure in pathogen-sensitive environments.

Proper quarantine measures should be followed and proper instructions should be given to the farmers of uninfected herds that they should buy any replacement animals from test-negative herds with good records and management practices. All animals should be quarantined and tested before mixing them into the herd.

Farmers must be educated about the benefits of Johne's disease control programmes and about losses related to paratuberculosis; such practices have helped to lower the prevalence of disease (Carter, 2012).

Animals shed plenty of MAP on grazing areas in faeces, which is a potential source of disease transmission. Affected pastures should be reseeded and preferably not used for grazing by unaffected animals, because MAP may persist on grass and soil for 1–4 years and remains viable to find the host. Sources of water supplies should be uncontaminated, as MAP survives in rivers and ponds for a period of 5 months (Al-Ghamdi, 2013).

18.11.2 Test and culling

Proper clinical evaluation with diagnostic facility should be performed for the prevention of these diseases. Control of paratuberculosis will be easier and the efficiency of overall control programme will be enhanced if animals that are shedding large numbers of organisms are removed (Bennett *et al.*, 2012). Proper 'test and cull' method should be applied for the economic benefits of the farmers and for the effective strategies to control paratuberculosis in various herds of goats (Kirkeby *et al.*, 2016).

18.11.3 Zoning

This is the general approach to disease control in animals, where zones are made on the basis of severity and prevalence of disease and movement is restricted in them. Disease-free, protected and control areas are managed accordingly. However, zoning may be a barrier in trading and marketing (Ayele *et al.*, 2001).

18.11.4 Vaccination

Vaccination protocol is the most important cost-effective strategy as compared with other preventive strategies and it is helpful for delaying the onset of shedding, slowing progression from low shedding to high shedding, reducing infectiousness of shedders and extending the length of the latent period towards infected animals. Nowadays promising new effective approaches to combat interference with the skin test for tuberculosis have been assessed successfully, by applying proteinic and peptidic cocktails in skin tests rather than the traditional test reagents (Serrano *et al.*, 2017). Singh *et al.* (2011) vaccinated goats and found recovery rates of 85% under optimal conditions of nutrition while 15% could not recover because of clinical stage. Thakur *et al.* (2013) suggested that an appropriate age of vaccination should be considered in vaccination protocols. Both live (attenuated and non- attenuated) as well as killed whole-cell vaccines have been used against paratuberculosis (Knust *et al.*, 2013).

In a few cases, subunit vaccines amalgamating sonicated bacteria, bacterial cell fractions and/or recombinant MAP antigens have been implicated for lowering the degree of protection (Kathaperumal *et al.*, 2009). DNA vaccines have also been used with better success rates (Park *et al.*, 2008). In addition, dairy goats in infected herds in the Netherlands are generally vaccinated once in the first month of life (Luttikholt *et al.*, 2019).

References

Al-Ghamdi, G.M. (2013) *Mycobacterium avium* subspecies *paratuberculosis* in camels; clinical aspects and control suggestions. *Egyptian Academic Journal of Biological Sciences* 5(1), 11–15.

Almujalli, A.M. and Al-Ghamdi, G.M. (2012) Clinicopathological findings of *paratuberclosis* in camels: Possible steps for control strategy. *Research Journal of Biological Sciences* 7(3), 128–131.

Ansari, M.M., Peer, F.U. and Wani, S.A. (2013) Studies on clinic-therapeutic management of paratuberculosis in bovine. *Blue Cross Book* 29, 60–61.

Ayele, W.Y., Machackova, M. and Pavlik, I. (2001) The transmission and impact of paratuberculosis infection in domestic and wild ruminants. *Veterinary Medicine – Czech* 46(7–8), 205–224.

Bauman, C.A., Jones-Bitton, A., Menzies, P., Toft, N., Jansen, J. *et al.* (2016) Prevalence of paratuberculosis in the dairy goat and dairy sheep industries in Ontario. *Canadian Veterinary Journal* 57, 169–175.

Bennett, R., McClement, I. and McFarlane, I. (2012) Modelling of Johne's disease control options in beef cattle: A decision support approach. *Livestock Science* 146(2–3), 149–159.

Borody, T.J., Bilkey, S., Wettstein, A.R., Leis, S., Pang, G. *et al.* (2007) Anti-mycobacterial therapy in Crohn's disease heals mucosa with longitudinal scars. *Digestive and Liver Disease* 39(5), 438–444.

Bryant, J.M., Thibault, V.C., Smith, D.G., McLuckie, J., Heron, I. *et al.* (2016) Phylogenomic exploration of the relationships between strains of *Mycobacterium avium* subspecies paratuberculosis. *BMC Genomics* 17, 79.

Carter, M.A. (2012) Prevalence and prevention of paratuberculosis in North America. *Japanese Journal of Veterinary Research* 60(Supplement), S9–S18.

CFSPH (Centre for Food Security and Public Health) (2007) Paratuberculosis. Available at: http://www.cfsph.iastate.edu/ Factsheets/pdfs/paratuberculosis.pdf (accessed 1 September 2014).

Clarke, C.J. and Little, D. (1996) The pathology of ovine paratuberculosis: Gross and histological changes in the intestine and other tissues. *Journal of Comparative Pathology* 114, 419–437.

Cocito, C., Gilot, P., Coene, M., De, M., Poupart, P. *et al.* (1994) Paratuberculosis. *Clinical Microbiology Reviews* 7, 328–345.

Collins, M.T., Eggleston, V. and Manning, E.J. (2010) Successful control of Johne's disease in nine dairy herds: Results of a six-year field trial. *Journal of Dairy Science* 93, 1638–1643.

Corpa, J.M., Garrido, J., Marin, J.F.G. and Perez, V. (2000) Classification of lesions observed in natural cases of paratuberculosis in goats. *Journal of Comparative Pathology* 122, 255–265.

Donat, K., Schlotter, K., Erhardt, G. and Brandt, H.R. (2014) Prevalence of paratuberculosis in cattle and control measures within the herd influence the performance of ELISA tests. *Veterinary Record* 174(5), 119.

Eda, S., Elliott, B., Scott, M.C., Waters, W.R., Bannantine, J.P. *et al.* (2005) New method of serological testing for *Mycobacterium avium* subsp. paratuberculosis (Johne's disease) by flow cytometry. *Foodborne Pathogens and Disease* 2(3), 250–262.

Fawcett, A.R., Goddard, P.I. and McKelvey, W.A.C. (1995) Johne's in a herd of farmed red deer. *Veterinary Record* 136, 165.

Fernandez-Silva, J.A., Correa-Valencia, N.M. and Ramirez, N.F. (2014) Systematic review of the prevalence of paratuberculosis in cattle, sheep, and goats in Latin America and the Caribbean. *Tropical Animal Health and Production* 46, 1321–1340.

Ferreira, R., Fonseca, L.S. and Lilenbaum, W. (2002) Agar gel immunodiffusion test (AGID) evaluation for detection of bovine paratuberculosis in Rio de Janeiro, Brazil. *Letters in Applied Microbiology* 35(3), 173–175.

Fiorentino, M.A., Gioffré, A., Cirone, K.C., Morsella Alonso, B., Delgado, F. *et al.* (2012) First isolation of *Mycobacterium avium* subsp. *paratuberculosis* in a dairy goat in Argentina: Pathology and molecular characterization. *Small Ruminant Research* 108, 133–136.

Ghosh, P., Hsu, C., Alyamani, E.J., Shehata, M.M., Al-Dubaib, M.A. *et al.* (2012) Genome-wide analysis of the emerging infection with *Mycobacterium avium* subspecies *paratuberculosis* in the Arabian camels (*Camelus dromedarius*). *PLoS ONE* 7, e31947.

Grewal, S.K., Rajeev, S., Sreevatsan, S. and Michel, F.C. (2006) Persistence of *Mycobacterium avium* subsp. *paratuberculosis* and other zoonotic pathogens during simulated composting, manure packing, and liquid storage of dairy manure. *Applied and Environmental Microbiology* 72(1), 565–574.

Gupta, A., Rani, S.M., Agrawal, P. and Gupta, P.K. (2012) Sero–prevalence of paratuberculosis (Johne's disease) in cattle population of South-Western Bangalore using ELISA kit. *Open Journal of Veterinary Medicine* 2, 196–200.

Henderson, D.C., Caldow, G. and Low, C.J. (2000) Paratuberculosis in cattle: Pathology and clinical disease. In: *Assessment of Surveillance and Control of Johne's Disease in Farm Animals in GB*. Scottish Agricultural College, Veterinary Science Division, Edinburgh, UK, pp. 15–19.

Herrold, R.D. (1931) Egg yolk agar medium for the growth of organisms would be *M. paratuberculosis* strain 18 or tubercle bacilli. *Journal of Infectious Diseases* 48, 236–241.

Kathaperumal, K., Kumanan, V., McDonough, S., Chen, L.-H., Park, S.-U. *et al.* (2009) Evaluation of immune responses and protective efficacy in a goat model following immunization with a cocktail of recombinant antigens and a polyprotein of *Mycobacterium avium* subsp. paratuberculosis. *Vaccine* 27, 123–135.

Kirkeby, C., Græsbøl, K., Nielson, S.S., Christiansen, L.E., Toft, N. *et al.* (2016) Adaptive test schemes for control of paratuberculosis in dairy cows. *PLoS ONE* 11, e0167219.

Knust, B., Patton, E., Ribeiro-Lima, J., Bohn, J.J. and Wells, S.J. (2013) Evaluation of the effects of a killed whole-cell vaccine against *Mycobacterium avium* subsp. *paratuberculosis* in 3 herds of dairy cattle with natural exposure to the organism. *Journal of the American Veterinary Medical Association* 242(5), 663–669.

Kostoulas, P., Browne, W.J., Nielsen, S.S. and Leontides, L. (2013) Bayesian mixture models for partially verified data: Age- and stage-specific discriminatory power of an antibody ELISA for paratuberculosis. *Preventive Veterinary Medicine* 111, 200–205.

Liapi, M., Leontides, L., Kostoulas, P., Botsaris, G., Iacovou, Y. *et al.* (2011) Bayesian estimation of the true prevalence of *Mycobacterium avium* subsp. paratuberculosis infection in cypriot dairy sheep and goat flocks. *Small Ruminant Research* 95(2–3), 174–178.

Luttikholt, S., Lievaart-Peterson, K., Gonggrijp, M., Aalberts, M., van Schaik, G. *et al.* (2019) *Mycobacterium avium* subsp. *paratuberculosis* ELISA responses in milk samples from vaccinated and nonvaccinated dairy goat herds in the Netherlands. *Veterinary Science* 6, 58.

Lybeck, K.R., Storset, A.K., Djønne, B., Valheim, M. and Olsen, I. (2011) Faecal shedding detected earlier than immune responses in goats naturally infected with *Mycobacterium avium* subsp. *paratuberculosis*. *Research in Veterinary Science* 91, 32–39.

Manning, J.B.E. and Collins, M.T. (2001) *Mycobacterium avium* subsp. *paratuberculosis*: Pathogen, pathogenesis and diagnosis. *Revue Scientifique et Technique. Office international des épizooties* 20(1), 133–150.

Manning, J.B.E., Steinberg, H., Krebs, V. and Collins, M.T. (2002) Diagnostic testing patterns of natural *Mycobacterium paratuberculosis* infection in pygmy goats. *Canadian Journal of Veterinary Research* 67, 213–218.

McNees, A.L., Markesich, D., Zayyani, N.R. and Graham, D.Y. (2015) *Mycobacterium paratuberculosis* as a cause of Crohn's disease. *Expert Review of Gastroenterology and Hepatology* 9, 1523–1534.

Mercier, P., Baudry, C., Beaudeau, F., Seegers, H. and Malher, X. (2010) Estimated prevalence of *Mycobacterium avium* subspecies *paratuberculosis* infection in herds of dairy goats in France. *Veterinary Record* 167(11), 412–416.

Milner, A.R., Wendy, N., Mack, K.J., Coates, J.H., Ian, G. *et al.* (1990) The sensitivity and specificity of a modified ELISA for the diagnosis of Johne's disease from a field trial in cattle. *Veterinary Microbiology* 25, 193–198.

Nielsen, S.S. and Toft, N. (2008) Ante mortem diagnosis of paratuberculosis: A review of accuracies of ELISA, interferon-g assay and faecal culture techniques. *Veterinary Microbiology* 129, 217–235.

Park, H.-T., Park, H.-E., Cho, Y.-I., Kim, E.-H., Jung, M. *et al.* (2017) Potential biomarkers as an indicator of vertical transmission of Johne's disease in a Korean native cattle farm. *Journal of Veterinary Science* 18, 343–349.

Park, S.U., Kathaperumal, K., McDonough, S., Akey, B., Huntley, J. *et al.* (2008) Immunization with a DNA vaccine cocktail induces a Th1 response and protects mice against *Mycobacterium avium* subsp. *paratuberculosis* challenge. *Vaccine* 26, 4329–4337.

Quinn, P., Markey, B., Carter, M. and Carter, G.R. (2013) *Clinical Veterinary Microbiology*. Mosby International, Edinburgh.

Rathnaiah, G., Zinniel, D.K., Bannantine, J.P., Stabel, J.R., Gröhn, Y.T. *et al.* (2017) Pathogenesis, molecular genetics, and genomics of *Mycobacterium avium* subsp. *paratuberculosis*, the Etiologic agent of Johne's disease. *Frontiers in Veterinary Science* 4, 187.

Robbe-Austerman, S. (2011) Control of paratuberculosis in small ruminants. *Veterinary Clinics of North America – Food Animal Practice* 27, 609–620.

Robbe-Austerman, S., Gardner, I.A., Thomsen, B.V., Morrical, D.G., Martin, B.M. *et al.* (2006) Sensitivity and specificity of the agar–gel– immunodiffusion test, ELISA and the skin test for detection of paratuberculosis in United States Midwest sheep populations. *Veterinary Research* 37, 553–564.

Salgado, M., Kruze, J. and Collins, M.T. (2007) Diagnosis of paratuberculosis by fecal culture and ELISA on milk and serum samples in two types of Chilean dairy goat herds. *Journal of Veterinary Diagnostic Investigation* 19, 99–102.

Saxegaard, F. and Fodstad, F.H. (1985) Control of paratuberculosis (Johne's disease) in goats by vaccination. *Veterinary Record* 116, 439.

Serrano, M., Elguezabal, N., Sevilla, I.A., Geijo, M.V., Molina, E. *et al.* (2017) Tuberculosis detection in paratuberculosis vaccinated calves: New alternatives against interference. *PLoS ONE* 12, e0169735.

Singh, K., Chandel, B.S., Dadawala, A.I., Singh, S.V., Chauhan, H.C. *et al.* (2013) Incidence of *Mycobacterium avium* subspecies *paratuberculosis* in mehsana breed of goats from South Gujarat using multiple tests. *Advances in Animal and Veterinary Sciences* 1, s28–s31.

Singh, S.V., Singh, P.K., Singh, M.K., Singh, A.V. and Sohal, J.S. (2011) Therapeutic potential of Johne's disease vaccine: A follow up post vaccination study in a goatherd of endangered Jamunapari breed, naturally infected with *Mycobacterium avium* subspecies paratuberculosis. *International Journal of Livestock Production* 2(13), 192–204.

Slana, I., Bartoš, M., Roubal, P., Babák, V. and Pavlík, I. (2009) *Mycobacterium avium* subsp. *paratuberculosis* and *M. a. avium* detected by culture, Is900 and Is901 highly sensitive PCR in bulk tank milk from dairy herds in the Czech republic between 2002 and 2004. *Czech Journal of Food Science* 27(5), 372–378.

Sting, R., Hrubenja, M., Mandl, J., Seemann, G., Salditt, A. *et al.* (2014) Detection of *Mycobacterium avium* subsp. *paratuberculosis* in faeces using different procedures of pre-treatment for real-time PCR in comparison to culture. *Veterinary Journal* 199(1), 138–142.

Thakur, A., Aagaard, C., Stockmarr, A., Ersen, P. and Jungersen, G. (2013) Cell-mediated and humoral immune responses after immunization of calves with a recombinant multiantigenic *Mycobacterium avium* subsp. *paratuberculosis* subunit vaccine at different ages. *Clinical and Vaccine Immunology* 20(4), 551–558.

Twort, F.W. and Ingram, G.L.Y. (1912) A method for isolating and cultivating *Mycobacterium enteritis* chronic *Pseudotuberculosis bovis*, Johne, and some experiments on the preparation of A diagnostic vaccine for pseudotuberculosis enteritis of bovines. *Proceedings of the Royal Society of London, Series B* 84, 517–542.

Verdugo, C., Jones, G., Johnson, W., Wilson, P., Stringer, L. *et al.* (2014) Estimation of flock/herd-level true *Mycobacterium avium* subspecies paratuberculosis prevalence on sheep, beef cattle and deer farms in New Zealand using a novel Bayesian model. *Preventive Veterinary Medicine* 117, 447–455.

Whittington, R.J. and Sergeant, E.S. (2001) Progress towards understanding the spread, detection and control of *Mycobacterium avium* subsp. *paratuberculosis* in animal populations. *Australian Veterinary Journal* 79, 267–278.

Whittington, R.J., Marsh, I.B., Taylor, P.J., Marshall, D.J., Taragel, C. *et al.* (2003) Isolation of *Mycobacterium avium* subsp. *paratuberculosis* from environmental samples collected from farms before and after destocking sheep with paratuberculosis. *Australian Veterinary Journal* 81(9), 559–563.

Windsor, P.A. and Whittington, R.J. (2010) Evidence for age susceptibility of cattle to Johne's disease. *Veterinary Journal* 184(1), 37–44.

19 Leptospirosis

J. Jyothi[1]* and M. Bhavya Sree[2]
[1]Department of Veterinary Medicine, P.V. Narasimharao Telangana Veterinary University, Hyderabad; [2]P.V. Narasimharao Telangana Veterinary University, Hyderabad

Abstract

Leptospirosis is a typical zoonotic illness affecting both humans and agricultural animals. Even though sheep and goats with leptospiral infection do not show any symptoms, they are especially important in the spread of *Leptospira* bacteria through urine. Young animals are frequently affected by severe disease, which is linked to accidental serovars. The main signs of subclinical infection include reproductive issues such as infertility, abortion, stillbirths and weak lambs or goat kids. For a precise infection diagnosis, laboratory testing is necessary. The most typical indirect diagnostic for leptospirosis is the microscopic agglutination test. Leptospirosis in small ruminants should be diagnosed using the PCR technique. Leptospirosis control measures include locating and treating carriers and other infection sources, keeping acquired animals in isolation and routine inoculation with commercial vaccines.

Keywords: leptospirosis, spirochaetes, micro agglutination test, serovars, urine, vaccination

19.1 Introduction

Small ruminants (sheep and goats) are ubiquitous and important for subsistence and for economic (income generation) and social sustenance (poverty alleviation) of the human population, mainly in developing countries (Pugh, 2001).

According to the Food and Agriculture Organization (FAO) in 2011, there were 875.5 million goats and one billion sheep in the world. Approximately 80% of the sheep and goats are in developing countries, many of them located in tropical regions, representing more than 70% of the production of these species (FAOSTAT, 2011).

These species can survive in a variety of climatic and geographical environments. Sheep and goats are small, have high reproductive rates and can eat a wide variety of foods. Developing countries offer a favourable environment for the expansion of sheep and goat breeding.

Despite the large population of small ruminants in emerging nations in recent decades, their production has remained low. Poor reproductive performance, insufficient management techniques and nutritional deficits are cited as major contributing reasons (Constable *et al.*, 2017).

Leptospirosis is brought on by pathogenic spirochaetes of the genus *Leptospira*, and the disease can be identified by anoestrum, recurrent oestrus, early embryonic mortality, abortion, retained placenta and delayed sexual maturity. The two inter-organ serovars that are most frequently involved with caprine abortion

*Corresponding author: jyothirvm1027@gmail.com

DOI: 10.1079/ 9781800622852.0019

are *Leptospira kirschneri* serovar Grippotyphosa and *Leptospira interrogans* serovar Pomona. Sheep have a low leptospirosis risk.

19.2 Aetiology

Worldwide, the serovars Guaricura (*Leptospira santarosai*) in the Americas and Hardjo (*L. interrogans*) predominate as members of the serogroup Sejroe. Poor management methods and the environment are more likely to be the source of transmission for these strains.

Sheep and goats are the main targets of serovars such as Pomona and Icterohaemorrhagiae (*L. interrogans*) and the *L. kirschneri* serovar Grippotyphosa.

19.3 Epidemiology

Leptospirosis in small ruminants is frequently linked to the serogroup Sejroe, especially the serovar Hardjo. For many years, small ruminants were thought of as inadvertent hosts of leptospiral infection, being affected only by incidental serovars carried by other domestic and wild species (Leon-Vizcaino *et al.*, 1987).

Leptospirosis in sheep and goats is caused by a variety of risk factors. Compared with younger animals, adult goats have a three times higher relative risk (RR) of contracting leptospirosis.

19.4 Reproductive Performance Due to Leptospirosis

Sheep and goats with leptospirosis might appear with acute infection or subclinical infection.

Symptoms of acute illness include loss of appetite, agitation, diarrhoea, opaque coats and epidemic abortions. Reproductive issues like infertility, additional procedures required for conception, delayed birthing intervals, abortion, stillbirths and poor lambs or goat kids are linked to subclinical infection. The most significant symptom of serovar Hardjo leptospirosis in goats is persistent infection of the reproductive tract. The most prevalent causes of severe sickness seen in lambs and young goats are Pomona, Ballum, Icterohaemorrhagiae, or Grippotyphosa serovars.

Sheep and goats become ill when they come into contact with polluted tissues or urine, whether directly or indirectly. The leptospiral organisms are localized and present in a variety of tissues following the incubation period, which is 7–10 days after infection.

19.5 Clinical Findings

Acute leptospirosis with incidental strains is seen less frequently and usually presents as an outbreak. The main characteristics of this syndrome include abortions at any stage of pregnancy and the birth of feeble offspring. Blood-tinged milk in lactating cows has also been documented.

Contrarily, a chronic, silent infection linked to repeated oestrous cycles and reproductive failure as seen in embryo losses is the most common manifestation. Serovars Hardjo and Guaricura are more strongly associated with the chronic reproductive form of infection, because they can colonize and stay in the genital tract of infected cows and bulls. The primary leptospirosis condition affecting cattle is now understood to be this genital leptospirosis presentation.

19.6 Diagnosis

Diagnosis is by means of serology, bacterial culture, or PCR assay. Bacterial culture is the gold-standard diagnostic technique, although it is rarely used, because of technical and financial constraints.

Infected animals produce elevated levels of the infectious serovar during the acute disease; a microagglutination test (MAT) antibody titre of 800 or less is regarded as proof of leptospirosis. In similar circumstances, immunofluorescence, PCR tests and immunohistochemistry can also be used to demonstrate leptospires in the placenta and fetus. In contrast, it is more challenging to diagnose persistent or subclinical infections brought on by Sejroe strains.

There is a lack of apparent clinical symptoms and characteristic lesions in leptospiral infection in small ruminants. Laboratory tests are essential to achieve an accurate diagnosis of the infection (Limmathurotsakul *et al.*, 2012).

19.6.1 Collection of blood and serum samples

- Animals are separated into clinically ill and seemingly healthy goats at the time of sample collection based on history and clinical observations, such as pale or icterus mucous membrane, anorexia, fever, agalactia, mastitis, or miscarriage.
- Jugular vein blood and serum samples are aseptically obtained using K3 ethylenediaminetetraacetic acid (EDTA).
- To send samples to the pathology laboratory, a cold chain method is used.

19.6.2 Collection of urine samples

- Random urine samples are taken at the same time as blood samples from the same population of goats.
- After cleaning the vulva or preputial orifice, midstream urine samples are obtained and placed in plastic containers. Each animal has sufficient urine (30–50 ml) collected from it. As quickly as feasible, all urine samples are brought to the laboratory.

19.6.3 Haematological analysis

- Blood samples are subjected to various haematological analyses. For example, haemoglobin estimation (Hb), packed cell volume (PCV), total erythrocyte count (TEC), mean corpuscular volume (MCV), mean corpuscular Hb (MCH), MCH concentration (MCHC) and total leukocyte count (TLC) are analysed using automatic whole-blood analyser.
- Differential leukocyte count (DLC) on Giemsa-stained smears is performed manually.

19.7 Treatment, Control and Prevention of *Leptospira*

A combined programme of antimicrobials, management adjustments and immunization is frequently advised. It is also frequently advised to use an integrated treatment that combines vaccination, certain management changes and antibiotics. According to reports, antimicrobial therapy stops abortions and other reproductive issues. The renal carrier status is normally eliminated by streptomycin (25 mg/kg, IM, single dose). Tulathromycin, ceftiofur and oxytetracycline are also equally efficient.

It has been shown that dividing animals into smaller batches, soil sealing and routine cleaning of milking sectors will considerably lower the exposure of animals to leptospires when environmental and management conditions are taken into account.

A study reported on the control of a leptospirosis outbreak in goats in Brazil. In this herd, a broad-based management approach was conducted, including serological and molecular diagnostic methods, vaccination, antibiotic treatment and correction of some environmental aspects. That approach was critical to the control of this outbreak, thereby minimizing subsequent reproductive failures and economic losses (Martins *et al.*, 2012).

19.8 Discussion

Because of its variable clinical presentations in animals, leptospirosis is now the most neglected or glaringly underreported disease with a diagnostic conundrum. Animal sickness can range from minor insignificant symptoms to severe forms that present with reproductive and productive issues.

Since leptospirosis is an infectious zoonotic illness that can occur everywhere in the world and is brought on by various *L. interrogans* serotypes, knowledge of the serotypes present in a particular area may aid in making a more accurate diagnosis of the disease's epidemiology and aetiology.

Since the 1990s, a number of PCR detection techniques for leptospiral DNA have been established. In fact, PCR is a quick and accurate diagnostic method that can find leptospiral DNA in body fluids and tissues.

19.9 Conclusion

In conclusion, described clinicopathological abnormalities can be useful in leptospirosis diagnosis and therapeutic management in goats that appear healthy or sick. Current findings suggest liver injury in seropositive goats based on elevated levels of ALT, AST, total bilirubin and lower levels of TP.

The lack of information regarding leptospirosis in small ruminants is still disproportionate to the risks that the condition poses to farmers around the world. Additional trials revealing the true function of goats and sheep as leptospire reservoirs, notably Hardjo, as well as wider research with proper sampling and risk factor analysis must be conducted in different countries. Small-ruminant control is still empirical and nothing is understood about the specifics of those animals.

References

Constable, P.D., Hinchcliff, K.W., Done, S.H. and Grünberg, W. (eds) (2017) *Veterinary Medicine*, 11th edn. Saunders Elsevier, St Louis, Missouri.

FAOSTAT (2011) FAOSTAT Database (FAO Statistical Databases). Food and Agriculture Organization of the United Nations, Rome. Available at: http://faostat.fao.org

Leon-Vizcaino, L., De Mendoza, M.H. and Garrido, F. (1987) Incidence of abortions caused by leptospirosis in sheep and goats in Spain. *Comparative Immunology, Microbiology, and Infectious Diseases* 10, 149–153.

Limmathurotsakul, D., Turner, E.L., Wuthiekanun, V., Thaipadungpanit, J., Suputtamongkol, Y. *et al.* (2012) Fool's gold: Why imperfect reference tests are undermining the evaluation of novel diagnostics: A re-evaluation of five diagnostic tests for leptospirosis. *Clinical Infectious Diseases* 55, 322–331.

Martins, G., Penna, B., Hamond, C., Leite, R.C.-K., Silva, A. *et al.* (2012) Leptospirosis as the most frequent infectious disease impairing productivity in small ruminants in Rio de Janeiro, Brazil. *Tropical Animal Health and Production* 44, 773–777.

Pugh, D.G. (2001) Sheep and goat medicine, 2nd edn. Saunders, Maryland Heights, Missouri.

20 Streptococcosis

Mahmuda Malik*
Dept of Pathology, Apollo College of Veterinary Medicine, Jaipur, Rajasthan

Abstract
Streptococcosis is a very common disease condition in both goats and humans. As humans and domestic animals reside close to each other, they commonly share aetiological agents that may be responsible for zoonotic diseases. Various strains of streptococcus have been reported to cause mastitis. *Streptococcus canis* results in mastitis, pneumonia, septicaemia and streptococcal toxic shock-like syndrome, lymphadenitis, omphalophlebitis, chronic cough, uncontrolled fasciculations, rigidity of muscles, intense pain and haemorrhages, blood in sputum, bleeding from the nose, dysentery and death. In humans it can result in throat infection, arthritis, septicaemia, renal diseases, endocarditis, meningitis and autoimmune reactions. The most common mode of transmission of streptococcus from goats to humans is direct or indirect contact with the animal or with an animal's excretions and secretions. Another way of contracting streptococcosis from goats is to handle and consume infected milk, meat or other animal products. Modern science has several tools to diagnose streptococcosis, like the application of molecular techniques, antigen–antibody-based techniques, conventional morphology and colony characteristics, which may aid in quick and efficient diagnosis of streptococcosis in both humans and animals.

Keywords: Streptococcus, human, goat, zoonosis, endocarditic, pyelonephritis, rheumatic fever

20.1 Introduction

Streptococcus species are a group of Gram-positive bacteria that reside in human and animal bodies. The bacteria grow in pairs and chains (Fig. 20.1). The incubation period of streptococcal infection may vary from a few days to a week.

20.2 Aetiology

There are about 55 recognized *Streptococcus* species (Pisoni *et al.*, 2009), but only a few of them are responsible for causing disease in cattle, sheep, goats, pigs, horses, dogs, cats, poultry and humans. They cause a wide variety of pathogenic conditions, affecting the genital tract, lymphatic system, cardiac system, nervous system, synovial membrane and fluid, and mammary glands. They also cause septicaemia (Minces *et al.*, 2011) (Fig. 20.2). One of the common examples of a streptococcal infection is strangles in horses.

Streptococcal organisms have the ability to ferment sugars without producing gas and are catalase-negative and oxidative-negative. These bacteria grow best on media containing blood or tissue extracts. Depending upon their growth on blood agar medium, streptococci are divided into three haemolytic types: alpha, beta and gamma. Alpha-haemolytic streptococci do not show any lysis of erythrocytes but may produce a zone of discoloration around the colonies as they change

*Corresponding author: drmahmudamalik@gmail.com

DOI: 10.1079/ 9781800622852.0020

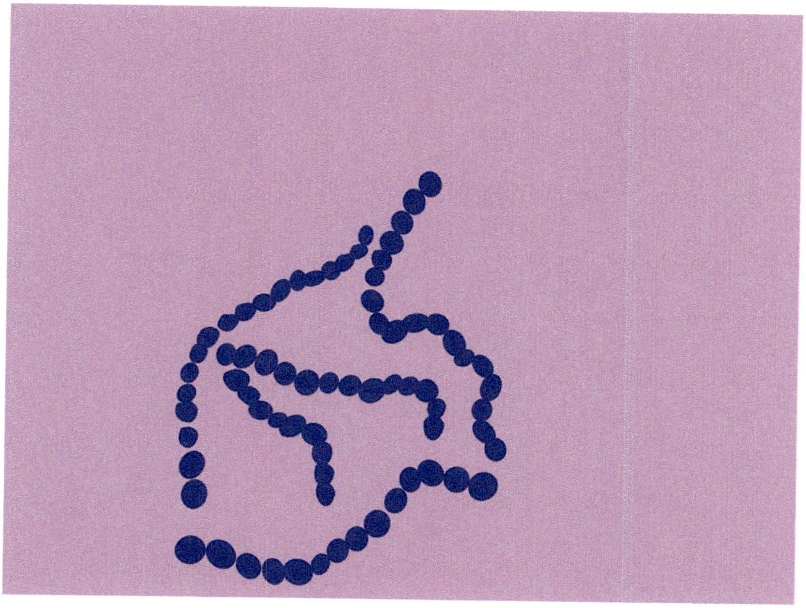

Fig. 20.1. Gram-positive *Streptococcus* appearing as long chain of round cocci. (Author's own image.)

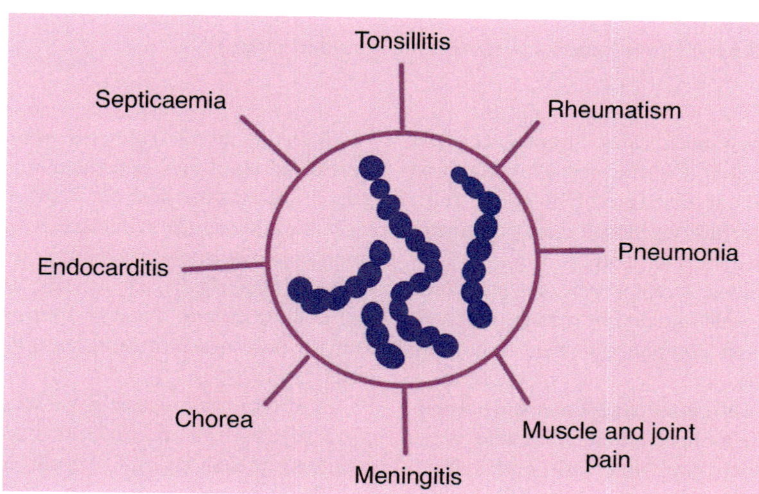

Fig. 20.2. Different clinical conditions due to *Streptococcus* spp. (Author's own image.)

the haemoglobin into methaemoglobin. A number of commensal streptococci are grouped under alpha-haemolytic streptococci and are called viridans streptococci (Kuusi *et al.*, 2006).

Beta-haemolytic streptococci can cause lysis of the erythrocytes, which can be seen as a clear zone around the growing colonies in blood agar medium. Gamma-haemolytic streptococci do not cause haemolysis.

Streptococci are spherical to short bacillary organisms of about 1 μm in diameter (Fig. 20.3). They have a Gram-positive cell wall composed of

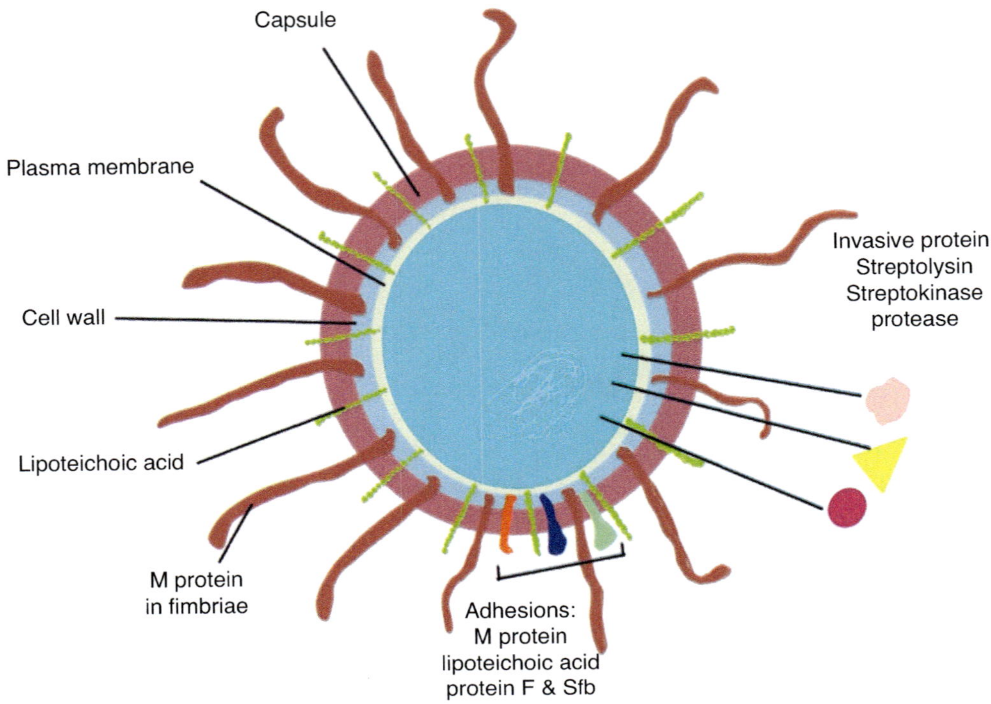

Fig. 20.3. Structure of *Streptococcus pyogenes*. (Author's own image.)

protein and polysaccharides. Streptococci may produce a number of surface proteins that bind with extracellular matrix protein of the host, like fibronectin, fibrinogen, collagen, vitronectin and laminin (Gibbs *et al.*, 1981).

Encapsulated streptococci are composed of hyaluronic acid and do not readily bind with the complement components; hence they are antiphagocytic.

The cell wall contains proteins and polysaccharides such as lipoteichoic acids and peptidoglycan, which can bind with macrophage, resulting in the release of proinflammatory cytokines (Dudas and Serwint, 2006) (Fig. 20.3).

Suppuration or pus formation occurs as a result of action of neutrophils on the bacterial products.

In animals, *Streptococcus agalactiae* causes subclinical mastitis in cattle, sheep and goats. In dogs it causes endocarditis and infection of the heart, whereas in humans the carrier remains asymptomatic.

Infection by *Streptococcus canis* results in mastitis, pneumonia, septicaemia (Las Heras *et al.*, 2002; Hashikawa *et al.*, 2004) and streptococcal toxic shock-like syndrome, lymphadenitis, omphalophlebitis, chronic cough, uncontrolled fasciculations, rigidity of muscles, intense pain and haemorrhages, blood in sputum, bleeding from the nose, dysentery and death within hours (Shah *et al.*, 2001).

Streptococcus dysgalactiae subsp. *dysgalactiae* can lead to both clinical and subclinical mastitis, cellulitis and toxic shock-like syndrome.

Streptococcus equi subsp. *zooepidemicus* affects the upper respiratory tract of horses and the lymph nodes, resulting in pleuropneumonia, dry cough, death due to pneumonia and septicaemia (Philpott *et al.*, 2004). In pigs, *S. equi* subsp. *zooepidemicus* affects the lymph nodes, genital system and respiratory system, and infection results in abscesses and inflammation in the respective organs (Albarraein *et al.*, 1998). In certain cases, *Streptococcus* infection results in severe respiratory affliction with copious exudation and torticollis in the neck (Soedarmanto *et al.*, 1996). In canines, *Streptococcus* organisms mostly cause septicaemia, septic shock, haemorrhagic nasal discharge and haematemesis. *S. equi* subsp. *zooepidemicus* has been reported in human cases in which the individuals are immunocompromised and are already suffering from chronic disease.

Streptococcus halichoeri seems to enter the body through wound infection and has been reported to cause the fur-animal epidemic, necrotic pyoderma, in farmed canines like raccoon-dogs and foxes. In humans, *S. halichoeri* affects older people.

Streptococcus iniae causes meningo-encephalitis (Low *et al.*, 1980; Downar *et al.*, 2001) in fish. Handling of these infected fish and products increases the chances of zoonosis in humans.

Streptococcus suis causes polyarthritis, meningitis (Ural *et al.*, 2003), ear infection, endocarditis, abortion and multifocal abscesses in the visceral organs of pigs. In humans, *S. suis* results in septicaemia, toxic shock syndrome and meningo-encephalitis (Eyre *et al.*, 2010).

20.3 Transmission

Streptococcal organisms normally reside on the skin, in the mucous membrane of the respiratory tract, or in the uro-genital tract and mammary glands. Transmission of streptococcal infection may occur due to close contact with humans or animals. Direct contact might involve either faecal–oral transmission or skin-to-skin contact or via the mucous membranes. The viable organism may be carried by air or wind to a distance of about 10 miles or more. Dissemination of the bacteria through aerosol is an important source of infection.

Droplet infection is another mode of transmission when an infected person or animal in close vicinity sneezes or coughs and the bacteria are disseminated in the air. As the size of an infectious droplet is about 5 μm in diameter, it cannot travel more than 1 m. Hence the spread of infection occurs in close vicinity (Daya *et al.*, 2005).

Consumption of unpasteurized milk, milk products, meat products and undercooked meat is another potent source of infection (Fig. 20.4). Handling of infected milk, milk products, meat and meat products may result in infection (Krauss *et al.*, 2003). Milk may serve as an important source of bacterial infection if milk has been drawn from animal with subclinical bacterial infection. Hence milk should be pasteurized and kept at 5–10°C during transportation. Before milk is consumed by humans it is advisable to boil the milk properly to avoid the risk of getting an infection.

Streptococcal infection may also enter the body by open wound, injury, cut or laceration on the skin. Another very important and common source of streptococcal infection is use by both

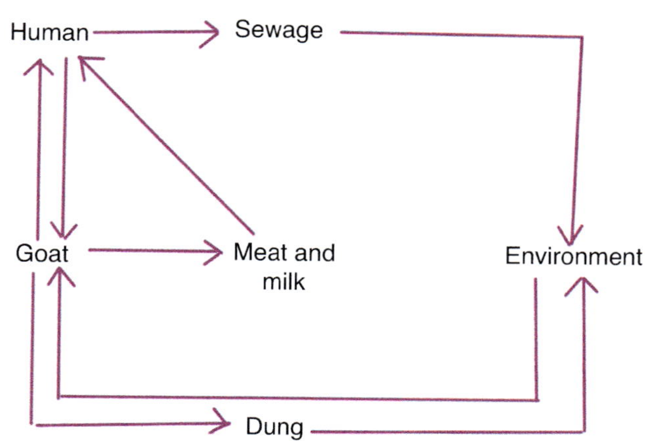

Fig. 20.4. Transmission of *Streptococcus* spp. in humans. (Author's own image.)

humans and animals of the same water body that has been contaminated with disposal of an infected carcass or waste from an infected farm.

Arthropods can act as a mechanical carrier of bacteraemia from one place to another. Likewise, mosquitoes can suck blood from an infected patient and can transmit the bacteria to a healthy patient while subsequently feeding. Similarly, flies can settle on excretions and secretions containing bacteria and may directly spread the organism by contaminating food and drink. Streptococcal organisms can also be spread from fomites, dust, environment, rotting carcasses, faecal material and aborted fetuses with infected uterine discharges. Vehicular transmission of bacteria may occur via contaminated water, food or feed and infected fomites (Lord *et al.*, 2022). Bacteria may adhere to the hands or body surface whenever a person or animal comes in contact with a contaminated surface or object and then transferred to the mucous membranes when the person touches their face or takes food without washing their hands. Similarly infection may occur when an animal licks a contaminated body part. Transmission of viable bacteria from animals may occur via handling of infected faeces, urine, animal hide and fetal membranes.

Medical and veterinary personnel should use proper personal protection equipment while attending clinically ill patients and animals. Precautions should be should be taken to avoid any direct contact during examination, treatment or vaccination.

Identification, isolation, culling and proper disposal of any diseased animal should be practised to reduce the risk of transmission. Proper measures should be taken to minimize the population of rodents and arthropods, which spread bacteria either by biting or by acting as a mechanical vector. Farmers should examine the body surface of their farm animals for presence of any ticks or mites (Harkani *et al.*, 2011).

20.4 Zoonotic Significance of Streptococcal Infection

Streptococcal infection can result in asymptomatic or very mild infections, like tonsillitis, red sores on the skin, or life-threatening conditions like streptoccocal toxic shock (Wasissa *et al.*, 2021). Severe symptoms of streptococcal infection are diarrhoea, vomiting, pyrexia, sepsis of wounds, pain in connective tissue, impetigo and cellulitis. Untreated cases of streptococcosis can result in the spread of the organism from the primary location to the secondary organs. Children having frequent throat infections at a young age may develop endocarditis in their later age with the organism being deposited in the valves of the heart. Similarly, streptococcal organisms from chronic infection can localize in joints, kidney and brain, resulting in arthritis, glomerulonephritis, meningitis and encephalitis (Kasahara *et al.*, 2001).

In humans, streptococcal infection may result in abscesses, cellulitis, pyoderma, pharyngitis, pneumonia and other respiratory diseases, arthritis, osteomyelitis, endocarditis, meningitis, septicaemia and shock-like syndromes (Wasniewska *et al.*, 2022). *Streptococcus* subsp. *zooepidemicus* has been isolated from a wide range of mild or moderate to severe illnesses. Streptococcal organisms could be isolated from skin lesions, blood in septicaemic conditions and various visceral organs containing foci of streptococcosis. Streptococcosis in the early phase of life may lead to autoimmune disease.

20.5 Pathology

20.5.1 Post-streptococcal glomerulonephritis

Post-streptococcal glomerulonephritis is an uncommon pathological condition affecting kidneys, caused by group A beta-haemolytic streptococci, also known as nephrogenic streptococci (Balter *et al.*, 2000; Abdel-Haq *et al.*, 2006). It is considered to be an immune response to an earlier streptococcal infection which is manifested as sore throat, scarlet fever, tonsillitis, pharyngitis or impetigo. These streptococcal infections result in the formation of antigen and antibody complex. Normally, after killing the foreign bodies, the antibody is cleaned out of the body by phagocytic cells. But when the size of these antigen–antibody complexes is too small, they can escape the vigilance of the phagocytic cells of the body (Blyth *et al.*, 2007).

As a result, these minute antigen–antibody complexes start to accumulate on the various visceral organs and initiate Type-III hypersensitivity. These antigen–antibody complexes, which are being carried by blood, remain adhered to the glomeruli and act as foreign particles. Sometimes there may be *in situ* aggregation of these antigen–antibody complexes in the glomerular basement membrane. The formation of these antigen–antibody complexes is due to two main reasons. First, there is reaction of the body's immune system streptococci, which were either already present or were deposited along the glomerular basement membrane. Secondly, the antibody formed during the early phase of streptococcal infection might react with glomerular cell components and cross-react with the streptococcal antigen due to molecular mimicry. The immune complexes adhere in the glomerular basement membrane, and initiate the activation of the complement pathway (Rammelkamp and Weaver, 1953).

Due to the action of leukocytes and proliferation of mesangial cells, the normal function of glomeruli is impaired. The capillaries cannot perform perfusion efficiently, resulting in reduced glomerular filtration rate, anuria, oliguria, imbalance of acid-balance and abnormalities in electrolyte concentration. When the glomerular filtration is obstructed, it leads to retention of sodium and water, which results in oedema and hypertension. A patient with post-streptococcal glomerulonephritis (Balter *et al.*, 2000; Pinto *et al.*, 2022) exhibits clinical sign of oedema, haematuria and hypertension, with a history of frequent throat infection, tonsillitis and impetigo. Most of the patients with post-streptococcal glomerulonephritis may suffer from hyperkalaemia, high blood pressure and acid–base imbalance. Generalized oedema is very common, while in severe cases oedema fluid may accumulate in the lungs, resulting in pneumonia and severe respiratory distress (Pinto *et al.*, 2022).

20.5.2 Streptococcal meningitis

Streptococcal meningitis is an acute inflammation of the meninges surrounding the brain and spinal cord. Numerous *Streptococcus* Group B species have been reported to cause meningitis in children but the most common causative organism is *Streptococcus pneumonia*, which is beta-haemolytic in nature (Baracco, 2019). *Streptococcus* meningitis occurs when the bacteria cross the blood–brain barrier via the blood circulation. As the streptococcal organism infects and colonizes the nasal mucosae, the organism multiplies and it reduces the immunity of the body, resulting in invasion by the bacteria into the meninges (Mungul and Meharaj, 2019). During this infectious phase the complement system is stimulated and the inflammatory mediators are released into the bloodstream, due to which the permeability of the blood–brain barrier increases, resulting in effective crossing of the bacteria into the blood–brain barrier. Patients affected by streptococcal meningitis might present stiffness of the neck muscles, fever, headache, alteration of mental behaviour and decision making and sometimes convulsion. These signs are found in adult patients, while clinical signs of lethargy and neck rigidity are common in young patients. In babies, there may be swelling of the fontanels due to severe infection of the meninges. Children may appear very sick, with inappetence, vomiting, diarrhoea, chills and sometimes unconsciousness (Carapetis *et al.*, 2005).

20.5.3 Streptococcal arthritis

Post-streptococcal arthritis is commonly found in patients who have a history of throat infection with streptococcal beta-haemolytic bacteria. In some patients with streptococcal arthritis there is a history of skin infection or heart disease. Many children may exhibit acute rheumatic fever with or without manifestation of post-streptococcal arthritis (Hunt and Somers, 2019). A constant factor regarding streptococcal arthritis is that patients do not respond to acetylsalicylic acid with minimal improvement of the condition. Post-streptococcal arthritis is generally seen with other clinical signs like endocarditis, skin nodules, chorea, pyrexia and acute rheumatic fever. Post-streptococcal arthritis is a lingering and persistent condition affecting the small and large joints, which includes upper limb joints, lower limb joints, hip, knee, ankle and wrist joints (Alber *et al.*, 2004). The nature of post-streptococcal arthritis may be migratory or non-migratory. Diagnosis can be made on the basis on recurring, persistent joint pain that might be acute in nature and does not respond well to non-steroidal anti-inflammatory drugs. The patient will always have a recent history of Group A streptococcal infection. Serology can be performed to detect a recent Group A streptococcal infection and detection of genetic markers like D8/17 antigens. HLA/DR is an MHC class II cell surface receptor that is identified as a marker of T-cell activation, which is found to be increased in autoimmune disease. D8/17, a monoclonal antibody, is helpful in detection of B-lymphocyte antigen associated with rheumatic fever (Bessen and Fischetti, 1992).

20.5.4 Streptococcal endocarditis

The most common aetiology of endocarditis is alpha-haemolytic streptococci and beta-haemolytic streptococci in the *Streptococcus bovis* group. But amongst these beta-haemolytic streptococci are the well-known causative organisms for endocarditis. Group beta streptococci infection can result in endocarditis in patients with a previous history of streptococcal infection. It has been documented that the patients have a common history of pharyngitis and arthritis, necrotizing fascitis and streptococcal shock syndrome. Later on, these patients may suffer from aortic failure, myocardial abscess and cardiac failure (Anderson *et al.*, 2014). Another *Streptococcus pyogenes* is known to produce exotoxins, which can stimulate the production of cytokines, resulting in tissue damage. This bacterium gets attached to various tissue surfaces, starts colonizing and has the special ability to resist the innate immune resistance, thereby causing degradation of tissue barriers and facilitating the spread and invasion of the *S. pyogenes* bacteria all over the body. The M surface protein found on *S. pyogenes* is believed to be involved in the attachment of the bacteria with the host membrane and to inhibit phagocytosis (Beachey *et al.*, 1974; Manjula *et al.*, 1991). The M surface protein of some strains, like *S. pyogenes* strain G773, has been reported to bind with C4b-binding protein and antibody, resulting in the production of bacteriocin. Bacteriocin has a bactericidal activity and the ability to eliminate the other commensal bacteria colonizing the same host (Lancefield, 1962). *S. pyogenes* has been recorded to express fibronectin and fibrinogen-binding genes which cause endovascular streptococcal infection (Chalker *et al.*, 2003).

Patients with endocarditis manifest a variety of clinical signs, like valvular regurgitation, with mobile, echo-dense masses adhered to the valves or with the presence of abscesses.

20.5.5 Toxic shock syndrome

Streptococcal toxic shock syndrome is caused by Group A *S. pyogenes*. This group of bacteria produces exotoxin, which results in the activation of cytotoxin, leading to initiation of shock (Valve and Vuento, 1992).

S. pyogenes is a Gram-positive bacterium that causes complete haemolysis of blood agar (Schneewind *et al.*, 1993). The most common clinical signs manifested by a patient affected with toxic shock syndrome are septicaemia, low blood pressure, tachycardia and increased rate of respiration.

Streptococci may enter the body through a skin injury or mucous membrane. The bacteria then multiply in the local lymph nodes and may enter the blood circulation. They may enter the body through any injury of the skin, including post-surgical wounds (Miles *et al.*, 2021). Direct or indirect contact with the patient or people associated with the patient, like health care workers and professionals, may also lead to infection. The incubation period of *S. pyogenes* is about 24–48 hour (Mobeen *et al.*, 2020). *S. pyogenes* is reported to affect people of about 65 years or older due to immunosuppression or due to senility. It is also common in immunocompromised patients suffering from chronic diseases like diabetes and fungal disease (Barrett, 1984). Streptococcal toxic shock syndrome has been reported in adults and children. It is reported that the Group A streptococcal infection associated with toxic shock syndrome ultimately results in death when it becomes invasive. Streptococcal toxic shock syndrome occurs due to secretion of super-antigen exotoxins, which cross-links the major histocompatibility class II and T-cells present on antigen-presenting cells and T-lymphocytes (Barnham *et al.*, 1983). The interaction of Group A streptococcal antigen with the immune cells of the body results in pro-inflammatory cytokines and vasodilating mediators, leading to shock. Group A streptococcal infection accompanies necrosis of muscles and subcutaneous tissue (Huang *et al.*, 2017). Streptococcal toxic shock syndrome has also been reported to manifest in three phases, where the first phase comprises the onset of severe hypotension with headache, muscle pain, pyrexia, chills and flu-like symptoms (Ferrandiere *et al.*, 1998). Some patients may also exhibit gastrointestinal tract problems with nervous symptoms. Soft-tissue infection is a common finding in Group A streptococcal infections (Gaglani and Edwards, 1995). Patients may show insignificant abrasion with redness and formation of haematoma. The second phase of streptococcal toxic shock syndrome is associated with tachycardia and increased respiration with pyrexia. Pain may be present in the thorax, abdomen and limbs. The third phase of streptococcal toxic shock syndrome manifests as shock-like symptoms, which ultimately results in multiple organ failure. The super-antigen present on the surface of the streptococcus stimulates the T-cell, which in turn activates the pro-inflammatory cytokines (Lancefield, 1959). These cytokines act in the vascular endothelium and increase the vascular permeability. This results in capillary leaking of plasma fluid, leading to decreased arterial blood volume and blood pressure.

20.6 Diagnosis

Streptococcus organisms can be diagnosed in stained smears of tissues, exudates and CSF fluid by demonstration of Gram-positive cocci that appear in pairs or chain. Clinical signs of pale mucous membranes, cold skin and bradycardia are indications of streptococcal toxic shock-like syndrome, which can be confirmed by isolation and identification of the organism (Yuen *et al.*, 1990; Mitchell *et al.*, 2020).

Streptococcus infection can also be determined by the colony-characteristic pattern of haemolysis on the blood agar, and the colour and morphology of the colony (Turner *et al.*, 2019).

Biochemical testing is another way to identify streptococcal infection, as the organisms are catalase-negative.

As for the serology, the capillary precipitation test is used to identify the streptococcal organism.

The presence of haemolysis of streptococcal organisms in a blood agar plate is another way to diagnose the disease.

Modern techniques like polymerase chain reaction can be performed for a confirmatory diagnosis (Salmenlinna *et al.*, 2000). Immunological tests like the immune-fluorescent antibody test can be done to identify the streptococcal antigen in impression smears, and nasal and throat swabs.

20.7 Disinfection

Streptococcal organisms are sensitive to chemicals and disinfectants like 1% sodium hypochlorite, formaldehyde, 70% ethanol, 6% hydrogen peroxide, ammonia compounds, phenyls and gluteraldehyde.

20.8 Detection of *Streptococcus* Organisms in Milk

Physical characteristics of the affected mammary gland include swelling of the udder, with pain on palpation (Brandt and Spellerberg, 2009). The mammary glands appear red in colour and are hot to touch. Milk from an affected udder may show characteristic alterations like formation of milk clots, flakes, presence of blood or discoloration. Animals with subclinical mastitis do not show any specific lesion, so confirmation can be made by identification of a bacterial colony where the samples are inoculated with eosine-methylene blue agar with 5% blood agar or in mannitol salt agar.

Biochemical tests widely used to detect *Streptococcus* organisms are coagulase test, oxidase test, triple sugar iron and the Christie, Atkins and Munch-Peterson (CAMP) test.

Antibiotic susceptibility/sensitivity tests involve growing a colony of *Streptococcus* in Mueller Hinton broth to achieve a definite bacterial concentration, which is further cultured in Mueller Hinton agar and incubated with different antibiotics to determine the sensitivity (Edward *et al.*, 1988).

Polymerase chain reaction (PCR) is a modern technique to detect *Streptococcus* (Elliott *et al.*, 1998). It amplifies the nucleic acid by thermal cycling but it is not suitable on a farm. Isolation and identification amplification is an effective diagnostic technique, cheaper than PCR and can be performed in farms. Isolation and identification DNA is another way to confirm the presence of bacteria in milk (Pancholi and Fischetti, 1988).

Microscopic examination of fresh samples of milk or sediment may be helpful in detection of the chains of streptococci. Growth of bacteria on blood agar plate is another conventional and commonly used technique (Mitchell *et al.*, 2020).

References

Abdel-Haq, N.M., Harasheh, A. and Asmar, B.I. (2006) Retropharyngeal abscess in children. The emerging role of group A beta hemolytic *Streptococcus*. *Southern Medical Journal* 99, 927–931. DOI: 10.1097/01.smj.0000224746.39728.ed.

Albarraein, C., Rosencrance, G., Boland, J. and Hernandez, J.E. (1998) Bacteremia due to *Streptococcus zooepidemicus* associated with an abdominal aortic aneurysm. *West Virginia Medical Journal* 94, 90–92.

Alber, J., El-Sayed, A., Lammler, C., Hassan, A.A., Weiss, R. *et al.* (2004) Multiplex polymerase chain reaction for identification and differentiation of *Streptococcus equi* subsp. *zooepidemiscus* and *Streptococcus equi* subsp *equi*. *Journal of Veterinary Medicine B, Infectious Diseases and Veterinary Public Health* 51, 1455–1458.

Anderson, E.L., Cole, J.N., Olsen, J., Rylan, B., Ghosh, P. *et al.* (2014) The fibrinogen-binding MI protein reduces pharyngeal cell adherence and colonization phenotypes of MiT1 young A *Streptococcus*. *Journal of Biological Chemistry* 289(6), 3539–3546.

Balter, S., Bonin, A., Pinto, S.W., Teixeira, L.M., Alvim, G.G. *et al.* (2000) Epidemic nephritis in Nova Serrani, Brazil. *Lancet* 9217, 1776–1780. DOI: 101016/s0140-6736(00)02265-0.

Baracco, G.J. (2019) Infections caused by group C and G streptococcus (*Streptococcus dysgalactiae* subsp. *equisimilis* and others): Epidemiological and clinical aspects. *Microbiology Spectrum* 7(2), GPP3-0016-2018. DOI: 10.1128/microbiolspec.GPP3-0016-2018.

Barnham, M., Thornton, T.J. and Lange, K. (1983) Nephritis caused by *Streptococcus zooepidemicus* (Lancefield group C). *Lancet* 1, 945–948. DOI: 10.1016/S0140-6736(83)92078-0.

Barrett, N.J. (1984) Communicable disease associated with milk and dairy products in England and Wales. *Journal of Infection* 12, 265–272. DOI: 10.1016/S0163-4453(86)94320-3.

Beachey, E.H., Campbell, G.L. and Ofek, I. (1974) Peptic digestion of Streptococcal M protein. II. Extraction of M antigen from group A Streptococci with pepsin. *Infection and Immunity* 9(5), 891–896.

Bessen, D.E. and Fischetti, V.A. (1992) Nucleotide sequence of two adjacent M and M-like protein genes of group A Streptococci: Different RN transcript levels and identification of A unique IgA-binding protein. *Infection and Immunity* 6(1), 124–135.

Blyth, C.C., Robetson, P.W. and Rosenberg, A.R. (2007) Post-streptococcal glomerulonephritis in Sydney, a 16 year retrospective review. *Journal of Pediatric Child Health* 433(6), 446–450.

Brandt, C.M. and Spellerberg, B. (2009) Human infections due to *Streptococcus dysgalactiae* subspecies *equisimilis*. *Clinical Infectious Diseases* 49(5), 766–772. DOI: 10.1086/605085.

Carapetis, J.R., Steer, A.C., Mulholand, E.K. and Weber, M. (2005) The global burden of group A streptococcal disease. *The Lancet Infectious Diseases* 5(11), 685–694.

Chalker, V.J., Brooks, H.W. and Brownlie, J. (2003) The association of *Streptococcus equi* subsp. *zooepidemicus* with canine infectious respiratory disease. *Veterinary Microbiology* 95, 1499–1506. DOI: 10.1016/S0378-1135(03)00155.

Daya, H., Lo, S., Papsin, B.C., Zachariasova, A., Murray, H. *et al.* (2005) Retropharyngeal and parapharyngeal infections in children: The Toronto experience. *International Journal of Pediatric Otorhinolaryngology* 69, 81–86. DOI: 10.1016/j.ijporl.2004.08.010.

Downar, J., Wiley, B.M., Sutherland, J.W., Mathew, K. and Low, D.E. (2001) Streptococcal meningitis resulting from contact with an infected horse. *Journal of Clinical Microbiology* 39(6), 2358–2359.

Dudas, R. and Serwint, J.R. (2006) In brief: Retropharyngeal abscess. *Pediatrics In Review* 27, 45–46. DOI: 10.1542/pir.27.6.e45.

Edward, A.T., Raulson, M. and Ironside, M.J. (1988) A milk-borne outbreak of serious infection due to *Streptococcus zooepidemicus* (Lancefield group C). *Epidemiology and Infection* 101, 43–51.

Elliott, J.A., Farmer, K.D. and Facklam, R.R. (1998) Sudden increase in isolation of group B streptococci, serotype V is not due to emergence of new pulsed-field gel electrophoresis type. *Journal of Clinical Microbiology* 36, 2115–2116.

Eyre, D.W., Kenkre, J.S., Bowler, I.C. and McBride, S.J. (2010) *Streptococcus equi* subspecies *zooepidemicus* meningitis – a case report and review of the literature. *European Journal of Clinical Microbiology and Infectious Diseases* 29(12), 1459–1463.

Ferrandiere, M., Cattier, B., Dequin, P.F., Hazouard, E., Legras, A. *et al.* (1998) Septicemia and meningitis due to *Streptococcus zooepidemicus*. *European Journal of Clinical Microbiology and Infectious Disease* 17, 290–291. DOI: 10.1007/BF01699990.

Gaglani, M.J. and Edwards, M.S. (1995) Clinical indicators of childhood retropharyngeal abscess. *American Journal of Emergency Medicine* 13(3), 333–336. DOI: 10.1016/0735-6757(95)90214-7.

Gibbs, H.C., McLaughlin, R.W. and Cameron, H.J. (1981) Meningoencephalitis caused by *Streptococcus zooepidemicus* in a goat. *Journal of American Veterinary Medical Association* 178, 735.

Harkani, A., Hassani, R., Ziad, T., Aderdour, L., Nouri, H. *et al.* (2011) Retropharyngeal abscess in adults: Five case reports and review of the literature. *The Scientific World Journal* 11, 1623–1629. DOI: 10.1100/2011/915163.

Hashikawa, S., Linuma, Y., Furushita, M., Ohkura, T., Nada, T. *et al.* (2004) Characterization of group C and G streptococcal strains that cause Streptococcal toxic shock syndrome. *Journal of Clinical Microbiology* 42, 186–192. DOI: 10.1128/JCM.42.1.186-192.2004.

Huang, C.M., Huang, F.L. and Chen, P.Y. (2017) Deep neck infections in children. *Journal of Microbiology, Immunology and Infection* 50, 627–633. DOI: 10.1016/j.mii.2015.08.020.

Hunt, E.A.K. and Somers, M.J.G. (2019) Infection-related glomerulonephritis. *Pediatric Clinics of North America* 66(1), 59–72.

Kasahara, T., Hayakawa, H., Okubo, S., Okugawa, T., Kabuki, N. *et al.* (2001) Prognosis of Acute Post Streptococcal Glomerulonephritis (APSGN) is excellent in children, when adequately diagnosed. *Pediatrics International* 43(4), 364–367.

Krauss, H., Weber, A., Appel, M., Enders, B., Isenberg, H.D. *et al.* (2003) *Zoonoses: Infectious Diseases Transmissible from Animals to Humans*, 3rd edn. ASM Press, Washington, DC.

Kuusi, M., Lahti, E., Virolainen, A., Hatakka, M., Vuento, R. *et al.* (2006) An outbreak of *Streptococcus equi* subspecies *zooepidemicus* associated with consumption of fresh goat cheese. *BMC Infectious Disease* 6, 36. DOI: 10.1186/1471-2334-6-36.

Lancefield, R.C. (1959) Persistence of type-specific antibodies in man following infection with group A streptococci. *Journal of Experimental Medicine* 110(2), 271–272.

Lancefield, R.C. (1962) Current knowledge of type specific M antigen of group A streptococci. *Journal of Immunology* 89(3), 307–313.

Las Heras, A., Vela, A.L., Fernandez, E., Legaz, E., Dominguez, L. *et al.* (2002) Unusual outbreak of clinical mastitis in dairy sheep caused by *Streptococcus equi* subsp. *zooepidemicus*. *Journal of Clinical Microbiology* 40, 1106–1108. DOI: 10.1128/JCM.40.3.1106-1108.2002.

Lord, J., Carter, C., Smith, J., Locke, S., Phillips, E. *et al.* (2022) Antimicrobial resistance among *Streptococcus equi* subspecies *zooepidemicus* and *Rhodococcus equi* isolated from equine specimens submitted to a diagnostic laboratory in Kentucky, USA. *Peer J* 10, e13682. DOI: 10.7717/peerj.13682.

Low, D.E., Young, M.R. and Harding, G.K. (1980) Group C streptococcal meningitis in an adult. Probable acquisition from a horse. *Archives of Internal Medicine* 140, 977–978. DOI: 10.1001/archinte.1407.977.

Manjula, B.N., Khande, K.M., Fairwell, T., Relf, W.A. and Sriprakash, K.S. (1991) Heptad motif within the distal subdomain of the coiled-coil rod region of M protein from rheumatic fever and nephritis associated serotypes of group A streptococcus are distinct from each other nucleotide sequence of the M57 gene and relation of the deduced amino acid sequence to other M protein. *Journal of Protein Chemistry* 10(4), 369–384.

Miles, B., Toumela, K. and Sanchez, J. (2021) Severe group C streptococcus infection in a veterinarian. *ID Cases* 23, 1036. DOI: 10.1016/j.idcr.2020.e01036.

Minces, L.R., Brown, P.J. and Veldkamp, P.J. (2011) Human meningitis from *Streptococcus equi* subsp. *zooepidemicus* acquired as zoonoses. *Epidemiology and Infection* 139, 406–410. DOI: 10.1017/S095026881000-1184.

Mitchell, C.M., Johnson, L.K., Crim, M.J., Wiedmeyer, C.E., Pugazhenthi, U. *et al.* (2020) Diagnosis surveillance and management of *Streptococcus equi* subspecies *zooepidemicus* infections in chinchillas (*Chinchilla lanigera*). *Comparative Medicine* 70(4), 370–375. DOI: 10.30802/AALAS-CM-20-000012.

Mobeen, K.M., Carter, J., Ahmed, Z. and Minton, J. (2020) Disseminated septic arthritis caused by *Streptococcus equi* infection. *BMJ Case Reports* 13(6), 234188. DOI: 1136/bcr-2019-234188.

Mungul, S. and Meharaj, S. (2019) Microbiology of pediatric deep neck space infection. *International Journal of Pediatric Otorhinology* 123, 116–122. DOI: 10.1016/j.ijporl.2019.04.042.

Pancholi, V. and Fischetti, V.A. (1988) Isolation and characterization of the cell-associated region of group A streptococcal M6 protein. *Journal of Bacteriology* 170(6), 2618–2624.

Philpott, C., Selvadurai, D. and Banerjee, A.R. (2004) Paediatric retropharyngeal abscess. *Journal of Laryngology and Otology* 118(12), 919–926. DOI: 10.1258/0022215042790538.

Pinto, S.W., Lima, H.N., Abreu, T.T., Otoni, A., Nogueira, P. *et al.* (2022) Twenty year follow up of patients with epidemic glomerulonephritis due to *Streptococcus zooepidemicus* in Brazil. *Kidney International Report* 7(9), 2029–2038. DOI: 10.1016/j.ekir.2022.06.11.

Pisoni, G., Zadoks, R.N., Vemerkati, C., Locatelli, C., Zomoni, M.G. *et al.* (2009) Epidemiological investigation of *Streptococcus equi* subspecies *zooepidemicus* involved in clinical mastitis in dairy goats. *Journal of Dairy Science* 92(3), 943–951. DOI: 10.168/jds.2008-1548.

Rammelkamp, C.H. and Weaver, R.S. (1953) Acute glomerulonephritis, the significance of the variation in the incidence of the disease. *Journal of Clinical Investigation* 32(4), 345–358.

Salmenlinna, S., Lyytikäinen, O., Kotilainen, P., Scotford, R., Siren, E. *et al.* (2000) Molecular epidemiology of methicillin-resistant *Staphylococcus aureus* in Finland. *European Journal of Clinical Microbiology and Infectious Diseases* 19, 101–107. DOI: 10.1007/s100960050438.

Schneewind, O., Mihaylova-Petkov, D. and Model, P. (1993) Cell wall sorting signals in surface proteins of gram-positive bacteria. *EMBO Journal* 12(12), 4803–4811. DOI: 10.1002/j.1460-2075.1993.tb06169.x.

Shah, S.S., Mathews, R.P. and Cohen, C. (2001) Group C Streptococcal meningitis: Case report and review of the literature. *Pediatric Infectious Disease Journal* 20, 445–448. DOI: 10.1097/00006454-200104000-00016.

Soedarmanto, I., Pasaribu, F.H., Wibawan, I.W. and Lammbu, C. (1996) Identification and molecular characterization of serological group C streptococci isolated from diseased pigs and monkeys in Indonesia. *Journal of Clinical Microbiology* 34, 2201–2204.

Turner, C.E., Bubba, L. and Efstratiou, A. (2019) Pathogenicity factors in group C and G streptococci microbiology spectrum. *Microbiology Spectrum* 7(3). DOI: 10.1128/microbiolspec.GPP3-0020-2018.

Ural, O., Tuncer, I., Dikici, N. and Aridogan, B. (2003) *Streptococcus zooepidemicus* meningitis and bacteraemia. *Scandinavian Journal of Infectious Diseases* 35, 206–207. DOI: 10.1080/00365540310000076.

Valve, K. and Vuento, R. (1992) *Streptococcus zooepidemicus* sepsis in an elderly woman. *Duodecim* 108, 1270–1274.

Wasissa, M., Lestari, F.B. and Salasia, S.I.O. (2021) *Streptococcus equi* subsp. *zooepidemicus* finding in confirmed feline infectious peritonitis cat patient. *Heliyon* 7(6), 07268. DOI: 10.1016/j.heliyan.2021.e07268.

Wasniewska, W.A., Pepas, R., Janowicz, R. and Kanopka, W. (2022) *Streptococcus equi* subsp. *equi* in retropharyngeal abscess: Case report and review of literature. *Microorganisms* 10, 10. DOI: 10.3390/microorganism10102032.

Yuen, K.Y., Seto, W.H., Choi, C.H., Ng, W., Ho, S.W, *et al.* (1990) *Streptococcus zooepidemicus* (Lancefield group C) septicemia in Hong Kong. *Journal of Infection* 21, 241–250. DOI: 10.1016/0163-4453(90)93885-V.

21 Listeriosis

Ranbir Singh Jatav[1]*, Sumit Kumar Patel[2], Shashi Pradhan[1] and Supnesh Jain[1]
[1]Department of Veterinary Medicine; [2]School of Wildlife Forensic and Health Nanaji Deshmukh Veterinary Science University, Jabalpur, MP

Abstract

Listeria monocytogenes is a bacterial disease that causes listeriosis in goats and humans. It mainly causes encephalitis, a blood infection and abortion. Goats are infected by ingesting mouldy or spoiled hay or silage, as the organism is commonly found in the environment. The bacterium can be located in the soil, the gut, food sources and faeces of healthy animals. Generally, people are infected with this disease by ingesting raw meat or unpasteurized dairy products. Goats can shed *L. monocytogenes* in the faeces, milk and uterine discharges. Pregnant women, as well as immunocompromised people, are the worst sufferers of the disease. The bacterium can grow in cold temperatures, including in the refrigerator. Skin infection of the disease can also occur in people who handle sick animals.

Keywords: Listeriosis, ingestion, goats, zoonosis, immunocompromised patients, food

21.1 Introduction

Listeriosis is an infectious and fatal bacterial disease caused by the pathogen *Listeria monocytogenes* (Fig. 21.1). It affects a wide range of animals, including goats.

Listeriosis in goats can be a significant concern for livestock farmers as it can lead to severe illness and, in some cases, mortality. It arises mainly from the ingestion of contaminated food (Barbuddhe *et al.*, 2012). It is also known as silage disease, circling disease and meningoencephalitis. It is a disease where septicaemia, meningoencephalitis, spontaneous abortions, subclinical mastitis and endometritis may be predominantly observed (Dhama *et al.*, 2015). The bacterium is commonly found in soil, water and decaying plant material, and animals can be exposed to it through contaminated feed, water, or the environment. Listeriosis can be transmitted through the ingestion of food or of silage made from poorly fermented or spoiled crops, and water contaminated with saliva, faeces, nasal secretions and aborted material from infected animals. In India, cases of listeriosis have been reported in the animal population as sporadic as well as outbreak forms. The bacteria can multiply in the gastrointestinal tract and in some cases they can enter the bloodstream and spread to other parts of the body, leading to more severe forms of the disease.

The clinical manifestations vary with the species affected. Symptoms of listeriosis in goats may include depression, loss of appetite, fever, circling, head pressing and sometimes drooping of one ear. In more severe cases, the infection can affect the nervous system, causing paralysis and even death.

Preventing listeriosis in goats involves proper management practices, including good sanitation, proper storage and handling of feed,

*Corresponding author: hindoliya.rambir@gmail.com

DOI: 10.1079/ 9781800622852.0021

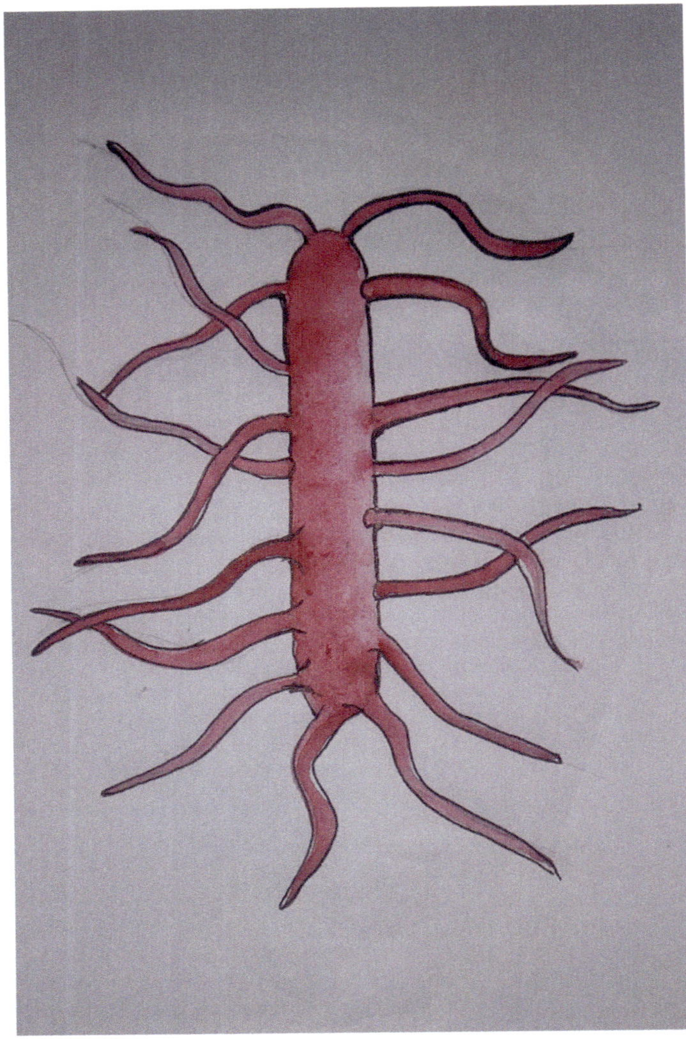

Fig. 21.1. *Listeria monocytogenes*. (Courtesy of Dr Anushka Upadhyay.)

and avoiding feeding spoiled or mouldy forage. The disease can be tentatively diagnosed based on clinical signs and its confirmation is achieved by isolating the pathogen from appropriate specimens. Characteristic neurological signs or abortion in association with silage feeding may suggest listeriosis (Quinn *et al.*, 2002).

Treatment of listeriosis may be a difficult task, because *L. monocytogenes* can invade virtually all cell types. The time period of treatment may vary according to the level of infection. Vaccination with killed vaccines, which do not induce an effective cell-mediated response, is not protective because *L. monocytogenes* is an intracellular pathogen. Live attenuated vaccines, which are available in some countries, are reported to reduce the prevalence of listeriosis.

21.2 Epidemiology

The epidemiology of goat listeriosis is not extensively documented in scientific literature compared with other animal species. However, it is known that listeriosis can affect goats, and the disease shares similar epidemiological patterns with listeriosis in other livestock and humans.

Although the organism is widespread in nature, clinical diseases in animals occur mainly in the northern and southern latitudes and are much less common in tropical and subtropical than in temperate climates. In the northern hemisphere, listeriosis has a distinct seasonal occurrence, probably associated with seasonal feeding of silage, with the highest prevalence in the months of December through May (Radostits *et al.*, 2007). Listeriosis is generally considered a sporadic disease in goats, meaning it occurs as individual cases or small outbreaks rather than widespread epidemics. The disease can occur at any time of the year, but there might be seasonal variations with a higher incidence during warmer months when bacterial growth in contaminated feed and forage is more favoured.

Preventive measures, such as proper feed and forage management, good hygiene practices and stress reduction, can help minimize the risk of listeriosis in goats. Several factors influence the prevalence of listeriosis in goat herds, including the presence of *L. monocytogenes* in the environment, herd size, feeding and forage practices, herd health management and overall biosecurity measures.

The first confirmed case of listeric abortion in any species of domesticated animal in India was reported by Dhanda *et al.* (1959) in a ewe. Most of the cases of listeriosis in India are reported from the states of Jammu and Kashmir, Himachal Pradesh, Maharashtra and Andhra Pradesh (Barbuddhe *et al.*, 2012). Listeriosis is considered a relatively uncommon disease in goats compared with other livestock species. However, it can still occur, particularly in regions with certain environmental conditions and management practices that favour the growth and transmission of *L. monocytogenes*.

21.3 Aetiology

Listeriosis is a serious and life-threatening disease caused by members of the genus *Listeria*. The genus totals 17 species, including *Listeria monocytogenes*, *L. ivanovii*, *L. innocua*, *L. welshimeri*, *L. seeligeri*, *L. grayi*, *L. marthii* and *L. rocourtia*. *Listeria* species are small, Gram-positive, non-acid-fast, non-spore-forming and non-capsulate coccobacilli measuring 0.5–2 mm × 0.4–0.5 mm. They are facultative, anaerobic, intra-cellular bacteria that are ubiquitously distributed in the environment and grow over a wide range of pH and temperature (Quinn *et al.*, 2002). Of these, *L. monocytogenes* is an opportunistic pathogen in human beings and various animal species, whereas *L. ivanovii* mainly affects ruminants, causing abortion and only occasionally occurring in humans (Barbuddhe *et al.*, 2012). *L. monocytogenes* has been divided into 13 serotypes (namely 1/2 a, 1/2b, 1/2 c, 3 a, 3b, 3 c, 4 a, 4ab, 4b, 4 c, 4d, 4e and 7) on the basis of somatic and flagellar antigens. Serotypes 1/2 a, 1/2b and 4b are commonly reported in humans, and serotypes 1/2 a and 4b in animals.

The bacterium can tolerate a wide range of pH and temperature. Optimum growth occurs at 30–37°C, but the organism can multiply at 4–45°C. A typical tumbling motility is observed around 25°C (Dhama *et al.*, 2015). The organism can tolerate pH values between 5.5 and 9.6. In such circumstances, *L. monocytogenes* may reach 10^7 colony-forming units (CFUs) per kilogram of silage (Fentahun and Fresebehat, 2012).

L. monocytogenes can infect a wide variety of animal species, including cattle, sheep, goats and birds, and has also been isolated from fish and crustaceans. Adult pigs are easily infected but rarely develop the disease, and birds are often asymptomatic carriers. Ruminants usually represent a reservoir for the bacterium; and raw milk (as well as meat) serves as a major source of transmission from dairy farms to humans (Ferreira *et al.*, 2014).

21.4 Transmission

Goats may become infected with the bacterium through ingestion of contaminated feed, water, or forage. The bacterium can also enter the body through wounds or damaged mucous membranes, allowing it to spread to other organs (Fig. 21.2). Listeriosis transmission in goats primarily occurs through the ingestion

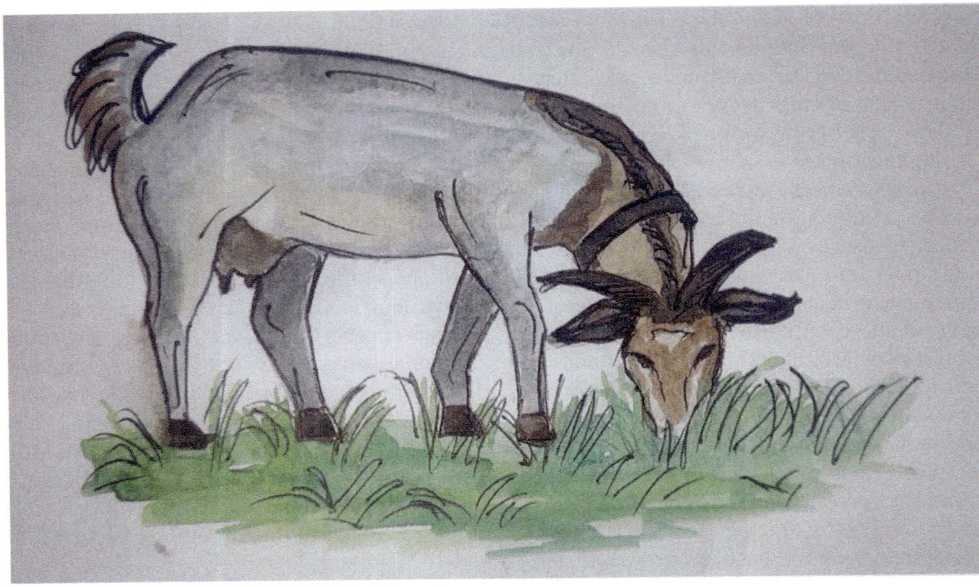

Fig. 21.2. Feeding decayed silage. (Courtesy of Dr Anushka Upadhyay.)

of feed or forage contaminated with *L. monocytogenes*. The bacterium is commonly found in the environment, including in soil, water and decaying plant material. When goats consume contaminated feed, especially silage or haylage made from poorly fermented or spoiled crops, they can become infected with *L. monocytogenes*. If contaminated feed is ingested by goats while grazing or drinking, the bacterium can survive in the gastrointestinal tract and potentially lead to infection. Vertical transmission can occur when an infected pregnant goat passes the bacterium to her offspring during gestation. This can result in infections in newborn kids.

Goat listeriosis can be transmitted through various routes, including the following.

- **Ingestion of contaminated feed or forage:** The most common route of transmission is through the consumption of feed, forage, or silage contaminated with *L. monocytogenes*. The bacteria can contaminate these food sources during harvesting, storage, or feeding practices.
- **Contaminated water:** Goats can acquire listeriosis by drinking water contaminated with *L. monocytogenes*.
- **Direct contact with infected animals:** Listeria can be shed in the faeces, nasal secretions and other body fluids of infected goats. Direct contact with infected animals can lead to transmission of the bacteria.
- **Vertical transmission:** Listeria can cross the placenta and infect the fetus during pregnancy, leading to abortion, stillbirth, or the birth of weak or infected kids.
- **Environmental exposure:** Listeria is widespread in the environment, including in soil, decaying vegetation and manure. Goats can become infected by coming into contact with contaminated surfaces or materials.
- **Zoonotic transmission:** While the main concern is the health of the goats, it is important to note that listeriosis is a zoonotic disease, meaning it can be transmitted from animals to humans. People handling infected goats or consuming contaminated goat products (e.g. unpasteurized milk or cheese) are at risk of infection.

To reduce the risk of transmission and prevent listeriosis in goats, it is crucial to practise good herd management, including the following.

- Ensure proper hygiene and sanitation in barns, feeders and water sources.
- Properly handle and store feed and forage to minimize bacterial contamination.
- Avoid overcrowding and stressful conditions for goats.
- Monitor the health of the herd regularly and promptly isolate and treat any sick animals.
- Provide a balanced and nutritious diet to support a healthy immune system.
- Practise good biosecurity measures to prevent the introduction of the bacteria to the herd.

Soil contamination and ingestion of contaminated feed (faecal-oral route; 80–90%) are the primary modes of transmission of *Listeria*. Poor-quality silage, with a pH greater than 5.5, is commonly implicated and accounts for listeriosis often being referred to as 'silage disease' (Hirsh and Zee, 1999). Kids that develop septicaemic disease may acquire infection from contamination on the doe's teat, from the ingestion of milk containing the organism from does with subclinical bacteraemia, through the navel from the environment and also as a congenital infection. The encephalitic form of the disease results from infection of the terminals of the trigeminal nerve consequent to abrasion of the buccal mucosa from feed or browse or from infection of tooth cavities (Radostits *et al.*, 2007).

Listeriosis transmission to humans occurs primarily through the consumption of contaminated food, especially ready-to-eat foods that have not undergone proper cooking or pasteurization. *L. monocytogenes* is commonly found in the environment, including soil, water and vegetation, and in the gastrointestinal tracts of many animals. The bacterium can contaminate food at various stages of production, processing and distribution, leading to potential outbreaks of listeriosis.

Listeriosis transmission in goats can be prevented by the following.

- **Proper feed management:** Ensure that feed, particularly silage and haylage, is properly fermented and stored to minimize the risk of *Listeria* contamination.
- **Good husbandry practices:** Maintain a clean and hygienic environment for goats, including their living area, barns and feeding equipment.
- **Uncontaminated water sources:** Provide access to clean and uncontaminated water sources to minimize the risk of environmental exposure to *Listeria*.
- **Regular health monitoring:** Monitor the health of goats regularly and promptly identify and isolate any sick animals to prevent the spread of infections.
- **Biosecurity:** Limit the movement of animals between different farms and quarantine newly introduced goats to prevent the introduction of infectious agents.
- **Veterinary care:** Early detection and intervention are essential for successful treatment.

By implementing these preventive measures and maintaining good management practices, goat farmers can reduce the risk of listeriosis transmission and help ensure the health and well-being of their herds.

21.5 Risk Factors

The risk factors for listeriosis in goats are similar to those for other livestock and include the following.

- **Contaminated feed and water:** Listeria bacteria can be found in the environment and may contaminate feed and water sources. Goats can become infected by consuming contaminated food or water.
- **Poor sanitation:** Inadequate cleaning and maintenance of barns, feeders, water troughs and milking equipment can lead to the build-up of *Listeria* bacteria and increase the risk of infection.
- **Overcrowding and stress:** Overcrowded or stressed goats are more susceptible to infections, including listeriosis. Proper management practices and providing adequate space can help reduce stress and minimize the risk of disease.
- **Pregnancy and lactation:** Pregnant and lactating goats are at a higher risk of listeriosis. The bacteria can cross the placenta and infect the developing fetus, leading to abortion or stillbirth.

- **Weakened immune system:** Goats with compromised immune systems due to other health conditions, such as concurrent infections or nutritional deficiencies, are more vulnerable to listeriosis.
- **Season and climate:** Listeriosis cases may increase during warmer months when bacteria growth is favoured. Additionally, exposure to silage contaminated with *Listeria* is more common during these periods.
- **Contaminated bedding material:** Bedding contaminated with *Listeria* can be a potential source of infection for goats, as they may come into contact with the bacteria through ingestion or skin abrasions.

To reduce the risk of listeriosis in goats, it is essential to maintain good hygiene practices, provide a clean and sanitary environment and ensure proper nutrition and stress management. Regular veterinary monitoring and prompt treatment of any health issues can also help prevent and control listeriosis outbreaks in goat herds. If there are suspected cases of listeriosis, it is crucial to seek veterinary advice and implement appropriate measures to protect the health of the goats and prevent further spread of the disease.

21.5.1 Season

Listeriosis in goats can occur throughout the year, but there are certain seasons when the risk may be higher due to environmental factors that favour the growth and transmission of *L. monocytogenes*. Generally, the incidence of listeriosis tends to increase during warmer months, particularly in late spring, summer and early fall. The reasons for the seasonal pattern of listeriosis in goats include the following.

- **Contaminated feed and forage:** During the warmer months, the temperature and humidity can promote the growth of *Listeria* bacteria in contaminated feed, silage and forage. Silage made from crops like maize and grass can be a common source of *Listeria* if not properly handled and stored.
- **Ingestion of spoiled feed:** In hot weather, feed and forage may spoil more quickly, providing an opportunity for *Listeria* bacteria to proliferate. Goats can become infected with *Listeria* by consuming spoiled feed or forage contaminated with the bacteria.
- **Increased environmental exposure:** During the warmer seasons, goats are more likely to graze in pastures or forage areas where *Listeria* bacteria may be present in the soil, water sources, or decaying organic matter.
- **Pregnancy and kidding season:** In some regions, late spring and early summer coincide with the kidding season for goats. Pregnant and lactating goats are more susceptible to listeriosis, and the stress associated with kidding can make them more vulnerable to infections.

While listeriosis cases may be more common during the warmer months, it is important to remember that the disease can occur at any time of the year. Proper management practices, good sanitation and careful handling of feed and forage can help minimize the risk of listeriosis in goats, regardless of the season.

21.5.2 Consumption of contaminated silage

Listeriosis cases increased when animals were fed silage, whereas sharp decreases in the numbers of reported cases were observed as soon as pasture was available (Ryser and Marth, 2007).

Consumption of contaminated silage is a well-known risk factor for listeriosis in goats. Silage is a fermented feed made from crops such as maize, grass, or other forages. When not properly handled, harvested, or stored, silage can become contaminated with *L. monocytogenes* and other harmful bacteria, which can pose a significant health risk to goats.

Silage management practices to minimize the risk of listeriosis from contaminated silage are as follows.

- **Harvesting high-quality crops:** Use fresh and healthy crops for silage preparation to reduce the initial bacterial load.
- **Proper ensiling:** Ensure proper fermentation and anaerobic conditions during the

ensiling process, including adequate compaction and sealing to prevent the growth of harmful bacteria.

- **Feed hygiene:** Use clean feeders and troughs and avoid feeding spoiled or mouldy silage to goats.
- **Monitoring and testing:** Regularly monitor the quality of silage for any signs of spoilage or contamination. If there are concerns about the presence of *Listeria*, consider testing the silage for bacterial content.
- **Good management practices:** By implementing good silage management practices and maintaining overall herd health, goat owners can help reduce the risk of listeriosis and other health issues associated with contaminated silage consumption.

21.5.3 Immunosuppression

Immunosuppression in goats can increase their susceptibility to listeriosis, making them more prone to infection and more severe disease outcomes. Immunosuppression refers to a weakening of the immune system, which can be caused by various factors. When goats have a compromised immune response, their ability to effectively fight off infections, including *L. monocytogenes*, is impaired. Several factors, including sudden changes in ration, climatic changes (e.g. extremely cold weather), or prolonged periods of transportation, have been associated with the onset of clinical listeriosis in ruminants. Other stressors, including pregnancy, parturition and lactation, may also suppress host immunity, leaving animals to be more susceptible to the disease.

Several factors can contribute to immunosuppression in goats, including the following.

- **Age:** Very young goats (kids) and elderly goats may have less robust immune systems, making them more susceptible to infections like listeriosis.
- **Stress:** Stressful conditions, such as overcrowding, transportation, abrupt changes in management, or exposure to extreme weather, can weaken the goat's immune system and increase its susceptibility to diseases like listeriosis.
- **Concurrent infections:** Goats suffering from other infections or diseases may experience immunosuppression, which can open the door for secondary infections like listeriosis.
- **Nutritional deficiencies:** Inadequate nutrition or deficiencies in essential nutrients can impair the goat's immune system, leaving it more vulnerable to infections.
- **Chronic health conditions:** Goats with chronic health issues or underlying diseases may have compromised immune systems, increasing their risk of listeriosis.
- **Medications:** Certain medications, particularly immunosuppressive drugs used to manage other health conditions, can weaken the goat's immune response.

When goats experience immunosuppression, *L. monocytogenes* can more easily evade the immune system's defences, leading to increased bacterial growth and a higher likelihood of severe disease, such as encephalitis, septicaemia, or abortion. Prevention measures should focus on minimizing stress, providing a balanced and nutritious diet, ensuring proper management practices and promptly addressing any health issues in the goat herd. Additionally, proper vaccination protocols can help strengthen the goat's immune response and reduce the risk of listeriosis and other infectious diseases.

21.5.4 Contact with infected animals

Animals may be exposed by direct contact with infective material from same or other animal species. Faeces, urine, aborted fetuses, uterine discharge and milk should be considered as infectious.

21.5.5 Use of H_2 blockers

Most *Listeria* species are destroyed by gastric acids. Use of antacids and histamine type-2 receptor antagonists (H_2 blockers) increases survival rate and they are considered as risk factors for developing listeriosis.

21.6 Zoonotic Potential

Listeriosis is a zoonotic disease, which means it can be transmitted from animals to humans. People can become infected by consuming contaminated food, including unpasteurized dairy products, and by direct contact with infected animals or their secretions. In humans, listeriosis can lead to severe illness, particularly in vulnerable populations such as pregnant women, the elderly, and individuals with weakened immune systems. Humans can acquire listeriosis from direct contact with infected goats or their environment, particularly if the goats are shedding the bacterium in their faeces.

21.7 Pathogenesis

The pathogenesis of goat listeriosis, caused by the bacterium *L. monocytogenes*, involves a series of steps that lead to infection and disease development. Here is a general overview of the pathogenesis of goat listeriosis.

- **Ingestion and colonization:** The initial step in the pathogenesis is the ingestion of *L. monocytogenes* by the goat. The bacteria can be present in contaminated feed, forage, silage, or water. Once ingested, the bacteria pass through the digestive system and can attach and colonize the intestinal lining.
- **Invasion of the intestinal wall:** *L. monocytogenes* has the ability to invade and penetrate the intestinal wall, allowing the bacteria to enter the bloodstream. This invasion is facilitated by several virulence factors produced by the bacterium.
- **Systemic spread:** Once in the bloodstream, *L. monocytogenes* can rapidly disseminate throughout the body. The bacteria are capable of surviving and multiplying within various immune cells, including macrophages.
- **Crossing the blood–brain barrier (neurolisteriosis):** In some cases, *L. monocytogenes* can cross the blood–brain barrier, leading to infection of the central nervous system. This form of the disease is known as neurolisteriosis and is characterized by neurological symptoms, such as circling, head pressing, paralysis and loss of balance.
- **Placental crossing (abortion):** In pregnant goats, *L. monocytogenes* can cross the placenta and infect the developing fetus. This can lead to abortion, stillbirth, or the birth of weak or infected kids.
- **Immune evasion:** *L. monocytogenes* is adept at evading the host's immune response. It can resist destruction by immune cells, enabling the bacteria to persist and spread throughout the body.
- **Disease outcome:** The clinical manifestations of listeriosis in goats can vary depending on the affected organs and tissues. The disease can present as encephalitis (brain inflammation) in cases of neurolisteriosis, abortion or stillbirth in pregnant goats, or as septicaemia (blood infection) in systemic cases (Fig. 21.3). The severity of listeriosis in goats can be influenced by factors such as the strain of *L. monocytogenes*, the immune status of the goat, stress levels and overall health status (Fig. 21.4).

21.8 Clinical Signs

The three primary forms of listeriosis in goats recognized are septicaemic, encephalitic and reproductive. Incubation periods vary with the pathogenesis of the disease. Thus, 1–2 days are usual for septicaemic disease or a gastrointestinal form, 2 weeks for abortion and longer for the encephalitic form (4–6 weeks).

- Clinical signs may arise secondary to immunocompromise, predisposing disease, or excessive environmental stress.
- Goats are often found acutely dead because they typically do not develop clinical signs secondary to septicaemic listeriosis. Uterine infections typically cause abortions in pregnant dams with few other systemic signs.
- Encephalitis and meningoencephalitis are perhaps the most common and well-recognized presentations of listeriosis. Affected goats become depressed, ataxic and often paralytic. Ocular disease is a fourth presentation of listeriosis.

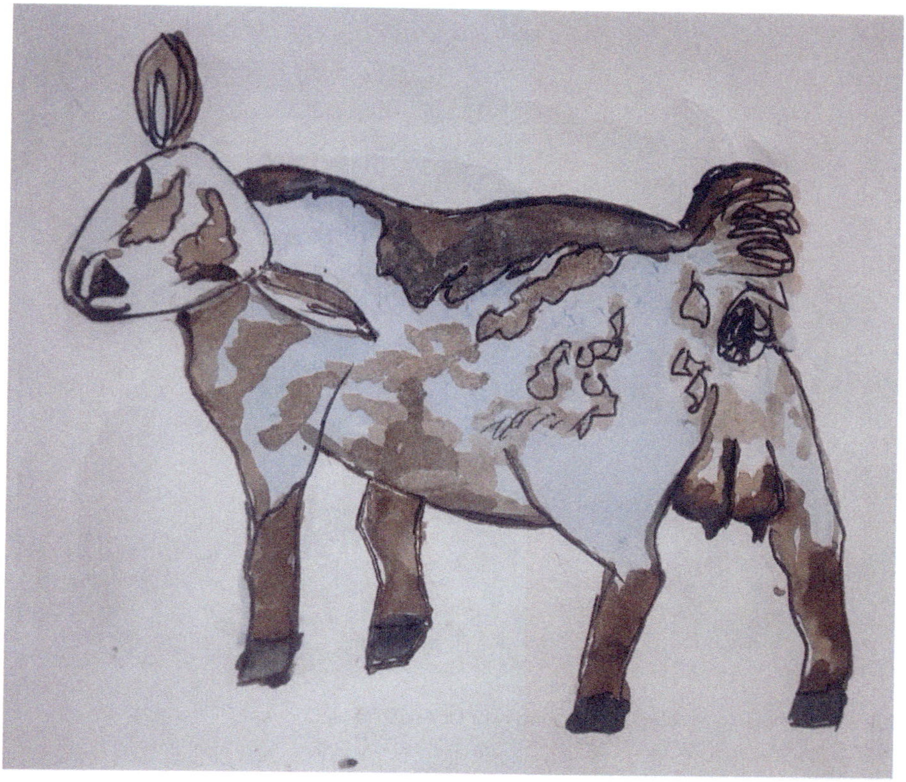

Fig. 21.3. Head tilt in listeriosis. (Courtesy of Dr Anushka Upadhyay.)

21.8.1 Septicaemic form

Goats infected with the septicaemic form may show sudden onset of fever, depression, anorexia, weakness, dyspnoea, loss of appetite and rapid deterioration of health. They may also experience diarrhoea and abortion in pregnant goats. In the septicaemic form of listeriosis, the bacteria spread through the bloodstream, leading to systemic infection.

21.8.2 Encephalitic form

In the encephalitic form, goats may exhibit neurological signs, including circling, head tilt (torticollis), facial paralysis and loss of coordination (ataxia). Muscle tremors and difficulty standing or walking may also be observed. The encephalitic form, sometimes called 'circling disease', is the most common form in ruminants. The course of the disease is more acute and frequently fatal in sheep and goats (Hirsh and Zee, 1999). The encephalitic form affects the central nervous system and the bacteria can invade the brain, leading to neurological signs.

21.8.3 Reproductive form

Pregnant goats infected with *L. monocytogenes* can experience abortions or stillbirths, or deliver weak and unthrifty kids. The bacteria can cross the placental barrier and infect the fetus, leading to fetal death. Abortion is common in ruminants usually in late term. The fetus may be macerated or delivered weak and moribund. Retained placenta and metritis may result (Hirsh and Zee, 1999). Outbreaks of abortion occur more commonly in sheep and goats and there will be a blood-stained vaginal discharge for several days. In both species,

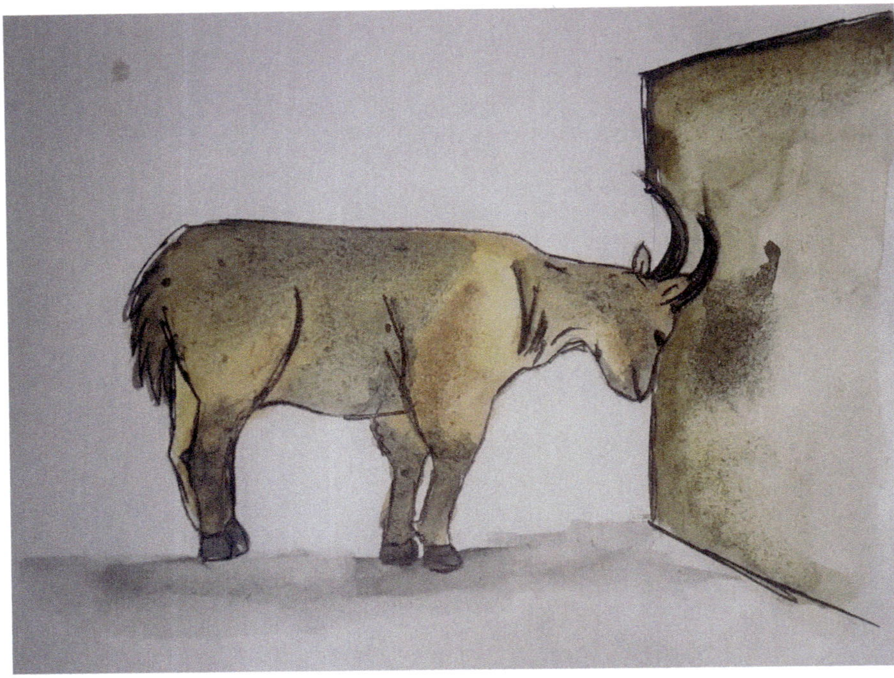

Fig. 21.4. Head pressing in listeriosis. (Courtesy of Dr Anushka Upadhyay.)

the rates of abortion in a group are low but may reach as high as 15%. On some farms, abortions recur each year (Scanlan, 1988).

21.9 Diagnosis

A veterinarian can diagnose listeriosis in goats based on clinical signs, history of exposure and laboratory tests, which may include blood analysis, cerebrospinal fluid analysis and postmortem examination.

21.9.1 Direct microscopy

Smears from cotyledons or from liver lesions may reveal Gram-positive coccoid bacillary bacteria. Histopathological examination of fixed (10% formalin) brain tissue can often give a presumptive diagnosis of neural listeriosis.

21.9.2 Isolation and identification

Isolating *Listeria* from goats involves obtaining samples from suspected cases and conducting specific laboratory tests to identify the presence of *L. monocytogenes*. Here is an overview of the process.

1. **Sample collection:** The first step is to collect appropriate samples from suspected cases of listeriosis in goats. Samples may include blood, cerebrospinal fluid (CSF), or tissues from affected organs like the brain. If the goat has succumbed to the disease, a post-mortem examination can be performed to collect tissue samples.
2. **Bacterial culture:** Once the samples are collected, they are sent to a diagnostic laboratory for bacterial culture. In the case of listeriosis, the laboratory will attempt to isolate *L. monocytogenes* from the samples. This involves placing the samples in specific nutrient media that promote the growth of

Listeria bacteria while inhibiting the growth of other bacteria.

3. **Identification:** After incubation, if *L. monocytogenes* is present in the samples, it will grow and form characteristic colonies on the culture plates. These colonies will then undergo further tests for identification, such as Gram staining and biochemical tests. *L. monocytogenes* is a Gram-positive bacterium and exhibits specific biochemical reactions that differentiate it from other bacteria.
4. **Confirmatory tests:** To confirm the identity of *L. monocytogenes*, additional tests may be conducted, such as agglutination tests or molecular methods like polymerase chain reaction (PCR). These tests can provide a definitive identification of the bacterium.

It is essential to handle and transport samples properly to maintain their viability and accuracy during testing. Working with a qualified veterinary diagnostic laboratory is crucial to ensure accurate and reliable results.

It should be kept in mind that the isolation of *Listeria* from clinical samples is not always straightforward, and sometimes other bacteria with similar characteristics may be present. In such cases, a combination of culture, biochemical tests and molecular methods is used to accurately identify the causative agent.

Specimens from cases of abortion and septicaemia can be inoculated directly onto blood agar, selective blood agar containing 0.05% potassium tellurite (inhibitory to Gram-negative bacteria) and MacConkey agar. The plates are incubated aerobically at 37°C for 24–48 hour (Quinn *et al.*, 2002). Commercial selective and indicator media are available, such as *Listeria*-selective agar (Oxoid), and these are designed mainly for the isolation of *Listeria* from human foodstuffs.

A 'cold-enrichment' procedure is necessary for brain tissue. Small pieces of spinal cord and medulla are homogenized and a 10% suspension is made in a nutrient broth. The suspension is held at 4°C in the refrigerator and sub-cultured onto blood agar once weekly for up to 12 weeks (Quinn *et al.*, 2003). Small transparent colonies with smooth borders appear on blood agar in 24 hour, becoming greyish-white in 48 hour. All the *Listeria* species hydrolyse esculin (esculin broth). *L. monocytogenes*, particularly, shows the characteristic 'tumbling motility' when a 2–4 hour broth is cultured, incubated at 25°C and examined by the hanging-drop method. Catalase test is positive for *Listeria* species.

21.9.3 PCR and PCR-coupled LCR

For the specific detection of *L. monocytogenes*, a nested PCR- reverse dot blot (PCR-RDB) assay is used. To allow fast detection of *L. monocytogenes* in the feed and environmental samples from the outbreak in goats, a PCR-RDB assay on a crude lysate from a 1 ml aliquot of the second enrichment in LEB is performed.

21.9.4 Animal inoculation

Most isolates of animal origin are virulent, a characteristic that can be confirmed by animal inoculation. The Anton test uses inoculation of a drop of broth culture into conjunctiva of a rabbit or guinea pig. Only *L. monocytogenes* causes purulent keratoconjunctivitis within 24–36 hour of inoculation. Both *L. monocytogenes* and *L. ivanovii* are pathogenic for mice. Intra-peritoneal inoculation of mice with a 24 hour broth culture results of their death within 5 days with necrotic lesions in the liver (Fentahun and Fresebehat, 2012).

For listeriosis in goats, serological tests are not recommended in veterinary practices due to prominent cross-reactivity with enterococci and *Staphylococcus aureus*, low assay sensitivity and specificity, and the presence of high titres that confound results in healthy goats.

21.9.5 Key steps in diagnosis

Here is a summary of the key steps involved in the diagnosis.

1. **Clinical signs and history:** The first step in diagnosing listeriosis is to observe the clinical signs exhibited by the affected goats. Common symptoms include depression, loss of appetite, fever, circling, head pressing and drooping of one ear. The veterinarian will

also inquire about the goat's history, including recent changes in feed, environment, or exposure to potentially contaminated sources.

2. **Physical examination:** The veterinarian will conduct a thorough physical examination of the affected goat, paying particular attention to any neurological symptoms, abnormal behaviour, or other signs of illness.
3. **Laboratory tests:** To support the diagnosis, the veterinarian may recommend various laboratory tests. These may include the following.

    - **Blood tests:** Complete blood count and serum chemistry tests can provide valuable information about the goat's overall health status and help rule out other diseases.
    - **CSF analysis:** In cases with severe neurological symptoms, a sample of CSF may be collected through a lumbar puncture. CSF analysis can help detect inflammation and signs of infection in the central nervous system.
    - **Bacterial culture:** A sample of tissue, blood, or CSF may be sent for bacterial culture to identify the presence of *L. monocytogenes* and determine the most effective antibiotic treatment.

4. **Response to treatment:** A positive response to treatment with antibiotics (e.g. penicillin or ampicillin) can further support the diagnosis of listeriosis.
5. **Necropsy (post-mortem examination):** If a goat succumbs to the disease, a necropsy (autopsy) may be performed to examine the organs and tissues. This can help confirm the diagnosis and identify any other potential underlying issues.

21.10 Differential Diagnosis

It is important to note that listeriosis in goats can have similar clinical signs to other diseases, such as rabies or other neurological infections. Therefore, a proper diagnosis is crucial to ensure appropriate treatment and management.

21.11 Treatment

Treatment involves administration of antibiotics, such as penicillin or ampicillin, to combat the infection. Supportive care, including fluid therapy and nutritional support, may also be necessary for maintaining hydration and nourishment to aid recovery. The treatment of listeriosis in goats involves a combination of medical interventions to control the bacterial infection and supportive care to manage the neurological symptoms. It is important to note that the success of treatment depends on the stage of the disease, the severity of symptoms and the overall health of the affected goat. Early detection and prompt veterinary intervention increase the chances of a positive outcome. Prevention is always better than treatment.

Sulfonamides, penicillin and tetracycline may be used as prophylactics. Chlortetracycline at 10 mg/kg body weight (BW) per day administered for 5 days intravenously is effective in encephalitis cases in goats. Penicillin at 44,000 IU/kg BW IM can be given daily for 7 days along with supportive therapies such as rehydration with electrolytes.

Listeriosis in animals can sometimes be cured with antibiotics when diagnosed early. Goats can be treated if showing facial paralysis, but it is generally fatal.

Quaternary ammonium compounds, povidone iodine, chlorhexidine, 7.0% ethanol, glutaraldehyde and sodium hypochlorite are typically effective disinfectants.

Anti-inflammatory medications may be needed to reduce brain swelling and alleviate neurological symptoms. Rest is also essential, to give the affected goat time to recover and heal. Since goats with listeriosis may have a compromised immune system, they are more susceptible to secondary infections. To prevent these complications, proper wound care and hygiene are essential. Goats with listeriosis may have difficulty eating and drinking, due to neurological impairment. Providing gentle nursing care, such as assisting with feeding and watering, can improve their chances of recovery. Regular monitoring of the goat's condition is crucial during treatment.

21.12 Prevention and Control

Implementing good husbandry practices, such as maintaining clean and hygienic living conditions, providing high-quality feed and avoiding feeding spoiled or contaminated forage, can help reduce the risk of listeriosis in goat herds. Infected goats should be isolated from the rest of the herd to prevent the spread of the disease. Listeriosis is a significant concern for goat farmers, as it can lead to severe illness and economic losses. Regular herd health checks and a proactive approach to animal welfare can help ensure the well-being of goats and reduce the risk of disease outbreaks. Additionally, vaccination against listeriosis may be available in some regions and can be considered as a preventive measure for susceptible herds.

Identifying spoiled feed is crucial to ensure goats' health and well-being. Spoiled feed can emit a musty, sour, or rancid smell, which is often a sign of mould or bacterial growth. Mouldy feed often appears fuzzy and discoloured, or has visible patches of green, blue, white, or black growth. Spoiled feed may feel sticky or excessively dry, or have an abnormal texture due to mould growth. A sudden decrease in feed intake can be a sign that the feed has gone bad or is unpalatable.

References

Barbuddhe, S.B., Malik, S.V.S., Kumar, J.A., Kalorey, D.R. and Chakraborty, T. (2012) Epidemiology and risk management of listeriosis in India. *International Journal of Food Microbiology* 154(3), 113–118.

Dhama, K., Karthik, K., Tiwari, R., Shabbir, M.Z., Barbuddhe, S. *et al*. (2015) Listeriosis in animals, its public health significance (food-borne zoonosis) and advances in diagnosis and control: A comprehensive review. *Veterinary Quarterly* 35(4), 211–235.

Dhanda, M.R., Lall, J.M., Seth, R.N. and Chandrasekhariah, P. (1959) A case of listeric abortion in an ewe with a small scale survey of the incidence of agglutinins of listeria in the sera of sheep. *Indian Veterinary Journal* 36, 113–124.

Fentahun, T. and Fresebehat, A. (2012) Listeriosis in small ruminants: A review. *Advances in Biological Research* 6(6), 202–209.

Ferreira, V., Wiedmann, M., Teixeira, P. and Stasiewicz, M.J. (2014) Listeria monocytogenes persistence in food-associated environments: Epidemiology, strain characteristics, and implications for public health. *Journal of Food Protection* 77(1), 150–170.

Hirsh, C.D. and Zee, C.Y. (eds) (1999) *Veterinary Microbiology*. Blackwell Science, Malden, Massachusetts, USA.

Quinn, P.J., García Sánchez, J. and Markey, B.K. (2003) *Concise Review of Veterinary Microbiology*, 3rd edn. Blackwell Science, Oxford, UK.

Quinn, P.J., Markey, B.K., Carter, M.E., Donnelly, W.J.C. and Leonard, F.C. (2002) *Veterinary Microbiology and Microbial Disease*. Blackwell Science, Oxford, UK.

Radostits, O.M., Gay, C.C., Blood, D.C., Hinchliff, K.W. and Constable, P.D. (2007) *Veterinary Medicine: A Textbook of the Diseases of Cattle, Sheep, Pigs, Goats and Horses*, 10th edn. Elsevier Health Science, pp. 805–810.

Ryser, E.T. and Marth, E.H. (2007) *Listeria, Listeriosis, and Food Safety*, 3rd edn. CRC Press, New York.

Scanlan, C.M. (1988) *Introduction to Veterinary Bacteriology*. Iowa State University Press, Ames, Iowa.

22 Q Fever (Queensland Fever)

Nourhan Eissa*
Department of Animal Hygiene and Zoonoses, Faculty of Veterinary Medicine, University of Sadat City, Egypt

Abstract
The disease 'Query fever' (Q fever), which is expanding globally and both emerging and re-emerging, is broadly described in this chapter. It can spread randomly or in outbreaks of 100–1000 cases. Despite the fact that Q fever cases are on the rise worldwide, the illness is still viewed as a somewhat underappreciated anthropozoonosis because 60% of acute cases are asymptomatic and can go undiagnosed, while in goats some cases may show signs of depression and decreased appetite before developing late-term abortions and decreased reproductive effectiveness. Q fever is still a highly mysterious zoonosis, due to its widespread occurrence, challenging epidemiology, variety of reservoirs and vectors, and paucity of studies describing the dynamic interaction between these variables.

Keywords: *Coxiella burnetii*, epidemiology, goats, Q fever, zoonosis

22.1 Introduction

Except for the Antarctic and New Zealand, Query fever (or Q fever, also known as Queensland fever) is a serious anthropozoonosis that is widespread and is dangerous, needing early detection and poorly understood. *Coxiella burnetii*, the bacterium that causes Q fever, is a highly contagious member of the Gammaproteobacteria class. It has been demonstrated that it may live for long periods of time in the environment, where it has been found to infect humans, a wide variety of domestic and wild animal species, domestic and wild birds, reptiles, ticks and marine animals. Storms of late-term abortions, stillbirths, neonatal mortality and infertility are just a few of the disease's severe manifestations in goats (Angelakis and Raoult, 2010).

The difficulty of diagnosing Q fever is exacerbated by the inability to isolate the bacterium and the need for specialized facilities with biosafety level 3 (BSL-3) for growing the bacteria, as well as the lack of economical, accurate and exact laboratory diagnostic procedures. Yet, laboratory testing is the only way to definitively diagnose Q fever (Oyston and Davies, 2011). This chapter aims to provide a comprehensive overview of zoonotic Q fever in goats and to shed light on its aetiology, risk factors, routes of transmission, hazards, epidemiology and disease control strategies.

22.2 Synonyms

Synonyms for Q fever include Query fever, Australian Q fever, coxiellosis, abattoir fever, Derrick-Burnet disease, hibernovernal bronchopneumonia, Balkan grippe, Queensland fever,

*Corresponding author: vet_noura@yahoo.com

DOI: 10.1079/ 9781800622852.0022

Nine-Mile fever, pneumorickettsiosis, quadrilateral fever and goat flu (Hadush *et al.*, 2016).

22.3 Historical Background

Derrick (1937) used the name 'Q fever' to describe an unusual, unidentified agent that caused febrile symptoms in slaughterhouse workers in Brisbane, Queensland, Australia. No one has attempted to change the disease's 'Query fever' name, despite the fact that its presence is no longer in question and its epidemiology and aetiology are well known. Subsequently, Burnet and Freeman (1937) proposed that the agent's origins were rickettsial. Derrick (1939) later gave the bacterium the name *Rickettsia burnetii*, and Philip (1948) gave it the name *Coxiella burnetii* (*C. burnetii*) in honour of Cox and Burnet's work in isolating and spreading the infection. *Rickettsia diaporica* was initially discovered by Cox (1939) as the cause of Q fever. The Centres for Disease Control and Prevention (CDC) classified *C. burnetii* as a potential class B bioterrorism agent because of its widespread development under multiple biological warfare initiatives by the USA and the former Soviet Union (CDC, 2000).

Since the 1980s, hundreds to thousands of instances of Q fever have been documented in numerous countries, including Greece, Italy, the United States, Spain, Switzerland, Great Britain (i.e. England, Scotland and Wales) and Germany. Between 2007 and 2010, the Netherlands experienced the world's greatest Q fever outbreak, resulting in more than 4000 human cases. This outbreak was blamed on the expansion of dairy goat rearing (Roest *et al.*, 2011).

22.4 Bacteriology

22.4.1 Aetiology

C. burnetii, a 2.5% coccobacillus bacterium that is obligate intracellular, non-motile, non-sporulated and pleomorphic (0.4 to 1 mm long and 0.2 to 0.4 mm wide), is the culprit behind Q fever. Despite having a Gram-negative membrane, it is typically difficult to stain using the Gram method. Moreover, the bacterium is regarded as having a low infectious dosage (one to ten organisms can infect a person) (Heppell *et al.*, 2017).

22.4.2 Taxonomy

According to Walter *et al.* (2014):

Kingdom: Bacteria
Phylum: Proteobacteria
Class: Gammaproteobacteria
Order: Legionellales
Family: Coxiellaceae
Genus: *Coxiella*
Species: *C. burnetii*

C. burnetii, according to Eldin *et al.* (2017), differs from other rickettsial agents in that it can spread with or without the aid of an invertebrate vector, is highly filterable, is resistant to physical and chemical agents, does not produce agglutinins in the Weil–Felix test and rarely causes a cutaneous rash.

22.4.3 *C. burnetii* antigenic phases

The naturally virulent phase I of *C. burnetii*, which can be found in ticks, animals and people, is one of the two antigenic phases of the organism. Phase II is created through multiple iterations in cell culture or chicken embryos (ECE). Phase II cells are thought to be avirulent and are swiftly eliminated by the host phagolysosomal pathway because they lack glucuronic acid, and the genes for lipopolysaccharide (LPS) synthesis produce truncated rough LPS devoid of an O-antigen side chain. The high virulence of phase I organisms is due to their lengthy, complete, smooth LPS, which contains glucuronic acid, glucose and galactose. Phase II antibodies would initially be created (in acute infections) in animals and people infected with *C. burnetii*, whereas phase I antibodies would be produced (or potentially not produced at all) in chronic infections. Phase II may also be successively transmitted through guinea pigs to reach phase I (Beare *et al.*, 2018).

22.4.4 *C. burnetii* forms (life cycle stages)

Natural variations of *C. burnetii* include the large cell variant (LCV), the small cell variant (SCV), and a spore-like form that cannot be taken seriously as a true spore because only Gram-positive bacteria produce true spores, whereas *C. burnetii* is a Gram-negative one. During logarithmic development, LCV is the replicative form that predominates (2 mm in length). When the bacterial growth is close to reaching the stationary phase, the spore-like shape begins to form inside LCV. After the giant cell releases the endospore, it changes into SCV (0.45 mm in length), which has less metabolic activity and is more resistant to osmotic and physical stressors. The characteristic Gram-negative cell wall, which comprises two different layers divided by a periplasmic gap, is present in both LCV and SCV. However, unlike LCV, the SCV's periplasmic space is occupied by proteins and peptidoglycan, which explains why SCV is more resilient to environmental challenges than LCV. Both phases allow for any form (Stead *et al.*, 2018).

22.5 Pathogenesis

22.5.1 Pathophysiology

After bacterial entrance into the host body, SCV adheres to the membranes of macrophages, internalizes into them through phagocytosis, and significantly differentiates to LCV within 1–2 days. Phase II cells of *C. burnetii* enter macrophages by binding to the leukocyte response integrin (v3) and the CR3 receptor, in contrast to phase I LPS, which inhibits the engagement of the CR3 receptor and binds by both v3 and the integrin-associated protein (IAP) complex. Sobotta *et al.* (2016) found that phase II phagocytosis occurs more frequently than phase I. Once phagosomes fuse with cellular acidic lysosomes, several intracellular phagolysosomes are produced, and they eventually combine to form a sizeable paracytopherous vacuole (PV). The survival, reproduction, absorption of nutrients inside acidic phagolysosomes (pH=4.5) and defence against various antibiotics of *C. burnetii* depend on the three proteins superoxide dismutase, catalase and macrophage infectivity potentiator (Cbmip) (Shaw and Voth, 2019).

After primary multiplication in the local lymph nodes in goats, the organism can be isolated from the liver, spleen, kidney, bone marrow, lymph nodes and intestine up to 13 weeks of pregnancy. However, the placenta does not turn positive until just before delivery, when it releases vast quantities of *C. burnetii* into the environment through the amniotic fluid. The bacterium then settles in the mammary glands. Some chronically infected goats shed *C. burnetii* during future parturitions due to immunomodulation, which increases the organism's ability to grow in the placenta. According to García-Ispierto *et al.* (2010), the contaminated environment induces the infection and weak clinical symptoms in newborn non-immune animals.

22.5.2 Immune response

The majority of the defence against *C. burnetii* depends on cell-mediated immunity. TLR4 recognizes LPS antigens, regulates the immune response to *C. burnetii* through granuloma formation and produces type one cytokines, whereas TLR2 recognizes peptidoglycan and lipopeptides and becomes involved in the production of type two cytokines (Schoenlaub *et al.*, 2015).

In a primary *C. burnetii* infection, the virulent organism is taken up by macrophages and dendritic cells, where it is then presented to T-cells and causes them to produce IFN-γ and TNF, which leads to the death of infected macrophages, the formation of granulomas and a reduction in the assimilation of iron by infected cells. In contrast, infected macrophages survive and their microbicidal function is decreased in immune-compromised individuals or pregnant women who are unable to develop a strong IFN-γ response, leading to persistent Q fever (Capo and Mege, 2012).

Regarding humoral immunity, a large amount of antibodies are generated against extracellular *C. burnetii* 3–4 weeks after infection. Chronic infection is associated with elevated levels of antibodies against phase I antigens, but the bulk of antibodies produced after the initial infection are against phase II antigens (immunogenic phase) and are also produced in response to the Q fever vaccination. IgM antibodies reactive with phase II antigens arise quickly, peak within 14 days, and remain for 10–12 weeks, whereas immunoglobulin M (IgM) antibodies against phase I antigens are frequently at lower titres during acute infection (Zhang *et al.*, 2012). IgG antibodies reactive with phase II antigens, on the other hand, reach higher titres 8 weeks after the onset of symptoms, but those that are reactive with phase I antigens increase slowly and remain at lower titres even after a year. In chronic Q fever, IgG titres against phases I and II antigens may both be high. Furthermore, phase I antigen (IgA) antibodies are frequently associated with ongoing illnesses (Angelakis and Raoult, 2010).

22.6 Epidemiology of Q Fever

22.6.1 Reservoir and sources

More than 30 different types of animals, including domestic and wild animals, birds, reptiles, ticks and marine mammals, are afflicted by Q fever. More than 40 hard and 14 soft tick species that naturally carry the *Coxiella* bacteria can spread the sickness from one continent to another by transstadial or transovarian ways (Knobel *et al.*, 2013).

Despite the species, *C. burnetii*-infected animals, tainted milk, aerosolized germs in baby items, excreta, vaginal mucus and semen of infected animals are the most likely causes of infection. The placenta has the most bacteria (109 bacteria/g), which after a late miscarriage increases to billions of bacteria (Koehler *et al.*, 2019).

22.6.2 Modes of transmission

C. burnetii enters goats primarily by the mouth, but it can also spread through sexual contact and transplacental (vertical) infection, according to Eldin *et al.* (2017). Diseases may also be spread by tick bites.

22.6.3 Associated risk factors

Host factors

- **Age:** It has been shown in numerous communities all over the world that age directly correlates with an increase in the seroprevalence of Q fever. According to González-Quijada *et al.* (2015), inflammatory and immune system changes brought on by ageing may be a factor in Q fever persistence or reactivation.
- **Sex:** The protective effect of the female sex hormone (17-beta-oestradiol), which regulates host responses to *C. burnetii*, was established by Chang *et al.* (2010). This could help to explain why Q fever is more common in males than females, with a rate ratio of 1.6:1 to almost 7.4:1.
- **Contact with water sources:** *C. burnetii* can live in free-living water amoebae, as well as in the soil around bodies of water, because infected animals may discharge their faeces onto water surfaces.
- **Exposure to ticks and other arthropods:** When feeding on Q fever-infected animals, ticks can become infected with *C. burnetii*, which multiplies in the ticks' middle gut and is expelled with saliva and faeces, where it can live for 18 months and be transmitted through aerosols or direct skin contact. Tick progeny may become germinatively infected when tick ovaries become infected, perpetuating *C. burnetii* infection in the tick population (Koka *et al.*, 2018). Ticks are not necessary for the disease's normal enzootic cycle in mammals. Nonetheless, they do play a substantial role in the dissemination of Q fever in wild rats, lagomorphs and birds. Moreover, Egyptian fleas and lice have both had *C. burnetii* DNA recovered from them (Loftis *et al.*, 2006).

Agent factors

- **The infectivity dose and the virulence of *C.burnetii*:** The two antigenic stages of *C. burnetii* are the virulent phase I and the avirulent phase II. It only takes one *C. burnetii* organism to infect someone. A large dosage would make the condition worse and shorten the period of incubation (Beare *et al.*, 2018).
- **Resistance of *C. burnetii against different stresses*:** The spore-like form of *C. burnetii* has been shown to be remarkably durable, capable of lasting for a long time outside, and resistant to a number of

physical and chemical challenges, including high temperatures and pressures, desiccation, osmotic stress and numerous chemical disinfectants. *C. burnetii* may live in contaminated food due to its physical resistance to acids (up to pH 4.5), heat (62°C for 30 min), UV light and pressure (up to 300,000 kPa). Moreover, according to Sidi-Boumedine *et al.* (2010), *C. burnetii* can survive for up to 30 months in preserved tap water, 4 months in dust at 15–20°C, 49 days in dry urine and 20 days in faeces. While gaseous formaldehyde is useless for sterilizing, 5% chloroform or 2% formaldehyde gas (with 80% relative humidity) may kill phase I and II cells in less than 30 min, and 5% formaldehyde for 5 min. In addition to heat treatments of 65°C for an hour, 72°C for 40 s, and even autoclaving at 131°C for 15 min, other substances that are effective at inactivating *C. burnetii* include 1% phenol, 5% hydrogen peroxide (H_2O_2), 5% sodium hydroxide, 5% chloroform, 0.5% sodium hypochlorite and 70% ethanol (Angelakis and Raoult, 2010).

Environmental factors

The ability of *C. burnetii* to survive in the open for weeks as well as in strong winds, dry heat, open terrain and other factors have all been connected to the spread of the bacteria. Moreover, transmission is more common in areas with low groundwater levels, high animal populations and low vegetation densities (Nusinovici *et al.*, 2017). Data of reported Q fever cases are frequently not very helpful in pinpointing the time of illness onset. However, information on the seasonality of infection reveals that the incidence increases in the lambing season during spring and early summer in many European countries (Roest *et al.*, 2011) as well as in Egypt, where the hot, dry climate with little total precipitation and open landscapes with high wind speeds may favour spreading of *C. burnetti* via contaminated aerosols (Angelakis *et al.*, 2014), whereas most Q fever cases were reported in winter in Japan (Ho *et al.*, 1995), and in autumn in Cyprus (Cantas *et al.*, 2011).

22.7 The Disease in Goats

Q fever is one of the major risks to underdeveloped countries. Because of their higher seroprevalence than that of goats and cattle, sheep were more frequently held responsible for being the main cause of Q fever epidemics in people (Johnson *et al.*, 2019). Clinical symptoms of *C. burnetii* infection in goats include decreased appetite and depression 1–2 days later, followed by outbreaks of abortion in the latter stages of pregnancy, decreased reproductive efficiency because of endometritis, infertility, stillbirths, premature delivery and delivery of weak offspring. Because the bacterium's primary favoured tissue is the female reproductive system, animal coxiellosis is often asymptomatic (De Oliveira *et al.*, 2018). The aborted fetus lacks any distinguishing characteristics, whereas the aborted placenta appears enlarged. Large amounts of *C. burnetii* were discharged in the fluids and materials that failed (Koehler *et al.*, 2019).

22.8 Diagnosis of Q Fever

The non-specific disease manifestations in various populations, the challenges in isolating the bacterium, the requirement for specialized laboratories with biosafety level three for culturing the bacterium, as well as the dearth of affordable, sensitive and specific laboratory diagnostic techniques all contribute to the difficulty of diagnosing Q fever. Nevertheless, the only way to confirm a Q fever diagnosis is by laboratory testing (Oyston and Davies, 2011). Both direct and indirect methods are used to study the diagnosis of Q fever in animals and humans. The direct methods of *C. burnetii* diagnosis involve identifying the presence of the pathogen inside the host by using culturing methods, immunohistochemistry (IHC), histology, or different molecular methods (Masala *et al.*, 2004). The common indirect serological techniques are immunofluorescence assay (IFA), enzyme-linked immunosorbent assay (ELISA), micro-agglutination test (MAT) and complement fixation test (CFT). A skin test and a gamma interferon release assay (IGRA) have been used to detect the cellular-mediated immunity against *C. burnetii* (Rousset *et al.*, 2007).

22.9 Prevention and Control Strategies for Q Fever in Goats

Notifying veterinary authorities of any animal population that has Q fever aids in preventing the zoonotic spread of the illness, its negative economic impacts and the spread of infection between populations. Under field conditions, it is essential to take precautions to control tick populations by using acaricidals like deltamethrin (1%), treating infected animals with ivermectin (0.2 mg/kg body weight, subcutaneously), separating sick animals from the rest of the herd and burning animal placentas to prevent the subsequent spread of *C. burnetii* (Sidi-Boumedine *et al.*, 2010). Additionally, the decontamination of faeces with calcium cyanide, the immediate use of hypochlorite or phenol to deal with contaminated material leaks in animal facilities and the disinfection of exposed surfaces with 2% formaldehyde, 1% lysol, 5% H_2O_2, 70% ethanol, or even 5% chloroform, are all options (Arricau-Bouvery *et al.*, 2001).

The greatest way to protect animals from sickness is through Q fever vaccine. One of the best vaccines on the market is the Cox-vac vaccine, which is excellent for immunizing goats. Phase I inactivated microorganisms are used to create it. Theoretically, this vaccination can lower the risk of human infection by stopping animal miscarriages, limiting the bacteria that sick animals shed and limiting the spread of the disease in the environment. Sero-negative herds or young animals ought to receive vaccinations (De Cremoux *et al.*, 2012).

22.10 Treatment of Q Fever in Goats

The biggest obstacle to effective treatment is the use of alkalinizing drugs such trimethoprim-sulfa, tetracycline, chloramphenicol and enrofloxacin against acidophilic *C. burnetii.* Goats that are pregnant are given oxytetracycline in the final trimester to reduce the possibility of abortion. Only the acute type of Q fever is effectively treated with antibiotics (Moodie *et al.*, 2008).

22.11 Conclusion

The information regarding *C. burnetii* infection in goats and their part in the epidemiology of infection, specifically their link to the prevalence of Q fever in people, has been reported in this chapter. Q fever is a widespread occurrence, and since its initial description, the risk it poses to humans has been understood. The traits of *C. burnetii* support its designation as a category B biological threat agent. International public health experts strongly advise global *C. burnetii* monitoring, particularly in light of the recent large-scale Q fever epidemics in the Netherlands that were caused by goat infection. To understand the dynamics of infection in an epidemiological analysis and to examine the involvement of goats in Q fever, an approach with the characterization of the bacteria, its tactics of infection and clinical patterns in goats is necessary.

References

Angelakis, E. and Raoult, D. (2010) Q fever. *Veterinary Microbiology* 140(3–4), 297–309.

Angelakis, E., Mediannikov, O., Socolovschi, C., Mouffok, N., Bassene, H. *et al.* (2014) *Coxiella burnetii*-positive PCR in febrile patients in rural and urban Africa. *International Journal of Infectious Diseases* 28, 107–110.

Arricau-Bouvery, N., Souriau, A., Montoussamy, A., Ladenise, K. and Rodolakis, A. (2001) Study of *Coxiella burnetii* excretion in an experimental goat model and decontamination of dung with calcium Cyanamid. *Rencontre Recherche Ruminants* 8, 153–156.

Beare, P.A., Jeffrey, B.M., Long, C.M., Martens, C.M. and Heinzen, R.A. (2018) Genetic mechanisms of *Coxiella burnetii* lipopolysaccharide phase variation. *PLoS Pathogens* 14(3), e1006922.

Burnet, F.M. and Freeman, M. (1937) Experimental studies on the virus of Q-fever. *Reviews of Infectious Diseases* 5(4), 299–305.

Cantas, H., Muwonge, A., Sareyyupoglu, B., Yardimci, H. and Skjerve, E. (2011) Q fever abortions in ruminants and associated on-farm risk factors in Northern Cyprus. *BMC Veterinary Research* 7, 13.

Capo, C. and Mege, J.L. (2012) Role of innate and adaptive immunity in the control of Q fever. *Advances in Experimental Medicine and Biology* 984, 273–286.

CDC (2000) Biological and chemical terrorism: Strategic plan for preparedness and response. *Morbidity and Mortality Weekly Report* 49, 1–14.

Chang, C.C., Lin, P.S., Hou, M.Y., Lin, C.C., Hung, M.N. *et al.* (2010) Identification of risk factors of *Coxiella burnetii* (Q fever) infection in veterinary-associated populations in Southern Taiwan. *Zoonoses Public Health* 57(7-8), e95–e101.

Cox, H.R. (1939) Studies of a filter-passing infectious agent isolated from ticks: V. further attempts to cultivate in cell-free media. Suggested classification. *Public Health Reports* 54, 1822–1827.

De Cremoux, R., Rousset, E., Touratier, A., Audusseau, G., Nicollet, P. *et al.* (2012) Assessment of vaccination by a phase I *Coxiella burnetii*-inactivated vaccine in goat herds in clinical Q fever situation. *FEMS Immunology and Medical Microbiology* 64(1), 104–106.

De Oliveira, J.M., Rozental, T., De Lemos, E.R., Forneas, D., Ortega-Mora, L.M. *et al.* (2018) *Coxiella burnetii* in dairy goats with a history of reproductive disorders in Brazil. *Acta Tropica* 183, 19–22.

Derrick, E.H. (1937) Q fever, a new fever entity: Clinical features, diagnosis and laboratory investigation. *Medical Journal of Australia* 2(8), 281–299.

Derrick, E.H. (1939) *Rickettsia burnetii*: The cause of Q fever. *Medical Journal of Australia* 1, 14.

Eldin, C., Mélenotte, C., Mediannikov, O., Ghigo, E., Million, M. *et al.* (2017) From Q fever to *Coxiella burnetii* infection: A paradigm change. *Clinical Microbiology Reviews* 30(1), 115–190.

García-Ispierto, I., Nogareda, C., Almería, S., Martínez-Bello, D., Beckers, J. *et al.* (2010) *Neospora caninum* and *Coxiella burnetii* seropositivity are related to endocrine pattern changes during gestation in lactating dairy cows. *Theriogenology* 74(2), 212–220.

González-Quijada, S., Salazar-Thieroldt, E. and Mora-Simón, M.J. (2015) Persistent Q fever and ischaemic stroke in elderly patients. *Clinical Microbiology and Infection* 21(4), 362–367.

Hadush, A., Kandi, V. and Pal, M. (2016) Epidemiology and public health implications of Q fever. *Perspectives in Medical Research* 4(3), 42–46.

Heppell, C.W., Egan, J.R. and Hall, I. (2017) A human time dose response model for Q fever. *Epidemics* 21, 30–38.

Ho, T., Htwe, K.K., Yamasaki, N., Zhang, G.Q., Ogawa, M. *et al.* (1995) Isolation of *Coxiella burnetii* from dairy cattle and ticks and some characteristics of the isolates in Japan. *Microbiology and Immunology* 39(9), 663–671.

Johnson, S.A., Kaneene, J.B., Asare-Dompreh, K., Tasiame, W., Mensah, I.G. *et al.* (2019) Seroprevalence of Q fever in cattle, sheep and goats in the Volta region of Ghana. *Veterinary Medicine and Science* 5(3), 402–411.

Knobel, D., Maina, A., Cutler, S., Ogola, E., Feikin, D. *et al.* (2013) *Coxiella burnetii* in humans, domestic ruminants, and ticks in rural Western Kenya. *American Journal of Tropical Medicine and Hygiene* 88(3), 513–518.

Koehler, L.M., Kloppert, B., Hamann, H.P., El-Sayed, A. and Zschöck, M. (2019) Comprehensive literature review of the sources of infection and transmission routes of Coxiella burnetii, with particular regard to the criteria of "evidence-based medicine". *Comparative Immunology, Microbiology and Infectious Diseases* 64, 67–72.

Koka, H., Sang, R., Kutima, H.L. and Musila, L. (2018) *Coxiella burnetii* detected in tick samples from pastoral communities in Kenya. *BioMed Research International* 201, 8158102.

Loftis, A.D., Reeves, W.K., Szumlas, D.E., Abbassy, M.M., Helmy, I.M. *et al.* (2006) Surveillance of Egyptian fleas for agents of public health significance: *Anaplasma*, *Bartonella*, *Coxiella*, *Ehrlichia*, *Rickettsia*, and *Yersinia pestis*. *American Journal of Tropical Medicine and Hygiene* 75(1), 41–48.

Masala, G., Porcu, R., Sanna, G., Chessa, G., Cillara, G. *et al.* (2004) Occurrence, distribution, and role in abortion of *Coxiella burnetii* in sheep and goats in Sardinia, Italy. *Veterinary Microbiology* 99(3–4), 301–305.

Moodie, C.E., Thompson, H.A., Meltzer, M.I. and Swerdlow, D.L. (2008) Prophylaxis after exposure to *Coxiellaburnetii*. *Emerging Infectious Diseases* 14(10), 1558–1566.

Nusinovici, S., Hoch, T., Brahim, M.L., Joly, A. and Beaudeau, F. (2017) The effect of wind on *Coxiella burnetii* transmission between cattle herds: A mechanistic approach. *Transboundary and Emerging Diseases* 64(2), 585–592.

Oyston, P.C. and Davies, C. (2011) Q fever: The neglected biothreat agent. *Journal of Medical Microbiology* 60(1), 9–21.

Philip, C.B. (1948) Observations on experimental Q- fever. *Journal of Parasitology* 34(6), 457–464.

Roest, H.I., Tilburg, J.J., Van der Hoek, W., Vellema, P., Van Zijderveld, F.G. *et al.* (2011) The Q fever epidemic in The Netherlands: History, onset, response and reflection. *Epidemiology and Infection* 139(1), 1–12.

Rousset, E., Durand, B., Berri, M., Dufour, P., Prigent, M. *et al.* (2007) Comparative diagnostic potential of three serological tests for abortive Q fever in goat herds. *Veterinary Microbiology* 124(3–4), 286–297.

Schoenlaub, L., Elliott, A., Freches, D., Mitchell, W.J. and Zhang, G. (2015) The role of B cells in host defense against primary *Coxiella burnetii* infection. *Infection and Immunity* 83(12), 4826–4836.

Shaw, E.I. and Voth, D.E. (2019) *Coxiella burnetii*: A pathogenic intracellular acidophile. *Microbiology* 165(1), 1–3.

Sidi-Boumedine, K., Rousset, E., Henning, K., Ziller, M., Niemczuck, K. *et al.* (2010) Development of harmonised schemes for the monitoring and reporting of Q-fever in animals in the European Union. *EFSA Supporting Publications* 7(5), 48E.

Sobotta, K., Hillarius, K., Mager, M., Kerner, K., Heydel, C. *et al.* (2016) *Coxiella burnetii* infects primary bovine macrophages and limits their host cell response. *Infection and Immunity* 84(6), 1722–1734.

Stead, C.M., Cockrell, D.C., Beare, P.A., Miller, H.E. and Heinzen, R.A. (2018) A *Coxiella burnetii* phospholipase A homolog pldA is required for optimal growth in macrophages and developmental form lipid remodeling. *BMC Microbiology* 18(1), 33.

Walter, M.C., Öhrman, C., Myrtennäs, K., Sjödin, A., Byström, M. *et al.* (2014) Genome sequence of *Coxiellaburnetii* strain Namibia. *Standards in Genomic Sciences* 9(1), 22.

Zhang, G., Zhang, Y. and Samuel, J. (2012) Components of protective immunity. In: Toman, R., Heinzen, R., Samuel, J. and Mege, J. (eds) *Coxiella Burnetii: Recent Advances and New Perspectives in Research of the Q Fever Bacterium*. Springer, Dordrecht, Netherlands, pp. 91–104.

23 Tularaemia

Subir Singh*
Dept of Veterinary Medicine and Public Health, Faculty of Animal Science, Veterinary Science and Fisheries, Agriculture and Forestry University, Rampur, Chitwan, Nepal

Abstract
Goats and humans are usually considered accidental hosts for tularaemia. Ticks play a pivotal role in transmitting *Francisella tularensis*. In endemic areas, transmission to humans and goats usually occurs via bites from infected arthropods, or the bacterium may enter into scratches to infect animal tissues. It also contaminates through ingestion of infected tissues or contaminated water and inhalation of aerosolized particles. Human-to-human transmission is considered to be rare. In human beings, fever, chills, malaise, cephalalgia and myalgia are the most prominent clinical signs of tularaemia.

Keywords: tularaemia, goats, zoonosis, contamination, endemic

23.1 Introduction

Tularaemia is a highly contagious disease caused by *Francisella tularensis* that can infect more than 300 species of wild and domestic animals, birds, reptiles, fish and people (AVMA, 2003). Tularaemia has a wide geographical distribution in the northern hemisphere and is more limited elsewhere (Hopla and Hopla, 1994). It has been reported in parts of North America, Europe, the Mediterranean, Africa, Asia and Russia. The disease occurs in different clinical forms and the severity of the disease varies depending on the virulence of the disease, its dose and the site of vaccination. The disease is confirmed by culture, serology or PCR. Antibiotic treatment can be effective if started early. It is classified as a Category A bioterrorism agent because, if released, it can cause death, air pollution and social disruption (Foley, 2022).

The disease was first described as a disease of humans prior to the discovery of the causative agent and probably occurred in Japan before 1818 and in Norway since at least 1890 and may be as early as 1653 (Zidon, 1964). People can become infected in various ways, including tick and deer fly bites, and contact with infected animals (especially rodents, rabbits and hares, etc.).

Synonyms for tularaemia include plague-like disease of rodents, plague-like lymphadenitis, conjunctivitis tularensis, Francis' disease, deerfly fever, rabbit fever, cattle-fly fever, Pahvant Valley fever, Pahvant Valley plague, glandular-type tick fever, epidemic lymphadenitis, hare meat poisoning, and hare plague.

*Corresponding author: ssingh@afu.edu.np

DOI: 10.1079/ 9781800622852.0023

23.2 Aetiology

Tularaemia is caused by *Francisella tularensis*, a non-spore-forming, Gram-negative coccobacillus, and antigenically related to *Brucella* spp. It is a facultative intracellular parasite that can be killed by heat and appropriate disinfection, but the bacteria can survive for weeks or months in moist environmental conditions. The bacteria can be cultured directly on blood supplemented with cysteine; however, the culture must be differentiated from other Gram-negative bacteria on blood agar. The taxonomic status of *Francisella* spp. has been revised and debated. *F. tularensis* is divided into three subspecies (*F. t. tularensis*, *F. t. holarctica* and *F. t. mediasiatica*) with diverse hosts, life cycles and geographical distributions. Recent consensus suggests that *F. t. tularensis* is associated with tularaemia type A; *F. t. holarctica* causes tularaemia type B; and the third type C is due to *Francisella novicida*, which is less common and has lower virulence than the other two (Koh *et al.*, 2019). Type A is found mostly in North America and is more virulent and can cause mortality as high as 30% in humans, if untreated. Type B is less virulent.

23.3 Global Distribution

Tularaemia has a wide global distribution and has been reported in North America, Europe, the Mediterranean, Africa and parts of Asia. In North America, the disease is widespread, affecting the United States (except Hawaii), Canada and the Mexican states. Tularaemia is common in Europe and Mediterranean Africa, except for the Iberian Peninsula.

Reports of tularaemia in Asia include China, Iran, Israel, Japan, South Korea, Russia and Turkey. The situation varies in different regions and may be affected by factors such as climate, wildlife population, vector distribution and public health surveillance.

23.4 Host Susceptibility

Tularaemia prefers lagomorphs and rodents, probably due to their habitat and feeding behaviours. In North America, snowshoe hares, black-tailed jack rabbits and eastern and desert cotton-tail hares are the most commonly affected species. These animals often act as reservoir hosts for the bacteria, allowing the disease to spread in the environment and contributing to the its persistence in the environment.

Carnivores are also susceptible to tularaemia, but they typically require high doses of the bacterium to become infected and rarely express signs of the disease. Due to this typical characteristics, early detection and control measures usually become difficult. Domestic animals and humans are usually considered accidental hosts, as they may contract the infection through direct contact with infected animals or contaminated environments (Friend, 2006).

It is worth noting that in Canada, the United States and Russia, domestic animals such as goats and sheep as well as mink, beavers and wolves are infected with tularaemia and it causes significant mortality. Although infections in domestic cats are rare, their documentation raises concerns about potential transmission to humans. On the other hand, dogs emerge as being immune to the disease but can continue the cycle of infection by becoming reservoirs of the disease or as maintenance hosts for the tick vector, continuing the transmission cycle.

23.5 Transmission

Arthropods, especially ticks, can host the disease and act as biological vectors of *F. tularensis* to spread infection to humans and animals (Sjöstedt, 2007). Ticks are the most important vectors, infecting humans and animals as well as prolonging and maintaining the life cycle of the bacteria between the host and the environment (Koh *et al.*, 2019). The occurrence of *T. tularensis* in ticks varies worldwide and has been reported in different tick species and also in species such as *Dermacentor*, *Hyalomma*, *Haemahysalis*, *Ixodes* and *Rhipicephalus*. (Esmaeili *et al.*, 2021). It is also frequently associated with tularaemia in rabbits, hares and mice and serves as an interepizootic reservoir for animal infections. Horseflies, mosquitoes, sucking lice and mosquitoes are also vectors. Wild animals, livestock, birds, fish and arthropods are potential carriers of these diseases. *F. tularensis* is transmitted to humans through contact with skin and mucosa, or via the conjunctival route, or respiratory or gastrointestinal tract (Sjöstedt, 2007). In endemic areas, transmission to humans and other domestic animals usually occurs through the bites of arthropods, or the parasite can enter areas where an infectious disease is present through a scratch or cut. Tularaemia can also be transmitted through ingestion of contaminated tissue or water and inhalation of aerosolized material. Goats, sheep and domestic cats are potential sources of infection for humans. Human-to-human transmission is thought to be rare. The clinical form of tularaemia depends on how bacteria enter the body.

23.6 Clinical Signs of Tularaemia in Animals and Humans

Tularaemia in animals and humans has a wide host diversity and numerous clinical indices in different animal species.

- **In rodents, rabbits and hares:** Rats, rabbits and mice are frequently affected, and the symptoms in these animals are often poorly described because they are often found as dead animals. In experimental animals, fatigue, fever, ulcers, regional lymphadenopathy and abscesses occur, usually resulting in death within 8–14 days.
- **In goats and sheep:** Tularaemia often occurs during tick infection in goats and sheep and presents with symptoms such as fever, rigid gait, frequent urination, diarrhoea, weight loss and difficulty in breathing. Abortion may occur as well, as kids and lambs are more susceptible to death.
- **In cattle:** Cattle shows evidence of natural infection of the disease, but a clear picture is yet to be revealed.
- **In horses:** The disease is clinically limited and usually manifests itself in horses as fever, dyspnoea, depression and incoordination associated with extensive infestation of ticks.
- **In cats:** Domestic cats infected with *F. tularensis* can range from asymptomatic to severe clinical infestation. It may present with symptoms such as fever, depression, lymphadenopathy, abscesses, mouth or tongue ulcers, gastroenteritis, hepatomegaly, splenomegaly and jaundice, anorexia, weight loss, pneumonia and sepsis.
- **In dogs:** There are few reports of clinical signs of tularaemia in dogs, but there is evidence of seroconversion. Infection tends to be inapparent or mild, depending on the mode of transmission. The signs of infection include fever, mucopurulent oculonasal discharge, pustules at inoculation sites, lymphadenopathy and anorexia. This disease usually resolves with suppurative therapy.
- **In humans:** Symptoms in humans include fever, chills, malaise, cephalalgia, myalgia and vomiting. Specific symptoms depend on the route of infection, and the disease can progress to many forms, like ulcero-glandular, glandular, typhoidal, oropharyngeal, oculo-glandular, or pulmonary. Complications such as pleuropneumonia, meningitis, sepsis and shock can be fatal.

23.7 Diagnosis

The enzyme-linked immunosorbent assay (ELISA), haemagglutination, microagglutination and test tube agglutination are commonly used to detect agglutinating antibodies from serum. For confirmatory diagnosis of tularaemia, the organism must be isolated from clinical specimens, such as blood, exudate or biopsy samples. However, many laboratories are reluctant to do this because of the risks to laboratory personnel and thus, diagnostic procedure require biosafety laboratory facilities. Routine laboratory tests, including complete blood counts (CBCs) and serum chemistry tests, typically produce false-positive or non-specific results.

The diagnosis of tularaemia in wild animals is usually made by postmortem examination. Clinical confirmation in goats and sheep is based on serology or bacterial isolation. Presumptive diagnosis in humans is based on clinical signs and exposure history. A prevalence of 1:160 or higher in disease-free areas is considered diagnostic. In contrast, in endemic areas where patient and convalescent titres are required, it is estimated that a four-fold change in titre can be tested in samples taken 2–4 weeks apart.

23.8 Treatment

Streptomycin and tetracycline are the 'drug of choice' antibiotics in the treatment of livestock and wildlife. In humans, streptomycin is preferred, along with tetracyclines (especially doxycycline), gentamicin and chloramphenicol as alternatives. Fluoroquinolones also show promise in the treatment of tularaemia. Chloramphenicol has been used to treat cases associated with meningitis.

23.9 Control

Tick control plays an important role in prevention of the disease in humans and animals. It is important to avoid contact with untreated water when *F. tularensis* contamination is suspected. Also, wild game needs to be properly cooked before consumption. Contact with and handling dead and dying animals in the endemic area should be avoided. It is highly recommended to wear gloves when handling wild game, animal skins or carcasses. Equipment used to detect, monitor or record animals suspected or confirmed for infection should be properly disposed of as medical waste (sterilized) and disinfected.

As for laboratory workers and individuals at risk of exposure, attenuated live vaccines that were previously available at risk of infection are no longer available.

23.10 Zoonotic Significance

Infections in humans are not contagious. Humans usually become infected through contact with infected wild animals, eating, or exposure to contaminated water, or being bitten by ticks and other arthropods that have fed on infected wildlife.

The incubation period for human tularaemia usually lasts 3–5 days but can vary from 1 to 14 days. Initial symptoms include fever, chills, malaise, cephalalgia, myalgia and vomiting, followed by more specific signs such as ulcero-glandular, glandular, typhoidal, oropharyngeal, oculo-glandular, or pulmonary manifestations, depending on the route of entry. All forms of tularaemia can cause pleuropneumonia, meningitis, sepsis, shock and, potentially, death.

- **Ulcero-glandular tularaemia** is the most common type of disease (75–85% of reported cases). It is characterized by the appearance of ulcers at the point of entry, most often on the fingers or hands, that are associated with exposure to rabbits, hares or rodents. The ulceration progresses to necrosis and lymphadenopathy with suppuration, ulceration and sclerotic lymph nodes.
- **Glandular tularaemia** shows similar symptoms but without the skin ulcers.
- **Pulmonary tularaemia** accounts for approximately 30% of infectious diseases and is caused by inhalation of aerosolized pathogens. Common symptoms include pneumonia in one or both lungs.
- **Typhoid tularaemia** is caused by consuming contaminated food or water and is rare. Clinical signs include fever, prostration, dehydration, weight loss, gastroenteritis and sepsis. If left untreated, the mortality rate can reach 40–60%.
- **Oropharyngeal tularaemia** is a disease caused by ingestion of the bacteria and causes pharyngeal tonsillitis, which can be exudative or membranous and may be accompanied by cervical lymphadenopathy.
- **Oculo-glandular tularaemia** is caused by conjunctival contamination. It usually appears as ulcerative papules, typically found on the lower eyelid, accompanied by lymphadenopathy.

23.11 Prevention

Healthcare workers who care for animal and human patients should wear personal protective clothing, including gowns, gloves and masks. Since tularaemia is highly contagious, laboratories should be informed when sending samples and tularaemia should be taken into consideration in the potential differential diagnosis. Biosafety level two is recommended for diagnostic work on suspect material, while biosafety level three is required for culture procedures. In the United States, tularaemia is a reportable disease, but it is not considered a notifiable disease internationally.

F. tularensis is an agent of bioterrorism because of its high infectivity, easy transmission and its potential to cause severe disease. Potential sources of transmission include contamination of food or water and aerosolization.

23.12 Conclusion

Tularaemia is an important zoonotic disease with multiple hosts, primarily affecting rabbits and rats. Although infection is rare in birds, fish, amphibians and reptiles, infection occurs in domestic and wild animals. Humans are becoming infected with the bacteria more frequently, but accidentally, and the number of reports has decreased in recent years. However, continuing surveillance of tularaemia in different regions is important to understand its epidemiology, host–host interactions and potential risks to public health. Efforts to improve surveillance, diagnostic capabilities and public awareness are essential for effective disease control and prevention.

References

AVMA (2003) Tularemia facts. American Veterinary Medical Association. Available at: https://www.avma.org/tularemia-facts

Esmaeili, S., Rohani, M., Ghasemi, A., Gouya, M.M., Khayatzadeh, S. *et al.* (2021) *Francisella tularensis* human infections in a village of Northwest Iran. *BMC Infectious Diseases* 21(1), 310. DOI: org/10.1186/s12879-021-06004-y.

Foley, J.E. (2022) Tularemia in animals. *MSD Veterinary Manual*. Available at: https://www.msdvetmanual.com/generalized-conditions/tularemia/tularemia-in-animals

Friend, M. (2006) Tularemia. Circular 1297. US Geological Survey, Reston, Virginia.

Hopla, C.E. and Hopla, A.K. (1994) Tularemia. In: Steele, J.H. (ed.) *CRC Handbook of Zoonoses, Section A: Bacterial, Rickettsial and Mycotic Diseases*, 2nd edn. CRC Press Inc, Boca Raton, Florida, pp. 113–125.

Koh, F.X., Nurhidayah, M.N., Tan, P.E., Kho, K.L. and Tay, S.T. (2019) *Francisella* spp. detected in *Dermacentor* ticks in Malaysian forest reserve areas. *Veterinary Parasitology, Regional Studies and Reports* 17, 100315. DOI: 10.1016/j.vprsr.2019.100315.

Sjöstedt, A. (2007) Tularemia: History, epidemiology, pathogen physiology, and clinical manifestations. *Annals of the New York Academy of Sciences* 1105, 1–29. DOI: 10.1196/annals.1409.009.

Zidon, J. (1964) Tularemia. In: Van Der Hoeden, J. (ed.) *Zoonoses*. Elsevier Publishing Co, Amsterdam, pp. 74–94.

24 Dermatophilosis

Abbas Rabiu Ishaq*, Muhammad Mahadi, Naziru Mukhtar and Aminu Abubakar Zugu
Paws And Claws Specialists Veterinary Clinic, Anas bin Malik Street 3939, Alsahafa District Riyadh, KSA

Abstract
Dermatophilosis is also known as 'lumpy wool disease' in goats. It is a severe contagious skin disease that affects mainly goats, causing the development of matted tufts of hair, and it progresses to scabs with yellow-green pus beneath. The disease is caused by a bacterium, *Dermatophilus congolensis*, that infects the skin. It plays a major role in causing wart-like accumulations of damaged skin. The lesions can occur anywhere in the body but typically appear as dense scabs along the topline. The moist lesions can be seen in the rectum or vulva or adjacent to the udder, causing thickened, folded skin. Genetics can influence susceptibility to dermatophilosis. Immunosuppressive goats are prone to suffer severely through saliva secreted during tick bites. It can also infect humans when handling or treating infected animals. Therefore, it is highly recommended to wear gloves or other protective gear and to wash hands and arms properly with an antibacterial soap to prevent becoming infected from the disease.

Keywords: Dermatophilosis, goats, transmission, genetics

24.1 Introduction

Dermatophilosis is an infectious skin disease of goats, sheep, camels, cattle, buffalo and several wild animals (Gebreyohannes and Gebresselassie, 2013) caused by *Dermatophilus congolensis*, which is a Gram-positive, facultative anaerobic, filamentous, coccus bacterium with transverse and longitudinal fragments that are arranged mimicking railway tracks (Quinn and Markey, 2003). The disease is cosmopolitan in distribution with more economic losses in the tropics, seen as declined production, low hide quality and high culling rates (Abu-Samra and Walton, 1977). Ticks and biting flies exposing the skin (Quinn *et al.*, 2011) along with a humid environment (Yeruham *et al.*, 2003) and the enzymes; proteases, keratinases and ceramidases produced by *D. congolensis* are essential for the disease pathogenesis (Ellis *et al.*, 1987). Crusty cutaneous lesions resulting from inflammatory responses of the body to the bacterium (Yeruham *et al.*, 2003) are mostly seen on ears, distal extremities and backs of animals (Burd *et al.*, 2007).

24.2 Anatomy of Goat Skin

Skin is the largest organ in the body, serving as barrier between the external and internal body environment (Razvi *et al.*, 2015). It serves thermoregulatory, protective, sensory, immunological, excretory and several other functions

*Corresponding author: abbasrabiuishaq@gmail.com

 The Handbook of Zoonotic Diseases of Goats (ed. T. Rana)
DOI: 10.1079/ 9781800622852.0024

(Bhattacharya *et al.*, 2003; Dyce *et al.*, 2009). The skin anatomy varies from one species to another depending on their ecological niches, with multiple layers consisting of an array of fibres, glands, nerve endings, muscle (commonly erector pili) and blood vessels (Razvi *et al.*, 2015). The skin consists of an outer epidermis and an inner dermis (Kapadnis and Bhosle, 2004).

24.2.1 Epidermis

The epidermis is covered by a keratin layer, made up of keratinized stratified epithelium, and is subdivided, from within outwards, into *stratum basale* (basal layer), *stratum spinosum* (spinous layer), *stratum granulosum* (granular layer) and *stratum corneum* (cornified layer) (Razvi *et al.*, 2015).

Stratum basale comprises a single layer of columnar cells that are arranged on the basement membrane (Kapadnis and Bhosle, 2004). *Stratum spinosum* has two to three layers of polyhedral cells (Razvi *et al.*, 2015). *Stratum granulosum* so named due to its component single layer of elongated cells with compressed nuclei (Kapadnis and Bhosle, 2004). *Stratum corneum* comprises four to five layers of cells (Kapadnis and Bhosle, 2004) that are discontinuous and sloughed off in the form of scales (Banks, 1993). The fifth epidermal layer, *stratum lucidium*, is practically absent in Black Bengal goats (Mandage *et al.*, 2003), Osmanabadi goats (Kapadnis and Bhosle, 2004) and American goats (Gayen *et al.*, 1989).

There are variations in the epidermal thickness from one region of the body to another; with the dorsal neck, thorax and loin being thickest (Atlee *et al.*, 1997). It has been shown that the epidermis is moderately reactive to periodic acid Schiff (PAS) and is due to the presence of neural mucopolysaccharides (Baba *et al.*, 1990).

24.2.2 Dermis

The dermis comprises dense, irregular connective tissue with collagen, reticular fibres, hair follicles, sebaceous glands, nerve endings, muscles (erector pili) and sweat glands (Dellmann and Brown, 1976). The dermis is histologically divided into two layers: outer papillary and inner reticular layers (Razvi *et al.*, 2015).

The reticular layer has a higher percentage of fibrous tissues (Dellmann and Brown, 1976; Kapadnis *et al.*, 2005), while the papillary layer comprises more active cells (Kapadnis *et al.*, 2005).

As observed with the epidermis, thickness of the dermis is variable, being thicker around dorsal neck, thorax and loin (Atlee *et al.*, 1997; Razvi *et al.*, 2015).

Similar variations are seen with relation to age, and adults tend to have thicker dermis than younger ones of the same species (Fig. 24.1).

24.3 Epidemiology

24.3.1 Spread in animals

Spread is by direct contact with infected animals, arthropods such as ticks (Woldemeskel, 2000), biting flies and contaminated fomites alongside high humidity, heat and rainfall (Harman *et al.*, 2001). Ticks such as *Amblyomma variegatum*, *Rhipicephalus pravus*, *Rhipicephalus evertsi* (Msami *et al.*, 2001) and *Boophilus annulatus* are commonly implicated for the spread of the pathogen (Bayisa *et al.*, 2012).

24.3.2 Spread in humans

Infection is by close contact with infected animals through feeding or milking and by consuming their unpasteurized milk (Amor *et al.*, 2011).

24.4 Prevalence

Dermatophilosis has a worldwide distribution (Koney, 1996), with more cases witnessed in the tropics due to varied humidity (Koney, 1996), especially between June and August (Yakhchali and Hosseine, 2006). Its enzootic nature was reported in Ethiopia (de Castro, 1997), with prevalence of 3.13% in goats (Woldemeskel, 2000). In Nigeria, Oyejide *et al.* (1984) recorded a 23.4% sero-prevalence in goats that were meant to be slaughtered at Kaduna central

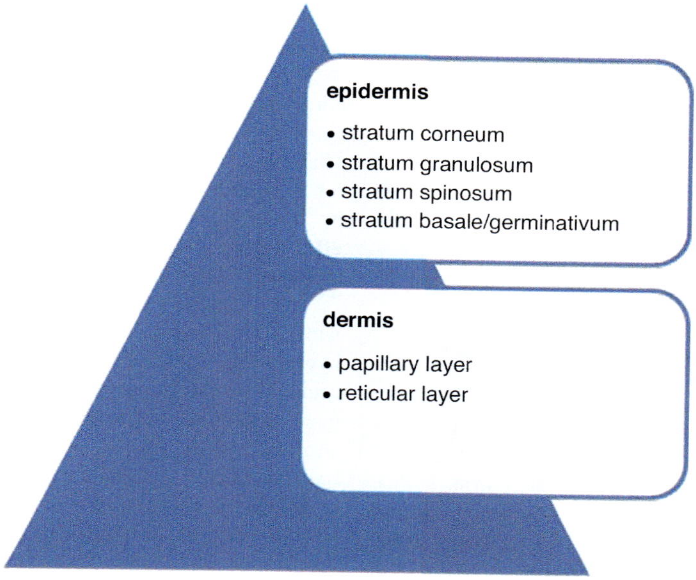

Fig. 24.1. The various skin layers of goats, the base of the triangle being the deepest aspect. (Author's own image.)

abattoir, 5.55% at Zaria and Jos, following its initial report by Henderson in 1927 (Harley *et al.*, 2017).

24.5 Vectors

Major arthropod vectors for the spread of *Dermatophilus* species include *Amblyomma variegatum* (Ndhlovu and Masika, 2015), *Dermacentor andersoni* and *Hyalomma* species (all hard ticks), and biting flies such as *Stomoxys* and *Lyperosia* species (Lloyd and Walker, 1993).

24.5.1 Life cycle of *Amblyomma variegatum*

Amblyomma variegatum, the tropical bont tick, is a large, brightly coloured (Pegram *et al.*, 2004) ixodid tick that has a small scutum covering only part of the dorsum, leaving it partially open when engorged after a blood meal (Georgi *et al.*, 1990). These ticks have convex eyes, long palps and posteriorly located festoons (Walker *et al.*, 2003). The entire life cycle depends on three hosts that are needed to support each of the larval, nymphal and adult stages for blood meals (Barré *et al.*, 1995). They show affinity for the host's ventral abdomen, perineum, ventral tail and towards the dewlap (Barré *et al.*, 1995; Prine and Hodges, 2012).

Pheromones secreted by the male ticks attract the females for mating (Popham *et al.*, 1996; Allan *et al.*, 1998); the presence of males is prerequisite for the female tick's attachment to the host and its maintenance for at least 2 weeks (Barré and Garris, 1990). The female ticks produce up to 30,000 eggs (Barré *et al.*, 1995; Prine and Hodges, 2012) that hatch within 50–100 days in warm weather to produce larvae that stay for some months (Pegram and Banda, 1990), congregated on vegetation prior to attachment to hosts (Barré *et al.*, 1995) for blood meal and subsequent moulting to the nymphal stage; the nymphal stage takes another blood meal and within approximately 45 days it moults to the adult stage (Yonow, 1995). The adults stay dormant for 4 weeks before questing for the next host (Pegram and Banda, 1990). It is found that the various developmental stages spend at most 15 days on a host (Yonow, 1995; Popham *et al.*, 1996) with potential tendencies to produce three generations within 2 years (Popham *et al.*, 1996) (Fig. 24.2).

Hosts of *A. variegatum* include goats, sheep, camels, cattle, horses, other wildlife (Gebreyohannes and Gebresselassie, 2013) and, uncommonly, humans (Amor *et al.*, 2011).

24.6 Aetiology

Dermatophilosis is caused by *Dermatophilus congolensis*, a facultative anaerobic (sometimes referred to as micro-aerobic) actinomycete (Zaria, 1993). *D. congolensis* is named after its country of origin (Van Saceghem, 1915, 1916); incorrect synonyms have included *Actinomyces dermatonomus* for British and Australian isolates (Bull, 1929) and *Polysepta pedis* (Thompson, 1954; Thompson and Bisset, 1957).

Disease–pathogen–host relationships include cutaneous streptothricosis by *D. congolensis* in goats, cattle, horses and sheep (Austwick, 1958; Macadam and Haalstra, 1971), strawberry foot rot by *Dermatophilus pedis* and mycotic dermatitis by *D. dermatonomus* in sheep (Denman *et al.*, 2021). *D. pedis* and *D. dermatonomus* are synonymous with *D. congolensis*.

D. congolensis yields tiny, smooth, creamy-white, haemolytic, adherent colonies with hyphae-like branches mimicking railway tracks under Gram staining upon growth on aerobic blood and chocolate agar at 32°C for 24 hours (Amor *et al.*, 2011).

Biochemical tests on pure isolates of *D. congolensis* reveal it to be β-haemolytic, catalase, urease and oxidase positive but negative for indole and nitrate reductase enzymes (Gordon, 1964; Amor *et al.*, 2011).

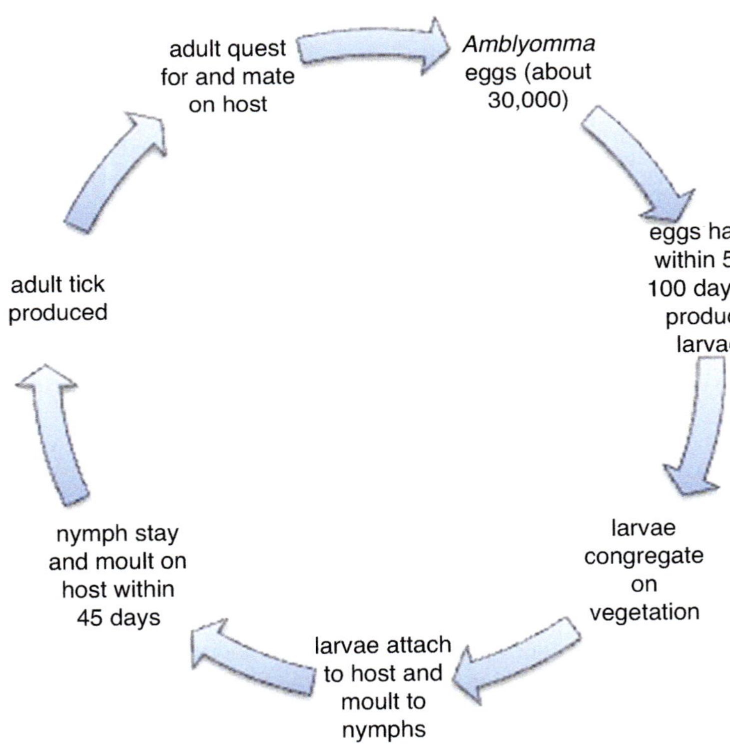

Fig. 24.2. Life cycle of *Amblyomma variegatum*. (Author's own image.)

24.7 Pathogenesis

Inoculation of *D. congolensis* zoospores via bites from ticks such as *Amblyomma* species or contact with contaminated formites which penetrate the upper layers of keratinized tissues, localize and grow to form hyphae, later maturing into zoospores (Tellam *et al.*, 2021). These zoospores, produced under high humidity and temperature concurrent with immunosuppression and starvation, precipitate the disease (Macêdo *et al.*, 2008). This is achieved by tampering with the integrities of skin (stratum corneum), hair follicles and sebaceous glands (Dalis *et al.*, 2009, 2010) (Fig. 24.3).

24.8 Clinical Signs

24.8.1 In animals

Two clinical forms exist, which include the localized epidermal forms presenting purulent, crusted and matted hair upon pustulation (Frye *et al.*, 2019); described more frequently as non-pruritic, exudative, proliferative, hyperkeratotic dermatitis with crustations and folliculitis (Zaria, 1993), or paintbrush appearance of wool, that are loose and easily removed without pain perception (Osman, 2015). The systemic form presents abortion, funiculitis, placentitis (Ambrose, 1996) and poor body condition (Osman, 2015).

24.8.2 In humans

Cutaneous forms have been reported with painful and itchy vesicular eruptions that progress to pustules and later crustations (Amor *et al.*, 2011). Other associated clinical signs include intertriginous lesions showing some fissuring and maceration of skin, and hairy leukopenia (Towersey *et al.*, 1993). Pitted keratolysis, seen under the soles (plantar), is named for the appearance of discrete pits (Lockwood *et al.*, 2010). They are opaque white alternating with black/brown with several arrangements and sizes accompanied by interrupted/discontinuous dermatoglyphic lines (Pattanaprichakul *et al.*, 2021).

24.9 Risk Factors

Humidity, living in the tropics, close contact with infected animals, low socioeconomic status, illiteracy, immunosuppression and starvation constitute the greatest risk factors

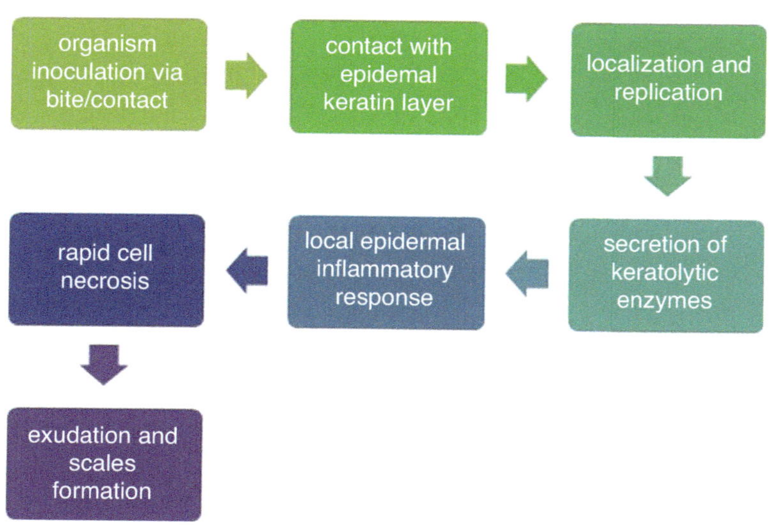

Fig. 24.3. Pathogenesis of dermatophilosis. (Author's own image.)

for dermatophilosis in humans (de Lorenzi *et al.*, 2021).

24.10 Pathology

24.10.1 Histopathology in animals

Cellular changes include epidermitis, hyperkeratosis, parakeratosis, keratosis and folliculitis (Msami *et al.*, 2001). Exudative crusty dermatitis with acanthosis and subcorneal abscessation has been reported (Bućek *et al.*, 1992).

Giemsa-stained specimens showing branched septate hyphae carrying zoospores are obtainable from direct smears of crusty wrinkled skin lesions (Osman, 2015).

24.10.2 Histopathology in humans

Erythematous, desquamative lesions of about 0.5 cm diameter with elevated edges have been reported (Amor *et al.*, 2011).

24.11 Diagnosis

24.11.1 In animals

Clinical signs

Clinical signs include hyperkeratotic dermatitis with exudation, proliferation, crust formation and folliculitis (Zaria, 1993) mostly over the dorsal midline of the body, which may be seen laterally and ventrally (Berry and Watt, 2017). Characteristic crusts appear to be hard, pyramidal and possibly discoloured (Bull, 1929; Roberts, 1965; Gardiner, 1971; Norris *et al.*, 2008).

Microbiology

For culture and isolation:

- Isolation of spherical/ovoid cocci with septate branching (Admassu and Alemu, 2011) that are Gram-positive (Mannan *et al.*, 2009) following culturing at 37°C in a 5–10% carbondioxide jar for 48–72 hour (Haalstra, 1965).

For seromolecular diagnosis:

- polymerase chain reaction (PCR) to demonstrate *D. congolensis* DNA gene sequences (Shaibu *et al.*, 2010);
- use of immunofluorescence to detect organism's specific antigens (Admassu and Alemu, 2011);
- exo-antigene containing hexosamine-galactose-xylose peptide detection via diffusion–precipitation, immuno-electrophoresis tests followed by chromatography (Kwapinski, 1966); and
- use of other advanced seromolecular diagnostics such as enzyme-linked immunosorbent assay (ELISA), counter-immunoelectrophoresis and haemagglutination (Martinez *et al.*, 1993).

24.11.2 In humans

Clinical signs include evidence of itchy erythematous vesicles that eventually desquamate to form crusts, with history of close contact with infected animals or consumption of unpasteurized milk (Amor *et al.*, 2011).

24.12 Differential Diagnoses

24.12.1 Animals (goats)

Contagious ecthyma (orf)

Orf is caused by parapoxvirus, which is a DNA virus (Ayhan and Aktaş, 2017; Rezende *et al.*, 2018). Parapoxvirus is epitheliotropic in nature and affects goats, sheep, wild ruminants, and rarely dogs and humans (Guo *et al.*, 2004; Haig, 2006). Orf is synonymous to cutaneous pustular dermatitis, scabby mouth and sore mouth (De La Concha-Bermejillo *et al.*, 2003). Presenting clinical signs include proliferative cauliflower-like outward growths, seen mainly on the lips, muzzle, nostrils and chin (Yeruham *et al.*, 1991). Other signs include exudative dermatitis of the pinna, scaling on the scrotum, ears and fetlock (Yeruham *et al.*, 1991).

Ruling out orf from a suspected case of dermatophilosis can be achieved clinically by thorough observation of the positioning and morphology of the lesions. Confirmatory ruling is achieved by culture and isolation of *D. congolensis* from exudates (Shaibu *et al.*, 2010).

Scrapie

Scrapie is caused by a prion (Monleón *et al.*, 2011) and is degenerative and usually fatal. Sheep and goats may exhibit signs such as itching, severe lymphadenomegaly, suppurative arthritis, vesicular lesions on the lips and nostrils (Ndikuwera *et al.*, 1992; De La Concha-Bermejillo *et al.*, 2003). Ruling out dermatophilosis can be achieved by observing presence of neurological signs such as uneven gait, grinding of teeth, trembling and stumbling (Taranukha *et al.*, 2020). Confirmatory rulings are achieved using immunohistochemistry to detect red granular immunoprecipitate (Monleón *et al.*, 2011).

Demodicidosis

Demodicidosis is caused by the mite *Demodex caprae*, which is a small, permanent, obligate parasite (Zhao *et al.*, 2013). It is synonymous (non-specific) with itch and scab (Rashid *et al.*, 2019) and has affinity for hair follicles and sebaceous glands (Mulugeta *et al.*, 2010). Major clinical signs of the disease are crusty pruritic dermatitis that results in alopecia (Arlian, 1989).

Ruling out dermatophilosis can be achieved by demonstrating the mite from skin scrapings treated with 10% potassium hydroxide under light microscopy (Seyoum *et al.*, 2015).

Psoroptes/ear mange

This is caused by *Psoroptes cuniculi*, popularly known as ear mite (Kumar *et al.*, 2016). Major presenting clinical signs include erythema, pyoderma, pruritus, crusting, alopecia, head shaking, ear scratching (Munro and Munro, 1980; Lofstedt *et al.*, 1994), otitis (Wilson and Brewer, 1984) and meningo-encephalitis (Yeruham *et al.*, 1984).

Trichophytosis

This skin disease is caused by the fungus *Trichophyton verrucosum* (Davidov *et al.*, 2018). It causes parakeratosis and inflammatory reaction by secreting exotoxins, proteolytic and parakeratolytic enzymes (Summerbell, 2000; Bojkovski *et al.*, 2013). These are about 10–50 mm ovoid scabs around the neck, forehead, eyes, forelimbs and chest (Seyfarth *et al.*, 2011). Confirmation is achieved by processing skin scrapings with 10% potassium hydroxide and subsequent fungus detection under light microscopy (Davidov *et al.*, 2018).

24.12.2 Humans

Tuberculosis verrucosa cutis

TBVC occurs as a sequel to bacterial penetration of skin (Franco-Paredes *et al.*, 2018). It presents dermatological symptoms such as yellow-orange spherical regions surrounded by yellowish/reddish epithelioid cell granuloma, thick scaling, papillomatosis and hyperkeratosis (Jakhar *et al.*, 2021).

Syphilis

Syphilis is caused by *Treponema pallidum* (Bakos *et al.*, 2022) characterized by epidermal scaling that progresses outwardly, in most cases surrounded by an erythematous halo, along with haemosiderosis (Errichetti and Stinco, 2017; Tognetti *et al.*, 2017), acanthosis (whitish to pinkish dermal regions) and macerated horny layers of the skin (Ikeda *et al.*, 2016).

Lichen scrofulosum

This is characterized by granulomatous infiltration, perifollicular lesions (Jassi *et al.*, 2020), follicular/perifollicular dots, marginal hypopigmentation and white scales (Jassi *et al.*, 2020; Garg *et al.*, 2021).

Peruvian wart

These warts are caused by *Bartonella bacilliformis*. Common clinical forms are with miliary scales (multiple red circular papules 1–4 mm in diameter), mular scales (blood-filled nodules) and diffuse lesions (groups of subdermal nodules > 5 mm in diameter), with vascular involvement and central depression (Durand *et al.*, 2017).

Trichobacteriosis

This is caused by *Corynebacterium* spp. (*C. flavescens*) that cause yellow, black or reddish adhesions of hair shafts around the axillar and pubic regions (Bakos *et al.*, 2022).

Human papilloma virus

Human papilloma virus infection, or warts, typically has palmoplantar, flat and anogenital forms (Zalaudek *et al.*, 2008; Dong *et al.*, 2012; Sonthalia *et al.*, 2021).

Sporothricosis

Caused by the fungus *Sporothrix schenckii* (Vinay *et al.*, 2020), sporothricosis presents as generalized erythema, white scar-like regions and pustules (Dabas *et al.*, 2019), superficial ulcers and haemorrhagic crustations (Vinay *et al.*, 2020).

Other differentials

Other differentials include molluscum contagiosum caused by poxvirus (Sonthalia *et al.*, 2021; Bakos *et al.*, 2022), milker's nodule caused by paravaccinia virus (Ayhan and Aktaş, 2017), blastomycosis caused by *Blastomyces dermatitidis* (Wang *et al.*, 2015; Elmas *et al.*, 2020), pityriasis versicolor caused by *Malassezia species* (Zhou *et al.*, 2015; Thomas and Malakar, 2019) and tiniasis caused by any of *Tinea nigra* (Zalaudek *et al.*, 2008; Bakos *et al.*, 2022), *Tinea corporis* (Vázquez-López *et al.*, 2004; Bhat *et al.*, 2019), *Tinea manum* (Errichetti and Stinco, 2018; Bhat *et al.*, 2019), or *Tinea incognito* (Singal *et al.*, 2019).

24.13 Treatment

24.13.1 Animals

Treatments with long-acting oxytetracycline, penicillin–dihydrostreptomycin combination (Osman, 2015), penicillin (Plant, 2007), or topical antiseptics present limited efficacy on hair follicle-localized hyphae (Dickson and de Elías Costa, 2010). Higher cure rates (100%) were seen following three doses of long-acting oxytetracycline 3 days apart, as well as a combination of penicillin and dihydrostreptomycin for five consecutive days in a low-humidity environment (Osman, 2015).

24.13.2 Humans

Treatment for humans is with 500 mg tetracycline (every 6 hour) alongside mupirocin topical cream (every 12 hour) for a period of 2 weeks (Harman *et al.*, 2001). Other systemic treatment options with some reported degrees of positive results include erythromycin, chloramphenicol and streptomycin (Zaria, 1993). Patients with classical pitted keratolysis respond to mupirocin, gentamicin sulfate, clindamycin phosphate, erythromycin and tetracycline hydrochloride topical preparations (Burkhart, 1980; Vazquez-Lopez and Perez-Oliva, 1996)

Also, cephalexin (500 mg every 6 hour) is an effective empirical therapy before appropriate culture and sensitivity is ready (Kaminski and Suter, 1976).

Dermatophilosis tends to be self-limiting in humans and regresses gradually, especially if the skin is not kept moist for a long period of time (Kaminski and Suter, 1976).

24.14 Vector Control Measures

Though mechanisms employed by the arthropod vectors in questing, identification and contact maintenance are complex (Adenubi *et al.*, 2016), the following techniques were reported to be effective for their control (Byford *et al.*, 1992).

- Use of organophosphate-based acaricides such as chloromethiuron, formamidines, clenpirin, potentiated chlordimeform (Fig. 24.3), though reported to be carcinogenic (Ware and Whitacre, 2004), and amitraz (Palmer *et al.*, 1973). Macrocyclic lactones (Burg *et al.*, 1979) of fungal origin comprising avermectins (eprinomectin and ivermectin) and milbemycins

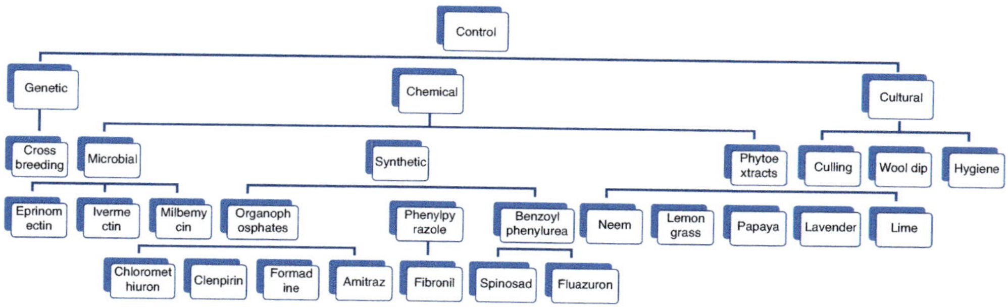

Fig. 24.4. Control methods for dermatophilosis. (Author's own image.)

(Lasota and Dybas, 1991), fibronil (phenylpyrazole compound), spinosad and fluazuron (benzoyl phenylurea) have all demonstrated acaricidal effects (Bull *et al.*, 1996).

- Phytoextracts from *Azadirachta indica* (Neem), *Cymbopogon* spp. (lemon grass), *Lavendula augustifolia* (lavender), *Gynandropsis gynandra* (chinsaga), *Pelargonium rostrum* (zonal/garden geranium) (Adenubi *et al.*, 2016), *Carica papaya* (papaya, papaw, pawpaw) and *Citrus aurantiifolia* (key lime, acid lime) offer some levels of acaricidal effects (Shyma *et al.*, 2022) (Fig. 24.4).

The following measures, among others, play a significant role in controlling the spread of dermatophilosis:

- avoidance of close contact;
- tick control (Chatikobo *et al.*, 2001);
- culling of chronically infected sheep and rearing genetically hardy ones (Roberts and Graham, 1966; Edwards, 1991);
- hygienic practices, isolation of infected animals;
- keeping in low humidity environment; and
- clipping of wool and use of antibacterial dips for the maintenance of hygiene (Gardiner, 1971; Smith *et al.*, 2010; Geenty *et al.*, 2013).

References

Abu-Samra, M.T. and Walton, G.S. (1977) Modified techniques for the isolation of *Dermatophilus* spp. from infected material. *Sabouraudia* 15(1), 23–27.

Adenubi, O.T., Fasina, F.O., McGaw, L.J., Eloff, J.N. and Naidoo, V. (2016) Plant extracts to control ticks of veterinary and medical importance: A review. *South African Journal of Botany* 105, 178–193.

Admassu, M. and Alemu, S. (2011) Study on clinical bovine dermatophilosis and its potential risk factors in North Western Ethiopia. *International Journal of Animal and Veterinary Advances* 3(1), 33–36.

Allan, S.A., Barré, N., Sonenshine, D.E. and Burridge, M.J. (1998) Efficacy of tags impregnated with pheromone and acaricide for control of *Amblyomma variegatum*. *Medical and Veterinary Entomology* 12(2), 141–150.

Ambrose, N.C. (1996) The pathogenesis of dermatophilosis. *Tropical Animal Health and Production* 28, 29S–37S.

Amor, A., Enríquez, A., Corcuera, M.T., Toro, C., Herrero, D. *et al.* (2011) Is infection by dermatophilus congolensis underdiagnosed? *Journal of Clinical Microbiology* 49(1), 449–451.

Arlian, L.G. (1989) Biology, host relations, and epidemiology of *Sarcoptes scabiei*. *Annual Review of Entomology* 34(1), 139–159.

Atlee, B.A., Stannard, A.A., Fowler, M.E., Willemse, T., Ihrke, P.J. *et al.* (1997) The histology of normal llama skin. *Veterinary Dermatology* 8(3), 165–176.

Austwick, P.K.C. (1958) Cutaneous streptothricosis, mycotic dermatitis, and strawberry foot rot and the genus *Dermatophilus* van saceghem. *Veterinary Reviews and Annotations* 4(1).

Ayhan, E. and Aktaş, H. (2017) Dermoscopic features and types of orf and milker's nodule. *Advances in Dermatology and Allergology/Postępy Dermatologii i Alergologii* 34(4), 357–362.

Baba, M.A., Sinha, R.D., Prasad, R. and Prasad, J. (1990) Comparative histological and histochemical-studies on the palpebral sweat glands of goat and sheep. *Indian Journal of Animal Sciences* 60(10), 1203–1205.

Bakos, R.M., Reinehr, C., Escobar, G.F. and Leite, L.L. (2022) Dermoscopy of skin infestations and infections (entomodermoscopy) – part I: Dermatozoonoses and bacterial infections. *Anais Brasileiros de Dermatologia* 96, 735–745.

Banks, W.J. (1993) *Applied Veterinary Histology*. Mosby-Year Book, St Louis, Missouri.

Barré, N. and Garris, G.I. (1990) Biology and ecology of *Amblyomma variegatum* (Acari: Ixodidae) in the Caribbean: Implications for a regional eradication program. *Journal of Agricultural Entomology* 7(1), 1–9.

Barré, N., Garris, G. and Camus, E. (1995) Propagation of the tick *Amblyomma variegatum* in the Caribbean. *Revue Scientifique et Technique (International Office of Epizootics)* 14(3), 841–855.

Bayisa, D., Berhanu, A., Fentahun, T. and Chanie, M. (2012) Occurrence of bovine dermatophilosis in Ambo town, West Shoa Administrative Zone, Ethiopia. *American-Eurasian Journal of Scientific Research* 7(4), 172–175.

Berry, W. and Watt, B. (2017) High prevalence mild dermatophilosis (lumpy wool) in unweaned Merino lambs following a wet spring. Available at: http://www. flockandherd. net.au/sheep/ireader/derma tophilosis

Bhat, Y.J., Keen, A., Hassan, I., Latif, I. and Bashir, S. (2019) Can dermoscopy serve as a diagnostic tool in dermatophytosis? A pilot study. *Indian Dermatology Online Journal* 10(5), 530.

Bhattacharya, M., Sheikh, I.U. and Rajkhowa, J. (2003) Epidermal thickness in the skin of Yak (*Poephagus poephagus*). *Indian Journal of Veterinary Anatomy* 15, 73–76.

Bojkovski, J., Giadinis, N., Rogožarski, D., Relić, R., Savić, B. *et al*. (2013) Prikaz kliničkih slučajeva trihoficije i papilomatoze kod visoko-mlečnih krava / Notice of clinical cases of dermatomycosis and papillomatosis at dairy cows. *Zbornik Naučnih Radova Instituta PKB Agroekonomik (Collection of Scientific Works of the Institute PKB Agroeconomics)* 19(3–4), 115–122.

Buĉek, J., Pospíŝil, L., Moster, M. and Skalka, B. (1992) Experimental dermatophilosis. *Journal of Veterinary Medicine, Series B* 39(1-10), 495–502.

Bull, L.B. (1929) Dermatomycosis of the sheep (lumpy or matted wool) due to *Actinomyces dermatonomus* (n. sp. *Australian Journal of Experimental Biology and Medical Science* 6(4), 301–314.

Bull, M.S., Swindale, S., Overend, D. and Hess, E.A. (1996) Suppression of *Boophilus microplus* populations with fluazuron – an acarine growth regulator. *Australian Veterinary Journal* 74(6), 468–470.

Burd, E.M., Juzych, L.A., Rudrik, J.T. and Habib, F. (2007) Pustular dermatitis caused by *Dermatophilus congolensis*. *Journal of Clinical Microbiology* 45(5), 1655–1658.

Burg, R.W., Miller, B.M., Baker, E.E., Birnbaum, J., Currie, S.A. *et al*. (1979) Avermectins, new family of potent anthelmintic agents: Producing organism and fermentation. *Antimicrobial Agents and Chemotherapy* 15(3), 361–367.

Burkhart, C.G. (1980) Pitted keratolysis: A new form of treatment. *Archives of Dermatology* 116(10), 1104–1104.

Byford, R.L., Craig, M.E. and Crosby, B.L. (1992) A review of ectoparasites and their effect on cattle production. *Journal of Animal Science* 70(2), 597–602.

Chatikobo, P., Kusina, N.T., Hamudikuwanda, H. and Nyoni, O. (2001) The effect of tick control on bovine dermatophilosis in a smallholder farming area of Zimbabwe. *Zimbabwe Veterinary Journal* 32(1), 32–40.

Dabas, G., Kaur, H., Vinay, K., Kumaran, M.S., Shivaprakash, M.R. *et al*. (2019) Dermoscopy in disseminated sporotrichosis. *Journal of the European Academy of Dermatology and Venereology* 33(1), e33–e35.

Dalis, J.S., Kazeem, H.M., Makinde, A.A. and Fatihu, M.Y. (2009) Distribution of lesions of dermatophilosis in cattle sheep and goats in Zaria and Jos, Nigeria. *Journal of Animal and Veterinary Advances* 8(2), 385–388.

Dalis, J.S., Kazeem, H.M., Makinde, A.A. and Fatihu, M.Y. (2010) Bacteria associated with bovine dermatophilosis in Zaria, Nigeria. *African Journal of Microbiology Research* 4, 1475–1476.

Davidov, I., Radinović, M., Kovačević, Z., Erdeljan, M., Galfi, A. *et al*. (2018) Trichophytosis in beef cattle. *Veterinary Journal of Republic of Srpska* 18(2).

de Castro, J.J. (1997) Sustainable tick and tickborne disease control in livestock improvement in developing countries. *Veterinary Parasitology* 71(2–3), 77–97.

De La Concha-Bermejillo, A., Guo, J., Zhang, Z. and Waldron, D. (2003) Severe persistent orf in young goats. *Journal of Veterinary Diagnostic Investigation* 15(5), 423–431.

de Lorenzi, C., Quenan, S. and Fontao, L. (2021) *Dermatophilus congolensis* dermatitis in a traveller from Thailand. *Journal of Travel Medicine* 28(6), taab017.

Dellmann, H.D. and Brown, E.M. (1976) *Textbook of Veterinary Histology*. Lea & Febiger, Philadelphia, Pennsylvania.

Denman, S., Tellam, R., Vuocolo, T., Ingham, A., Wijffels, G. *et al.* (2021) Fleece rot and dermatophilosis (lumpy wool) in sheep: Opportunities and challenges for new vaccines. *Animal Production Science* 62(4), 301–320.

Dickson, C. and de Elías Costa, M.R.I. (2010) Human and animal dermatophilosis. An unusual case report and review of the literature. *Dermatología Argentina* 16, 349–353.

Dong, H., Shu, D., Campbell, T.M., Frühauf, J., Soyer, H.P. *et al.* (2012) Correction: Dermatoscopy of genital warts (Journal of the American Academy of Dermatology (2011) 64, (859–564)). *Journal of the American Academy of Dermatology* 66(5).

Durand, D., Quijano, E. and Sanz, M.E. (2017) Clinical and dermoscopic characteristics of a patient with cutaneous and mucosal manifestations of Peruvian wart. *International Journal of Dermatology* 56(12), 1442–1444.

Dyce, K.M., Sack, W.O. and Wensing, C.J.G. (2009) *Textbook of Veterinary Anatomy – E-Book*. Elsevier Health Sciences, Amsterdam.

Edwards, J.R. (1991) Studies on the epidemiology of ovine dermatophilosis. Doctoral dissertation, Murdoch University.

Ellis, T.M., Robertson, G.M., Sutherland, S.S. and Gregory, A.R. (1987) Cellular responses in the skin of merino sheep to repeated inoculation with *Dermatophilus congolensis*. *Veterinary Microbiology* 15(1–2), 151–162.

Elmas, Ö.F., Uyar, B. and Kilitçi, A. (2020) A 25-year history of leg ulceration: Cutaneous blastomycosis. *Dermatology Practical & Conceptual* 10(3), e2020054.

Errichetti, E. and Stinco, G. (2017) Dermoscopy in differentiating palmar syphiloderm from palmar papular psoriasis. *International Journal of STD & AIDS* 28(14), 1461–1463.

Errichetti, E. and Stinco, G. (2018) Dermoscopy in *Tinea manuum*. *Anais Brasileiros de Dermatologia* 93, 447–448.

Franco-Paredes, C., Marcos, L.A., Henao-Martínez, A.F., Rodríguez-Morales, A.J., Villamil-Gómez, W.E. *et al.* (2018) Cutaneous mycobacterial infections. *Clinical Microbiology Reviews* 32(1), e00069-18.

Frye, C.C., Bei, D., Parman, J.E., Jones, J., Houlihan, A.J. *et al.* (2019) Efficacy of tea tree oil in the treatment of equine streptothricosis. *Journal of Equine Veterinary Science* 79, 79–85.

Gardiner, M.R. (1971) Mycotic dermatitis (lumpy wool) of sheep. *Journal of the Department of Agriculture, Western Australia, Series 4* 12(6), 183–185.

Garg, T., Kumar, P., Das, S., Singh, S. and Madan, S. (2021) *Lichen scrofulosorum* coexisting with phlyctenular keratoconjuctivitis: Dermoscopy and ocular findings. *Indian Dermatology Online Journal* 12(6), 941.

Gayen, S., Prasad, G. and Sinha, R.D. (1989) Comparative histological studies on the skin of Indian buffalo and Black Bengal goats. *Indian Journal of Animal Sciences* 59, 920–924.

Gebreyohannes, M. and Gebresselassie, M. (2013) An overview on dermatophilosis of animals: A review. *Journal of Animal Science Advances* 3(7), 337–344.

Geenty, K.G., Brien, F.D., Hinch, G.N., Dobos, R.C., Refshauge, G. *et al.* (2013) Reproductive performance in the sheep CRC information nucleus using artificial insemination across different sheep-production environments in Southern Australia. *Animal Production Science* 54(6), 715–726.

Georgi, J.R., Georgi, M.E. and Theodorides, V.J. (1990) *Parasitology for veterinarians*, 5th edn. W.B. Saunders, Philadelphia, Pennsylvania.

Gordon, M.A. (1964) The genus *Dermatophilus*. *Journal of Bacteriology* 88(2), 509–522.

Guo, J., Rasmussen, J., Wünschmann, A. and de La Concha-Bermejillo, A. (2004) Genetic characterization of orf viruses isolated from various ruminant species of a zoo. *Veterinary Microbiology* 99(2), 81–92.

Haalstra, R.T. (1965) Isolation of *Dermatophiliis congolensis* from skin lesions in the diagnosis of streptothricosis. *Veterinary Record* 77(28), 824–825.

Haig, D.M. (2006) Orf virus infection and host immunity. *Current Opinion in Infectious Diseases* 19(2), 127–131.
Harley, G.L., Maxwell, J.T., Larson, E., Grissino-Mayer, H.D., Henderson, J. *et al.* (2017) Suwannee river flow variability 1550–2005 CE reconstructed from a multispecies tree-ring network. *Journal of Hydrology* 544, 438–451.
Harman, M., Sekin, S. and Akdeniz, S. (2001) Human dermatophilosis mimicking ringworm. *British Journal of Dermatology* 145(1), 170–171.
Ikeda, E., Goto, A., Suzaki, R., Sawada, M., Dekio, I. *et al.* (2016) *Condylomata lata* on the ankle: An unusual location. *Dermatology Practical & Conceptual* 6(2), 49.
Jakhar, D., Gupta, R.K. and Sarin, N. (2021) Dermoscopy of tuberculosis verrucosa cutis. *Indian Dermatology Online Journal* 12(1), 206–207.
Jassi, R., Yadav, A. and Chander, R. (2020) Dermoscopy of lichen scrofulosorum. *Indian Dermatology Online Journal* 11(5), 876–877.
Kaminski, G.W. and Suter, I.I. (1976) Human infection with *Dermatophilus congolensis*. *Medical Journal of Australia* 1(13), 443–447.
Kapadnis, P.J. and Bhosle, N.S. (2004) Microscopic anatomy of the integument of Osmanabadi goat. *Indian Veterinary Journal* 81(8), 912–914.
Kapadnis, P.J., Bhosle, N.S. and Mamade, C.S. (2005) Study on connective tissue fibre in neck skin of goat. *Indian Journal of Animal Research* 39(1), 60–62.
Koney, E.B.M. (1996) Dermatophilosis in Ghana: Effect on the livestock industry. *Tropical Animal Health and Production* 28, 3S–8S.
Kumar, M., Pal, B., Purkayastha, R.D. and Roy, J. (2016) Clinico-pathological and therapeutic evaluation of Black Bengal goats (*Capra hircus*) infested with *Psoroptes cuniculi* mange. *Journal of Parasitic Diseases* 40(1), 41–45.
Kwapinski, J.B. (1966) Serological and chromatographic characterization of exo-antigens of the dermatophilus. *Australian Journal of Experimental Biology and Medical Science* 44(1), 87–92.
Lasota, J.A. and Dybas, R.A. (1991) Avermectins, a novel class of compounds: Implications for use in arthropod pest control. *Annual Review of Entomology* 36(1), 91–117.
Lloyd, C.M. and Walker, A.R. (1993) The systemic effect of adult and immature *Amblyomma variegatum* ticks on the pathogenesis of dermatophilosis. *Revue d'elevage et de medecine veterinaire des pays tropicaux* 46(1–2), 313–316.
Lockwood, L.L., Gehrke, S. and Navarini, A.A. (2010) Dermoscopy of pitted keratolysis. *Case Reports in Dermatology* 2(2), 146–148.
Lofstedt, J., White, S.D., Garlick, D.S. and Hanna, P. (1994) Severe psoroptic mange and endoparasitism in a Nubian doe. *The Canadian Veterinary Journal* 35(11), 716.
Macadam, I. and Haalstra, R.T. (1971) Bacteriology of Nigerian strains of *Dermatophilus congolensis*. *Tropical Animal Health and Production* 3, 225–231.
Macêdo, J., Riet-Correa, F., Dantas, A.F.M. and Simões, S.V.D. (2008) Skin diseases in goats and sheep in the Brazilian semi-arid region. *Brazilian Veterinary Research* 28, 633–642.
Mandage, S.T., Bhosle, N.S., Kapadnis, P.J. and Mamade, C.S. (2003) Microscopic anatomy of the integument of the Deccani sheep. *Indian Journal of Veterinary Anatomy* 15(1 & 2), 68–69.
Mannan, M.A., Khan, M.S.R., Rahman, M.M., Begum, F. and Uddin, M.Z. (2009) Isolation and identification of dermatophilus bacteria from the skin lesions of cattle. *Bangladesh Journal of Veterinary Medicine* 7(2), 342–347.
Martinez, D., Aumont, G., Moutoussamy, M., Gabriel, D., Tatareau, A.H. *et al.* (1993) Epidemiological studies on dermatophilosis in the Caribbean. *Revue d'Élvage et de Médecine Vétérinaire* 46(1–2), 323–327.
Monleón, E., Garza, M.C., Sarasa, R., Álvarez-Rodriguez, J., Bolea, R. *et al.* (2011) An assessment of the efficiency of PrPsc detection in rectal mucosa and third-eyelid biopsies from animals infected with scrapie. *Veterinary Microbiology* 147(3–4), 237–243.
Msami, H.M., Khaschabi, D., Schöpf, K., Kapaga, A.M. and Shibahara, T. (2001) *Dermatophilus congolensis* infection in goats in Tanzania. *Tropical Animal Health and Production* 33, 367–377.
Mulugeta, Y., Yacob, H.T. and Ashenafi, H. (2010) Ectoparasites of small ruminants in three selected agro-ecological sites of Tigray Region, Ethiopia. *Tropical Animal Health and Production* 42, 1219–1224.
Munro, R. and Munro, H.M. (1980) Psoroptic mange in goats in Fiji. *Tropical Animal Health and Production* 12(1), 1–5.

Ndhlovu, D.N. and Masika, P.J. (2015) Risk factors associated with clinical dermatophilosis in smallholder sector cattle herds of Zimbabwe at the *Amblyomma variegatum* and *Amblyomma hebraeum* interface. *Tropical Animal Health and Production* 47, 353–360.

Ndikuwera, J., Odiawo, G.O., Usenik, E.A., Kock, N.D., Ogaa, J.S. *et al.* (1992) Chronic contagious ecthyma and caseous lymphadenitis in two Boer goats. *The Veterinary Record* 131(25–26), 584–585.

Norris, B.J., Colditz, I.G. and Dixon, T.J. (2008) Fleece rot and dermatophilosis in sheep. *Veterinary Microbiology* 128(3–4), 217–230.

Osman, S.A. (2015) Clinical and therapeutic studies on dermatophilosis of sheep and goats in Quassim, Kingdom of Saudi Arabia. *Assiut Veterinary Medical Journal* 61(4), 51–55.

Oyejide, A., Makinde, A.A. and Ezeh, A.O. (1984) Prevalence of antibodies to *Dermatophilus congolensis* in sheep and goats in Nigeria. *Veterinary Quarterly* 6(1), 44–45.

Palmer, B.H., McCarthy, J.F., Kozlik, A. and Harrison, I.R. (1973) A new chemical group of cattle acaricides. In: *Proceedings of the 3rd International Congress of Acarology: Prague, August 31–September 6, 1971*, Springer, Dordrecht, Netherlands, pp. 687–691.

Pattanaprichakul, P., Kulthanan, K., Bunyaratavej, S., Eimpunth, S., Rungruang, T. *et al.* (2021) The correlations between clinical features, dermoscopic and histopathological findings, and treatment outcomes of patients with pitted keratolysis. *BioMed Research International* 2021(Oct 25), 3416643. DOI: 10.1155/2021/3416643.

Pegram, R., Indar, L., Eddi, C. and George, J. (2004) The Caribbean Amblyomma program: Some ecologic factors affecting its success. *Annals of the New York Academy of Sciences* 1026(1), 302–311.

Pegram, R.G. and Banda, D.S. (1990) Ecology and phenology of cattle ticks in Zambia: Development and survival of free-living stages. *Experimental & Applied Acarology* 8(4), 291–301.

Plant, J. (2007) Bacterial and fungal infections of the skin and wool. In: Aitken, I.D. (ed.) *Diseases of Sheep and Goats*, 4th edn. Blackwell Science, Oxford, UK, pp. 315–316.

Popham, T.W., Garris, G.I. and Barré, N. (1996) Development of a computer model of the population dynamics of *Amblyomma variegatum* and simulations of eradication strategies for use in the Caribbean. *Annals of the New York Academy of Sciences* 791, 452–465.

Prine, K.C. and Hodges, A.C. (2012) Tropical bont tick *Amblyomma variegatum* fabricius (Arachnida: Acari: Ixodidae): EENY-518/IN934, 6/2012 *EDIS* 2012(7). University of Florida IFAS Extension, Gainesville, Florida. DOI: 10.32473/edis-in934-2012.

Quinn, P. and Markey, B. (2003) Section II: Pathogenic bacteria, *Dermatophilus congolensis*. In: *Concise Review of Veterinary Microbiology*, 1st edn. Blackwell Publishing, Ames, Iowa.

Quinn, P.J., Markey, B.K., Leonard, F.C., Hartigan, P., Fanning, S. *et al.* (2011) *Veterinary Microbiology and Microbial Disease*. John Wiley & Sons, Hoboken, New Jersey.

Rashid, M., Malik, M.A., Singh, M. and Sharma, H.K. (2019) Mange infestation in sheep, goats and nomads of Jammu and Kashmir state. *Journal of Entomology and Zoology Studies* 7(5), 734–736.

Razvi, R., Suri, S., Sarma, K. and Sharma, R. (2015) Histomorphological and histochemical studies on the different layers of skin of Bakerwali goat. *Journal of Applied Animal Research* 43(2), 208–213.

Rezende, A.L.R.A., Bernardes Filho, F., de Paula, N.A., Towersey, L., Hay, R. *et al.* (2018) Clinical manifestation, dermoscopy, and scanning electron microscopy in two cases of contagious ecthyma (orf nodule). *Case Reports in Dermatological Medicine* 2018, 2094086.

Roberts, D. and Graham, N.P.H. (1966) Control of ovine cutaneous actinomycosis. *Australian Veterinary Journal* 42(3), 74–78.

Roberts, D.S. (1965) Penetration and irritation of the skin by *Dermatophilus congolensis*. *British Journal of Experimental Pathology* 46(6), 635.

Seyfarth, F., Roediger, C., Gräser, Y., Erhard, M., Burmester, A. *et al.* (2011) Case report: *Trichophyton verrucosum* infection after needlestick injury with an attenuated live vaccine against cattle ringworm. *Mycoses* 54(6), e870–e876.

Seyoum, Z., Tadesse, T. and Addisu, A. (2015) Ectoparasites prevalence in small ruminants in and around Sekela, Amhara Regional State, Northwest Ethiopia. *Journal of Veterinary Medicine* 216085.

Shaibu, S.J., Kazeem, H.M., Abdullahi, U.S. and Fatihu, M.Y. (2010) The use of polymerase chain reaction in the diagnosis of dermatophilosis from cattle, sheep and goats in Nigeria. *Journal of Infection* 41(3), 221–226.

Shyma, K.P., Singh, V., Parsani, H.R., Solanki, V., Pawar, M.M. *et al.* (2022) Acaricidal properties of herbal extracts against deltamethrin resistant multi-host cattle tick *Hyalomma anatolicum*. *Indian Journal of Animal Research* 56(5), 613–618.

Singal, A., Jakhar, D., Kaur, I., Pandhi, D. and Das, S. (2019) *Tinea pseudoimbricata* as a unique manifestation of steroid abuse: A clinico-mycological and dermoscopic study from a tertiary care hospital. *Indian Dermatology Online Journal* 10(4), 422.

Smith, W.J., Li, Y., Ingham, A., Collis, E., McWilliam, S.M. *et al*. (2010) A genomics-informed, SNP association study reveals FBLN1 and FABP4 as contributing to resistance to fleece rot in Australian Merino sheep. *BMC Veterinary Research* 6(1), 1–16.

Sonthalia, S., Agrawal, M., Bhatia, J., Zeeshan, M., Elsamanoudy, S. *et al*. (2021) Entodermoscopy update: A contemporary review on dermoscopy of cutaneous infections and infestations. *Indian Dermatology Online Journal* 12(2), 220.

Summerbell, R.C. (2000) Form and function in the evolution of dermatophytes. In: *Biology of Dermatophytes and Other Keratinophilic Fungi*. Revista Iberoamericana de Micología, Bilbao, Spain, pp. 30–43.

Taranukha, N., Bezgina, Y., Fedota, N., Gorchakov, E., Ozheredova, N. *et al*. (2020) Ensuring food security and control of sheep and goat scrapie. *E3S Web of Conferences* 210, 06020.

Tellam, R.L., Vuocolo, T., Denman, S., Ingham, A., Wijffels, G. *et al*. (2021) Dermatophilosis (lumpy wool) in sheep: A review of pathogenesis, aetiology, resistance and vaccines. *Animal Production Science* 62(2), 101–113.

Thomas, N. and Malakar, S. (2019) Dermoscopy: An easy way to solve the diagnostic puzzle in pityriasis versicolor. *Indian Journal of Dermatology, Venereology, and Leprology* 85(6), 664–664.

Thompson, R.E.M. (1954) A species of rhizobium isolated from strawberry foot-rot in the sheep. *The Journal of Pathology and Bacteriology* 68(2), 445–452.

Thompson, R.E.M. and Bisset, K.A. (1957) Polysepta: A new genus and sub-order of bacteria. *Nature* 179(4559), 590–591.

Tognetti, L., Sbano, P., Fimiani, M. and Rubegni, P. (2017) Dermoscopy of Biett's sign and differential diagnosis with annular maculo-papular rashes with scaling. *Indian Journal of Dermatology, Venereology and Leprology* 83, 270.

Towersey, L., Martins, E.D.C.S., Londero, A.T., Hay, R.J., Soares Filho, P.J. *et al*. (1993) *Dermatophilus congolensis* human infection. *Journal of the American Academy of Dermatology* 29(2), 351–354.

Van Saceghem, R. (1915) Dermatose contagieuse (impetigo contagieux). *Bulletin de la Société de pathologie exotique* 8, 354–359.

Van Saceghem, R. (1916) Étude complémentaire sur la dermatose contagieuse (impétigo contagieux). *Bulletin de la Société pathologie exotique* 9, 290.

Vazquez-Lopez, F. and Perez-Oliva, N. (1996) Mupirocine ointment for symptomatic pitted keratolysis. Infection 24(1), 55–55.

Vázquez-López, F., Kreusch, J. and Marghoob, A. (2004) Dermoscopic semiology: Further insights into vascular features by screening a large spectrum of nontumoral skin lesions. *British Journal of Dermatology* 150(2), 226–231.

Vinay, K., Bhattacharjee, R., Bishnoi, A., Chatterjee, D., Rudramurthy, S. *et al*. (2020) Dermatoscopic features of cutaneous sporotrichosis. *Journal of the European Academy of Dermatology and Venereology* 34(11), e718–e720.

Walker, A.R., Bouattour, J.-L., Camicas, A., Estrade-Peña, I.G., Horak, A.A. *et al*. (2003) *Ticks of Domestic Animals in Africa: A Guide to Identification of Species*. Bioscience Reports, Edinburgh.

Wang, S., Martini, M.C., Groth, J.V. and Hernandez, C. (2015) Dermatoscopic and clinicopathologic findings of cutaneous blastomycosis. *Journal of the American Academy of Dermatology* 73(5), e169–e170.

Ware, G.W. and Whitacre, D.M. (2004) An introduction to insecticides. In: *The Pesticide Book*, 6th edn. Meister Media Worldwide, Willoughby, Ohio.

Wilson, J. and Brewer, B.D. (1984) Vestibular disease in a goat [*Psoroptes cuniculi*]. *The Compendium on Continuing Education for the Practicing Veterinarian* 6, S179–S182.

Woldemeskel, M. (2000) Dermatophilosis: A threat to livestock production in Ethiopia. *Deutsche Tierarztliche Wochenschrift* 107(4), 144–146.

Yakhchali, M. and Hosseine, A. (2006) Prevalence and ectoparasites fauna of sheep and goats flocks in Urmia suburb, Iran. *Veterinarski Arhiv* 76(5), 431–442.

Yeruham, I., Elad, D. and Perl, S. (2003) Dermatophilosis in goats in the Judean foothills. *Revue de Médecine Vétérinaire* 154(12), 785–788.

Yeruham, I., Hadani, A. and Elad, D. (1991) Human dermatophilosis (*Dermatophilus congolensis*) in dairymen in Israel. *Israel Journal of Veterinary Medicine* 46(3), 114–116.

Yeruham, I., Hadani, A., Orgad, U., Rosen, S. and Ratner, D. (1984) Otocariasis caused by *Psoroptes cuniculi* (Delafond, 1859) accompanied by meningoencephalitis in a goat. *Refuah Veterinarith* 41(3), 89–90.

Yonow, T. (1995) The life-cycle of *Amblyomma variegatum* (Acari: Ixodidae): A literature synthesis with a view to modelling. *International Journal for Parasitology* 25(9), 1023–1060.

Zalaudek, I., Giacomel, J., Cabo, H., Di Stefani, A., Ferrara, G. *et al*. (2008) Entodermoscopy: A new tool for diagnosing skin infections and infestations. *Dermatology* 216(1), 14–23.

Zaria, L.T. (1993) *Dermatophilus congolensis* infection (dermatophilosis) in animals and man! An update. *Comparative Immunology, Microbiology and Infectious Diseases* 16(3), 179–222.

Zhao, Y.E., Hu, L. and Ma, J.X. (2013) Phylogenetic analysis of *Demodex caprae* based on mitochondrial 16S rDNA sequence. *Parasitology Research* 112, 3969–3977.

Zhou, H., Tang, X.H., De Han, J. and Chen, M.K. (2015) Dermoscopy as an ancillary tool for the diagnosis of pityriasis versicolor. *Journal of the American Academy of Dermatology* 73(6), e205–e206.

25 Vesicular Stomatitis

Shashi Pradhan*, Aditya Pratap, Pooja Dawar and Akansha Agnihotri
Department of Veterinary Medicine, College of Veterinary Science and Animal Husbandry, NDVSU, Jabalpur, Madhya Pradesh, India

Abstract
Vesicular stomatitis (VS) is caused by members of the *Vesiculovirus* genus (*Rhabdoviridae* family), two of which are called vesicular stomatitis viruses (VSVs). Clinical disease manifests as severe blisters or ulcers of the tongue, feet, oral mucosa and papillae. Vesiculoviruses are transmitted by arthropods and may actually be insect viruses adapted to infect mammals. Vesicular stomatitis viruses are classified according to serotypes that are similar in size and their morphology but produce different neutralizing antibodies in infected animals. The ecological conditions that support the inherent VSV cycle include forested tropical and subtropical regions with wet and dry seasons defined as wet and sub-swamp conditions. The incubation time could be a little longer in a natural environment. Vesicular stomatitis is an OIE List A disease that is important to the international pet trade because it can spread rapidly, impact public health and can be confused with foot-and-mouth disease.

Keywords: animal, arthropods, tropical, erosion, ulceration, OIE

25.1 Introduction

Vesicular stomatitis (VS) is an animal disease caused by members of the *Vesiculovirus* genus (*Rhabdoviridae* family), two of which are called vesicular stomatitis viruses (VSVs) (World Organisation for Animal Health, 2013). Clinical disease manifests as severe blisters or ulcers of the tongue, feet, oral mucosa and papillae, resulting in significant loss of productivity. It is clinically indistinguishable from foot-and-mouth disease, except in horses and donkeys (Mebus, 1998).

VS is a highly contagious and temporarily debilitating disease. It occurs seasonally every year in the south-eastern United States, southern Mexico, throughout Central America and in northern South America (Mason, 1984). It causes sporadic epidemics during the cool summer months in tropical regions. Other vesiculoviruses are endemic to India and Africa only. Vesiculoviruses are transmitted by arthropods and may actually be insect viruses adapted to infect mammals.

Recent advanced studies on VSVs have yielded many important and interesting fundamental discoveries in microbiology, but these findings have not resulted in safe and fully effective vaccines for humans and animals (Mead, 2000). In the absence of a vaccine, and with continuous intercontinental migration, increasing concentrations of susceptible animals, the plasticity of viral genomes and zoonotic infections, vesiculoviruses are seen by regulators and biomedical researchers as pathogens with potentially significant consequences (Letchworth *et al*., 1999).

*Corresponding author: shee1811@gmail.com

DOI: 10.1079/ 9781800622852.0025

VS is one of the most important viral diseases that primarily affects horses and cattle and occasionally other livestock. Humans can also contract the disease from handling infected animals, but this is rare. VS has been identified to be more prominent in the Western Hemisphere, according to the case data and research conducted. It is known to be endemic in temperate regions of North, Central and South America, with sporadic epidemics in other temperate regions of the hemisphere.

25.2 Aetiology

VS is caused by VSVs, which belong to the family *Rhabdoviridae* and genus *Vesiculovirus*. The disease primarily affects horses and cattle and occasionally it infects pigs, llamas, alpacas and goats. The virion is enveloped and consists of a globular ribonucleoprotein containing a single negative-sense strand of RNA of approximately 11 kb.

Vesiculoviruses are relatively simple, with a linear single-stranded negative-sense RNA genome surrounded by globular virions composed of five proteins. Upon infecting cultured cells, the viral product shuts down gene expression in the cell, maximizing the metabolic capacity of the cell. It also depolymerizes the cytoskeleton, causing rapid tissue destruction. Viral infection in animals produces interferon and nitric oxide responses that rapidly regulate viral replication and antibody responses that prevent further viral replication (Letchworth *et al.*, 1999).

Replication of the vesiculovirus genome is inaccurate and produces viral progeny containing many variants. This allows quick adjustments. However, the VSV genome sequences appear to be relatively stable within individual endemic regions and are increasingly variable on the north–south axis in the Western Hemisphere (Schmitt, 2002).

VSVs are classified according to serotypes that are similar in size and morphology but produce different neutralizing antibodies in infected animals. There are two main distinct serotypes: (i) New Jersey (VSV-NJ), which causes the majority of outbreaks in the United States, and (ii) Indiana (VSV-IN). Indiana serovars have been classified into three different serological complexes. The Indiana-1 subtype (VSV-IN1) includes the classic Indiana virus (VSIV), found from northern South America to the southern United States. The Indiana-2 subtype (VSV-IN2) has cocal virus (COCV) as the prototype virus, which was first isolated from ticks collected from rice mice in Trinidad in 1961. The Indiana-2 virus mostly causes disease in cattle and horses, usually reported in the broad geographical area of Brazil and Argentina. The Indiana-3 subtype (VSV-IN3), or Alagoas VSV (VSAV) was first isolated in 1964 from mules in Alagoas, Brazil. This subtype is the most common cause of bullous stomatitis in Brazilian livestock. Other than this there are many vesiculoviruses that infect mammals, some of which also cause disease in humans, like Piry virus, Isfahan virus and Chandipura virus (Rainwater-Lovett, 2007). Several viruses have been isolated from blood-sucking insects, but so far they are not known to cause any disease in vertebrates (e.g. Maraba virus and Carajas virus).

Four VSVs have been noted to cause outbreaks of vesicular disease in livestock. These viruses are serologically classified as VSV-NJ, VSV-IN1, VSV-IN2 and VSV-IN3. VSV-NJ and VSV-IN1 viruses are endemic to Northern and Central America to southern Mexico and occur sporadically in northern Mexico and the United States. VSV-IN2 and VSV-IN3 occur only in South America (Brazil, Argentina and Trinidad).

Piry, Chandipura, Jrona, Carajas, Maraba, Calchaqui, YugBogdanovac, Isfahan, Perinet and Porton-S vesiculoviruses have been isolated from arthropods and mammals. However, these have not been proven to cause spontaneous occurrence in livestock.

Fish vesiculoviruses include the spring viraemia of carp virus (SVCV), which has a single serotype. Antibodies to SVCV cross-react with other fish rhabdoviruses to varying degrees. Pike rhabdovirus (PFRV), grass carp virus (GrCRV) and tench rhabdovirus (TenRV) indicate that the viruses are closely related. Even though SVCV and PFRV have similar antigenic determinants on their G, N and M proteins, neutralization experiments have demonstrated that they may be distinguished from one another.

Serotyping of vesiculoviruses is based on neutralization patterns determined by epitopes on the viral G protein. G proteins also determine the protection of animals vaccinated with either inactivated whole-virus or subunit vaccines. The N protein is a cross-reactive antigen used in complement fixation assays that help to define members of the genus. Weak serological cross-reactivity can occur between viruses of different genera. One of the criteria used to classify VSVs is cross-reactivity through complement fixation.

VSV glycoprotein G triggers membrane fusion via low-pH-induced structural rearrangements. Despite the balance of pre- and post-fusion states, the structure of the pre-fusion morphology determined at 3.0 Å resolutions indicates that the fusogenic transition involves extensive structural rearrangements of G fusion (Tesh *et al.*, 1971, 1972). A comparison with the structure of the latter morphology suggests a pathway of nearly conformational change. In the pre-fusion form, G is tripod-shaped, with the fusion loop facing the viral membrane and the antigenic site located at the distal end of the molecule. Numerous G glycoproteins, presumably organized like crystals, act in concert to induce membrane fusion (Roche *et al.*, 2007).

The core of the nucleocapsid consists of the viral genome firmly wrapped around the viral N protein that forms an RNase-resistant nuclear environment. The P and L proteins combine to catalyse RNA-dependent RNA polymerization (RdRp) of genomic RNA and transcription of mRNA in the order N-P-M-G-L. For genome replication, RdRp initiates at different 3' ends to synthesize full-length positive-sense copies of the genome as templates of replication. Due to the low precision of RdRp, VSVs have a high error rate in RNA transcription, which results in large genetic diversity and quasi-species populations. VSV transcription and replication mechanisms are very complex and not yet fully understood. Laboratory and natural populations provide different information on genetic fitness and maintenance. Under laboratory conditions, VSVs show great capacity for genetic modification and rapid adaptation. Conversely, VSVs remain relatively stable under field conditions, and evolutionary patterns are defined by similar ecological conditions rather than geographical origin or immunological selection. Genetic fitness studies examining evolutionary pressures on VSV genomes in switching between cellular environments in insects and mammals suggest that field population stability is not due to the need for viruses to restrict adaptation between host cell types (Rozo-Lopez *et al.*, 2018).

25.3 Pathology and Epidemiology

VSVs appear to exist in a stable natural cycle, with the very same viral genotypes persisting for long periods in specific ecological zones. The natural maintenance cycle is poorly understood; insects such as sandflies carry the virus in native swarms and spread the infection to susceptible hosts without causing clinical symptoms. The presence of neutralizing antibodies is proof of widespread infection among the wild animals living in unique herds. The ecological conditions that support the inherent VSV cycle include forested tropical and subtropical regions with wet and dry seasons, defined as wet and sub-swamp conditions. Livestock living near these areas become infected during the season when insect populations are very high, generally in the rainy season (Tesh *et al.*, 1977).

VSV infection occurs mainly in domesticated cattle, horses and pigs, and rarely in llamas, sheep, goats and humans. Equine infection is of particular concern in the United States. Infections are usually short and self-limiting, although secondary bacterial infections such as mastitis can occur, especially in dairy cows and lactating mares. The incubation period varies from species to species, but clinical symptoms usually develop after 2–7 days. Viral transcription and replication occur within a few hours of infection, with peak viral replication occurring 24–48 hour after inoculation of infection. A viral growth phase with the detectable infectious virus has not been demonstrated in livestock, probably due to the inhibitory effects of serum proteins such as complement. However, VSV RNA persists for many months in various tissues of the body, including B lymphoid tissue (Tesh *et al.*, 1987).

Histologically, VSV infection can cause severe interstitial oedema with bleb formation, epithelial cell lysis and inflammatory cell infiltration. The clinical pathology of VSV infection includes the development and subsequent rupture of mucosal vesicles, resulting in cavities filled with cellular exudates. The pathway of VSV exposure influences host response and subsequent clinical disease, such as in the oral mucosa, porcine nose, bovine teat and coronary ligament of porcine, bovine and equine animals. Lesions are considered critically important for direct contact and vector-mediated infection due to high viral titres in follicular fluid, margins of damaged tissue and copious saliva from oral lesions.

VSV infection is prevalent in subtropical and tropical regions of the United States. However, it is well known to spread from the north of the United States and Canada into the temperate zone during the summer months, first appearing in the states along the Gulf of Mexico in April or May, and then as far as Manitoba, Canada. In Latin America, VS epidemics vary and are often associated with the transition between wet and dry seasons. In tropical and subtropical regions, VSV infection is most common at the end of the rainy season or the beginning of the dry season. In temperate regions, VS outbreaks occur seasonally in summer, often propagating along streams, upwind directions and following distinct ecological features, usually terminating after the first hard frost. The southern and south-eastern US states have seen the highest VSV cases recorded, but the incidence patterns in the two areas differ. Although yearly outbreaks were noted in the south-east until the middle of the 1970s, rare VS outbreaks continue to occur in the south-western states at intervals of around 10 years, with the most recent epidemic occurring in 2014–2015. The epidemic virus overwintered in an as yet unidentified natural reservoir, as it did in the 2004–2005 and 2014–2015 outbreaks, and the same viral genotype can cause illness over the 2 years.

VSV infection appears to have spread among animal caretakers and laboratory workers before the advent of modern biosafety procedures and equipment. According to several studies, 48–100% of Central Americans are seropositive, and one study found that in the 1950s, cattle epidemics were widespread in south-eastern Georgia, USA, and antibodies were found in 25% of people tested. In contrast, a subsequent study showed that the infectivity of the VSV-NJ virus was significantly higher than that for veterinarians, different laboratory workers and others during the 1982–1983 epidemic in the United States and was found to be relatively low for the risk group. Evidence of infection was detected in only 17 of the total 133 people who were exposed to the virus and appeared to require relatively close contact with the source of the virus.

The proportion of symptomatic human infections is unknown. Some sources suggest that clinical cases are very rare, while others suggest that human infections are likely to be underreported because they are easily misdiagnosed as influenza. In the above study, 31 of 54 seropositive laboratory workers or animal attendants had mild acute illness associated with the VS. In most cases, clinical cases had no serious sequelae. Laboratory infections resolved without complications in these cases and no deaths were reported. However, one reported case of severe encephalitis in a young child was attributed to VSV (Bezerra *et al.*, 2018).

According to the Pan American Center for Foot-and-Mouth Disease (PANAFTOSA), VS is endemic in northern South America, with an outbreak in Brazil mainly associated with VSV-IN3 serotype. The first isolation of the VSV in Brazil was in 1964 from the oral epithelium of a diseased horse in the state of Alagoas (Andrade *et al.*, 1980). Two years later, VSV-IN2 was identified in horses in the state of São Paulo, Brazil. According to the Ministry of Agriculture, Livestock and Supply (MAPA), 169 VS outbreaks have been reported in several states (Bahia, Ceara, Goias, Pernambuco, Maranhão, Mato Grosso and Minas), mainly due to VSV-IN3, sporadically VSV-IN2 (Gerais, Para, Paraíba, Piauí, Rio Grande do Norte, Rio de Janeiro, São Paulo and Tocantins) from 2005 to 2013.

The disease has a seasonal pattern, with a greater frequency during hot, humid months, even if the mechanisms of maintenance and transmission of VS are not entirely understood. Transmission can occur through direct contact between infected animals, healthy animals and carriers; consumption of infected vegetables can also transmit the disease. Due to its irregular spatial distribution in outbreak situations, it has been hypothesized to be spread by wind and birds (Zimmer *et al.*, 2013). The importance of insects in the epidemiology of VS has been reported under natural and experimental conditions. VSIV was first identified in *Aedes* sp. when VS occurred in cattle and horses in Mexico in 1965 (Sudia *et al.*, 1967; Tesh *et al.*, 1987). Subsequently, Shelokov and Peralta (1967) reported the first isolation of

VSIV from the Panama domesticated Warabyo (Diptera: Psychodidae). Mead *et al.* (1999, 2004), described the segregation of VSV-NJ in black-flies (Diptera: Simuridia) under experimental conditions.

VSVs are an important cause of clinical disease in livestock throughout the United States. There are endemic (5–10 year intervals) and epidemic (1 year) areas of VSV activity, depending on the interval between the onsets of clinical disease. Endemic activity is most common in northern South America to northern Mexico, whereas epidemic activity occurs mainly in southern South America, the United States and Canada. Extensive epidemiological studies in Costa Rica have identified two VSV-NJ epidemic foci in that country, one in dry lowland (tropical dry forest) and one in highland (premontane wet forest). Typically, more than 80–90% of cattle living in these areas have antibodies to VSV-NJ, and 9% experience clinical bullous disease in any given year. Antibodies to VSV-NJ are also found in captive wild animals (rodents and primates) in these areas (Rodriguez and NichoL, 1999).

25.4 Vectors and Mechanism of Transmission

Factors influencing transmission in the United States are not well understood, but may include the following.

- **Topography:** The virus is endemic to tropical and subtropical lowland forests and savannas. Eruptions occur along sides of rivers and in plains where trees provide shade and where natural surface water is present. The disease has not been reported in treeless dry plains or at high altitudes. This distribution may be related to the habitat of the vector.
- **Climate:** Outbreaks are more common in tropical and subtropical regions and less common in temperate regions. Typically, outbreaks start in the late summer or near the conclusion of the rainy season and disappear when frost sets in or the dry season has a good start. Despite the fact that there are significant outbreaks in the southern United States throughout the winter, these data are compatible with insect transmission.
- **Feed quality:** Transmission may be enhanced by abrasion of the oral mucosa by feed such as forage, seeds, stubble, hard pellets, coarse willow, or feed contaminated with awns, ridges, thorns or stems of plants.
- **Animal Husbandry:** Improper fitting, poor maintenance, or improper application of improper clusters, horse bits and feeding troughs that can damage teat skin, teat canals, or oral mucosa can facilitate transmission. In cattle and horses, the incidence and severity of disease are reportedly higher in pasture-raised animals than in farmed animals. In dairy herds, morbidity was observed to increase with decreasing quality of management (Hansen *et al.*, 1985). Identified risk factors included high stocking density, poor milking hygiene, poor floor condition, leftover feed materials and dirty troughs.
- **Age:** Older cows and calves get sick more often than cows of other ages (Goodger *et al.*, 1985; Hansen *et al.*, 1985).
- **Stress:** High-yielding cows show more severe disease symptoms than low-yielding cows.
- **Endoparasitism:** Experiments have shown that pigs fed roundworm and VSVs at the same time are more likely to develop disease.

During outbreaks, VSV infection spreads quickly within animal herds through direct touch and fomites. Animals with the virus salivate excessively and release between four and six lots of virus for every millilitre of saliva. Vesicular exudates and saliva contaminated with viruses easily infect buildings and the environment, allowing for animal-to-animal or fomite-to-animal transmission. Research has proven that bugs additionally play an extensive function in VSV dissemination in proposed ways, as mechanical vectors through both biting and non-biting flies, or as organic vectors through haematophagous biting flies. Currently, numerous factors of VSV transmission are not well understood, particularly the following:

- where and how the proposed insect vectors gather the virus in nature;

- if the virus removed from bugs captured in discipline collections at some stage in epizootics corresponds to organic or mechanical transmission and isepidemiologically relevant;
- if any of the presently incriminated or suspected insect species are concerned in VSV preservation at some stage in inter-epidemic periods; and
- if the low or regularly undetectable viraemia in inflamed mammals suggests that different transmission mechanisms can be concerned for vectors to become inflamed.

There are various routes of transmission which include insect vectors, contact carriers and bacterial carriers. Sandflies (*Lutzomyia* spp.), blowflies (*Simuliidae*), mosquitoes or culicoides (*Culicoides* spp.) are thought to play an important role in disease transmission during disease outbreaks. Viral replication and transovarial transmission occur in the insect groups listed above. The viral cycle cannot be sustained over the long term with transovarial infection, however, according to experimental evidence. Therefore, it has been hypothesized that there might be natural reserves that are still undiscovered. Experiments with blowflies co-feeding on a variety of mammalian hosts, including horses, pigs and cattle, have been used to demonstrate horizontal fly-to-fly transmission. This might be crucial to the growth of VSVs and explain insect transmission in the lack of a viral host.

The VSV has also been isolated from other insects, like mosquitoes (*Culex* spp. and *Aedes* spp.) and houseflies (*Musca domestica*). The importance of vectors is reflected in the fact that most outbreaks disappear after the first frost. Important contact infection sources include viruses found on mucosal surfaces when vesicles have burst. Urine, faeces and milk do not shed any viruses.

Clinical symptoms often occur 24–72 hour after an experimental infection during the incubation phase. The incubation time could be a little longer in a natural environment. Incidence is highly dependent on whether the area is endemic for VS, the number of infected vectors and the proximity of contact with animals once they have become colonized. In non-endemic areas, the disease usually occurs in an outbreak fashion with a prevalence of approximately 40–60%. In endemic areas, most natural VSV infections are asymptomatic, so the prevalence is likely to be much lower.

25.4.1 Mechanical vector transfer

Mechanical transmission happens in insects as well as diseases, and it is often characterized by physical viral transport with little insect specificity and no latency time. In the case of VSV infection, transient viraemia in pets during infection is low, complicating the dogma of the transmission cycle of vector-borne diseases. However, follicular lesions contain high viral titres and are clearly important for direct animal-to-animal contact transmission. Consequently, the high viral titres in the skin associated with bullous lesions may serve as a viral source for vector mechanical transmission. For blood-sucking pool flies, such as sandflies, blowflies and *Culicoides* mosquitoes, VSV may be acquired by eating intact skin at or near vesicular lesions or contaminated with virus-laden saliva. The potential for mechanical transmission of VSV is supported by many species that transmit the virus under natural conditions. During animal epidemics, VSVs have been isolated from non-blood-sucking insects such as the housefly, Chloropidae and Diptera flies. Furthermore, long-distance dissemination and outbreaks in pasture swarms remote from water supplies are made feasible by the capacity of locusts to infect and reproduce large titres of VSV after consuming virus-contaminated pasture plants. In laboratory experiments, fly species, including horseflies (*Tabanus*), deer flies (*Chrysops*), midges (*Aedes* and *Culex*) and stable flies (*Stomoxys*), caught in large numbers in barns, were affected by transmission. It has been shown that developing eggs can be easily injected with VSVs. Animals bitten by infected flies develop neutralizing antibodies to VSVs.

25.4.2 Biological vector transfer

High vector specificity and an extrinsic latency period (EIP), during which the virus replicates before getting to the organs involved in transmission (eggs, salivary glands), are the defining characteristics. Despite the undetectable viraemia in infected animals, several aspects of an outbreak suggest that VSV infection is mediated by blood-sucking insects. Seasonal outbreaks of VS in temperate regions peak in summer and autumn, when vector populations are highest, and reported cases usually cease after the first hard frost. Additionally, certain geographical regions are more likely to have recurring outbreaks than others, notably those close to flowing or still waterways, which are the ideal homes for blowflies and mosquitoes, respectively. Finally, the virus may be transported by flying insects due to the speed and method of propagation in the absence of animal migration. Only sandflies have been shown to transmit the vesicular stomatitis virus transovarially to offspring. As in most arbovirus infectious cycles, the vertebrate host typically acts as an amplification reservoir capable of producing sustained levels of viraemia. Serological studies have shown that species such as bats, deer and monkeys living in endemic areas produce neutralizing antibodies to the virus and that wild grass-eating rodents and deer mice may play a role in virus maintenance in small grass-eating rodents. However, a definitive natural viral host reservoir for VSVs has not yet been identified.

The absence of VSV viraemia in vertebrate hosts implies that blood-feeding biological vector species must be extremely susceptible to infection. However, there is insufficient data to show that low viraemias are unable to infect vectors. The vector species determines the number of hosts with that viraemia, the duration of the viraemia, the number of viral particles required to initiate a replicative infection with the vector, and the number of different vectors feeding on the host. Two alternative sources of viral uptake by feeding vectors other than blood from viraemic hosts have been proposed: infection by co-feeding with infected insects and in clinically infected animals. Probing or feeding on or near epidermal follicular lesions. Pool-eater mouthparts (sandflies, blowflies, beetles) that cut through the epidermis to pick up pooled blood from wounds naturally encounter more skin microbes than capillaries and insert the proboscis directly into blood vessels (mosquitoes). Therefore, a pool eater is likely to pick up more viruses on contaminated skin surfaces, so may play a more important role in transmitting the VSV from epidermal lesions than mosquitoes. Although the complex natural transmission cycle of VSVs is not yet fully understood, many laboratory studies have demonstrated the ability of certain haematophagous dipterans to transmit VSVs and epidemiological studies have demonstrated the ability to transmit VSV-associated clinical cases in cattle, horses and pigs with exposure to four major vector species: *Culicoides* biting midges, mosquitoes, sandflies and blackflies.

Sandflies are one of the earliest insect species to be infected with VSV in their natural habitat and have historically been the most common insects associated with natural infection. In the United States, VSV-NJ is endemic in wild boar populations on Ossabaw Island, Georgia, and several entomological collections isolated this serovar from *Lutzomyia shannoni* in the early 2000s. In tropical regions where VSV-IN is endemic, a large number of sandflies that are captured during surveillance for leishmaniasis also contribute to our knowledge of VSV infection from natural habitats.

Only sandflies have been proven to be capable of transovarial transmission (TOT), out of all the blood-sucking insects implicated in VSV infection. This generational manner of transmission raises the possibility of a method for preserving VSVs in the wild without a vertebrate host. With 1.1% of F1 offspring carrying VSV-NJ and 20% of F1 offspring infected with VSV-IN, TOT studies demonstrated VSV replication during sandfly development and F1 virus titres equivalent to those reported in wild-infected sandflies. The presence of the VSV was also detected in F2 larvae, indicating that the virus may be handed down over several generations.

Sandflies appear to be the most important vectors in endemic regions of Central and South America. However, several factors raise open questions about their ability to transmit VSVs and the contribution to outbreaks in the central and western regions of the United States. First, *Lutzomia* species often have very specific habitat requirements and are found only in areas with climates suitable for the species and host animals. Secondly, due to their limited flight range and sporadic activity patterns, sandflies are not thought to spread the virus over long distances. Finally, TOT rates of 20% for VSV-IN and 1.1% for VSV-NJ were associated with infected adults, gender-specific transmission by infected males, or hyper-viraemic reservoirs for *in situ* replenishment of the virus. The virus cannot be maintained indefinitely. VSV disappearance on sandfly-infested Ossabaw Island following the eradication of native boar is a good example of this.

25.5 Clinical Signs

Fever is a typical clinical symptom of experimental tongue infections. The mouth (gums, lips and tongue), nose, coronary bands of the foot, or teats of lactating ruminants can all develop blanching patches that eventually turn into vesicles. It is typical to have excessive salivation, a change in stride, lameness and unpleasant reactions when milking. Laminitis and possibly hoof loss can result from lesions on the coronary band in ruminants. Goats milking with teat sores are more susceptible to bacterial mastitis. Dehydration and malnutrition are risks associated with severe tongue lesions. Clinically ill animals often fully recover with the right treatment, although hoof loss or severe mastitis may necessitate culling.

Affected animals either reduce their food intake or stop eating and become ill. Lactating animals either have low milk production or stop lactating. Mastitis may develop as a result of secondary bacterial infection complicating a viral infection of the mammary epithelium and teat duct. A limited percentage of goats have central nervous system (CNS) symptoms, including voluntary head tremors and involuntary tongue and jaw movements.

Incidence varies widely but can reach 100%. Mortality is low and usually associated with other concomitant infections.

Various signs and lesions are similar in goats, pigs and deer. Additionally, the nasal turbinates, nasopharynx and larynx can be affected in horses, leading to nosebleeds and feeding and breathing difficulties. Coronary band lesions can lead to hoof deformities and abrasions. Lesions may occur on the breast or foreskin.

Human clinical illnesses are reported primarily among laboratory workers and veterinarians. Due to flu-like symptoms, undetected cases may occur more frequently in rural areas and up to 90% of farmers in endemic areas have antibodies to the VSV. Many VSV infections are asymptomatic. The very first clinical signs in livestock are fever, anorexia, excessive salivation, difficulty in feeding, smacking and lameness. Intact vesicles are usually not seen unless the animal is closely examined in the early stages of the disease (Fig. 25.1). Thin-walled, solitary or coalesced vesicles may appear on the tongue, lips, gums, coronary ligaments, interdigital skin and near the teat orifice. Such vesicles are transient and rupture easily. The resulting ulcer usually heals quickly over the next 10 days, but secondary infections can delay healing for weeks. Epithelial inflammation, oedema and necrosis occur in many animals but do not progress to severe blistering. The area will appear pale before forming a dry blemish. In each shed, lesions usually occur at only one site (mouth, feet, or teats).

A transient fever may be seen early in clinical cases. Excessive salivation is often the first noticeable sign. Closer examination may show whitened areas and characteristic raised vesicles (blisters). The size of the vesicles varies greatly; some are as small as peas, while others cover the entire surface of the tongue. They rupture rapidly and become eroded or ulcerated. The lips and tongue (especially the back) are commonly affected in the mouth. Lesions may also be present on the gingiva and palate. Oral ulcers and erosions often coalesce into large exposed areas of mucosa with epithelial appendages. Lesions can also develop on other parts of the nose and can swell as a result of tissue damage. When foot lesions are present, they are usually located in the coronary ligament or the interdigital space of the hoof. Crown inflammation with oedema that spreads to the lower legs is typical. In pigs, lesions may first appear on the legs, but the muzzle and the nose are also commonly affected. The condition can appear as crusts on the nose, lips, ventral abdominal wall, foreskin and udders in certain horses, where vesicles and erosions might go undetected. Vesicular stomatitis lesions are uncomfortable and can result in an animal losing its appetite, refusing to drink, becoming lame, bleeding from an ulcer or having bad breath. Loss of hooves and laminitis are also possible outcomes of coronary ligament damage. The secondary

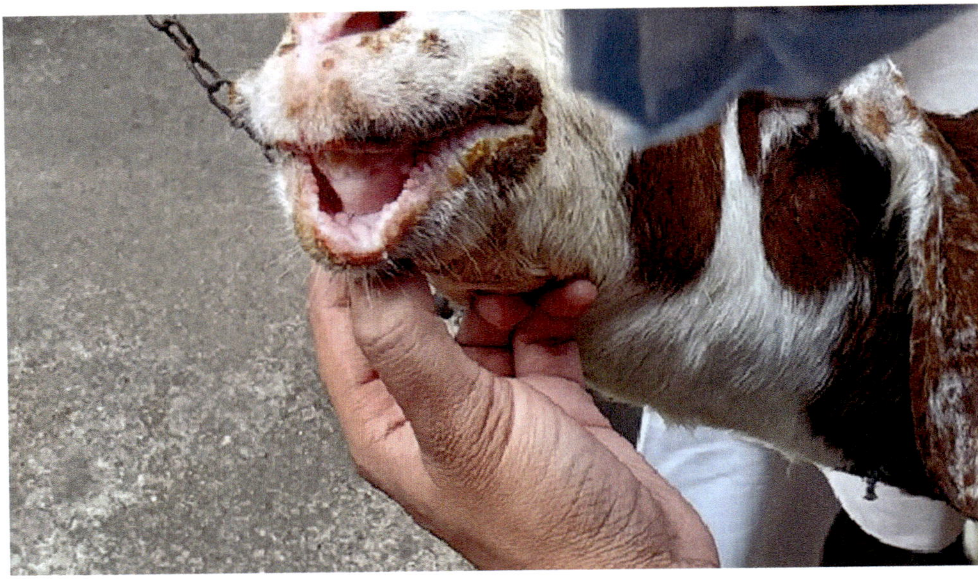

Fig. 25.1. Oral lesion (stomatitis) in goats. (Author's own image.)

infection that results from teat sores can cause mastitis. Goats that are milked may lose a lot of weight and produce less milk. There are reports of healthy yet anorexic goats among the affected animals. Animals usually recover in about 2–3 weeks, unless secondary bacterial infections or other complications develop. When convalescent animals are transported, stress can cause new lesions to develop.

There is little information about other species. Early research found that juvenile wild mice, hamsters, marmosets and opossums were all fatally affected by neurological illness after receiving experimental subcutaneous VSV-NJ inoculations. In these young animals, there were no follicular lesions to be noticed. Adults who received the same vaccination regimen remained symptom-free.

25.6 Post-Mortem Lesions

A coarse vesicle begins as a small hereditary area that develops into a fluid-filled bulge that ruptures to reveal a clinically or macroscopically assessed area of pain, erosion, or ulceration.

Vesicles in this disease are very similar to the other vesicular diseases, such as foot-and-mouth disease (FMD) or swine vesicular disease (SVD), in that they rupture quickly so the vesicular stage is often missed but a raw ulcerated area remains for longer. These erosions and ulcers are frequently seen on all species. In goats they are especially common on the teats and in the interdigital spaces of the feet. In pigs, lesions are more likely to occur on the snout, the coronary band and interdigital spaces. There are no significant lesions recorded in any internal organs.

Microscopic lesions associated with the vesicles do not differ from those of any other vesicular diseases of animals. Histologically, microvesicles form in the stratum spinosum of the epithelium soon after infection and then coalesce to form larger vesicles which progressively degenerate; necrosis occurs as the vesicles enlarge and fill with fluid. Mixed inflammatory cells infiltrate the lesion site and several distinct VSV antigen-containing cells with dendritic cell-like morphology are observed in the lower layers of the dermis. The virus can also be found and isolated from lymph nodes that drain from lesions, usually associated with cells of dendritic morphology.

25.7 Immune Response

In endemic locations, animals mount an immunological response to subclinical illness that is evidenced by relatively low neutralizing antibody titres. Neutralizing antibodies can persist for years, but lesions form at the insect inoculation site and reinfection can occur. Neutralizing antibodies may not be able to prevent the formation of this initial lesion. Low neutralizing activity is often reported in naive animals from non-endemic areas.

Several experimental vaccines are being tested against VSVs. Inactivated bivalent oil-adjuvanted vaccines for VSV-NJ and VSV-IN1 have been successfully used to control VSV outbreaks in South America, where the disease is endemic. Following an experimental challenge, these vaccinations produce large titres of disease-preventing antibodies.

25.8 Diagnosis

25.8.1 Field diagnosis

The presence of a vesicular disease in the field should always raise suspicion of FMD, hence laboratory confirmation is essential. Although there is the belief that FMD causes more severe form of diseases and affects a larger number of animals in a herd, this is not always the case. In susceptible populations, attack rates of 80–100% have been observed for vesicular stomatitis virus. Also, some FMD virus strains can cause only mild clinical infection in a small population of less susceptible animals (e.g. strain O-UK/2001 in sheep). For these reasons, it is very important to submit samples for diagnosis in a specified laboratory for confirmation of disease.

25.8.2 Laboratory diagnosis

Vesicular fluid or epitheliums from ruptured vesicles are generally sent to the laboratory, as both have ample amounts of virus and are good specimens for detecting the agent. Swab sample of lesions are also suitable. Even dried-up lesions can be used as laboratory samples, as the virus remains active in these lesions, and even if the virus is no longer infectious, viral antigens or RNA can be detected. For serology, blood is collected for serum. Serum can be extremely valuable, as recent infections are evidenced by the presence of VSV-specific IgM.

VSV is present in the vesicular fluid, swabs of ruptured vesicles, epithelium overlying unruptured vesicles and epithelial flaps of newly ruptured vesicles (e.g. epithelial appendages from the mouth). Lesions are very painful and sedation is recommended prior to specimen collection. Up to 7 days after infection, the VSV can be found in oral and nasal secretions. The ability to distinguish the VSV from other viruses that produce follicular lesions using tissue samples under electron microscopy is helpful. It is also possible to extract VSVs from other clinical specimens using a variety of additional cell lines. Fertilized eggs can be used to recover viruses, and animal (mouse) injection has been used in the past on occasion. The identity of cultured viruses can be confirmed using immunofluorescence, complement fixation or ELISA to detect viral antigens. Antigen-capture ELISA (indirect sandwich) is commonly used to distinguish virus serotypes. RT-PCR tests can also be used to distinguish between the New Jersey and Indiana serotypes of VSV. A Brazilian group reported that they used RT-PCR to confirm the isolation of VSV-AV and to distinguish these viruses from cocal viruses. VSV antigen can be detected in tissue samples or vesicle fluid using antigen-capture ELISA, complement fixation or virus neutralization. Descriptions of other antigen detection assays involving lateral flow devices have been published and some laboratories can use the RT-PCR test to directly detect viral nucleic acids in tissues sample. However, it does not seem to be common at this point. Genetic identification is complicated by the variability of the VSV. This includes variable changes that inculcate in the epidemic virus that continues to circulate. It might be necessary to standardize genetic testing for every area where these viruses are present. Numerous multiplex RT-PCR tests that have been described may recognize a wide variety of VSVs from both North and Central American serotypes. Unexpected loads may be overlooked. Bullous stomatitis can also be diagnosed serologically. A fourfold increase in titre is the diagnosis. Animals infected by the virus tend to develop serotype-specific antibodies to VSV 5–8 days after infection. ELISA and virus neutralization (VN) are the recommended serological tests, according to the World Organisation for Animal Health (WOAH, formerly OIE), but early antibodies can also be quantified by complement fixation. Complement fixation cannot detect antibody-like ELISA or VN. Some ELISAs for VSVs are quantitative (such as the liquid-phase blocking ELISA), while others only report the presence or absence of antibodies against this virus. Other serological tests have been described or used in the past, such as agar gel immunodiffusion and counter-immunoelectrophoresis.

25.9 Differential Diagnosis

VS can be differentially diagnosed from various disease conditions like FMD, SVD, bovine viral diarrhoea, rinderpest, malignant catarrhal fever, blue tongue, epizootic haemorrhagic disease, etc. Other diseases that can present with vesicular stomatitis like signs and lesions include the following.

- Epidemic infections: bovine ulcerative mastitis, pseudocowpox, bovine vulvovaginitis.
- Lameness: foot rot, hoof abscess, laminitis, poor floors, new concrete, mud.
- Dermatitis: burns, wetness, contact dermatitis, photosensitization.
- Phytophotodermatitis: certain plants, including furocoumarins (particularly members of the Umbelliferae family such as parsnips, celery and parsley), cause photosensitization.

25.10 Prevention and Control

No specific treatment is available for this viral disease but antibiotics may avoid secondary infection of abraded tissues sanitary prophylaxis. When a disease is suspected, animal movement must be restricted, and contaminated premises must be quarantined until a confirmatory laboratory diagnosis is made. Once confirmed, these precautions must be properly maintained. Additionally, vehicles and fomites need to be cleaned, and animals that are only sub-clinically affected need to be quarantined indoors for at least 21 days or until all lesions have healed. Controlling insect populations may help in preventing disease spread; breeding areas should be eliminated or reduced and insecticide sprays or insecticide-treated ear tags can be used on animals' medical prophylaxis. After all the healthy animals have been milked by various personnel, infected animals with lesions (or those suspected of having them) should be milked last in dairy operations. If done mechanically, milking machines should be fully decontaminated.

Due to the occurrence of natural cycles including insect and wild animal species, control and eradication may be challenging. Although inactivated and attenuated viral vaccines have undergone experimental testing, they are not yet commercially accessible.

As VSVs are widely studied at the molecular level, they are known to be transmitted directly via the transcutaneous or transmucosal route also. Specific VSVs have been isolated from various vectors like sandflies, blowflies, midges and other insects in ruminants. Seasonal variations (disappearance at the end of the rainy season in tropical regions and early frosts in temperate regions) also support the vector-borne transmission hypothesis that VSVs are grazing-plant viruses. When it comes to the endemic areas, the VSVs maintain a prolonged and stable cycle between potentially susceptible hosts and sandflies (the prominent vector).

25.10.1 Quarantine and movement control

The disease spreads rapidly and can cause up to 100% morbidity within affected flocks and herds. It is not highly contagious between flocks and herds. Nonetheless, the outbreak (specifically in horses) has been attributed to the movement of infected animals from one place to another. Therefore, it is crucial to regulate mobility and quarantine effectively. Movement control speeds up the process of viral eradication, enhances its chance of success, and lowers the expense of control measures and compensation payments. The transportation and build-up of ruminants should first be strictly regulated. After a thorough evaluation of the issue, they could be minimized. A defined region should be implemented at some level to impose quarantine, as follows.

- Dangerous Contact Premises (DCP): premises that have had direct or indirect contact with susceptible animals, or have infected animals – total of movement restrictions will be imposed.
- Suspicious Premises (SP): locations suspected of spreading disease. If there is no evidence of infection, the quarantine will be lifted.
- Restricted Areas (RAs): RAs are imposed around all infected premises (IPs) and DCPs and include as many SPs as possible; high levels of movement control and surveillance are applied to restricted areas.
- Control Area (CA): a CA is imposed around the RA and includes all remaining SPs. The purpose of a CA is to control the movement of susceptible animals and potentially contaminated equipment, such as vehicles, for the time required to conduct traceability and epidemiological studies. Less restrictive movement restrictions and surveillance apply. Once disease boundaries are firmly defined, CA boundaries and movement restrictions should be relaxed or removed.

In the field, vaccination studies in the species in which the vaccine is used will demonstrate the level of protection the vaccine provides.

Species used in challenges faced during vaccination against VSVs studies must be free of antibodies to VS. Vaccination studies should be conducted with laboratory animal models like rat or mice, using viruses produced by the intended production method, at the maximum permissible virus passage. The sensitivity, specificity, reproducibility, statistical significance and reliability of such experimental models should be verified properly.

In vitro measured post-vaccination antibody levels can be used to assess vaccine efficacy in animals if statistically significant correlation studies have been performed. For vaccines containing multiple viruses (e.g. VSNJV and VSIV), the efficacy of the different components of these vaccines should be demonstrated individually and also in combination, if there is interference between the different viruses. Duration of immunity and recommended vaccination frequency should be established before a product is approved. First, such information is collected directly using host-animal vaccination/challenge trials. The demonstrated duration of protection, measured by the ability of vaccinated animals in valid trials to withstand challenge, can be included in the labelling of vaccines. If the vaccine is to be used for ruminants and is intended for marketing and human consumption, a washout period (usually 21 days) suitable for the adjuvant used has to be submitted to the relevant regulatory authority for food safety.

25.10.2 Control

It should be highlighted that antibody responses in vaccinated animals might not be able to be distinguished from those infected with field viruses. To accurately identify vaccinated animals, it is required to employ serological approaches in conjunction with suitable clinical symptoms to determine exposure to field viruses.

Several insect species (as discussed earlier) from which the VSV was isolated have been found in different parts of the world. Regulation of the vector is important for the control of VS and may be essential for the eradication of the disease. In practice, it is difficult to monitor insects for the presence of the VSV and achieve effective insect control. However, it could be possible to control insect populations locally and limit the exposure of animals that could become ill from insect infection. Whether this is practical will depend on the kind of insects involved, their distribution and abundance, the climate and geography, and the accessibility of skilled workers and the necessary supplies.

25.11 Conclusion

VS in goats and sheep is a challenging condition to comprehend and manage. Since it may exhibit symptoms that are similar to FMD, producers may be understandably concerned. To keep people aware of the effects of the zoonotic risk of VSV infection and the necessary control measures, it is crucial to work closely with businesses and the media. Media campaigns should stress the value of routinely inspecting sensitive animals and reporting abnormal tumours or fatalities as soon as they occur. The general population should be made aware that animal products are safe and non-contagious. The media and veterinary authorities play a crucial role in maintaining consumer confidence in its goods. All persons working with infected animals must be informed that the virus can cause illness in humans (viral zoonoses). The public should be reassured that there is no risk of coming into contact with or consuming infected animal products.

VS is an OIE List A disease that is important to the international pet trade because it can spread rapidly, impact public health and can be confused with FMD. The strategy is to eradicate the disease, recognizing that the virus can be transmitted by a variety of insect vectors and that disease does not always follow predictable patterns of transmission and spread.

Strategies to be adapted for better results for the prevention of infection include the following.

- quarantine and movement control of animals, animal products and goods in declared areas to prevent the spread of infection;
- tracking and surveillance to identify the source and mode of transmission of infection;
- vector control to protect valuable individuals in declared areas and to prove freedom from disease and to reduce further transmission of the VSV;
- decontamination of products and goods to remove residual virus from infected buildings and equipment to prevent spread in declared areas;
- epidemiological investigation of whether insect or wildlife vectors are involved in the spread of infection;
- public awareness campaign to promote industry and community cooperation; and
- early diagnosis, which is important because FMD should be considered and delay in final diagnosis could have a significant impact on international trade in various commodities until FMD is ruled out.

References

Andrade, C.M., Rosas, C.E., Amorim, L.L., Mota, J.P., Teixeira, E.N. *et al.* (1980) Vesicular stomatitis in Brazil I – isolation and identification of the Alagoas strain. *Annals of Microbiology* 25, 81–87.

Bezerra, C.S., Cargnelutti, J.F., Sauthier, J.T., Weiblen, R., Flores, E.F. *et al.* (2018) Epidemiological situation of vesicular stomatitis virus infection in cattle in the state of Paraíba, semiarid region of Brazil. *Preventive Veterinary Medicine* 160, 68–75.

Goodger, W.J., Thurmond, M., Nehay, J., Mitchell, J. and Smith, P. (1985) Economic impact of an epizootic of bovine vesicular stomatitis in California. *Journal of the American Veterinary Medical Association* 186(4), 370–373.

Hansen, D.E., Thurmond, M.C. and Thorburn, M. (1985) Factors associated with the spread of clinical vesicular stomatitis in California dairy cattle. *American Journal of Veterinary Research* 46(4), 789–795.

Letchworth, G.J., Rodriguez, L.L. and Del Cbarrera, J. (1999) Vesicular stomatitis. *The Veterinary Journal* 157(3), 239–260.

Mason, J. (1984) *Vesicular stomatitis in Mexico*. Proceedings of an international conference on vesicular stomatitis, Mexico City, 24–27 September 1984.

Mead, D.G., Maré, C.J. and Ramberg, F.B. (1999) Bite transmission of vesicular stomatitis virus (New Jersey serotype) to laboratory mice by *Simulium vittatum* (Diptera: Simuliidae). *Journal of Medical Entomology* 36(4), 410–413.

Mead, D.G., Ramberg, F.B., Besselsen, D.G. and Mare, C.J. (2000) Transmission of vesicular stomatitis virus from infected to non-infected black flies co-feeding on nonviremic deer mice. *Science* 287, 485–487.

Mead, D.G., Gray, E.W., Noblet, R., Murphy, M.D., Howerth, E.W. *et al.* (2004) Biological transmission of vesicular stomatitis virus (New Jersey serotype) by *Simulium vittatum* (Diptera: Simuliidae) to domestic swine (*Sus scrofa*). *Journal of Medical Entomology* 41(1), 78–82.

Mebus, C.A. (1998) Vesicular stomatitis. In: Buisch, W.W., Hyde, J.L. and Mebus, C.A. (eds) *Foreign Animal Diseases*, 6th edn. Richmond (VA): United States Animal Health Association, Richmond, Virginia, pp. 419–423.

Rainwater-Lovett, K., Pauszek, S.J., Kelley, W.N. and Rodriguez, L.L. (2007) Molecular epidemiology of vesicular stomatitis New Jersey virus from the 2004–2005 U.S. outbreak indicates a common origin with Mexican strains. *Journal of General Virology* 88, 2042–2051.

Roche, S., Rey, F.A., Gaudin, Y. and Bressanelli, S. (2007) Structure of the prefusion form of the vesicular stomatitis virus glycoprotein G. *Science* 315(5813), 843–848.

Rodriguez, L.L. and NichoL, S.T. (1999) Vesicular stomatitis viruses. In: Webster, R.G. and Granoff, A. (eds) *Encyclopedia of Virology*, 2nd edn. Academic Press, London, pp. 1910–1919.

Rozo-Lopez, P., Drolet, B.S. and Londoño-Renteria, B. (2018) Vesicular stomatitis virus transmission: A comparison of incriminated vectors. *Insects* 9(4), 190.

Schmitt, B. (2002) Vesicular stomatitis. *Veterinary Clinics of North America: Food Animal Practice* 18, 453–459.

Shelokov, A. and Peralta, P.H. (1967) Vesicular stomatitis virus, Indiana type: An arbovirus infection of tropical sandflies and humans? *American Journal of Epidemiology* 86, 149–157.

Tesh, R.B., Chantiotis, B.N. and Johnson, K.M. (1971) Vesicular stomatitis virus, Indiana serotype: Multiplication in and transmission by experimentally infected sandflies (*Lutzyomyia trapidoi*). *American Journal of Epidemiology* 93(6), 491–495.

Tesh, R.B., Chantiotis, B.N. and Johnson, K.M. (1972) Vesicular stomatitis virus (Indiana serotype): Transovarial transmission by Phlebotomine sandflies. *Science* 175, 1477–1479.

Tesh, R., Saidi, S., Javadian, E., Loh, P. and Nadim, A. (1977) Isfahan virus, a new vesiculovirus infecting humans, gerbils, and sandflies (*Phlebotomus papatasi*) in Iran. *American Journal of Tropical Veterinary Medicine and Hygiene* 26, 299–306.

Tesh, R.B., Boshell, S.J., Modi, G.B., Morales, A.A., Young, D.G. *et al*. (1987) Natural infection of humans, animals, and phlebotomine sand flies with the Alagoas serotype of vesicular stomatitis virus in Colombia. *American Journal of Tropical Medicine and Hygiene* 36(3), 653–661.

World Organisation for Animal Health (2013) *Manual of Diagnostic Tests and Vaccines for Terrestrial Animals*. OIE, Paris.

Zimmer, B., Summermatter, K. and Zimmer, G. (2013) Stability and inactivation of vesicular stomatitis virus, a prototype Rhabdovirus. *Veterinary Microbiology* 162(1), 78–84.

26 Crimean–Congo Haemorrhagic Fever

Sina Salajegheh Tazerji[1,2*], Pouneh Hajipour[3], Natalia Pshenichnaya[4,5], Hafiz Muhammad Rizwan[6], Gulzhan N. Abuova[7] and Phelipe Magalhães Duarte[8]

[1]Faculty of Veterinary Medicine, Islamic Azad University, Tehran, Iran; [2]Islamic Azad University, Tehran, Iran; [3]Faculty of Veterinary Medicine, Shahid Bahonar University of Kerman, Kerman, Iran; [4]Central Institute of Epidemiology, Moscow, Russia; [5]Moscow Regional Research Clinical Institute, Vladimirsky, Moscow, Russia; [6]KBCMA College of Veterinary and Animal Sciences, Narowal, Lahore, Pakistan; [7]South-Kazakhstan State Pharmaceutical Academy, Shymkent, Kazakhstan; [8]Federal Rural University of Pernambuco (UFRPE), Recife, Pernambuco, Brazil

Abstract

Crimean–Congo haemorrhagic fever (CCHF) is a viral disease that can cause severe haemorrhagic fever in humans. This disease is caused by the Crimean–Congo haemorrhagic fever virus (CCHFV), which is transmitted to humans through tick bites or contact with the blood or tissues of infected animals. This chapter provides a systematic review and meta-analysis of post-exposure prophylaxis for the CCHFV among healthcare workers. It also discusses the immunopathogenesis, clinical, diagnostic and therapeutic perspectives of CCHFV infection. Other topics include the prevalence of post-traumatic stress disorder among CCHF survivors, the use of GP38-targeting monoclonal antibodies to protect against CCHFV infection, and the detection of CCHFV antibodies in humans and imported livestock in Saudi Arabia. The chapter provides an update on the current state of knowledge regarding the CCHFV and highlights the need for preparedness in the face of this emerging threat.

Keywords: Crimean–Congo haemorrhagic fever, CCHFV, postexposure prophylaxis, GP38-targeting monoclonal antibodies, prevalence of post-traumatic stress disorder, immunopathogenesis, preparedness

26.1 Introduction

Arbovirus is transmitted by multiple vectors to different susceptible hosts. The Crimean–Congo haemorrhagic fever virus (CCHFV), one of the members of genus *Arbovirus*, was first described between 1944 and 1945 by Russian soldiers (Khan *et al.*, 1995). Crimean–Congo haemorrhagic fever (CCHF) is one of the high-priority viral tick-borne diseases, affecting humans and animals and with the potential for nosocomial outbreaks. It is especially dangerous for humans, with a case fatality rate (CFR) ranging from 3% to 40%. Up to now, there have been many difficulties in its treatment and prevention.

The description of a case of a disease accompanied by haemorrhage in the territory of modern Tajikistan in AD 1100 may be the first known description of CCHF (Hoogstraal, 1979). It is the most widespread arthropod-borne virus distributed in many regions of Europe, Africa and Asia, with remarkable

*Corresponding author: sina.salajegheh@gmail.com

DOI: 10.1079/ 9781800622852.0026

zoonotic significance. Most livestock species such as goats, camels, cattle and sheep can be infected by this virus; however, the infection remains subclinical in them except for detectible viraemia. The CCHFV is persistent in the environment and can be transmitted horizontally and vertically (Cunningham *et al.*, 2017). Emergence and re-emergence of CCHF caused by vectors throughout the domain show a relationship among vectors, pathogens, humans and animals. Ticks are ectoparasites that are significant vectors of viral pathogens and play an important role in the transmission of diseases, such as tick-borne encephalitis and CCHF (Temur *et al.*, 2021). CCHF is transmitted by an infected *Hyalomma* tick bite, which is the chief reservoir and vector of CCHFV. CCHFV belongs to the family *Nairoviridae*, genus *Orthonairovirus*, and it was classified as an arbovirus in 1962. A schematic representation of the CCHFV is given in Fig. 26.1. Though animals remain asymptomatic, many can reproduce the virus and become the source of infection of hosts via ticks (Bente *et al.*, 2013).

Safe and effective vaccines are not yet available for humans or animals. Ribavirin has been commonly used in its treatment, but there is no evidence of its effectiveness (Soares-Weiser *et al.*, 2010) (Fig. 26.1).

26.2 Crimean–Congo Haemorrhagic Fever in Humans

26.2.1 Aetiology

The causative pathogen is the CCHFV, a member of the *Bunyaviridae* family of RNA viruses (genus *Nairovirus*). The CCHF orthonairovirus species comprises over 50 different CCHFV strains. From a public health perspective, CCHFV is considered to be the most significant orthonairoviruses (Adams *et al.*, 2017).

The CCHFV is an enveloped virus 90–100 nm in diameter. CCHFV virions contain small (S), medium (M) and large (L) genome segments of a single-stranded negative-sense RNA. The RNA genome of the CCHFV is encapsulated by the nucleoprotein and is associated with RNA-dependent RNA polymerase (RdRp).

The CCHFV is genetically diverse. Phylogenetic analyses based on the S-, M- or L-segment sequence analysis has led to differing conclusions about the number of distinct clades of CCHFV, because segment reassortment is observed in many viruses (Zivcec *et al.*, 2016). Seven distinct clades have been identified based on the S-segment or L-segment sequence analysis, whereas phylogenetic grouping of the M-segment sequences of the CCHFV

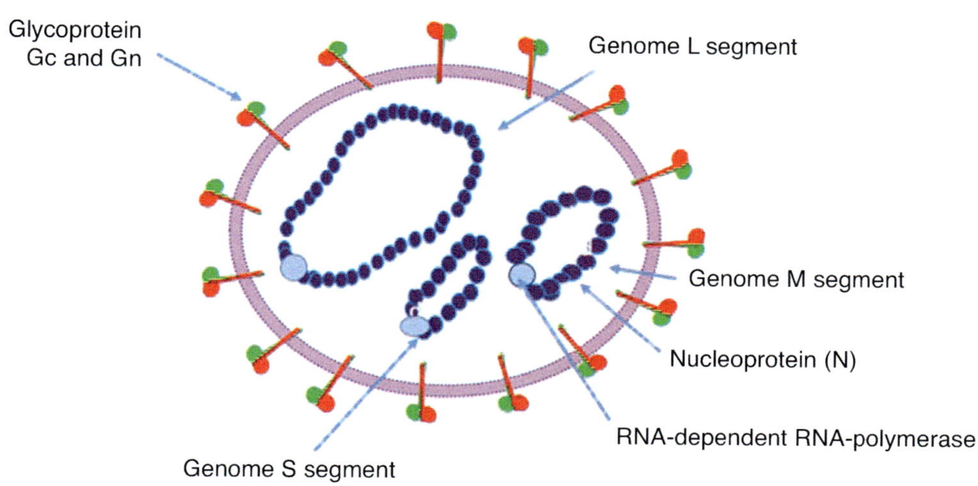

Fig. 26.1. Schematic representation of the Crimean–Congo haemorrhagic fever virus. (Authors own image.)

resulted in its division into six clades. Recently the International Committee on Taxonomy of Viruses (ICTV) Nairoviridae Study Group reclassified genogroup VI (also known as Europe-2 or AP-92-like) as a distinct virus, Aigai virus (AIGV) (Temur *et al.*, 2021). AIGV, previously classified as CCHFV genotype VI, Europe II, or AP92-like CCHFV, has recently been designated as a member of a new viral species within the genus *Orthonairovirus*. It has been postulated that AIGV and AIGV-related viruses may be less virulent than the original CCHFV despite their close phylogenetic relationship (Pickin *et al.*, 2022).

26.2.2 Epidemiology

CCHFV is maintained in a cycle between small mammals, sometimes including wild and domestic livestock and ixodid ticks, basically of the genus *Hyalomma*. Infection in animals is mild or asymptomatic. The geographical distribution of human infection matches the distribution of the principal tick vector (genus *Hyalomma*). CCHF is endemic throughout Africa, Asia, the Middle East and southern Europe, generally south of the 50th parallel north. In the 20th century the geographical range of the CCHFV appears to have extended to new regions (including Turkey and the Balkans), and in the 21st century, it has re-emerged in countries previously free from CCHF (including Georgia and Spain) (ProMED-mail, 2009, 2016), sometimes resulting in large outbreaks (Fig. 26.2). Probable explanations for the geographical spread are climate change favouring expansion of ixodid tick habitats, tick carriage on migratory birds, and transport of infected livestock and ticks. Disease incidence is usually highest during the spring and summer, when ticks consume blood for growth and reproduction (Bente *et al.*, 2013). Climatic factors, such as high humidity and favourable

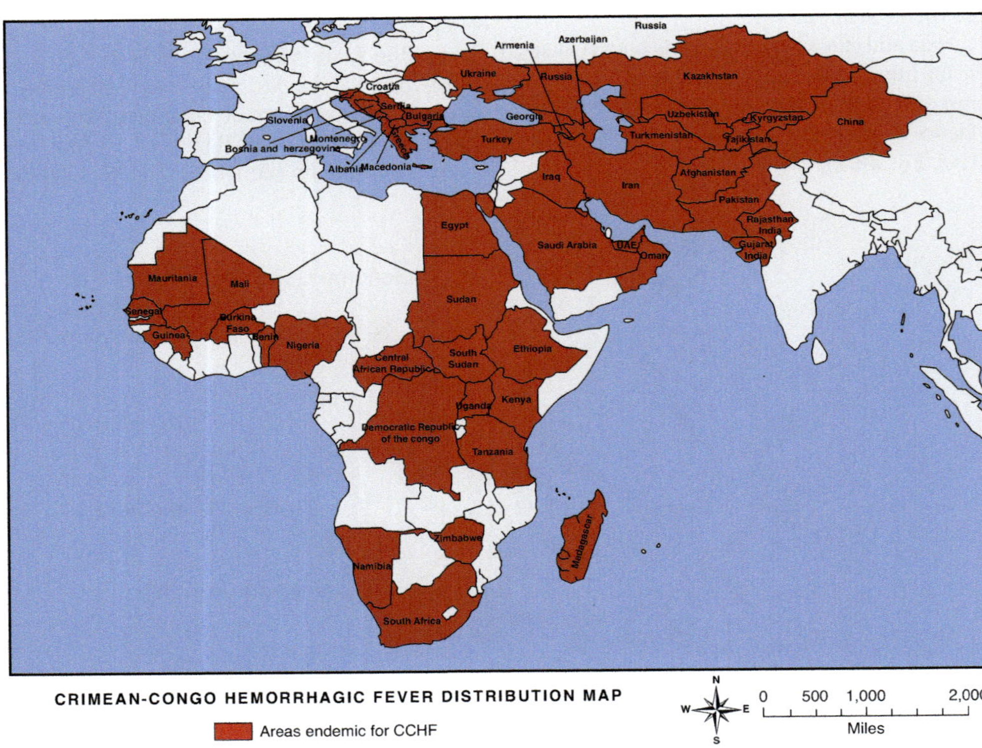

Fig. 26.2. CCHF. (CDC https://www.cdc.gov/crimean-congo-hemorrhagic/about/index.html)

temperatures (about 28°C), promote tick multiplication (Serretiello *et al.*, 2020).

26.2.3 Transmission

Transmission from ticks to humans occurs basically from bites or from handling or crushing ticks with the bare skin. Transmission to humans from infected animals occurs through direct contact with blood or other body fluids, especially during slaughter of livestock (Fig. 26.3). High-risk groups are slaughterhouse workers, agricultural workers, veterinarians and healthcare workers.

Human-to-human transmission occurs within families and in healthcare settings, including nosocomial clusters. The greatest risk of nosocomial exposure is from a needle stick injury (Leblebicioglu, 2016; Tsergouli *et al.*, 2020). Transmission may also occur through droplet exposure, exposure of skin or mucosal membranes to infected blood and airborne transmission from ventilated or oxygenated patients (Conger *et al.*, 2015; Pshenichnaya and Nenadskaya, 2015). There are a few case reports of possible sexual transmission at the end of the incubation period, during the mild course of disease or early convalescence (Pshenichnaya *et al.*, 2017). Vertical transmission occurs,

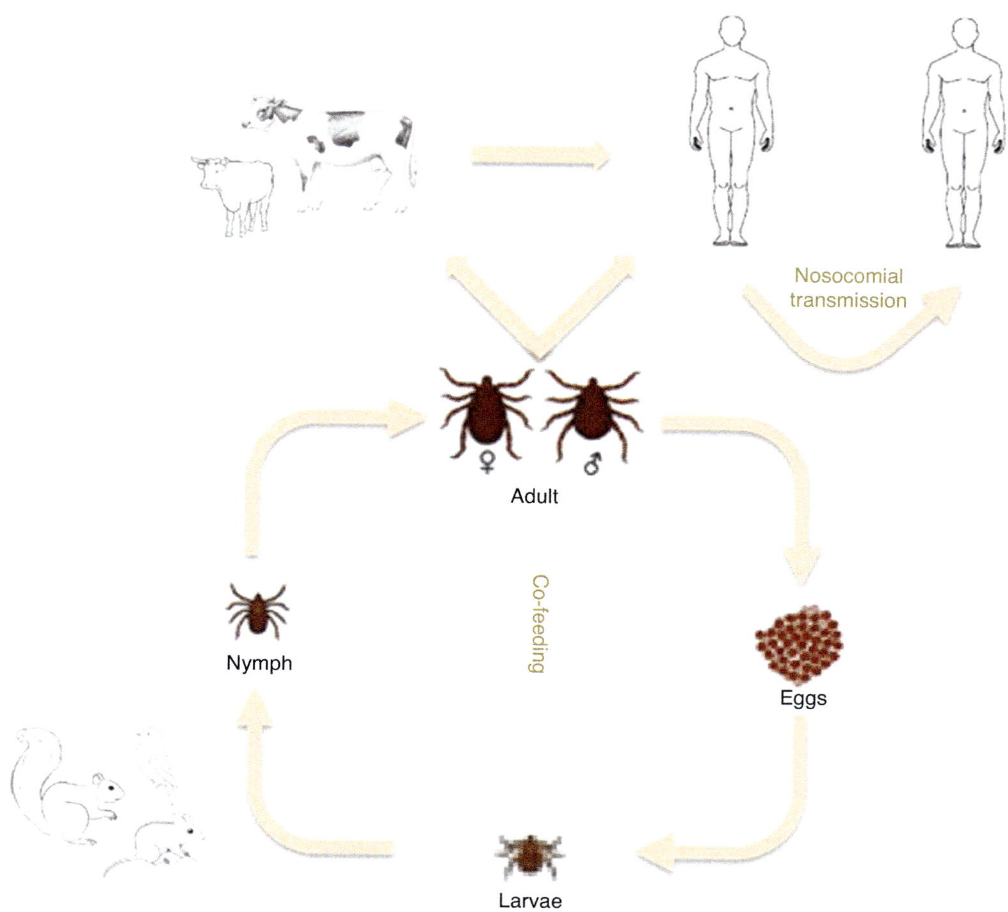

Fig. 26.3. CCHFV routes of transmission. (Author's own image.)

but whether it is perinatal or intrauterine is unknown (Ergönül *et al.*, 2010).

26.2.4 Pathophysiology

The pathophysiology of CCHF is still under investigation and is not fully understood. The main pathophysiological features of CCHF are coagulopathy and microvascular instability due to a combination of direct viral infection and indirect immune-mediated damage. CCHFV appears to weaken the immune response through a variety of approaches to facilitate unregulated viral replication. Disease severity commonly correlates with the viral level in the blood (Akıncı *et al.*, 2013).

After inoculation, the CCHFV first replicates in monocyte-derived dendritic cells and local tissues before disseminating widely in the lymphatic system. Although the virus has broad tissue tropism, the spleen, liver, bone marrow, endothelium and lymph tissue are commonly the most affected tissues. Infection of the liver can lead to significant necrosis (Burt *et al.*, 1997). Lymphocytes are not usually infected but may be diminished by apoptosis. Erythrocyte, platelet and leukocyte destruction is usually observed in bone marrow. Endothelial cell damage is connected directly with viral infection or indirectly with host-derived pro-inflammatory mediators (Schnittler and Feldmann, 2003).

The result is increased permeability and microvascular instability with extravasation of blood or plasma in severe cases of infection (Papa *et al.*, 2015). Endothelial damage may lead to platelet aggregation and subsequent activation of the intrinsic coagulation cascade, which lead to the development of clotting factor abnormalities causing disseminated intravascular coagulopathy and subsequent bleeding (Hamidinejad *et al.*, 2021).

26.2.5 Laboratory diagnosis

Identification of CCHFV RNA by RT-PCR is the standard diagnostic method. Virus-specific IgM and IgG can be detected by ELISA or IFA but, because anti-CCHFV antibodies are only detectable after 5–6 days of disease and may never appear in fatal cases, these diagnostic methods are not useful for early diagnosis or in patients who die. Virus is relatively easily isolated by cell culture but requires a laboratory BSL 3 + or BSL4 (Bente *et al.*, 2013). Past infection can be diagnosed by anti-CCHFV IgG using ELISA or IFA. Rapid tests are still under investigation (Baniasadi *et al.*, 2019) because they still have low sensitivity (less than 40%).

26.2.6 Clinical presentation

There are four phases of CCHF in humans: incubation, pre-haemorrhagic, haemorrhagic and convalescent periods (Fig. 26.4). Sometimes the phases of disease are not very clearly recognized in practice. The clinical course of disease varies from mild illness to rapidly developing fatal infectious disease.

The incubation period is usually shorter (2–7 days) after a tick bite and relatively longer (5–6 days) after exposure to infected biological fluids. The disease commonly presents as sudden onset of fever and non-specific constitutional symptoms (muscle pain, nausea and headache). During the next few days gastrointestinal symptoms (abdominal pain, vomiting and diarrhoea) may develop. Also lymphadenopathy, hepatomegaly and conjunctivitis are often noted. Jaundice is not typical.

After 3–5 days, the severe haemorrhagic phase of the illness with microvascular instability may develop in a small proportion of patients. The haemorrhagic phase generally manifests as conjunctival haemorrhage, petechial rash and the subsequent development of ecchymosis. Bleeding from the nasopharynx, gums, stomach, intestines, urinary tract and uterus is typical. Alveolar, retroperitoneal and intracranial haemorrhage may rarely develop in severe cases. Lethal outcome is usually recorded between 5 and 14 days of disease and is attributed to coagulopathy, shock, respiratory distress and kidney and liver insufficiency. The case fatality rate is about 30% in hospitalized patients (Leblebicioglu, 2010).

Maternal mortality is very high. During the first part of pregnancy it is about 9%, and after the 20th week of pregnancy it can reach 48%. Fetus mortality is up to 65% (Pshenichnaya *et al.*,

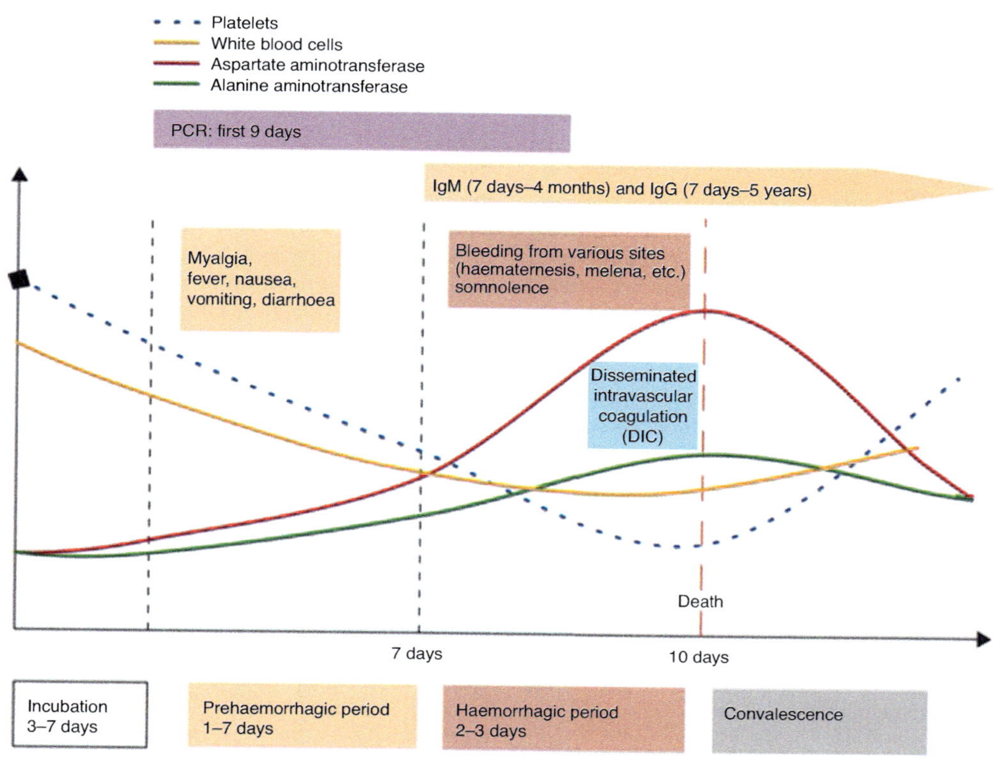

Fig. 26.4. Clinical and laboratory course of CCHF. (Adapted from Ergönül, 2006.)

2017). CCHF in children also may vary from mild to fatal cases (Keshtkar-Jahromi *et al.*, 2011).

During several months after recovery, surviving patients may complain of headache, weakness, anorexia, alopecia, post-traumatic stress disorder and hearing and visual impairments (Gul *et al.*, 2012; Bente *et al.*, 2013). There have been no reports of virus persistence or disease recurrence in CCHF in humans, but a recent experimental model has demonstrated the persistence of CCHFV in the testes and within the granulomas of non-human primates with concurrent latent tuberculosis (Smith *et al.*, 2019).

26.2.7 Clinical management

Routine supportive care basically includes the transfusion of blood products (fresh frozen plasma, packed red blood cells and platelets). Intravenous fluid replacement should be limited due to risk of pulmonary oedema. Antibiotics are not routinely prescribed without evidence of bacterial co-infection (Fillâtre *et al.*, 2019). A few reports published about usage of steroids for CCHF 5–7 days after symptom onset reported favourable results (Erduran *et al.*, 2013; Kouhpayeh, 2021). Meanwhile, more data are needed to recommend routine use.

Ribavirin, a guanosine analogue with broad antiviral activity, is sometimes used. The specific mechanism of antiviral activity is unclear. Recommended scheme of ribavirin administration is 2g loading dose, 1g four times per day in the first 4 days, and 0.5g four times per day in the next 6 days (WHO, 2014). Oral ribavirin (500 mg four times per day for 7 days) has sometimes been used as post-exposure prophylaxis with good results in cases with high risk of contamination due to direct unprotected contact with infected body fluids (Ergönül *et al.*, 2018).

Given the poor antibody response of patients with fatal CCHF, there is a theoretical rationale for the use of immunoglobulin or convalescent plasma therapy. Various immunoglobulin preparations have been used but in a small number of patients and without control groups, making interpretation of efficacy difficult (Vassilenko *et al.*, 1990; Ascioglu *et al.*, 2011; Kubar *et al.*, 2011; Fabara *et al.*, 2021).

In a small prospective interventional trial of intravenous immunoglobulin combined with ribavirin, symptom improvement was noted compared with ribavirin alone but there was no survival benefit (Salehi *et al.*, 2013). Further trials are needed.

In vitro data suggest that type I interferons have antiviral activity against the CCHFV but no efficacy data are available on animal models or humans (Andersson *et al.*, 2006).

Monoclonal antibodies against the CCHFV are still under development. At present only data about their efficiency on experimental models in animals are available (Golden *et al.*, 2019).

Favipiravir is now considered a potential antiviral drug for CCHF treatment. It has demonstrated efficiency in several experimental models (Hawman *et al.*, 2020).

26.2.8 Vaccines

There is no widely available vaccine for animals or humans. An inactivated mouse brain vaccine was developed by the former Soviet Union (SU) in the 1970s, but it is not used now in countries of the former SU. A similar vaccine (originated in the SU) has been used in Bulgaria since 1974, but safety and efficacy data are lacking.

CCHF human vaccine development has sped up in recent years and some vaccine studies have reported prospective results in animal models. Various experimental vaccines, including subunit vaccines, plant-based vaccines, DNA-vaccines, virus-like replicon particle systems, mRNA-vaccines, viral vectored vaccines and inactivated vaccines, are under development (Tipih and Burt, 2020).

26.2.9 Infection prevention and control

Patients should be isolated in a single room. There is no evidence of airborne transmission in the absence of aerosol-generating procedures such as endotracheal intubation and oxygenation. If aerosol-generating procedures are necessary, patients should be placed in negative-pressure rooms when possible. Healthcare workers should follow standard droplet and contact precautions to prevent exposure to blood and body fluids, and instruments and other materials in contact with the patient should be disinfected. During aerosol-generating procedures, respirators with at least the protection levels N95 and FPP2 should be used.

26.3 Crimean–Congo Haemorrhagic Fever in Goats

26.3.1 Epidemiology of CCHF in goats

CCHF was first identified during an outbreak in the Crimea in the year 1944 when 200 Soviet soldiers were infected. After that the same virus was reported in a 13-year-old male in the Congo in 1956. The topographical circulation of CCHF is associated with that of *Hyalomma* ticks, which are endemic in Asia, Africa, the Middle East and Eastern Europe. Ticks feed on specific animals, including wildlife and livestock, which function as asymptomatic pools of the CCHFV in endemic areas.

In Algeria (2009–2010), the CCHFV was reported in *Hyalomma aegyptium* ticks collected from tortoises. The adult *H. aegyptium* feeds on turtles, hedgehogs, or rabbits; however, larvae and nymphs can feed on mammals, humans, reptiles and birds, which increases the chances of the species functioning as a vector to contaminate humans, wildlife and livestock with CCHFV (Kautman *et al.*, 2016). Egypt has the highest number of tick species associated with the CCHFV. Birds during fall and spring migration southwards and northwards have been connected to the transference of vast numbers of ticks over Egypt, Africa and the Eurasian ranges (Darwish *et al.*, 1978).

In 2013, CCHFV was reported in *Hyalomma marginatum* ticks collected from migratory fowl in Zouala, Morocco. The presence of *H. marginatum* ticks and reservoir hosts (livestock) provides optimum conditions for the spread of CCHFV in different countries (Palomar *et al.*, 2013). Ticks collected from livestock in 1990 in Mecca, Saudi Arabia, were infected with the CCHFV, which may have been possible with the help of tick species like *H. onatoli*, *H. dromedarii* and *H. schulzei*. The CCHFV was detected in 0.8%, 4.1%, 3.2 and 0.6% of humans, sheep, goats and cattle, respectively (Hassanein *et al.*, 1997). Several species of ticks in Yemen are vectors for the CCHFV, which poses a major threat of the presence of CCHF in livestock (Bente *et al.*, 2013).

26.3.2 Transmission of CCHF in goats

CCHFV vectors belong to the family Ixodidae, i.e. hard ticks of the genus *Hyalomma*, ordinarily circulating between ticks and animals in an enzootic series. In this genus, trans-stadial, venereal and transovarian transmission take place. The most significant vector in Europe is *H. marginatum*, but in some cases, CCHFV can also be present in *H. anatolicum* and other species. Besides ixodid ticks, members of *Ixodes*, *Dermacentor*, *Rhipicephalus* and *Boophilus* may also transmit the virus. Birds seem to be resistant to infection, though they may act as mechanical vectors transporting CCHFV-infected ticks. Migrating birds might spread the virus between geographical regions (Yessinou *et al.*, 2018).

26.3.3 Pathogenesis of CCHF in goats

The virus arrives inside the cells because of receptor reliance on endocytosis via viral glycoproteins (Gn and Gc) that bind with the specific virus receptor cell surface in nucleolin. Due to the destruction of immune compartments, the virus quickly replicates and the resulting dysregulation of the vascular structure and lymphoid tissues leads to the production of pro-inflammatory cytokines, such as TNF, IL-10, and IL-6, which induce destruction of the endothelium. Because of this destruction, inherent clotting-initiation leads to the platelet accumulation resulting in obstruction of the endothelial lining. The resulting platelets travel through the body of the infected host and eventually result in dispersed intravascular coagulopathy (DIC) (Goswami *et al.*, 2014).

CCHFV infections are mostly asymptomatic in goats. The only common symptom in infected goats is mild transient rise in body temperature. Goats become viraemic for 1 week after the onset of infection and can transfer CCHFV infection in their tissues and blood (Shayan *et al.*, 2015).

26.3.4 Diagnosis of CCHF in goats

The CCHFV can be isolated from autopsy, blood/plasma and tissues. The virus is present in the spleen, brain, lungs, kidneys, bone marrow and liver. BHK-21, SW-13, Vero and LLC- MK2 are cell lines that can be used for the isolation of CCHFV. Cell cultures can be used to identify concentrations of the virus, which is most beneficial in the first 5 days of infection. The CCHFV can be analysed by inoculation into neonatal mice.

Reverse passive haemagglutination inhibition techniques, indirect immunofluorescence, complement fixation and agar gel diffusion assay are used to detect anti-CCHFV antibodies. Reverse transcription polymerase chain reaction (RT-PCR) on serum testers can be used in the early stages of CCHF disease development. Using enzyme-linked immunosorbent assay (ELISA) and immunofluorescence assay (IFA), IgM and IgG antibodies can be identified in infected goats. Immunohistochemistry can be used for the diagnosis of CCHFV in formalin-fixed tissue trials. The latest method for rapid diagnosis of CCHFV is reverse transcription loop-mediated isothermal amplification (Osman *et al.*, 2013).

26.3.5 Treatment of CCHF in goats

Domestic animals brought from CCHF-infected areas must be treated at entry points by the application of insecticides or acaricides directly to their bodies via liquid spraying with a hand compression sprayer or powder dusting via a nozzle-type duster (heavy dusting application must be avoided and the eyes, mouths and nostrils of animals must be protected). It is most important to treat the back of the head, belly and neck of animals. Insecticides must be used 12–15 days before animal slaughtering (Mourya *et al.*, 2012).

26.4 Prevention and Control of CCHF

Preventive measures used to control CCHF in livestock and animals include evasion of tick bites, use of acaricides and use of personal protective equipment (PPE). Acaricides are used for resistant ticks when smeared prior to animal butchery or in quarantine. Uncontrolled animal activities in endemic areas known as trans-border transmission must be circumscribed by regulations and punishments enforced by local establishments. Acaricides can be applied to animals to restrict unrestrained animal travel (Maltezou and Papa, 2011; Papa *et al.*, 2015).

26.4.1 Controlling infection in healthcare settings

The key to reducing the risk is to boost awareness of CCHF, which permits healthcare workers to adopt basic PPE, infection control and regulator practices (Mourya *et al.*, 2012). Recommended practices for CCHF prevention during animal care and slaughter in order to control infection in health care settings include the following.

1. Proper care should be taken of healthcare employees and abattoir staff. Proper training must be given about animal upkeep, well-being and slaughtering.
2. Unintentional exposure to the fluids and blood of animals must be avoided
3. Employees must take precautions to avoid injuring themselves or others.
4. Hands must be rinsed properly.
5. Gloves and additional protective clothes must be worn during animal slaughtering and animal management. The hide, fleshy tissue and body fluids must not be handled without gloves.
6. Tick bites should be avoided when skinning the animals and tanning the hides.
7. The animal's body should be examined every day for ticks and attached ticks removed from the skin with tweezers. Spraying may help rinse off unattached ticks.
8. Do not touch and press the tick with naked hands.
9. Do not eliminate the ticks with fingers.
10. Avoid the yard while the animal is being slaughtered.
11. Slaughtering must be done in a slaughterhouse or closed areas.
12. The blood of slaughtered animals must be washed out as soon as possible.
13. Rodents, fowls, insects and pets must be prevented from entering the slaughterhouse.

Training public health experts, animal health specialists and policymakers is essential.

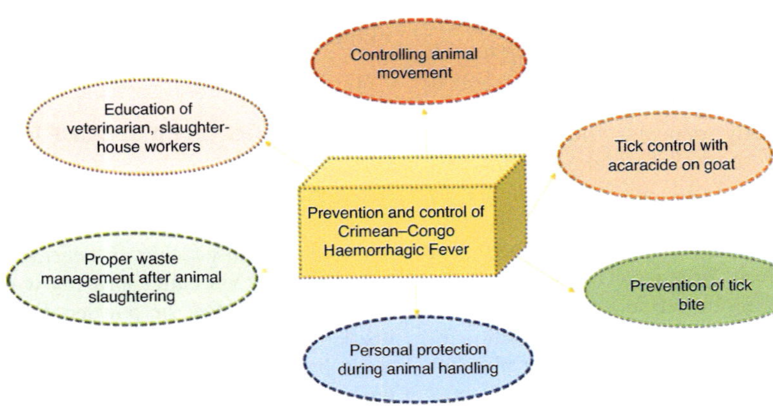

Fig. 26.5. Prevention and control of Crimean–Congo haemorrhagic fever. (Author's own image.)

Different strategies used to control and prevent CCHF are presented in Fig. 26.5.

26.5 Conclusions

CCHF is a tick-borne viral infection that is a zoonotic and public health issue. It is asymptomatic in goats and can sometimes lead to death. Its diagnosis is mostly done by cell culture, serological tests and molecular techniques. At present, there is no appropriate CCHF vaccine available and treatment is generally through symptomatic or supportive therapy. Tick-borne diseases can be controlled and prevented by avoidance of tick bites, using tick repellents. The geographical disease range is growing because of changes in climatic conditions, travel and trade of animals. Moreover, because of modification in the dissemination of the host variety, the conditions of *Hyalomma* ticks are expanding and, therefore, CCHFV disease risk is on the increase. Further action is required to create effective strategies and take strict preventive and regulatory measures in countries and regions where the disease is emerging.

References

Adams, M.J., Lefkowitz, E., King, A.M.Q., Barrach, B., Harrison, R.L. *et al.* (2017) Changes to taxonomy and the International Code of Virus classification and nomenclature ratified by the International Committee on Taxonomy of Viruses (2021). *Archives of Virology* 162, 2505–2538. DOI: 10.1007/s00705-017-3358-5.

Akıncı, E., Bodur, H. and Leblebicioglu, H. (2013) Pathogenesis of Crimean-Congo hemorrhagic fever. *Vector-Borne and Zoonotic Diseases* 13, 429–437. DOI: 10.1089/vbz.2012.1061.

Andersson, I., Lundkvist, A., Haller, O. and Mirazimi, A. (2006) Type I interferon inhibits Crimean-Congo hemorrhagic fever virus in human target cells. *Journal of Medical Virology* 78, 216–222. DOI: 10.1002/jmv.20530.

Ascioglu, S., Leblebicioglu, H., Vahaboglu, H. and Chan, K.A. (2011) Ribavirin for patients with Crimean–Congo haemorrhagic fever: A systematic review and meta-analysis. *Journal of Antimicrobial Chemotherapy* 66, 1215–1222. DOI: 10.1093/jac/dkr136.

Baniasadi, V., Pouriayevali, M.H., Jalali, T., Fazlalipour, M., Azadmanesh, K. *et al.* (2019) Evaluation of first rapid diagnostic kit for anti-Crimean-Congo hemorrhagic fever virus IgM antibody using clinical samples from Iran. *Journal of Virological Methods* 265, 49–52. DOI: 10.1016/j.jviromet.2018.12.015.

Bente, D.A., Forrester, N.L., Watts, D.M., McAuley, A.J., Whitehouse, C.A. *et al.* (2013) Crimean-Congo hemorrhagic fever: History, epidemiology, pathogenesis, clinical syndrome and genetic diversity. *Antiviral Research* 100, 159–189. DOI: 10.1016/j.antiviral.2013.07.006.

Burt, F.J., Swanepoel, R., Shieh, W.J., Smith, J.F., Leman, P.A. *et al.* (1997) Immunohistochemical and *in situ* localization of Crimean-Congo hemorrhagic fever (CCHF) virus in human tissues and implications for CCHF pathogenesis. *Archives of Pathology & Laboratory Medicine* 121, 839.

Conger, N.G., Paolino, K.M., Osborn, E.C., Rusnak, J.M., Günther, S. *et al.* (2015) Health care response to CCHF in US soldier and nosocomial transmission to health care providers, Germany, 2009. *Emerging Infectious Diseases* 21, 23. DOI: 10.3201/eid2101.141413.

Cunningham, A.A., Daszak, P. and Wood, J.L.N. (2017) One health, emerging infectious diseases and wildlife: Two decades of progress? *Philosophical Transactions of the Royal Society B: Biological Sciences* 372, 20160167. DOI: 10.1098/rstb.2016.0167.

Darwish, M.A., Imam, I.Z.E., Omar, F.M. and Hoogstraal, H. (1978) Results of a preliminary seroepidemiological survey for Crimean-Congo hemorrhagic fever virus in Egypt. *Acta Virologica* 22(1), 77.

Erduran, E., Bahadir, A., Palanci, N. and Gedik, Y. (2013) The treatment of crimean-congo hemorrhagic fever with high-dose methylprednisolone, intravenous immunoglobulin, and fresh frozen plasma. *Journal of Pediatric Hematology/Oncology* 35, e19–e24. DOI: 10.1097/MPH.0b013e3182706444.

Ergönül, Ö. (2006) Crimean-congo haemorrhagic fever. *The Lancet Infectious Diseases* 6(4), 203–214. Available at: https://www.thelancet.com/journals/laninf/article/PIIS1473-3099(06)70435-2/fulltext (accessed 20 October 2024).

Ergönül, Ö., Celikbas, A., Yildirim, U., Zenciroglu, A., Erdogan, D. *et al.* (2010) Pregnancy and Crimean-Congo haemorrhagic fever. *Clinical Microbiology and Infection* 16, 647–650. DOI: 10.1111/j.1469-0691.2009.02905.x.

Ergönül, Ö., Keske, S., Çeldir, M.G., Kara, I.A., Pshenichnaya, N. *et al.* (2018) Systematic review and meta-analysis of postexposure prophylaxis for Crimean-Congo hemorrhagic fever virus among healthcare workers. *Emerging Infectious Diseases* 24, 1642. DOI: 10.3201/eid2409.171709.

Fabara, S.P., Ortiz, J.F., Smith, D.W., Parwani, J., Srikanth, S. *et al.* (2021) Crimean-Congo hemorrhagic fever beyond ribavirin: A systematic review. *Cureus* 13(9), e17842. DOI: 10.7759/cureus.17842.

Fillâtre, P., Revest, M. and Tattevin, P. (2019) Crimean-Congo hemorrhagic fever: An update. *Medecine et Maladies Infectieuses* 49, 574–585. DOI: 10.1016/j.medmal.2019.09.005.

Golden, J.W., Shoemaker, C.J., Lindquist, M.E., Zeng, X., Daye, S.P. *et al.* (2019) GP38-targeting monoclonal antibodies protect adult mice against lethal Crimean-Congo hemorrhagic fever virus infection. *Science Advances* 5, eaaw9535. DOI: 10.1126/sciadv.aaw9535.

Goswami, T.K., Singh, D.K., Saminathan, M., Verma, A.K. and Dhama, K. (2014) An emerging threat of Crimean Congo hemorrhagic fever: Call for preparedness. *Advances in Animal and Veterinary Sciences* 2(1), 8–14. DOI: 10.14737/journal.aavs/2014.2.1.8.14.

Gul, S., Gul, E.U., Yesilyurt, M., Ozturk, B., Kuscu, F. *et al.* (2012) Health-related quality of life and the prevalence of post-traumatic stress disorder among Crimean-Congo hemorrhagic fever survivors. *Japanese Journal of Infectious Diseases* 65, 392–395. DOI: 10.7883/yoken.65.392.

Hamidinejad, M.A., Ghaleh, H.E.G., Farzanehpour, M., Bolandian, M. and Ruhollah, D. (2021) Crimean-Congo hemorrhagic fever from the immunopathogenesis, clinical, diagnostic, and therapeutic perspective: A scoping review. *Asian Pacific Journal of Tropical Medicine* 14, 254–265. DOI: 10.4103/1995-7645.315899.

Hassanein, K.M., El-Azazy, O.M.E. and Yousef, H.M. (1997) Detection of Crimean-Congo haemorrhagic fever virus antibodies in humans and imported livestock in Saudi Arabia. *Transactions of the Royal Society of Tropical Medicine and Hygiene* 91, 536–537. DOI: 10.1016/S0035-9203(97)90014-6.

Hawman, D.W., Haddock, E., Meade-White, K., Nardone, G., Feldmann, F. *et al.* (2020) Efficacy of favipiravir (T-705) against Crimean-Congo hemorrhagic fever virus infection in cynomolgus macaques. *Antiviral Research* 181, 104858. DOI: 10.1016/j.antiviral.2020.104858.

Hoogstraal, H. (1979) The epidemiology of tick-borne Crimean-Congo hemorrhagic fever in Asia, Europe, and Africa. *Journal of Medical Entomology* 15, 307–417. DOI: 10.1093/jmedent/15.4.307.

Kautman, M., Tiar, G., Papa, A. and Siroky, P. (2016) AP92-like Crimean-Congo hemorrhagic fever virus in Hyalomma aegyptium ticks, Algeria. *Emerging Infectious Diseases* 22, 354. DOI: 10.3201/eid2202.151528.

Keshtkar-Jahromi, M., Sajadi, M.M., Ansari, H., Mardani, M. and Naieni, K.H. (2011) Crimean-Congo hemorrhagic fever: Current and future prospects of vaccines and therapies. *Antiviral Research* 90, 85–92. DOI: 10.1016/j.antiviral.2011.02.010.

Khan, J.A., Rehman, S., Fisher-Hoch, S.P., Mirza, S., Khurshid, M. *et al.* (1995) Crimean Congo-haemorrhagic fever treated with oral ribavirin. *The Lancet* 346, 472–475. DOI: 10.1016/S0140-6736(95)91323-8.

Kouhpayeh, H. (2021) A systematic review of treatment strategies including future novel therapies in Crimean-Congo hemorrhagic fever. *International Journal of Infection* 8. DOI: 10.5812/iji.113427.

Kubar, A., Haciomeroglu, M., Ozkul, A., Bagriacick, U., Akinci, E. *et al.* (2011) Prompt administration of Crimean-Congo Hemorrhagic Fever (CCHF) virus hyperimmunoglobulin in patients diagnosed with CCHF and viral load monitorization by reverse transcriptase-PCR. *Japanese Journal of Infectious Diseases* 64, 439–443. DOI: 10.7883/yoken.64.439.

Leblebicioglu, H. (2010) Crimean–Congo haemorrhagic fever in Eurasia. *International Journal of Antimicrobial Agents* 36, S43–S46. DOI: 10.1016/j.ijantimicag.2010.06.020.

Maltezou, H.C. and Papa, A. (2011) Crimean-Congo hemorrhagic fever: Epidemiological trends and controversies in treatment. *BMC Medicine* 9, 1–5.

Mourya, D.T., Yadav, P.D., Shete, A.M., Gurav, Y.K., Raut, C.G. *et al.* (2012) Detection, isolation and confirmation of Crimean-Congo hemorrhagic fever virus in human, ticks and animals in Ahmadabad, India, 2010–2011. *PLoS Neglected Tropical Diseases* 6, e1653. DOI: 10.1371/journal.pntd.0001653.

Osman, H.A.M., Eltom, K.H., Musa, N.O., Bilal, N.M., Elbashir, M.I. *et al.* (2013) Development and evaluation of loop-mediated isothermal amplification assay for detection of Crimean Congo hemorrhagic fever virus in Sudan. *Journal of Virological Methods* 190, 4–10. DOI: 10.1016/j.jviromet.2013.03.004.

Palomar, A.M., Portillo, A., Santibáñez, P., Mazuelas, D., Arizaga, J. *et al.* (2013) Crimean-Congo hemorrhagic fever virus in ticks from migratory birds, Morocco. *Emerging Infectious Diseases* 19, 260. DOI: 10.3201/eid1902.121193.

Papa, A., Mirazimi, A., Köksal, I., Pena, A.E. and Feldmann, H. (2015) Recent advances in research on Crimean-Congo hemorrhagic fever. *Journal of Clinical Virology* 64, 137–143. DOI: 10.1016/j.jcv.2014.08.029.

Pickin, M.J., Devignot, S., Weber, F. and Groschup, M.H. (2022) Comparison of Crimean-Congo hemorrhagic fever virus and Aigai virus in life cycle modeling systems reveals a difference in I protein activity. *Journal of Virology* 96, e00599–22. DOI: 10.1128/jvi.00599-22.

ProMED-mail (2009) *Crimean-Congo hem. fever - Georgia, 1st case*. Available at: https://promedmail.org/promed-post/?id=290497 (accessed 26 November 2022).

ProMED-mail (2016) *Crimean-Congo hem. fever - Spain: (CL) autochthonous, 1st rep*. Available at: https://promedmail.org/promed-post/?id=20160901.4458484 (accessed 26 November 2022).

Pshenichnaya, N.Y. and Nenadskaya, S.A. (2015) Probable Crimean-Congo hemorrhagic fever virus transmission occurred after aerosol-generating medical procedures in Russia: Nosocomial cluster. *International Journal of Infectious Diseases* 33, 120–122. DOI: 10.1016/j.ijid.2014.12.047.

Pshenichnaya, N.Y., Leblebicioglu, H., Bozkurt, I., Sannikova, I.V., Abuova, G.N. *et al.* (2017) Crimean-Congo hemorrhagic fever in pregnancy: A systematic review and case series from Russia, Kazakhstan and Turkey. *International Journal of Infectious Diseases* 58, 58–64. DOI: 10.1016/j.ijid.2017.02.019.

Salehi, H., Salehi, M., Adibi, N. and Salehi, M. (2013) Comparative study between ribavirin and ribavirin plus intravenous immunoglobulin against Crimean Congo hemorrhagic fever. *Journal of Research in Medical Sciences* 18, 497.

Schnittler, H.J. and Feldmann, H. (2003) Viral hemorrhagic fever – a vascular disease? *Thrombosis and Haemostasis* 89, 967–972. DOI: 10.1055/s-0037-1613397.

Serretiello, E., Astorri, R., Chianese, A., Stelitano, D., Zannella, C. *et al.* (2020) The emerging tick-borne Crimean-Congo haemorrhagic fever virus: A narrative review. *Travel Medicine and Infectious Disease* 37, 101871. DOI: 10.1016/j.tmaid.2020.101871.

Shayan, S., Bokaean, M., Shahrivar, M.R. and Chinikar, S. (2015) Crimean-congo hemorrhagic fever. *Laboratory Medicine* 46, 180–189. DOI: 10.1309/LMN1P2FRZ7BKZSCO.

Smith, D.R., Shoemaker, C.J., Zeng, X., Garrison, A.R., Golden, J.W. *et al.* (2019) Persistent Crimean-Congo hemorrhagic fever virus infection in the testes and within granulomas of non-human primates with latent tuberculosis. *PLoS Pathogens* 15, e1008050. DOI: 10.1371/journal.ppat.1008050.

Soares-Weiser, K., Thomas, S. and Garner, P. (2010) Ribavirin for Crimean-Congo hemorrhagic fever: Systematic review and meta-analysis. *BMC Infectious Diseases* 10, 1–9.

Temur, A.I., Kuhn, J.H., Pecor, D.B., Apanaskevich, D.A. and Keshtkar-Jahromi, M. (2021) Epidemiology of Crimean-Congo hemorrhagic fever (CCHF) in Africa—underestimated for decades. *The American Journal of Tropical Medicine and Hygiene* 104, 1978. DOI: 10.4269/ajtmh.20-1413.

Tipih, T. and Burt, F.J. (2020) Crimean-Congo hemorrhagic fever virus: Advances in vaccine development. *BioResearch Open Access* 9, 137–150. DOI: 10.1089/biores.2019.0057.

Tsergouli, K., Karampatakis, T., Haidich, A.B., Metallidis, S. and Papa, A. (2020) Nosocomial infections caused by Crimean–Congo haemorrhagic fever virus. *Journal of Hospital Infection* 105, 43–52. DOI: 10.1016/j.jhin.2019.12.001.

Vassilenko, S.M., Vassilev, T.L., Bozadjiev, L.G., Bineva, I.L. and Kazaroy, G.Z. (1990) Specific intravenous immunoglobulin for Crimean-Congo haemorrhagic fever. *The Lancet* 335, 791–792. DOI: 10.1016/0140-6736(90)90906-L.

WHO (2014) *Clinical management of patients with viral haemorrhagic fever: A pocket guide for the front-line health worker: Interim emergency guidance-generic draft for West African adaptation 30*. World Health Organization, Geneva.

Yessinou, R.E., Adoligbe, C., Akpo, Y., Adinci, J., Karim, I.Y.A, *et al.* (2018) Sensitivity of different cattle breeds to the infestation of cattle ticks *Amblyomma variegatum*, *Rhipicephalus microplus*, and *Hyalomma* spp. on the natural pastures of Opkara Farm, Benin. *Journal of Parasitology Research* 2018, 2570940. DOI: 10.1155/2018/2570940.

Zivcec, M., Scholte, F.E.M., Spiropoulou, C.F., Spengler, J.R. and Bergeron, E. (2016) Molecular insights into Crimean-Congo hemorrhagic fever virus. *Viruses* 8, 106. DOI: 10.3390/v8040106.

27 Rabies

Amita Tiwari[1]*, Salil Pathak[1], Brejesh Singh[1] and Shivangi Udainiya[2]
[1]Department of Veterinary Medicine, College of Veterinary Science & Animal Husbandry, NDVSU, Jabalpur; [2]Veterinary Polytechnic College, Bhopal

Abstract
Rabies occurs in goats infrequently but should be taken into consideration if an animal is exhibiting any behavioural changes or signs of paralysis. Signs include drooling of saliva, inability to swallow any food, dullness and depression, stupor, weakness, aggression, excitation, circling movement, blindness or any repetitive action. Rabies is fatal when the animal has been infected. The usual route of infection is from bites by infected animals. The main reservoirs of the virus are bats, foxes, skunks and raccoons. Vaccination is recommended by veterinarians for rabies prevention in goats living in endemic rabies areas.

Keywords: Rabies, vaccination, endemic areas, fatality

27.1 Introduction

Rabies is a viral disease that affects warm-blooded animals and is almost always fatal. It is caused by an RNA virus of the family *Rhabdoviridae* and genus *Lyssavirus*. The origin of the word 'rabies' is the Latin word *rabere*, which means 'to rage or rave' or 'to be mad'. *Rabere* may have originated from Sanskrit word *rabhas*, which means 'violence' (Drew, 2004). In Greek, the word *lyssa* is used, which means 'madness'.

The disease has been around the world from very early times. Although rabies is a vaccine-preventable viral zoonosis, it remains an important public health issue in developing countries. The disease is responsible for more than 60,000 human deaths worldwide annually (Wilde *et al.*, 2013). Despite global efforts and the implementation of extensive control schemes and public health awareness programmes, over 95% of deaths occur in Asia and Africa, where canine rabies is enzootic, and 99% in the endemic regions (WHO, 2013).

Rabies has been known since around 2000 BC. The first written record of rabies is in Mesopotamia (*c.* 1930 BC). The Greeks had a special god in their mythology to counteract the effects of rabies: Aristaeus, the son of Apollo. Artemis is portrayed as a rabies healer.

Rabies appears to have originated in the Old World, the first epizootic in the New World occurring in Boston, Massachusetts, in 1768. There was so much fear of the disease that a person bitten by a dog merely suspected of being rabid used to commit suicide or ask to be killed by others. There were many myths associated with the disease. In ancient times the attachment membrane of the tongue was cut and removed, as this was where rabies was thought to originate. This practice ceased with the discovery of the actual cause of rabies.

*Corresponding author: amitasandhu@gmail.com

DOI: 10.1079/ 9781800622852.0027

27.2 Aetiology

A virus with a single-stranded RNA genome from the *Lyssavirus* genus of the *Rhabdoviridae* family is the cause of rabies. These are enveloped viruses with a single-stranded, negative-sense RNA genome of about 12 kb in size. Rabies virus is a member of the order *Mononegavirales*, which includes viruses with non-segmented and negative-stranded RNA genomes. They target the central nervous system (CNS). They are bullet-shaped and approximately 180 nm long and 75 nm wide. Nucleoprotein (N), phosphoprotein (P), matrix protein (M), glycoprotein (G) and large protein (L) are the five proteins encoded by the genome. The ordination and placement of these proteins encoding genes in the genome affect the virus's structure.

The genus contains six so-called rabies-related viruses, including the classical rabies virus (genotype 1), the Lagos bat virus (genotype 2), the Mokola virus (genotype 3), the Duvenhage virus (genotype 4), the European bat lyssaviruses 1 and 2 (genotypes 5 and 6) and the recently discovered Australian bat genotype 7. The Mokola virus, Lagos bat virus, Duvenhage virus, European bat virus 1 and 2 and Australian bat Lyssavirus are all members of the genus *Lyssavirus*, which also includes the rabies virus and other closely related viruses from Africa, Europe and Australia. Each of these viruses is thought to be capable of inducing rabies-like disease in both animals and humans. Sodium hypochlorite, 45–75% ethanol, iodine preparations, quaternary ammonium compounds, formaldehyde, phenol, ether, trypsin, propiolactone and some other detergents can all inactivate the rabies virus. It is also inactivated by extremely low pH (below 3.00) or extremely high pH (above 7.00). This virus is sensitive to ultraviolet light. It is rapidly deactivated by sunlight and drying, and it does not survive in the environment for long periods of time (in dried blood and secretions) (Balcha and Abdela, 2017).

27.3 Epidemiology

Rabies is found in 150 countries and on every continent except Antarctica. In many parts of Asia and Africa, stray dogs are a major source of human infections (ECDC, 2016). The disease is less common in goats. Several countries, including Australia, Canada, Japan and the United States, as well as Western Europe and island nations, are free of rabies (CDC, 2014).

Rabies is a neglected zoonotic disease and is almost always fatal after the onset of symptoms. Dogs are responsible for the spread of rabies in 95% of cases in places like Asia and Africa. In rabies-endemic areas, dogs alone are responsible for 99% of disease transmission. However, in nature, rabies is transmitted and maintained in two interconnected cycles: the urban cycle, which involves domesticated and stray dogs, and the sylvatic cycle, which involves wildlife such as foxes, wolves, jackals, mongoose, raccoons, skunks and bats. In some areas, the sylvatic and urban rabies cycles coexist, while in others, the sylvatic cycle predominates. Although rabies cases are typically sporadic, epizootic outbreaks are possible.

Rabies is indigenous to a reservoir species in a locality in an enzootic state and has a relatively stable incidence rate. An epizootic occurs when the incidence of disease in the reservoir species increases significantly. The term spillover refers to rabies that spreads sporadically from a reservoir to non-reservoir species. Dogs are the primary reservoir hosts in South-east Asian countries such as Bangladesh, India and Nepal, while wolves (*Canis lupus*), jackals (*Canis aureus*) and foxes (*Vulpes bengalensis*) are the wildlife reservoirs.

27.4 Transmission

Rabies is primarily transmitted by rabid-animal bites, but in rare cases a rabid animal licking into an open wound may also transmit the virus. Virus transmission via organ transplant has also been reported on very rare occasions. Although bodily fluids such as tears and nervous tissues can potentially transmit the disease, the virus has not been found in faeces or blood. The disease's oral transmission, transmission through abrasions in the oral mucosa and transplacental transmission have all been experimentally documented. Transmission via milk and cooked meat has not yet been reported, but consumption of raw milk and meat from rabid animals is discouraged. Previously, only a few cases of disease transmission via aerosol have been reported (Pantha *et al.*, 2020).

Various species of insectivorous bats inhabiting caves are reported to have spread rabies naturally via the inhalation route. Although this route of infection is still under suspicion, it is now accepted that inter-bat spread and the spread from bats to other species are principally by bites, but infection by inhalation also occurs. Bats are the most important species in which subclinical carriers occur. Multiplication of the virus without invasion of the CNS is known to occur in fatty tissues in bats and it may be the basis of making this species a reservoir for the disease.

27.5 Economic Importance

Rabies is not of major economic concern in goats, although individual goats and flocks may suffer from fatalities. The economic costs of rabies in a country are always associated with the vaccination of pet populations of the country, animal bite investigations, quarantine rules and their strict follow-ups, etc. of domestic animals that bite humans or that are suspected of exposure to rabid animals. The infrastructure of laboratories for rabies diagnosis, the costs of pre-exposure and post-exposure prophylaxis and treatment and consultation, public education, etc. also play major roles in the occurrence of rabies.

27.6 Pathogenesis

The rabies virus enters the body via wounds or direct contact with mucosal surfaces. It cannot pass through intact skin. Rabies virus replicates in the bitten muscle (local viral proliferation in non-neural tissue) and gains access to the CNS via viral attachment to motor endplates and motor axons. Virions are carried in transport vesicles and only travel to the CNS via fast retrograde transport along motor axons, with no uptake by sensory or sympathetic endings. The salivary glands become infected as a result of centrifugal transport along efferent cranial nerves, and virus particles are shed in the saliva. Infection of the brain frequently results in behavioural changes that cause the host to bite other animals, allowing the virus to spread. The widespread infection of the CNS almost always results in death, usually through respiratory paralysis, but also through secondary circulatory, metabolic, or infectious processes (Fig. 27.1). Viruses can also enter peripheral nerve motor axons directly during a penetrating injury. Depending on the amount of virus in the inoculum, the density of motor endplates at the wound site and the proximity of virus entry

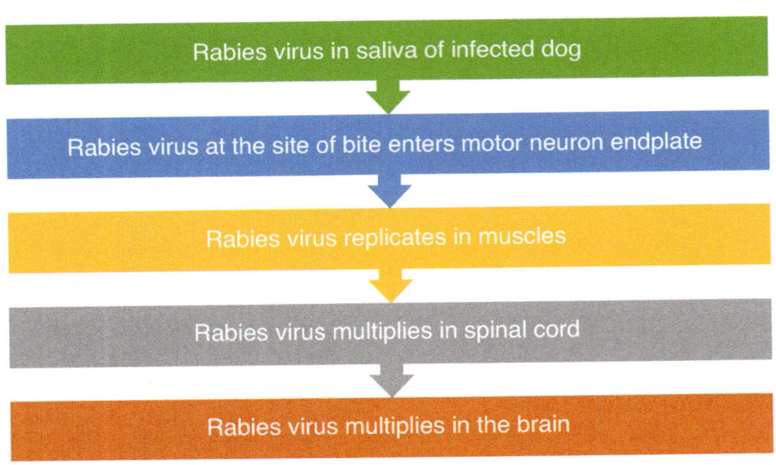

Fig. 27.1. Diagrammatic representation of the pathogenesis of rabies virus. (Author's own image.)

to the CNS, the incubation period can range from a few days to several months (usually 2–3 months; rarely more than 1 year) (Hemachudha *et al.*, 2013). If the animal is bitten on the head or neck, or if a large inoculum is transferred through multiple bites, deep wounds or large wounds, the incubation period is less than 50 days. The incubation period for rabies in goats is 2–17 weeks and the disease lasts from 5 to 7 days (Fig. 27.1).

27.7 Clinical Signs

The disease occurs in cattle, sheep, horses and pigs in most countries. The clinical picture can vary greatly between species, individuals within the same species and even within the course of the disease. Animals with rabies may exhibit unusual behaviour as the disease progresses. Laboratory testing is required to confirm any clinical suspicion of rabies (Blackmore, 2014).

There are three possible manifestations of rabies: furious, dumb and paralytic. The most commonly reported manifestation in goats is the furious form. However, it may be because most of the cases reported worldwide are from Asia or Africa, where furious rabies affects dogs. The common symptoms include aggression, excitability, restlessness, excessive crying, difficulty swallowing and excessive salivation or drooling.

The dumb form of the disease is exhibited by the depressed animal, which lies down and is not interested in eating or drinking, and drooling saliva is observed. However, the behaviour and temperaments of 'dumb' animals frequently change and they may become unusually aggressive or unusually affectionate.

In the prodromal stage, clinical symptoms appear after a certain period of incubation. Minor behavioural changes, such as aggressiveness in tame animals, daytime activities in nocturnal animals, no fear of humans in wild animals, or abnormalities in appetite, may occur during this first stage, which usually lasts about 1–3 days (Balcha and Abdela, 2017).

During the excitement (furious) phase, the prodromal stage is eventually followed by a period of severe agitation and aggression. The animal frequently bites anything. Even without the paralytic stage of the disease, death can occur as a result of convulsions. Restlessness, wandering, howling, polypnea, drooling and attacks on other animals, people, or inanimate objects characterize the furious form. Foreign objects, such as sticks and stones, are frequently swallowed by affected animals. Wild animals frequently lose their fear of humans and may attack humans or other animal species that they would otherwise avoid (e.g. porcupines). During the day, nocturnal animals may be visible. Unusual alertness in animals can also be a sign of this form (Balcha and Abdela, 2017).

Progressive paralysis characterizes the 'dumb' form of rabies (Fig. 27.2). The throat and masseter muscles become paralysed in this form; the animal may be unable to swallow and may salivate excessively. Laryngeal paralysis can result in a change in vocalization. There may also be facial paralysis or the lower jaw dropping.

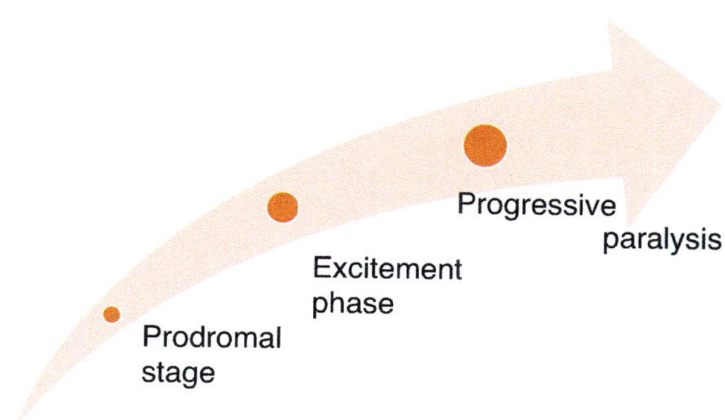

Fig. 27.2. Developmental stages of clinical signs. (Author's own image.)

Ruminants can become somnolent or depressed if they become separated from the herd. Rumination is suspended. Ataxia, incoordination and ascending spinal paresis or paralysis are also observed. This stage is distinguished by the inability to swallow, which results in the typical sign of foaming saliva around the mouth. Some animals may develop paralysis beginning in the hind limbs. Eventually, complete paralysis occurs (WHO, 2013) (Fig. 27.2).

27.8 Diagnosis

In most cases, rabies is diagnosed primarily on the basis of clinical symptoms and signs and a corroborative anamnesis or evidence of an animal bite, death of an animal and incomplete or no vaccination following exposure. For timely post-exposure prophylaxis, laboratory diagnosis of rabies is essential. Rabies can be diagnosed *in vivo* or post-mortem. Ante-mortem rabies virus infection can be difficult to detect. Despite the fact that hydrophobia is highly suggestive of rabies, no clinical signs of the disease are pathognomonic. Because of low sensitivity, historical reliance on the detection of Negri bodies accumulations is no longer regarded as suitable for diagnostic assessment, and alternative laboratory-based tests have been developed to conclusively confirm infection.

Most rabies virus diagnostic tests in animals require brain material for diagnosis, which is often only available after death. Any part of the affected brain can be used to diagnose rabies in animals. However, to rule out rabies, the test must include tissues from at least two different parts of the brain: the brainstem and the cerebellum.

There are numerous rabies detection methods in animals, including direct fluorescent antibody, mouse inoculation technique, tissue culture infection technique and polymerase chain reaction. The clinical samples used for ante-mortem diagnosis include cerebrospinal fluid (CSF), saliva, swabs from the nasal mucosa, eye and throat, impression smears from the eyeball and cornea, biopsies from the skin on the face and nuchal regions of the body and brain tissues (brainstem, cerebellum and hippocampus) from dead animals. The first recommended diagnostic procedure for rabies is an intra-vitam test, which can be used on either dead or alive patients. For the intra-vital diagnosis of rabies, a new technique has been developed: the cornea test. Transporting samples for diagnosis should be done at low temperatures and with glycerol or saline. Skin biopsies can be used to diagnose rabies in humans and animals both before and after death. The viral antigen was found in the peripheral nerves surrounding the hair follicles, and the positive diagnosis rate increased as the infection progressed (Singh *et al.*, 2017).

Brain samples can be obtained most easily by breaching the skull and sampling directly. For both human and animal samples, brain smears or touch impressions are used for the detection of virus antigen with the fluorescent antibody test (FAT). The direct fluorescent antibody test (dFAT) is the recommended diagnostic test in animals and it is used routinely by all the laboratories engaged in the diagnosis of rabies. The dFAT is the most widely recommended test for diagnosis of rabies by both OIE (2009) and WHO (2013). In fresh brain tissues, the sensitivity of the dFAT is 100% and confirmative diagnosis can be made within 2 hour. The dFAT has been found suitable to detect 100% rabies-positive cases even in formalin-fixed, paraffin-embedded materials and compared with PCR targeting a short region of the N gene in the fresh tissue samples from dogs, cats, foxes, racoon dogs and badgers, which also detected 100% of cases. The highest sensitivity of 99.6% was observed by FAT in the brainstem compared with in the cerebellum (99.3%), cerebrum (98.9%) and hippocampus (98.7%) (Tepsumethanon *et al.*, 1997).

Reverse transcription polymerase chain reaction (RT–PCR), direct rapid neuro immunohistochemistry test (dRIT) and serological tests are among the other diagnostic techniques (fluorescent antibody neutralization test, rapid fluorescent focus inhibition test). An immunochromatographic technique using lateral flow principle facilitated the diagnosis of different rabies virus strains (RABV species 1, 5, 6 and 7) and showed 100% specificity and more than 88% sensitivity when compared with RTCIT and FAT (Servat *et al.*, 2012).

In the brains of humans and animals, RABV can directly be detected by rapid immunochromatographic test using a monoclonal antibody (Ahmed *et al.*, 2012). A direct rapid immunohistochemical test (dRIT) for quick detection of rabies in humans and animals has been developed (Madhusudana *et al.*, 2012).

Serological tests are rarely used to diagnose rabies because the animals do not survive the disease long enough to produce enough antibodies. Post-infection antibodies, on the other hand, can persist in some cases. These tests are primarily used to evaluate the efficacy of various rabies vaccines (Wasniewski *et al.*, 2014). The counter-current immuno-electrophoresis (CCIE) test has been used for rabies diagnosis but has not been found to be as specific and sensitive as FAT and MIT.

Several nucleic acid (NA)-based tests (*in situ* hybridization, PCR, genomic sequencing, etc.) have been developed and are used for rabies diagnosis (WHO or OIE reference laboratories) (Meng *et al.*, 2013). These methods detect highly specific molecular subunits of rabies RNA in either experimental or routine brain material. As a result, the NA hybridization technique outperforms all other tests in terms of sensitivity and specificity.

27.9 Differential Diagnosis

The differential diagnosis of the disease is one of the most challenging jobs for a veterinarian. In most of the cases there is always a probability of human exposure, and if not recognized appropriately on time, the human life may be at risk. It is not always true that every animal showing nervous signs is rabid, and nervous signs may not be evident for some days after the illness commences. In addition, many animals suffering from other diseases will be left untreated. The best way is to handle all suspect animals with extreme care but treatment must be continued for other diseases as well. If the animal is rabid, it will die and the diagnosis can then be confirmed by laboratory examination.

Rabies in goats may be differentially diagnosed from various other conditions. such as lead toxicity, vitamin A deficiency, polioencephalomalacia, listeriosis, enterotoxaemia, pregnancy toxaemia, etc.

27.10 Prevention and Control

Once symptoms of rabies infection appear, there is no cure and the infection is fatal. The management of animals is currently the key to preventing and controlling rabies (Rupprecht *et al.*, 2008). Animal rabies control primarily consists of vaccinating dogs and cats, along with eradication and sterilization of stray animals, spreading public health awareness, etc. Bats act as a wildlife reservoir apart from carnivore species on which control measures are focused traditionally.

Rabies is nearly 100% fatal in humans (Mazigo *et al.*, 2010), but it is also 100% preventable (Tekki *et al.*, 2013). The first and most important part of a rabies control programme is to define a case by identifying the rabid animal after diagnosis by a qualified laboratory. Confirmation in the laboratory should be accomplished through dFAT or RABV isolation in cell culture.

Rabies prevention and control programmes necessitate increased surveillance based on laboratory and variant typing. For this, accurate and timely information and reporting are necessary for the management of potentially exposed animals aiding in emerging pathogen discovery. There is always the possibility of virus introduction through the entry of infected animals (Castrodale *et al.*, 2008). This aids in describing disease epidemiology and determining the need for effective immunization programmes for both wild and domestic animals.

27.10.1 Pre-exposure management

As rabies is quite rare in goats, pre-exposure vaccination in goats is generally not recommended. Moreover, no rabies vaccine is labelled for use in goats. However, rabies vaccination is mandated in pet cats and dogs, so as to ensure that these pets are properly vaccinated for the safety of other animals. Goats must be provided with adequate housing and fencing for keeping out wildlife and other nocturnal animals.

27.10.2 Post-exposure management

Any goat that has been exposed to a confirmed or suspected rabid animal must be quarantined. Rabies vaccine should be administered upon admission to isolation or 1 month before release. The severity of the exposure, the time period since the last vaccination, the number of prior vaccinations, the animal's current health status and the local rabies epidemiology must all be considered when evaluating animals. After exposure, vaccination is required. Animals that are showing signs of rabies should be put to death and their brain samples must be sent for laboratory testing (Green, 1997).

27.10.3 Immunization (rabies vaccine)

For veterinary use, a number of recently developed and highly effective thermostable inactivated vaccines are now available. The duration of immunity ranges between 1 to 3 years. Most veterinary vaccines are only approved for use in certain species, such as dogs. All rabies vaccines approved for human and animal use must achieve potency standards. It is necessary to have a minimum antigenic potency of 2.5 IU per dose (WHO, 2013). Cattle, goats and sheep can be vaccinated once a year or every 2–3 years, depending on the manufacturer's recommendations. It is highly advised that animals without obvious bite wounds should receive vaccination after an outbreak in domestic livestock (Murray *et al.*, 2009).

There are currently 17 parenteral animal rabies vaccines approved for use in dogs, cats, sheep, cattle, horses or ferrets by the US Department of Agriculture (USDA).

Rabies vaccines for animal use include live attenuated virus (such as Flury high egg passage, Flury low egg passage, Street-Alabama-Dufferin, and Kelev), chemically or physically inactivated virus, and recombinant vaccines. For virus cultivation, embryonated eggs, CNS tissues from newborn animals and cell cultures are preferred. Rabies vaccines are typically lyophilized, but can be inactivated with an adjuvant and stored in liquid form. The advent of genetic engineering has influenced vaccine development by providing more opportunities to produce inactivated antigens and attenuate different viruses through direct mutation (Yang *et al.*, 2013). Several novel approaches, such as the use of vectors, lipopeptide vaccines, plasmid DNA and plant virus-based rabies vaccines, are also being investigated (Ohara *et al.*, 2013). Injectable vaccine preparations have limitations, particularly in carnivores and wildlife. As a result, oral vaccine formulation has been continuously attempted, with significant results in both laboratory and field trials (Cliquet *et al.*, 2007). Oral vaccines are primarily based on avirulent mutants or the use of recombinant vaccines. In order of improving antibody response induction ability in large mammals, for that purpose DNA vaccine must be a better alternative to the conventional vaccine (Ullas *et al.*, 2012).

27.10.4 Quarantine

The most effective method of preventing rabies in an area or a country free of the disease is to impose a quarantine period of about 4–6 months on all imported dogs. If the rabies in dogs is controlled, then there are fair chances of rabies eradication in a country. As the incubation period of rabies is variable, vaccination on two occasions with an inactivated vaccine when the animal is in quarantine for 6 months is the current recommendation for its control. Where there is high risk, attention must be given to mass vaccination of wildlife, because wildlife are the breach in the defences against the disease. Mass oral vaccination of rabies in terrestrial wild animals is an effective control method that is very effective and internationally accepted. It is based on the concept of herd immunity and vaccines are effective when fed as vaccine baits. Sufficient trials have been conducted successfully.

27.10.5 Economics of prevention and control

In most countries, rabies is an endemic disease and a major public health concern. In India, annual human deaths from rabies are estimated to be around 20,000, with an annual incidence of animal bites of 1.7% (17.5 million per year). To prevent rabies transmission in a dog population, it is theoretically necessary to vaccinate at least 60–70% of the dogs. Even countries with potentially adequate resources do not always meet and maintain these rates. One reason for such failure could be that individual dog owners believe that vaccinating their pets is too expensive. Lethal methods of dog population control are even more expensive, and reducing dog populations to control rabies has not worked for a long time. The most expensive aspect of wildlife rabies is the cost of vaccinating domestic animals, large and small. The advantages of immunizing a specific wildlife population with vaccine-infused baits may be overestimated if the entire cost of vaccinating domestic animals is attributed to one species. For instance, using oral vaccines in Europe to control fox rabies has proven challenging, despite a noticeable decrease in the number of rabid foxes. Other authors assert that using oral vaccines to prevent fox rabies is cost-effective, but there is not any solid evidence to back up that assertion. It is also highly debatable whether using oral vaccine to try to eradicate raccoon rabies in areas where it is present would be cost-effective, given that vaccinating raccoons with an oral vaccine requires roughly four times as many vaccine-laden baits as vaccinating foxes (Meltzer and Rupprecht, 1998).

27.11 Zoonotic Importance

The disease is always considered as a fatal disease in unvaccinated and untreated humans. The prime importance of rabies is its transmissibility to humans, with veterinarians and animal handlers being at highest risk. Humans who have contracted the disease are likely to have been exposed to a rabid domestic animals and not wild animals. Human rabies is extremely rare in countries where canine rabies is controlled by regular vaccination.

27.12 Conclusion

Rabies is one of the most important zoonoses that is a vaccine-preventable disease. Various studies suggest that the single effective way to control the disease is to vaccinate dogs and control the disease in wildlife. Medical and veterinary professionals must be aware of the route of rabies transmission in order to raise public awareness about precautionary measures for people living in rural areas as well as those working in abattoirs, thereby reducing the chances of disease spread. The disease is incurable, but it can be prevented. Rabies prevention in animals needs to rely on vaccination and avoiding contact with infected animals. The vast majority of rabies exposures in animals and humans can be avoided by increasing public awareness of rabies transmission routes and avoiding contact with wildlife. It is critical to raise community awareness about the mode of transmission, prevention and control of rabies. The use of international law should aid in the control of communicable diseases. Regulations for stray dog management should be implemented, as should strict control of free-roaming dogs and mandatory rabies vaccination. All in-contact individuals must report to the physicians and personal protection equipment must be prioritized.

References

Ahmed, K., Wimalaratne, O., Dahal, N., Khawplod, P., Nanayakkara, S. *et al.* (2012) Evaluation of a monoclonal antibody-based rapid immunochromatographic test for direct detection of rabies virus in the brain of humans and animals. *American Journal of Tropical Medicine and Hygiene* 86(4), 736.

Balcha, C. and Abdela, N. (2017) Review of rabies preventions and control. *International Journal of Public Health Science* 6(4), 343–350.

Blackmore, C. (2014) *Rabies Prevention and Control in Florida*. Division of Disease Control and Health Protection, Florida Department of Health, Tallahassee, Florida, p. 122.

Castrodale, L., Walker, V., Baldwin, J., Hofmann, J. and Hanlon, C. (2008) Rabies in a puppy imported from India to the USA, March 2007. *Zoonoses and Public Health* 55(8-10), 427–430.

CDC (2014) Rabies-Free Countries and Political Units. Available at: https://www.cdc.gov/importation/rabies-free-countries. html

Cliquet, F., Gurbuxani, J.P., Pradhan, H.K., Pattnaik, B., Patil, S.S. *et al.* (2007) The safety and efficacy of the oral rabies vaccine SAG2 in indian stray dogs. *Vaccine* 5(17), 3409–3418.

Drew, W.L. (2004) Rabies. In: Ryan, K.J. and Ray, C.G. (eds) *Sherri's Medical Microbiology*, 4th edn. McGraw-Hill, pp. 597–600.

ECDC (2016) Annual Epidemiological Report 2016 – Rabies. Available at: http://ecdc.europa.eu/en/healthtopics/rabies/Pages/Annual-epidemiological-report-2016.aspx

Green, S.L. (1997) Rabies. *Veterinary Clinics of North America Equine Practice* 13, 1–11.

Hemachudha, T., Ugolini, G., Wacharapluesadee, S., Sungkarat, W., Shuangshoti, S. *et al.* (2013) Human rabies: Neuropathogenesis, diagnosis, and management. *The Lancet Neurology* 12(5), 498–513.

Madhusudana, S.N., Subha, S., Thankappan, U. and Ashwin, Y.B. (2012) Evaluation of a direct rapid immunohistochemical test (dRIT) for rapid diagnosis of rabies in animals and humans. *Virologica Sinica* 27, 299–302.

Mazigo, H.D., Okumu, F.O., Kweka, E.J. and Mnyone, L.L. (2010) Retrospective analysis of suspected rabies cases reported at Bugando Referral Hospital, Mwanza, Tanzania. *Journal of Global Infectious Diseases* 2(3), 216.

Meltzer, M.I. and Rupprecht, C.E. (1998) A review of the economics of the prevention and control of rabies: Part 2: Rabies in dogs, livestock and wildlife. *Pharmacoeconomics* 14, 481–498.

Meng, S., Lv, W., Wu, J., Wang, J., Xu, G. *et al.* (2013) Comparison of three strategies for sequencing rabies viral G gene. *Journal of Applied Virology* 2(1).

Murray, K.O., Holmes, K.C. and Hanlon, C.A. (2009) Rabies in vaccinated dogs and cats in the United States, 1997–2001. *Journal of the American Veterinary Medical Association* 35(6), 691–695.

Ohara, S., Sato, S., Oyama, K., Tsutsui, K.I. and Iijima, T. (2013) Rabies virus vector transgene expression level and cytotoxicity improvement induced by deletion of glycoprotein gene. *PloS ONE* 8(11), e80245.

OIE (2009) Rabies. Chapter 2.1.13. In: *Manual of Diagnostic Tests and Vaccines for Terrestrial Animals 2009*.

Pantha, S., Subedi, D., Poudel, U., Subedi, S., Kaphle, K. *et al.* (2020) Review of rabies in Nepal. *One Health* 10, 100155.

Rupprecht, C.E., Barrett, J., Briggs, D., Cliquet, F., Fooks, A.R. *et al.* (2008) Can rabies be eradicated? *Developments in Biologicals* 131, 95–121.

Servat, A., Picard-Meyer, E., Robardet, E., Muzniece, Z., Must, K. *et al.* (2012) Evaluation of a rapid immunochromatographic diagnostic test for the detection of rabies from brain material of European mammals. *Biologicals* 40(1), 61–66.

Singh, R., Singh, K.P., Cherian, S., Saminathan, M., Kapoor, S. *et al.* (2017) Rabies – epidemiology, pathogenesis, public health concerns and advances in diagnosis and control: A comprehensive review. *Veterinary Quarterly* 7(1), 212–251.

Tekki, I.S., Okewole, P.A., Ekong, S.P., Kumbish, P.R., Shamaki, D. *et al.* (2013) Control of rabies and rabies related viruses in Nigeria: Perspectives from the national Veterinary Research ilstitute, Vom, Nigeria. *Epizootiology and Animal Health in West Africa* 9(1), 59–69.

Tepsumethanon, V., Lumlertdacha, B. and Mitmoonpitak, C. (1997) Sensitivity of fluorescent rabies antibody testing on samples taken from brain stem, cerebellum, cerebrum and hippocampus. *Thai Journal Veterinary Medicine* 27, 335–340.

Ullas, P.T., Desai, A. and Madhusudana, S.N. (2012) Rabies DNA vaccines: Current status and future. *World Journal of Vaccines* 2, 36–45.

Wasniewski, M., Labbe, A., Tribout, L., Rieder, J., Labadie, A. *et al.* (2014) Evaluation of a rabies ELISA as an alternative method to seroneutralisation tests in the context of international trade of domestic carnivores. *Journal of Virological Methods* 195, 211–220.

WHO (2013) Expert consultation on rabies. Second report. WHO Tech. Rep. Ser., 982 1–139.

Wilde, H., Hemachudha, T., Wacharapluesadee, S., Lumlertdacha, B. and Tepsumethanon, V. (2013) Rabies in Asia: The classical zoonosis. In: *One Health: The Human–Animal–Environment Interfaces in Emerging Infectious Diseases*. Springer, Berlin, pp. 185–203.

Yang, D.K., Kim, H.H., Lee, K.W. and Song, J.Y. (2013) The present and future of rabies vaccine in animals. *Clinical and Experimental Vaccine Research* 2(1), 19–25.

28 Kyasanur Forest Disease (KFD)

Alok Kumar Chaudhary*, Mukesh Kumar Srivastava, Pradeep Kumar, Renu Singh and Shruti Bhatt

Department of Veterinary Medicine, COVAS, DUVASU, Mathura, India

Abstract

Kyasanur Forest disease (KFD), or monkey fever, is caused by a zoonotic virus transmitted by ticks, first observed in Karnataka, India, in 1957. The virus sporadically re-emerges in the Western Ghats range, causing febrile illness and potential haemorrhagic complications in primates and humans, with mortality rates of 2–10%. Environmental factors like climate change and deforestation, along with the distribution of animal and human hosts and reservoirs, impact its spread. It mainly circulates among small mammals, birds and larger animals, with *Haemaphysalis* ticks acting as key vectors. Monkeys amplify the virus, while humans serve as accidental dead-end hosts. The virus's pathogenesis involves entry and immune evasion, particularly interfering with interferon responses. Preventive measures include tick avoidance, vaccination, public awareness, vector control and surveillance. Immunization of domestic animals may reduce virus reservoirs. Understanding these facets is vital for surveillance and control efforts.

Keywords: forest, climatic stress, vector, vaccine, tick

28.1 Introduction

Kyasanur Forest disease (KFD), commonly known as monkey fever, is a tick-borne viral zoonotic disease caused by the Kyasanur Forest disease virus (KFDV), an arbovirus belonging to the *Flaviviridae* family (Work, 1958). KFD is placed in the Biosafety Risk Group four category as per the guidelines of the Centers for Disease Control and Prevention (CDC) (Mourya *et al.*, 2014). The first outbreak of KFD was recorded in 1957 in the Kyasanur Forest region of Shimoga district in Karnataka, southern India (Work and Trapido, 1957). Subsequently, sporadic outbreaks have occurred in various parts of India, particularly in the Western Ghats range, including Karnataka, Kerala, Tamil Nadu, Goa and Maharashtra. The disease primarily affects two species of monkeys: red-faced bonnet monkeys (*Macaca radiata*) and black-faced langur (*Semnopithecus entellus*), which serve as the primary reservoir hosts (Pattnaik, 2006) (Fig. 28.1).

In goats, KFD manifests as fever, lethargy, reduced appetite, diarrhoea and haemorrhages. Infected goats may also exhibit neurological signs such as tremors, ataxia (loss of coordination) and paralysis, with severe cases leading to fatality. Humans visiting forests during outbreaks have also been affected by the disease (Mehla *et al.*, 2009). KFD outbreaks have been observed in new regions such as Wayanad and Malappuram districts of Kerala during 2014–2015 (Sadanandane *et al.*, 2017), and more recently in Goa, India (Patil *et al.*, 2017). In humans, KFD causes acute febrile illness that

*Corresponding author: dr.alokvet@gmail.com

 The Handbook of Zoonotic Diseases of Goats (ed. T. Rana)
DOI: 10.1079/ 9781800622852.0028

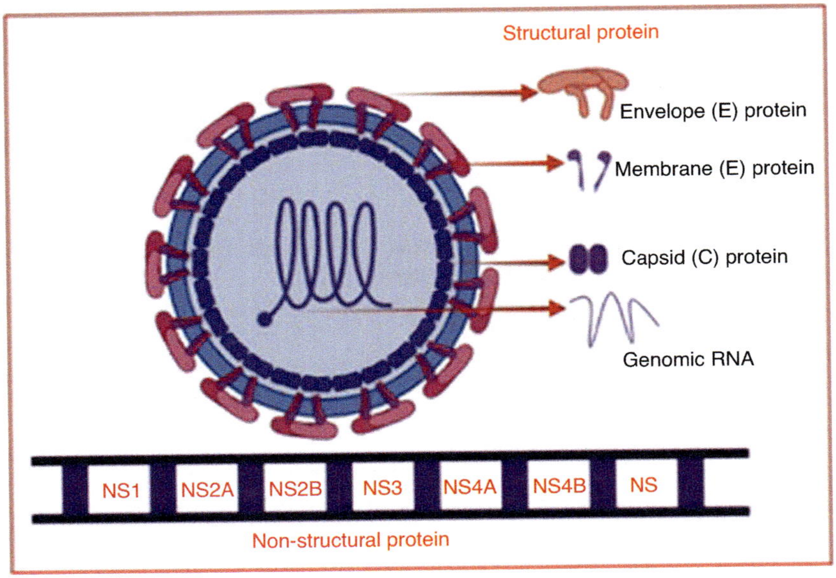

Fig. 28.1. Proposed possible pathogenesis mechanism of the KFDV. (Author's own image.)

can progress to haemorrhages, with mortality rates ranging from 2% to 10%. The virus also circulates in small animals such as rodents and shrews and also birds and other animals, including goats. Initially, KFD was localized to a specific geographical area. The spread of the disease to a wider range of areas can be attributed to the complex interplay of climate change, deforestation (Sadanandane *et al.*, 2018), tick populations and the distribution of animal and human hosts and reservoirs (Ogden *et al.*, 2013). Understanding these intricate interactions is crucial for implementing effective surveillance and control measures. Incorporating climate factors into disease modelling and management strategies can help mitigate the impact of climate change on KFD epidemics and enable the development of proactive measures to protect both human and animal populations.

28.2 Aetiology

KFD is caused by the Kyasanur Forest disease virus (KFDV), a spherical virus belonging to the *Flaviviridae* family. The KFDV has an envelope and a single-stranded RNA genome with a positive sense. It falls under the genus *Flavivirus*, along with other well-known viruses like the dengue fever, Zika and yellow fever viruses. The antigenic characteristics of KFDV are similar to those of other flaviviruses. KFDV possesses structural proteins, including the envelope (E) protein, membrane (M) protein and capsid (C) protein. These proteins are vital for viral replication, assembly and immune recognition.

The E protein is the main target for neutralizing antibodies and enables viral entry into host cells while also evading the host immune response (Fuzik *et al.*, 2018). The M protein contributes to viral envelope formation and participates in viral assembly. The C protein encloses the viral RNA genome and is involved in viral replication. In addition to the structural proteins, the KFDV has seven non-structural proteins: NS1, NS2A, NS2B, NS3, NS4A, NS4B and NS5 (Dodd *et al.*, 2011). These non-structural proteins play various roles in viral replication, immune evasion and modulation of host-cell functions (Kuzmenko *et al.*, 2016). Understanding the structure and functions of these viral proteins is crucial for studying KFDV infection and immune responses, and for developing potential interventions and vaccines. The genome of KFDV is very similar (> 92% homologous) to that of the Alkhurma haemorrhagic fever virus (ALKV), which is primarily found in Saudi Arabia.

28.3 Host

28.3.1 Natural host or reservoir host

The natural hosts or reservoir hosts of the KFDV are primarily small mammals and birds. These animals can become infected with the virus but do not usually develop a high level of viraemia (presence of virus in the bloodstream) or show symptoms of the disease. However, they can serve as a sufficient source of infection for ticks that feed on them. The reservoir hosts for the KFDV include porcupines, rats, squirrels, mice and certain bird species (Munivenkatappa, 2018).

28.3.2 Amplifying host

Primates such as black-faced hanuman langurs (*Presbytis entellus*) and red-faced bonnet monkeys (*Macaca radiata*) play a crucial role in amplifying the viral load (Work and Trapido, 1957). In infected monkeys, the virus multiplies within their bodies and they develop a high level of viraemia, thereby facilitating its transmission to other ticks.

28.3.3 Maintenance host

Larger animals such as goats, sheep and cattle can become infected with the KFDV, but their role in the transmission of the disease to humans is limited. They play an important ecological role in maintaining and distributing the tick population. Ticks, which act as vectors for the KFDV, can infest these animals and use them as hosts for feeding and reproduction (Pattnaik, 2006). As a result, the animals help sustain the tick population and provide a habitat for the ticks to thrive. The animals do not suffer from the disease, nor do they amplify the KFDV within their bodies. However, they have shown the presence of antibodies to the virus, indicating previous exposure (Fig. 28.2)

28.3.4 Dead-end/accidental host

Humans act as dead-end or accidental hosts for the KFDV. After infection, they do not

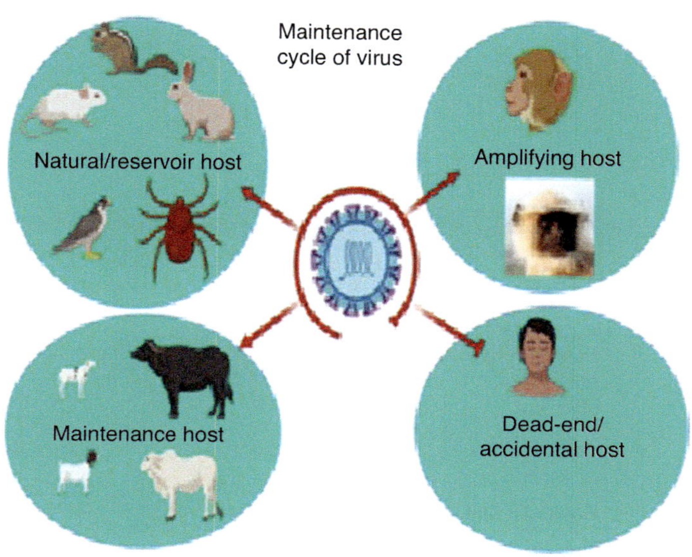

Fig. 28.2. Maintenance cycle of the KFDV. (Author's own image.)

actively contribute to the spread of the virus in the natural environment or to other humans (Chakraborty *et al.*, 2019). Human infections typically occur due to accidental exposure to infected ticks in forested areas or other tick-infested regions, leading to the individual suffering from the disease. There is no documented evidence of human-to-human transmission of the KFDV.

28.4 Vector

Ticks play a vital role as vectors in the transmission, maintenance and spread of the KFDV. Ticks belong to the family Ixodidae of the order Acarina, which falls under the subclass Acari and class Arachnida. In KFD-affected areas, a total of 41 species of ticks have been recorded (Muraleedharan, 2016). Among these, the KFDV has been isolated from 16 species. The genus *Haemaphysalis* comprises ten species from which the virus has been isolated, followed by two species from the genus *Ixodes*, and one species each from the genera *Dermacentor*, *Amblyomma*, *Rhipicephalus* and *Ornithodoros*. Within the KFD region, approximately 95% of the virus isolations have been obtained from *Haemaphysalis* ticks. Among them, *Haemaphysalis spinigera* is the most predominant species and has yielded the maximum number of virus isolates (Table 28.1).

28.5 Transmission

The wild monkeys *Semnopithecus entellus* and *Macaca radiata* get the disease through the bite of infected ticks. These hosts act as amplification hosts, allowing the virus to multiply within their bodies. When infected monkeys die, the ticks fall off their bodies and contribute to the further spread of the disease. Anthropogenic activities have increased the interaction between humans and domestic animals, resulting in infected ticks also biting domestic animals, which act as maintenance hosts for the virus, and humans also can get the disease from an infected tick bite or by contact with an infected animal (Fig. 28.3). Human-to-human transmission has still not been reported (Babu, 2019).

In humans, people with occupational exposure to rural or outdoor settings (e.g. hunters, herders, forest workers, farmers) in these districts are potentially at risk for infection if they come into contact with infected ticks. Some small mammals also can be infected through tick bites and play an important role in transmission of the virus as reservoir host. There is no evidence of disease transmission via the unpasteurized milk of any of these animals. The epidemic period usually begins in October or November and peaks from January to April, then declines by May and June. Epidemics and outbreaks relate to the activity of tick nymphs, which is very high during November to May.

Table 28.1. The most common species of ticks that play a role in virus transmission. (Author's own table.)

Genus	Species	References
Haemophysalis	*H. spinigera*, *H. turturis*, *H. kinneari*, *H. kyasanurensis*, *H. minuta*, *H. wellingtoni*, *H. cuspidata*, *H. bispinosa*, *H. intermedia*, *H. shimoga*	Muraleedharan, 2016 Anand, 2020
Ixodes	*I. petauristae*, *I. ceylonensis*	
Dermacentor	*D. auratus*	
Amblyomma	*Amblyomma* species	
Rhipicephalus	*R. haemophysaloides*	
Ornithodorous	*O. chiropterphite*	

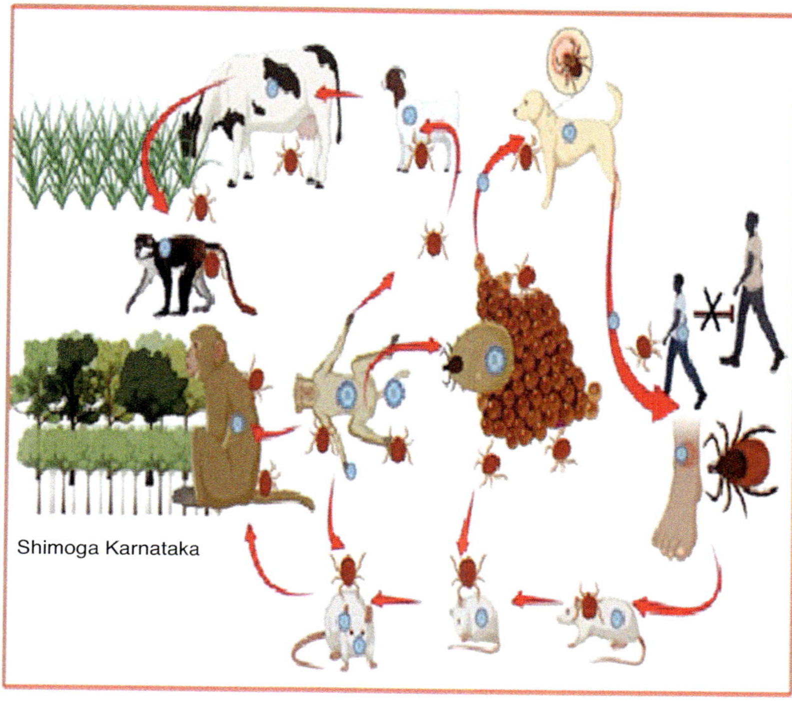

Fig. 28.3. Transmission cycle of the KFDV. (Author's own image.)

28.6 Distribution

The KFDV was endemic during 1957–2012, but its activity was limited to the coastal state of Karnataka in India. In 1957, KFD was reported around the Sagar and Sorab taluks in the Shimoga district of Karnataka (Work and Trapido, 1957; Work *et al.*, 1959; Bhatt *et al.*, 1966); subsequently it spread to other districts of Karnataka such as Chikmagalur, Uttara Kannada, Dakshina Kannada and Udupi. After that, in 2012 it was found in the Nilgiris district of Tamil Nadu state. During 2013–2015, confirmed cases were reported from Wayanad, Malappuram, Palakkad and Nilambur districts of Kerala State in the Sindhudurg district in Maharashtra (Awate *et al.*, 2016; Sadanandane *et al.*, 2017) (Fig. 28.4). Antibodies against the virus have also been detected in humans in areas of Gujarat state, parts of West Bengal, and the Andaman and Nicobar Islands (Pattnaik, 2006). Important outbreaks are listed in Table 28.2.

28.7 Proposed Possible Pathogenesis Mechanism of KFDV

There are various pathological mechanisms governing this multisystemic illness in monkeys and humans. Some clinical and laboratory findings have helped in the understanding of the pathobiology of KFD but it is still not clear, due to the lack of suitable *in vivo* and *in vitro* models of the disease. Some mechanisms underlying pathogenesis are common to all flaviviruses (Pastorino *et al.*, 2010). Based on published knowledge of the immunopathology of KFDV and closely related tick-borne flavivirus or haemorrhagic fever viruses, a hypothesized elucidation of the pathogenesis of KFDV infection has been presented in this section (Fig. 28.4). The virus enters the body of the host via a tick bite or via contact with an infected animal. The virus initially targets antigen-presenting cells (macrophages and dendritic cells). Multiplication of the virus occurs in these hosts (Fig. 28.5).

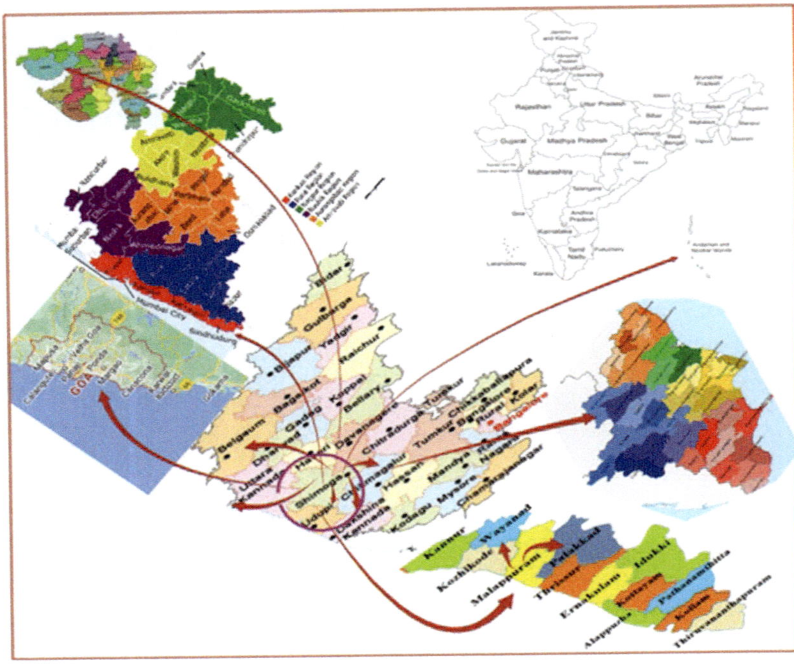

Fig. 28.4. Spreading potential of KFD in India. (Author's own image.)

The virus transmits through general body circulation and enters into the cell (viraemia) leading to systemic spread of the virus to spleen, liver and other tissue. Replications of virus in these sites produce disease symptoms. The infected antigen-presenting cells (macrophages and dendritic cells) revealed that viral antigens to T-cells release large numbers of pro-inflammatory cytokines early after KFV infection and also inflect host immune response by dint of type one interferon production. Activated T-cells might also produce IFN-1. Humoral immune response produced via antibodies formed by activated B-cells might also boost clearance of the virus from the body. To reverse the host immune response, the KFDV employs its NS5 non-structural protein to counteract the cytokine interferon gamma response by inhibiting JAK-STAT pathway (Best, 2017). The phenomenon results in abandoned viral replication and poor immune response in the host (Hollidge *et al.*, 2011). By inducing disseminated intravascular coagulation (DIC), neurological disorders and vascular dysfunction that reveal haemorrhagic manifestations, multiple organ failure and shock, the multisystemic disturbances like immunosuppression and disease progression might be associated with the pro-inflammatory cytokine storm. These complications combined will finally result in death.

28.8 Clinical Symptoms

28.8.1 In humans

The clinical manifestations of KFD can vary significantly at different stages of the disease's progression. Here is a detailed breakdown of the clinical symptoms in four stages.

1. **Incubation stage or initial prodromal stage:**
    - This stage lasts for about 3–8 days after the tick bite.
    - Most individuals remain asymptomatic during this period, showing no visible signs or symptoms.

Table 28.2. Important outbreaks of KFD in India. (Author's own table.)

Year	Outbreak location
1957	Shimoga, Karnataka
1975	Uttara Kannada, Karnataka
1990	Chikkamagalore, Uttara Kannada
2002	Shimoga, Uttara Kannada, Chikkamagalore, Udupi, Mangalore, Karnataka
2002	Andman nicobar
2005	Shimoga, Uttara Kannada, Chikkamagalore, Udupi, Mangalore, Karnataka
2010	Shimoga, Uttara Kannada, Chikkamagalore, Udupi, Mangalore, Karnataka
2012	Niligiris, Tamilnadu
2012	Bandipur national Tiger Reserve, Karnataka
2013	Wayanad, Kerala
2014	Kannangi and Konandur, Thirthahalli, Shimoga, Karnataka
2014	Wayanad, Kerala
2014	Malappuram, Kerala
2014	Palakkad and Wayanad, Kerala
2015	Nalambur and Malappuram, Kerala
2015	Wayanad, Kerala
2015	Shimoga, Karnataka
2015	Sattri taluk Goa
2016	Dobamarg, Sindhudrug, Maharashtra
2016	Khanapur, Belgaum, Karnataka
2016	Dharbandora taluk Goa
2017	Dobamarg, swantanwadi Sindhudrug, Maharashtra
2017	Valpoli taluk, Prenem taluk, Dharbandora taluk Goa
2018	Shivamogga, Maharashtra
2018	Karnataka
2019	Karnataka
2020	Karnataka

2. **Febrile stage:**

- The febrile stage typically follows the incubation period and lasts for 2–10 days.
- The most common manifestation is a sudden onset of high-grade fever, often exceeding 101°F (38.3°C).

Other symptoms that have been reported during the febrile stage include the following.

- Chills, severe headache, muscle and extremity pain, fatigue, conjunctivitis, decreased blood pressure, increased heart rate, headache and sore throat are generally observed.
- Nausea, vomiting, abdominal pain and diarrhoea are the main observable abdominal manifestations.
- Common ophthalmic manifestations are haemorrhages in conjunctiva, retina and vitreous humor, keratitis, opacity of the lens and mild iritis (Jhon, 2018).
- With pancytopenia, in haematological parameters mainly, low levels of platelet count, white

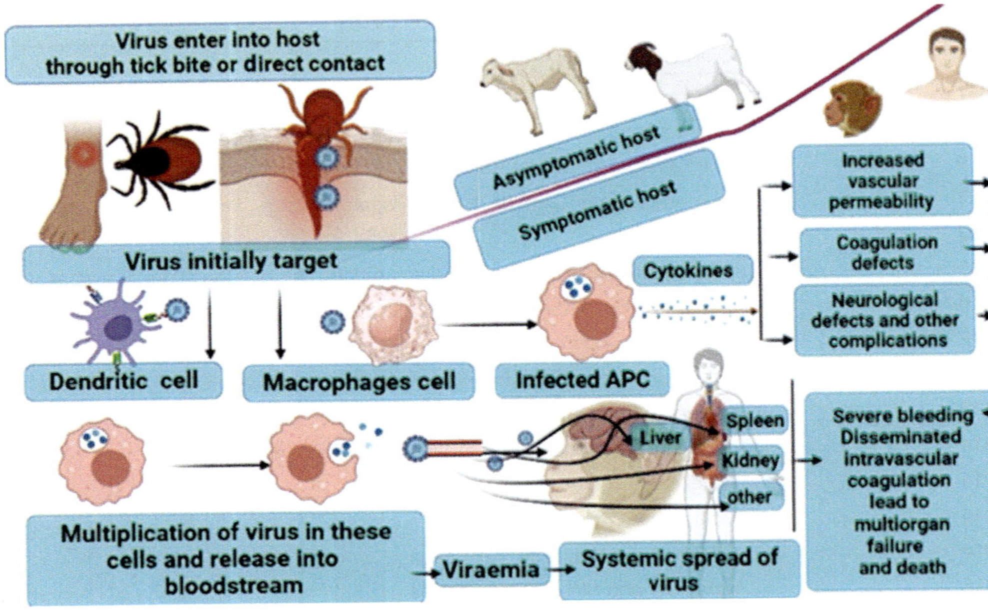

Fig. 28.5. Proposed possible pathogenesis mechanism of the KFDV. (Author's own image.)

blood cell count and red blood cell count are found.

3. Haemorrhagic stage:

- In some cases, after the febrile stage, patients may progress to the haemorrhagic stage, which usually begins around the second week.
- Haemorrhagic manifestations may include bleeding from the nose, gums and gastrointestinal tract.
- Small red or purple spots on the skin (petechiae) and larger areas of bruising (ecchymosis) may also appear.
- Patients may develop bleeding disorders and may experience heavy menstrual bleeding or bleeding into the urine.

4. **Recovery stage:**

- Following the haemorrhagic stage, patients usually enter a recovery phase.
- Symptoms gradually subside, and patients begin to show signs of improvement.
- Convalescence can take several weeks, with fatigue and weakness being common during this period.
- Some patients may exhibit various neurological complications, such as abnormal reflexes, confusion and tremors (Heymann, 2004; Pattnaik, 2006).

28.8.2 In monkeys

The disease manifestation in monkeys is more or less similar to that in human beings (Webb and Chaterjea, 1962) and is characterized by a high fatality rate, particularly in bonnet macaques, which has been reported as approximately 85%. It is also known as monkey disease or monkey fever because of its association with monkey deaths. In experiments, the KFDV has shown 100% case fatality rate (Kenyon *et al.*, 1992). High mortality of monkeys (epizootics) has been observed during the months of December to June, which coincides with the seasonal activity of nymphal stages of

Haemaphysalis ticks. Infected macaques show haematological changes such as thrombocytopenia and leukopenia, elevated alkaline phosphatase (ALP) and alanine transaminase (ALT) enzyme levels as well as phagocytosis of nuclear material in the peripheral blood and reticulo-endothelial system. Systemically, necrosis has been observed in the liver, spleen, kidney and occasionally the gastrointestinal tract. Neurological signs have been noted in bonnet macaques during the second febrile stage of experimental KFDV infection (Webb and Burston, 1966).

28.8.3 Domestic animals

In domestic animals, including goats, infections are generally asymptomatic.

28.9 Diagnosis

The diagnosis of KFD is primarily based on clinical manifestations, laboratory investigation, imaging and postmortem findings.

28.9.1 Clinical manifestations

The presence of characteristic clinical symptoms is important for suspecting KFD. Typically, the initial symptoms of KFD appearing within 3–8 days after a person is bitten by an infected tick include flu-like symptoms and may include high fever, headache, muscle pain and chills. Other symptoms that may develop in the later stages include bleeding manifestations (such as nosebleeds or gastrointestinal bleeding), vomiting, diarrhoea and altered mental status. A thorough assessment of the patient's medical history, including potential exposure to ticks or tick-infested areas, is also taken into account.

28.9.2 Laboratory investigations

Laboratory investigations play a crucial role in confirming the diagnosis of KFD. For the laboratory procedure some basic steps must be followed.

1. **Sample collection from infected patients**: Collect 4–5 ml of blood in a plain vial and separate the serum while adhering to standard biosafety precautions.
2. **Collection of monkey viscera:** Collect the different visceral organs from deceased monkeys and store them separately in labelled bottles while following standard biosafety precautions.
3. **Tick collection:** Collect nymph ticks from the endemic or infected areas and place them in an airtight, sterilized container.
4. **Sample storage:** If processing (or sending to a reference laboratory) is to be done within 48 hour, refrigerate the serum from human cases, viscera from monkeys and tick samples at 2–8°C. If processing is to be done after 1 week, freeze them at −10 to −20°C.
5. **Transportation:** For transportation to the reference laboratory, always use triple-layer packaging and ship the samples within 48 hour of collection under cold chain conditions (using dry ice or cooling gels at the very least). Pack, label and mark the original samples appropriately. Include a fully completed clinical and epidemiological record.

Laboratory tests

Laboratory tests include the following.

1. **Isolation of virus:** Virus can be isolated by inoculation into infant mice or in cell culture (Vero E6, BHK-21 or Chick embryo cells). Virus isolation from KFDV-positive samples should be carried out in a BSL-3 laboratory.
2. **Serological tests:** Blood samples are tested to detect antibodies against the KFDV.
    - Haemagglutination inhibition: antibodies if present react with viruses and inhibit agglutination of red blood cells.
    - Complement fixation: measuring amount of complement available in serum to bind with an antigen–antibody complex.
    - Neutralization test: neutralization of viruses by specific antibodies performed on 2–3-day-old mice.

3. **ELISA and IFA:** Enzyme-linked immunosorbent assay (ELISA) or indirect fluorescent antibody (IFA) tests are commonly used. A significant increase in antibody levels between acute and convalescent phase samples can help confirm the diagnosis. The KFD IgM antibody can be detected from 5th day of onset of symptoms until 3 months.
4. **Molecular testing:** Polymerase chain reaction (PCR) tests are used to detect the genetic material of the KFDV in blood or tissue samples. PCR is highly specific and sensitive in confirming the presence of the virus.

    - Reverse transcription polymerase chain reaction (RT–PCR) and real-time PCR are variants of PCR that allow for the continuous monitoring of the amplification process. RT–PCR can detect the virus in samples after onset of febrile illness up to the 8th day. It provides rapid and accurate detection of the KFDV by measuring the fluorescence emitted during the amplification. Real-time PCR is known for its high sensitivity and specificity.
    - Next-generation sequencing (NGS) technologies allow for the rapid and comprehensive sequencing of the entire genetic material of the KFDV. NGS can provide valuable insights into the viral genome, genetic variations and evolution of the virus.

5. **Complete blood count (CBC):** Blood tests may reveal abnormalities such as a decrease in platelet count (thrombocytopenia) and an increase in white blood cell count (leukocytosis).

28.9.3 Imaging

In severe cases or when neurological symptoms are present, imaging studies such as computed tomography (CT) scan or magnetic resonance imaging (MRI) may be conducted to assess brain involvement and rule out other possible causes.

28.9.4 Differential diagnosis

The symptoms of KFD can resemble those of other infectious diseases such as dengue fever, malaria, or other tick-borne illnesses. Differential diagnosis helps exclude other potential causes and narrow down the specific disease.

28.10 Treatment

Currently, no specific antiviral treatment exists for KFDV in humans. Early hospitalization and supportive treatment become more essential. Treatment should be planned according to individual complication and severity.

28.11 Prevention and Control

Prevention and control measures for KFD primarily involve reducing exposure to infected ticks and implementing public health interventions. Here are some key strategies.

- **Tick avoidance:** Minimize exposure to tick-infested areas, particularly during peak tick activity seasons. Wear appropriate clothing such as long sleeves, long trousers and closed-toe shoes to reduce exposed skin. Tuck in clothing and use insect repellents containing DEET (*N,N*-diethyl-*meta*-toluamide) on exposed skin.
- **Tick checks:** Perform regular tick checks on yourself, family members and pets after potential exposure to tick habitats. Promptly remove any attached ticks using fine-tipped tweezers, grasping the tick close to the skin's surface and pulling straight upwards with steady pressure.
- **Vaccination:** Vaccination is available for KFD in endemic areas. Consult with healthcare professionals or local health authorities to determine if vaccination is recommended for individuals at risk. An inactivated/killed tissue culture vaccine has been used in endemic areas of Karnataka, India, since 1990. Initially two doses were used in people aged 7–65 years, at an interval of 4 weeks. Revaccination is required

after 6–9 months for 5 years (Kasabi *et al.*, 2013).

- **Awareness and education:** Promote public awareness campaigns about KFD, its symptoms, transmission and preventive measures. Educate communities, health-care providers and veterinary professionals about the disease to enhance early detection and appropriate management.
- **Vector control:** Implement measures to control tick populations in endemic areas, such as environmental modification, use of acaricides (tick-killing agents) and targeted treatment of domestic animals to reduce tick infestations.
- **Surveillance and reporting:** Establish active surveillance systems to monitor KFD cases in humans and animals. Encourage reporting of suspected cases to local health authorities for timely response and implementation of control measures.
- **Hygiene practices:** Encourage personal hygiene practices, such as regular hand-washing with soap and water, especially after outdoor activities in tick-prone areas.
- **Animal vaccination:** Consider vaccination programmes for domestic animals, such as cattle, dogs and goats, in endemic regions to reduce the reservoir of the virus and minimize transmission to humans.

References

Anand, K.J. (2020) Ticks and its vectorial potentiality for outbreak of kyasanur forest disease in Shivamogga: A malnad region of Karnataka. In: *XVII AZRA International Conference on 'Frontier Research in Applied Zoology and Insect Pest Management Strategies: A Way Forward for Food and Nutritional Security'*, Raichur, Karnataka, 12-14 February 2020.

Awate, P., Yadav, P., Patil, D., Shete, A., Kumar, V. *et al.* (2016) Outbreak of Kyasanur forest disease (monkey fever) in Sindhudurg, Maharashtra State, India, 2016. *The Indian Journal of Medical Research* 62(4), 497–510.

Babu, N.N., Jayaram, A., Kumar, H.H., Pareet, P., Pattanaik, S. *et al.* (2019) Spatial distribution of *Haemaphysalis* species ticks and human Kyasanur forest disease cases along the Western Ghats of India, 2017–2018. *Experimental and Applied Acarology* 77, 435–447.

Best, S.M. (2017) The many faces of the flavivirus NS5 protein in antagonism of type I interferon signaling. *Journal of Virology* 91(3), 10–11.

Bhatt, P.M., Work, T.H., Varma, M.G., Trapido, H., Murthy, D.P. *et al.* (1966) Tracing of viruses of tick-borne and Japanese encephalitis in cultures of transplanted cells using the fluorescent antibody method. *Indian Journal of Medical Sciences* 20(5), 316–320.

Chakraborty, S., Andrade, F.C.D., Ghosh, S., Uelmen, J. and Ruiz, M.O. (2019) Historical expansion of Kyasanur forest disease in India from 1957 to 2017: A retrospective analysis. *GeoHealth* 3(2), 44–55.

Dodd, K.A., Bird, B.H., Khristova, M.L., Albarino, C.G., Carroll, S.A. *et al.* (2011) Ancient ancestry of KFDV and AHFV revealed by complete genome analyses of viruses isolated from ticks and mammalian hosts. *PLoS Neglected Tropical Diseases* 5(10), 1352.

Fuzik, T., Formanová, P., Ruzek, D., Yoshii, K., Niedrig, M. *et al.* (2018) Structure of tick-borne encephalitis virus and its neutralization by a monoclonal antibody. *Nature Communications* 9(1), 1–11.

Heymann, D.L. (2004) *Control of Communicable Diseases Manual*, 18th edn. American Public Health Association, Washington, DC.

Hollidge, B.S., Weiss, S.R. and Soldan, S.S. (2011) The role of interferon antagonist, non-structural proteins in the pathogenesis and emergence of arboviruses. *Viruses* 3(6), 629–658.

Jhon, N.S. (2018) Kyasanur forest disease: A case series from Wayanad, Kerala, India. *Indian Journal of Critical Care Medicine* 22(11), 811–813.

Kasabi, G.S., Murhekar, M.V., Sandhya, V.K., Raghunandan, R., Kiran, S.K. *et al.* (2013) Coverage and effectiveness of Kyasanur Forest Disease (KFD) vaccine in Karnataka, South India, 2005–10. *PLoS Neglected Tropical Diseases* 7(1).

Kenyon, R.H., Rippy, M.K., McKee, K.T.J., Zack, P.M. and Peters, C.J. (1992) Infection of *Macaca radiata* with viruses of the tick-borne encephalitis group. *Microbial Pathogenesis* 13, 399–409.

Kuzmenko, Y.V., Smirnova, O.A., Ivanov, A.V., Starodubova, E.S. and Karpov, V.L. (2016) Nonstructural protein 1 of tick-borne encephalitis virus induces oxidative stress and activates antioxidant defense by the Nrf2/ARE pathway. *Intervirology* 59, 111–117.

Mehla, R., Kumar, S.R., Yadav, P., Barde, P.V., Yergolkar, P.N. *et al.* (2009) Recent ancestry of Kyasanur Forest disease virus. *Emerging Infectious Diseases* 15(9), 1431.

Mourya, D.T., Yadav, P.D. and Patil, D.Y. (2014) Highly infectious tick borne viral diseases: Kyasanur forest disease and Crimean–Congo hemorrhagicfever in India. *WHO South–East Asia Journal of Public Health* 3(1), 8–21.

Munivenkatappa, A., Sahay, R.R., Yadav, P.D., Viswanathan, R. and Mourya, D.T. (2018) Clinical & epidemiological significance of Kyasanur forest disease. *Indian Journal of Medical Research* 148(2), 145–150.

Muraleedharan, K. (2016) Wildlife arthropods of Karnataka with special reference to KFD endemic area of Shivamogga District: Those parasitic on small and large mammals. *Veterinary Research International* 04(04), 114–123.

Ogden, N.H., Samir, M. and Gabriele, M. (2013) Changing geographic ranges of ticks and tick-borne pathogens: Drivers, mechanisms and consequences for pathogen diversity. *Frontiers in Cellular and Infection Microbiology* 3, 46.

Pastorino, B., Nougairède, A., Wurtz, N., Gould, E. and de Lamballerie, X. (2010) Role of host cell factors in flavivirus infection: Implications for pathogenesis and development of antiviral drugs. *Antiviral Research* 87, 281–294.

Patil, D.Y., Yadav, P.D., Shete, A.M., Nuchina, J., Meti, R. *et al.* (2017) Occupational exposure of cashew nut workers to Kyasanur forest disease in Goa, India. *International Journal of Infectious Diseases* 61, 67–69.

Pattnaik, P. (2006) Kyasanur forest disease: An epidemiological view in India. *Reviews in Medical Virology* 16(3), 151–165.

Sadanandane, C., Elango, A., Marja, N., Sasidharan P.V., Raju, K.H.K. and Jambulingam, P. (2017) An outbreak of Kyasanur forest disease in the Wayanad and Malappuram districts of Kerala, India. Ticks and Tick-borne Diseases 1, 25–30.

Sadanandane, C., Gokhale, M.D., Elango, A., Yadav, P., Mourya, D.T. *et al.* (2018) Prevalence and spatial distribution of Ixodid tick populations in the forest fringes of Western Ghats reported with human cases of kyasanur forest disease and monkey deaths in South India. *Experimental and Applied Acarology* 75(1), 135–142.

Webb, H.E. and Burston, D. (1966) Studies on Kyasanur Forest disease in monkeys. II. The early viraemic phase. *Indian Journal of Medical Research* 54(1), 77–90.

Webb, H.E. and Chaterjea, P.N. (1962) Studies on Kyasanur Forest disease in monkeys. I. Clinical and pathological findings in naturally and experimentally infected animals. *Indian Journal of Medical Research* 50(6), 947–963.

Work, T.H. (1958) Kyasanur forest disease. II. Pathologic studies. *The American Journal of Tropical Medicine and Hygiene* 7(5), 594–600.

Work, T.H. and Trapido, H. (1957) Kyasanur forest disease, a new virus disease in India. *Indian Journal of Medical Sciences* 11(5), 341–345.

Work, T.H., Roderiguez, F.R. and Bhatt, P.N. (1959) Virological epidemiology of the 1958 epidemic of Kyasanur forest disease. *American Journal of Public Health and the Nation's Health* 49(7), 869–874.

29 Cryptosporidiosis

Shashi Pradhan*, Aditya Pratap, Pooja Dawar and Akansha Aguihotri
Department of Veterinary Medicine, College of Veterinary Science and Animal Husbandry, NDVSU, Jabalpur, MP, India

Abstract

Cryptosporidium, a genus of single-celled parasites, is widely distributed in vertebrates and causes mainly gastrointestinal disease in mammals and reptiles, and intestinal, renal and respiratory disease in birds. Diarrhoea in neonatal ruminants is thought to be caused in part by *Cryptosporidium parvum*, which is associated with significant direct and indirect economic losses. It is acquired orally through contaminated water and is often spread through faeces. Weather-resistant oocysts are shed in the faeces of infected animals and are transmitted via the faecal–oral route by ingestion of contaminated feed or drinking water. Young animals are a major source of environmental pollution. The highest shedding rates have been reported in lambs aged 8–14 days. In outbreaks of cryptosporidiosis in goat kids the morbidity varies from 80% to 100% and the mortality rate may exceed 50% in young kids. The diagnosis of cryptosporidiosis is usually done by using microscopic detection of the parasite. Microscopically, oocysts (morphology) or oocyst antigens or oocyst DNA in stool samples can also be used to detect the infective organism.

Keywords: diarrhoea, economic loss, faecal–oral route, morbidity, lambs

29.1 Introduction

Members of the genus *Cryptosporidium*, an obligate intracellular protozoan belonging to the phylum Apicomplexa, are responsible for the diarrhoeal disease known as cryptosporidiosis. It acutely and briefly infects the intestines of newborns, causing diarrhoea (Xiao *et al.*, 2004). *Cryptosporidium*, a single-celled parasite, is widely distributed in vertebrates and causes mainly gastrointestinal disease in mammals and reptiles, and intestinal, renal and respiratory disease in birds. Respiratory diseases in mammals, including humans, are also observed, though very rarely. Although infections have been reported in fish and amphibians, the disease is poorly characterized.

In human cryptosporidiosis, symptoms can last up to 3 weeks but usually resolve on their own. However, the disease can be protracted and life-threatening in immunocompromised patients. Transmission is faecal–oral through direct contact with an infected host or through multiple vehicles, including recreational and drinking water, food, or carriers (Giles *et al.*, 2009).

Understanding the host, source of infection and mode of transmission is critical for controlling this parasite, for which specific therapeutic options are limited and vaccines are scarce. Zoonotic transmission has long been known. The first human case was reported in 1976.

Diarrhoea in neonatal ruminants is thought to be caused in part by *Cryptosporidium*

*Corresponding author: shee1811@gmail.com

 The Handbook of Zoonotic Diseases of Goats (ed. T. Rana)
DOI: 10.1079/ 9781800622852.0029

parvum and is associated with significant direct and indirect economic losses. It is acquired orally through contaminated water and is often spread through faeces. Weather-resistant oocysts are shed in the faeces of infected animals. After ingestion, the oocysts are believed to excyst and invade the intestinal epithelium. Cryptosporidia, which do not require vectors or intermediate hosts, can complete their life cycle in a single host and can also infect themselves. Neonatal animals less than 3 months old usually show clinical symptoms for 5–15 days. Mild to severe diarrhoea is the main symptom of cryptosporidiosis, but it can also cause additional clinical symptoms such as depression, dehydration, anorexia, lethargy, lack of thrift and abdominal pain (Paul *et al.*, 2014).

One of the first domesticated animals, goats are used worldwide for their milk, meat, hides and wool. Goats are now one of the most popular and valuable animals for those without money. Small-scale goat production provides great benefits to families and communities around the world in a variety of climates and conditions (Utaaker *et al.*, 2021).

In a world where our future is increasingly determined by adaptation to climate change, goat farming is critical not only to maintain production levels but also because it has a relatively low climate impact. According to the Food and Agriculture Organization (FAO), more than 90% of goats live in developing countries. Asia accounts for the largest share of the world's goat population, followed by Africa (Utaaker *et al.*, 2021).

Goats are traditionally raised differently than cattle, with herds grazing in spacious pens or unfenced rather than being kept indoors. Goats are also popular backyard livestock for needy homes with few supplies. These environments weaken the barriers to animal-to-human transmission of zoonotic diseases. Therefore, when promoting and supporting goat farming, it is important that efforts are also made to minimize the transmission of pathogens between goats and their owners (Utaaker *et al.*, 2021).

In low-income countries, for example in Asia, Africa and Latin America, locally adapted goat breeds are bred for milk and meat; and in dry, drought-prone regions, goat's milk is the only protein source in children's diets. In countries where goats are the most abundant, most goat owners are of low socioeconomic class (Utaaker *et al.*, 2021), and in rural areas goats are mainly kept to earn a basic living for the household. In many texts, goats are rightly regarded as more important than cattle in rural areas (Pumipuntu and Piratae, 2018).

Cryptosporidium infection in goats has an impact on growth and production and has been found to cause anorexia and diarrhoea in goat kids, with morbidity and mortality reaching 50% and 100%, respectively, with accompanying economic consequences, impacting especially marginal farmers. Reduced growth, with and without diarrhoea, has also been associated with *Cryptosporidium* infections in goats aged between 9 and 15 months, including in asymptomatic goats, raising further questions regarding the long-term effects of apparently asymptomatic infections. Some studies have reported asymptomatic shedding of *Cryptosporidium* oocysts in adult goats, but the long-term effects of chronic asymptomatic infections remain unclear, and goat health protocols recommend screening for *Cryptosporidium* infections after weaning, even in the absence of diarrhoea (Utaaker *et al.*, 2021).

Cryptosporidium infection is distributed worldwide but its impact on human health is seen to be greater in developing countries. Although global health is steadily improving, diarrhoeal disease remained the third most common cause of disability-adjusted life-years (DALYs) in the under-10-years age group in 2019.

Due to the high prevalence of cryptosporidiosis among people living in resource-poor areas, this pathogen was included in the World Health Organization's (WHO) Neglected Diseases Initiative in 2004. *Cryptosporidium* infections in humans are associated with diarrhoea, especially in children, but play a minor role in causing diarrhoea in the elderly population. Significant mortality in children under 5 years of age (7.6 deaths per 100,000) from cryptosporidiosis has been reported. This likely reflects that cryptosporidiosis is acute and that explosive and profuse diarrhoea is likely to have a large and direct impact on infant survival. Cryptosporidia damage intestinal cells and reduce nutrient absorption. A meta-analysis suggests that the true burden of cryptosporidiosis was probably underestimated in previous reports. This is because the post-acute phase effects of infection (reduced growth and subsequent increased risk of infection) are not considered (Utaaker *et al.*, 2021).

29.2 *Cryptosporidium*: Taxonomy and Life Cycle

The genus *Cryptosporidium* is classified under the family Cryptosporidiidae and order Eucoccidiorida. A member of the phylum Apicomplexa and of the class Sporozoasida, this protozoan genus was previously thought to be closely associated with coccidia, owing to the morphological similarities and presence of organelles resembling mitochondria. *Cryptosporidium* species parasitize the microvillous border of the gastrointestinal (GI) epithelium of a broad range of vertebrates, including cattle, buffalo, sheep, goats, reptiles and humans (Paul *et al.*, 2014).

Cycles of infection generate robust encapsulated oocyst stages that are shed in billions in the faeces of infected hosts. Transmission of the parasite can be via the faecal–oral route or directly through contamination of the water supply with oocysts, the infectious stage of the parasite (Xiao *et al.*, 2004).

Development of genetic tools for the taxonomic characterization of *Cryptosporidium* allows direct assessment of the potential for human infection with environmental *Cryptosporidium* oocysts. Currently, the identification of the oocysts in environmental samples is primarily based on immunofluorescence assays (IFA) through an enrichment process. The IFA detects all types of oocysts, but cannot assess the species distribution in environmental samples. Although many surface-water samples contain oocysts, it is unlikely that all of these oocysts originated from a human pathogenic species or genotype.

C. parvum, *C. hominis*, *C. meleagridis*, *C. canis* and *C. felis* are responsible for most human cryptosporidial infections. Accurate water pollution risk assessment requires information on the identification of *Cryptosporidium* oocysts. Assignment of oocysts to species and genotypes is therefore of public health importance. Several methods of species identification and genotyping are used. The SSU-rRNA-based nested PCR–RFLP method has been successfully used to detect and differentiate *Cryptosporidium* oocysts present in rainwater, raw surface water and wastewater. In one study, 29 rainwater samples were collected from streams serving the New York City water supply system and analysed. Twelve wild-animal *Cryptosporidium* genotypes were detected in 27 of the 29 positive samples. None of these genotypes has been found in humans, so they are unlikely to infect humans (Xiao *et al.*, 2004).

A major reason for the long controversy in *Cryptosporidium* taxonomy is the difficulty in meeting the definition of biological species. The classical definition of species defined as a group of outbred natural populations reproductively isolated from other groups is difficult to apply to many organisms, including *Cryptosporidium*. Although *Cryptosporidium* has a sexual stage and intraspecific sexual recombination has been demonstrated in *C. parvum*, the parasite's enormous reproductive potential results in large numbers of genes in localized regions. Mating is therefore usually between siblings. Consequently, *Cryptosporidium* has a strong propensity for clonal population structure, as shown by multilocus analyses (Xiao *et al.*, 2004).

Different *Cryptosporidium* oocysts look morphologically similar. Differentiating oocyst morphometry can play an important role in the identification of several *Cryptosporidium* species; for example, established species in birds and reptiles are easily distinguished by oocyst size and shape. There are also large differences in morphometry among mammalian gut species. A species description, therefore, includes a series of morphological measurements of a population of oocysts (usually 20–100 oocysts), along with the mean, range and possibly standard deviation or confidence limits. Whenever possible, oocysts should be collected and sporozoite sizes measured.

Cycles of infection result in the generation of robust cystic oocyst stages, which are shed in billions in the faeces of infected hosts. The oocysts are fully sporulated upon elimination. There are two types of oocysts: thick-walled and thin-walled. Thick-walled oocysts are excreted in the faeces and infect other hosts, whereas thin-walled oocysts rupture in the gut and the released sporozoites carry out endogenous autoinfection, a unique feature of the genus *Cryptosporidium*. After ingestion by the host, the oocysts excyst and release four motile sporozoites that subsequently invade and parasitize epithelial cells of the gastrointestinal tract (they rarely parasitize extraintestinal sites). Successive endogenous developmental stages are commonly found on the microvillus surface of epithelial host cells, usually in intracellular but also extracytoplasmic locations (Paul *et al.*, 2014).

Sporozoites are nucleated, spindle-shaped and 5.0 μm × 0.5 μm. The apical complex plays a role in gliding movements to access target cells. The nucleus is in the centre of the cell. Sporozoites recognize and invade target host cells, including in the stomach (*C. muris* and *C. andersoni*) and intestine (such as *C. parvum* and *C. hominis*). Invading sporozoites arise near the parasitic cytoplasmic vacuole (PCV), where they differentiate to form the trophozoite stages, about 1.5–2.5 μm in diameter, within the parasitic cytoplasmic vacuole (Pumipuntu and Piratae, 2018).

Trophozoites initiate three merogonies and produce type I meronts containing eight merozoites (morphologically resembling rod-shaped 0.4 × 1.0 μm sporozoites). Type I merozoites can re-invade host cells and reproduce asexually from type I meronts containing eight merozoites or from type II meronts containing only four merozoites. Merozoites that are released from type II meronts are likely to be less uniform in shape, slightly larger and less agile than the merozoites released from type I meronts. The released merozoites may develop into microgamonts (males) or macrogamonts (females) that will further undergo the process of gametogenesis. Each microgamont produces 16 microgametes that are rod-shaped, devoid of flagella, and 1.4 × 0.5 μm in size. They fertilize with unicellular adjacent macrogamonts, which are globular to ovoid structures 4–6 μm in diameter with a large central nucleus. After two rounds of mitosis, the fertilized egg develops as either thin-walled oocysts covering only a monolayer or thick-walled oocysts containing a bilayer membrane. Thick-walled oocysts are released through faeces, whereas thin-walled oocysts can be re-released in the same host's gastrointestinal tract by rupturing and releasing infectious sporozoites.

29.3 Epidemiology of Caprine Cryptosporidiosis

Neonatal deaths are seen as a major development hurdle that negatively impacts the economy of goat farming. The widely held belief that *Escherichia coli* is the primary cause of diarrhoea in goats and in children contrasts with several reports in which large-scale laboratory analyses have revealed the genus *Cryptosporidium*. It was previously overlooked as one of the most common pathogens of neonatal diarrhoea. The first case of *Cryptosporidium* infection in goats was reported from Australia, where a 2-week-old Angora goat kid died following a short clinical course characterized by diarrhoea. Caprine cryptosporidiosis has been reported all over the globe, including in Australia, South America, France, Spain and other European countries. The disease has been reported in Sri Lanka and, lately, cryptosporidiosis in goats has also been reported in India (Paul *et al.*, 2014).

During an epidemiological study of the possible animal source of sporadic human cases of cryptosporidiosis in south-west England (Giles *et al.*, 2009), a pygmy goat (*Capra hircus*) was found to be excreting a moderate number of *Cryptosporidium* oocytes (5×10^5 oocysts per gram of faeces). The oocysts were identified by a modified Ziehl–Nielsen microscope. The *Cryptosporidium* species was tested using a nested PCR restriction fragment length polymorphism (RFLP) assay targeting the small subunit (SSU) rRNA gene (Xiao *et al.*, 2004) and a multiple allele-specific PCR assay. The species was determined as *Cryptosporidium hominis*. This was independently confirmed by PCR–RFLP of the COWP locus and sequencing of an 830 base-pair (BP) fragment of SSU rRNA genes (Xiao *et al.*, 2004). The pygmy goat came from a petting farm which had a variety of species, including goats, sheep and cows. PCR analysis of faecal samples from some animals on the farm showed that *C. parvum* was also present. A 10-month-old child who visited the petting farm weeks before the onset of symptoms was screened for *Cryptosporidium* sp. after being diagnosed with *C. hominis* infection (Giles *et al.*, 2009).

It is well known that young animals and humans are most at risk of *Cryptosporidium* infection and most likely to develop symptomatic disease when infected. Other epidemiological aspects concern routes of exposure and geographical, meteorological, cultural and other environmental factors that may influence transmission patterns. In relation to the epidemiological pressure of transmission between goats and humans, it is interesting to examine where zoonotic transmission from goats to humans has been documented. We know that populations in Africa, Asia and Latin America bear the brunt of the global cryptosporidiosis burden, but high infection rates make it difficult to identify specific transmission opportunities or outbreaks in these countries. However, outbreaks can also be detected in other countries, some associated with direct or indirect contact between goats (and their produce) and humans. For example, an outbreak of cryptosporidiosis in the United States was associated with the consumption of unpasteurized goat's milk. An outbreak of cryptosporidiosis in Norwegian schoolchildren was associated with tourism farms, with the same subtype associated with exposure of lambs and children – *C. parvum* is found in lambs as well as children. It is also worth noting that in studies in which *Cryptosporidium* species were identified, surveys detected all but two zoonotic species of particular relevance to human health in relation to goats and cryptosporidiosis and that children are most affected in countries where cryptosporidiosis is a particular burden as described above. It is also children who most often have contact with goats in the same part of the world. The grazing habits of goats, which generally eat shrubs and weeds rather than grasses, may indicate that they are less likely to ingest parasites (Utaaker *et al.*, 2021). However, in many environments, particularly urban and suburban areas with sparse shrubbery, the animals are forced to forage for nutrients close to the ground, where they are more likely to ingest the parasite. The oocysts contaminating the environment may have been shed by human children caring for the goats, or by baby goats foraging nearby. Similarly, children caring for a herd of young goats can be exposed to the infectious stage of the parasite found in goat droppings. In cooler climates of temperate regions, cattle, especially calves, are often considered a zoonotic source of *Cryptosporidium*. In other parts of the world, goats appear to be an even more likely source (Utaaker *et al.*, 2021).

29.3.1 *Cryptosporidium* as a one health model pathogen

Oocysts are the environmental stages of parasites responsible for transmission between humans and animals. Although oocysts contain wall structures that are highly resistant to chemicals, including disinfectants, the four sporozoites within the oocyst wall are sensitive to temperature changes and desiccation, probably due to the presence of the stress protectant trehalose. For these reasons, *Cryptosporidium* oocysts are a major environmental contaminant responsible for numerous waterborne outbreaks of cryptosporidiosis worldwide. Long-surviving oocysts are transported in water and soil to different locations around the world, interacting with humans and animals, adapting to new environments and hosts, and contributing to the evolution of cryptosporidiosis epidemiology and population structure. Therefore, *Cryptosporidium* serves as one of the One Health model pathogens that affect human, animal and environmental health on a regional and global scale.

Exposure to *Cryptosporidium* parasites early in life may be relevant for limiting future infection (as with older children responsible for herding small ruminants, for example), including with zoonotic species. Other associated risk factors may support the prevalence of the infection in Africa. These could include concurrent infections or conditions that may limit the robustness or effect of an immune response against future challenges. It is well known that most people living with HIV reside in Africa, with 25.7 million estimated by the WHO in 2018, compared with 3.8 million in South-east Asia and 3.5 million in the Americas. Cryptosporidiosis is known as one of the major causes of diarrhoea in patients with HIV, and is associated with significant morbidity and mortality in the AIDS population; a recent systematic review and meta-analysis indicated that the pooled prevalence of *Cryptosporidium* in HIV-positive patients in Africa was around 11.9% (CI: 8.8–16.0%), only marginally below that of South-east Asia, which topped the list at 12.7% (CI: 9.7–16.4%). It is not surprising that reports on zoonotic *Cryptosporidium* infections in Africa with species other than *C. parvum* are common in immunocompromised people, especially those with HIV. Other human health disorders, including malnutrition and other infectious diseases, which are more common in some African countries, not only exacerbate symptoms but also make individuals susceptible to infectious diseases, partly by suppressing immunity. It is also clear that it can make it easier to get sick (Robertson *et al.*, 2020).

In addition to the effects of infection on the immune system and other factors, genetic variation within the population itself can render individuals or populations more or less susceptible to particular infectious diseases. For cryptosporidiosis, candidate genetic studies suggesting an increased risk of cryptosporidiosis include variations within human leukocyte antigen (HLA) class I and II genes, mannose-binding lectin (MBL) gene single nucleotide polymorphisms (SNPs), and protein kinase C alpha (PRKCA) genes. Some of these variations are of particular importance to Africans; for example, average blood MBL protein concentrations in Africans have been found to be significantly lower than in other racial groups. In contrast, a relatively high number of 'at-risk' T alleles in the PRKCA gene have been reported. It is common in Africa and least common in West Africa. Whether these genetic variants affect zoonotic transmission (zoonotic *C. parvum* infection) remains to be investigated (Robertson *et al.*, 2020).

29.4 Sources and Transmission of Infection

Being a monoxenous parasite with a direct life cycle, *Cryptosporidium* is therefore transmitted via the faecal–oral route by ingestion of contaminated feed and oocysts via feed or drinking water. Young animals are a major source of environmental pollution because they shed *Cryptosporidium* oocysts. The rate of oocyst shedding depends on the severity of the infection and the age of the animal. Adult animals also excrete oocysts into the environment, but to varying degrees. Nevertheless, the main burden on the environment is caused by small children. Newborns have a very low infectious dose, and the minimum infectious dose in gnotobiotic lambs varies from one to five oocysts (Paul *et al.*, 2014).

When humans or animals ingest oocysts, sporozoites are released from the oocysts, enter intestinal epithelial cells, and begin intracellular development. In humans and other mammals, the ileum is the primary site of infection for intestinal *Cryptosporidium* species (Zhu *et al.*, 2021).

Parasites primarily infect intestinal epithelial cells and are separated from the host-cell cytosol by electron-dense (ED) bands and associated structures, whereas host-cell-derived parasitophorous vacuole membrane (PVM). *Cryptosporidium* species are localized in the epicytoplasm in comparison to other apicomplexan parasites such as *Eimeria*, *Toxoplasma* and *Plasmodium* that reside in the host-cell cytosol.

The age of the animal has a significant effect on the frequency of *Cryptosporidium* isolates. The highest shedding rates have been reported in lambs aged 8–14 days, of whom 76% shed oocysts. In naturally infected children, shedding of *Cryptosporidium* oocysts begins at 4 days of age, peaks at 7 days of age, and declines at 3 weeks of age (Paraud *et al.*, 2010).

Of the 19 currently active *Cryptosporidium* species, 13 infect mammals, 3 infect birds, 2 infect reptiles and 1 infects amphibian. (There is no valid species name for the fish cryptosporidia.) Species identification requires sufficient information on morphological characteristics, host range, genetic data and more. Genetically distinct isolates for which there is insufficient data are called genotypes. These are commonly named after the animals in which they were first discovered. Some adaptation to the host is evident. *Cryptosporidium* species that infect reptiles, amphibians and fish do not appear to infect mammals or birds. Two of the three species that infect birds are confined to birds. Interestingly, the only intestinal avian species, *Cryptosporidium meleagridis*, infects many mammalian hosts, including humans. Among the *Cryptosporidium* species that infect mammals, several exhibit some degree of host adaptation, with rare reports of aberrant infections, limited numbers of oocysts detected, and persistence in populations. The lack of evidence of normal transmission suggests that cross-infection under normal circumstances is possible but not typical. Species and genotypes with the widest host range include *C. parvum*, *C. meleagridis*, *C. muris* and a *Cryptosporidium* deer genotype. The biological mechanisms of host adaptation and virulence are not yet fully understood.

Cryptosporidium infection is transmitted by ingestion of oocysts, direct licking of contaminated material, or ingestion of contaminated food or drinking water. Prevalence in diarrhoea-free, pre-weaned animals varies widely, ranging from 2% to 85% in lambs and 5 to 30% in kids. Diarrhoeic kids excrete very high numbers of oocysts between 7 and 21 days of age.

29.5 Pathogenesis

The pathogenesis of cryptosporidiosis is rather unclear. The characteristic diarrhoea results from dyspepsia and malabsorption due to a reduction in both the enzymatic activity and absorptive area of the gastrointestinal tract as a result of reduced microvillus size and parasite destruction of the intestinal epithelium. The mucosal damage inflicted by cryptosporidia is linked with an increase in paracellular permeability of the gastrointestinal tract and destruction of the functional mucosal barrier system. Studies of *C. parvum* infection in calves have shown that the jejunum and ileum are mainly affected and the diarrhoea occurs either due to the hindrance in sodium absorption coupled with increased prostaglandin production in the intestinal mucosa or due to the increase in mucosal permeability. There are no pathognomonic lesions of cryptosporidiosis. The intracellular and extracytoplasmic location of the endogenous stages are characteristic in the intestinal mucosa. Macroscopic lesions may include catarrhal enteritis. Histological examination may show atrophy and fusion of villi and replacement of enterocytes by immature cells. The characteristic *Cryptosporidium* oocysts of are found in the microvillus epithelium of the jejunum and ileum (Paul *et al.*, 2014).

29.6 Clinical Signs

In outbreaks of cryptosporidiosis in goat kids the morbidity varies from 80% to 100% and the mortality may exceed 50% in young kids. Flock mortality may increase with additional infections with other pathogens. The condition may deteriorate due to existing nutritional deficiencies and unhygienic managemental practices. Unhygienic conditions do facilitate contamination and propagation of oocysts in the environment that automatically reach the susceptible being. Other aggravating factors like transportation stress and infective dose may play a role. A positive correlation exists between the rate of excretion of oocysts and the severity of clinical symptoms. Caprine cryptosporidiosis is mainly associated with young kids aged 0–2 months. The prepatent period for young small ruminants is around 4 days and clinical symptoms are more pronounced at an early age. As per the recorded data from various geo-climatic zones of different countries, the predominant symptom of cryptosporidiosis remains mild to moderate-intensity diarrhoea or even cases of severe diarrhoea (Paul *et al.*, 2014) (Fig. 29.1).

Other clinical symptoms that are present along with diarrhoea are depression, dehydration, unthriftiness, abdominal ache, anorexia, listlessness and losing condition. The diarrhoeic faeces colour is yellow and consistency is pasty to liquid. Also, faeces have an offensive odour and contain a huge quantity of oocysts, likely 10^5–10^7 oocysts per gram (OPG) of faecal sample. The infection subsides with the attainment of immunological maturity; the recovered animal becomes a carrier, thereby serving as a potential source of infection to the susceptible population. Cryptosporidiosis-associated disease in adults is usually chronic in nature and characterized by progressive loss in body weight. An animal in this chronic course remains mostly asymptomatic. The analysed rate of OPG counts is found to be considerably higher in goat kids below 6 months of age. This OPG decreases further in kids above 12 months of age (Paul *et al.*, 2014).

29.7 Diagnosis

There is no specific technique for diagnosing *Cryptosporidium* infection in goats, but several methods are available. Staining techniques are often used in prevalence studies, and molecular techniques provide species and subtype information. The choice of diagnostic technique depends on available equipment and reagents, analyst experience, and time and cost of

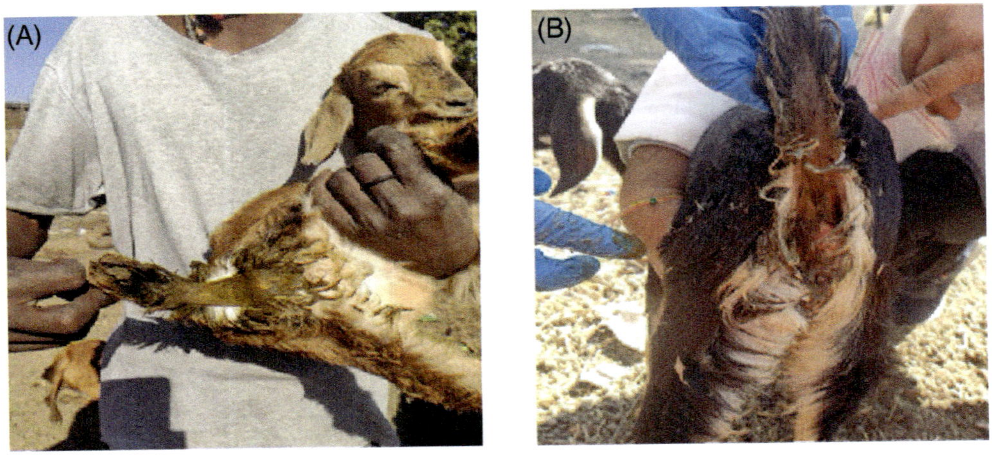

Fig. 29.1. Diarrhoea in goats infected with cryptosporidiosis. (Author's own image.)

analysis. Molecular techniques are usually not routine diagnostics in resource-poor settings, but specific diagnostics with high sensitivity are important everywhere, especially when positive findings lead to appropriate interventions such as improved hygiene and better farm management. Targeted pre-diagnostic sampling and preparation and dual use of staining and molecular techniques can provide the best possible results in terms of prevalence and epidemiological investigations (Utaaker *et al.*, 2021).

The diagnosis of cryptosporidiosis is usually done by using microscopic detection of the parasite. Microscopically, oocysts (morphology) or oocyst antigens or oocyst DNA in stool samples can also be used to detect the infective organism. The most common symptom of cryptosporidiosis in small ruminants is a watery diarrhoea associated with the causal signs of depression and gradual loss in body condition.

Differential diagnosis for *Cryptosporidium* includes infections caused by all pathogens of the neonatal ruminant diarrhoea complex – bacteria, viruses and parasites that are enteric pathogens associated with acute diarrhoea, such as rotaviruses, coronaviruses and bacteria (*Escherichia coli*, *Salmonella* spp., *Clostridium perfringens*). Multiple enteric pathogens can coexist with *Cryptosporidium* infection in the same animal. However, gastrointestinal disorders may also have non-infectious causes, such as inflammatory bowel disease in humans.

Diagnosis of cryptosporidiosis is usually made by microscopically identifying the presence of oocysts of 4–6 μm in diameter in the stool of the infected subjects. Since the detection of *Cryptosporidium* oocysts can be difficult, three faecal samples collected on separate days should be microscopically examined for detection of oocysts prior to excluding a *Cryptosporidium* infection in subjects with severe diarrhoea. In addition, for the detection of oocysts in the stool, the sample must be concentrated using the formalin-ether sedimentation method prior to microscopic examination. *Cryptosporidium* oocysts are visible by the use of acid-fast (modified Ziehl–Neelsen staining method) or phenol–auramine staining method on unconcentrated faecal smears. By these two methods, the oocysts stain red and bright yellow, respectively, but they may also appear as 'ghost' cells. Additionally, *Cryptosporidium* oocytes are half the size of those of *Cyclospora cayetanensis* (nearly 4–5 μm in diameter compared with 9–10 μm), another coccidian protozoan parasite that infects the intestine of humans, causing acute diarrhoea. Care should be taken when evaluating stool samples since the oocysts of both parasites are auto-fluorescent and acid-fast. In addition, although *Cyclospora cayetanensis* has a life cycle similar to that of *Cryptosporidium* species, its oocysts are unsporulated and not infective when shed in the faeces, therefore direct faecal–oral transmission cannot occur. Routine diagnosis of cryptosporidiosis is generally based on microscopic detection of oocysts in stool swabs, but unfortunately this method has low sensitivity (≤ 30%) despite its ease of use and low cost. Moreover, the exact diagnosis of cryptosporidiosis using the microscopic identification technique is dependent on the experience of the microscopist. Sensitivity can be improved by performing modified acid-fast stain, a staining generally performed if there are structures that are suspicious for *Cryptosporidium*, which has been reported to be associated with a sensitivity of 55%. However, these methods cannot distinguish between different *Cryptosporidium* species. In addition to the methods described above, laboratory diagnosis of cryptosporidiosis can use a variety of techniques, such as enzyme-linked immunosorbent assay (ELISA) and immunochromatography, to examine watery or thick stools (Editorial, 2021).

29.7.1 Detection of *Cryptosporidium* antigen

Commercially available kits have higher sensitivity and specificity than microscopic methods (ranging from 58% to 95%), but previous studies have shown that these antigen/antibody-based detection methods are effective for parasites in patients below the minimum threshold. Moreover, these methods are more expensive than polymerase chain reaction (PCR), which is currently considered by most laboratories to be the gold standard for detecting this parasite in stool. Previous studies have shown that microscopy, ELISA and immunochromatography (ICT) are inconvenient and time-consuming in terms of cost, sensitivity and specificity, compared with PCR. Although important advances have been made in diagnostic tools (such as the availability of multiplex PCR assays to detect intestinal protozoa), access to this molecular technology has been limited in some laboratories and it does not exist in other laboratories. In addition, costs and the need for technical expertise limit its use, especially in high-prevalence areas such as developing countries (Editorial, 2021) (Fig. 29.2).

29.7.2 Molecular diagnosis

Molecular tools provide a better understanding of the genus *Cryptosporidium*. Genotyping and subtyping data clearly demonstrate the occurrence of anthropogenic and zoonotic *Cryptosporidium* species in humans in industrialized countries. In contrast, the transmission of cryptosporidiosis in some developing countries appears to be largely manmade. For example, in Africa, despite frequent human–animal contact, transmission appears to be primarily anthropogenic, and human *Cryptosporidium* infections are most commonly caused by *C. hominis* or *C. parvum anthroponosum*. However, since many *Cryptosporidium* species infect both humans and goats, it is clear that transmission between the two host species is possible (Utaaker *et al.*, 2021).

C. parvum is probably the best-studied *Cryptosporidium* zoonotic species. For example, in China the IId subtype of *C. parvum* has been found in most studies. It appears to have a unique distribution in China, prevalent in *C. parvum* infections in humans, domestic animals and rodents. The IId subtype has also been detected in European, Asian and Oceanian goats. However, the role of the rodent hosts, possibly additional intrinsic reinforcers, remains unclear in these areas (Utaaker *et al.*, 2021).

In Africa, human *C. parvum* dominating infections are of the Iic subtype, and the role of small ruminants such as goats in transmission remains mostly unknown. The IIa subtype appears to be present in *C. parvum* infections in goats in many parts of the world and has been reported from all continents except Africa (Utaaker *et al.*, 2021).

29.8 Treatment

Since cryptosporidiosis is associated with major common symptoms like depression, anorexia, listlessness and foul-smelling diarrhoea, its treatment must be combined with effective supportive therapy that includes rehydration, administration of anti-diarrhoeals and nutritive feed supplements. There is no specific cure for cryptosporidiosis in goats, but several drugs have been analysed for their cryptosporicidal activities, including a-cyclodextrin, b-cyclodextrin, decoquinate, nitazoxanide, tilmicosin, halofuginone lactate and paromomycin sulfate (Paul *et al.*, 2014).

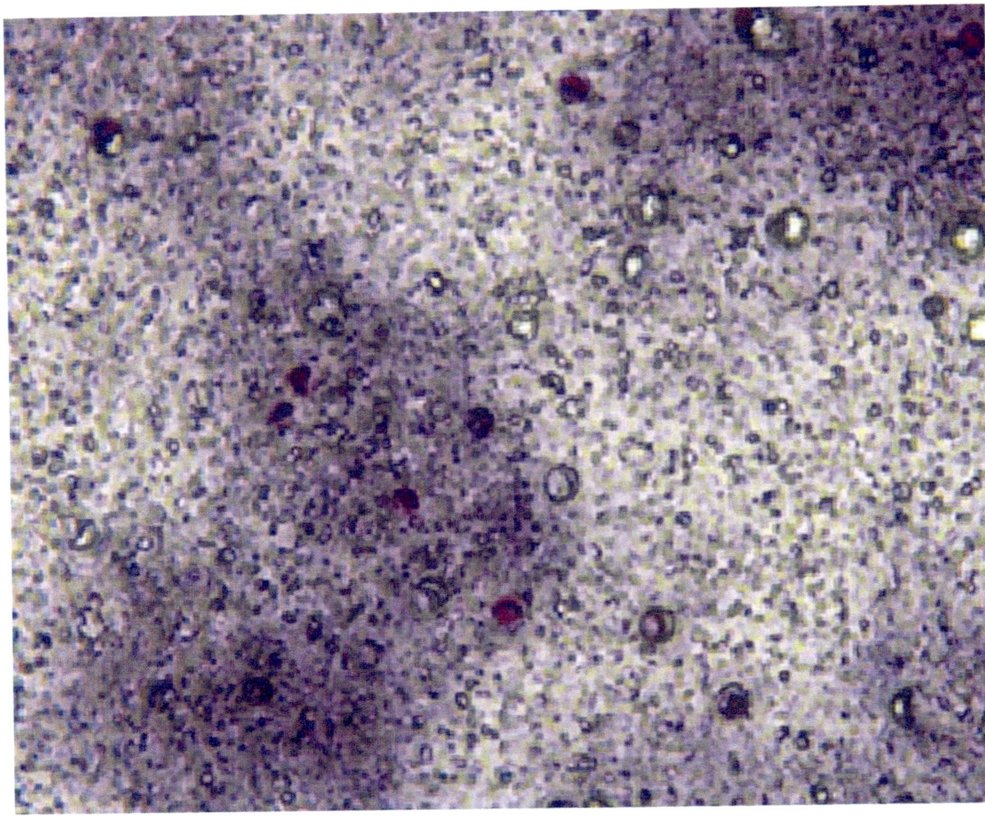

Fig. 29.2. Stained *Cryptosporidium* oocysts under microscope. (Author's own image.)

29.8.1 Limited treatment options

Despite its medical and veterinary importance, current options for treating cryptosporidiosis in humans and animals are limited. Only nitazoxanide is approved by the US Food and Drug Administration (FDA) for the treatment of cryptosporidiosis in immunocompetent persons, but not in immunocompromised individuals such as those with AIDS. However, nitazoxanide is not completely efficacious and its mechanism of action is poorly defined. There are also no FDA-approved drugs to treat cryptosporidiosis in animals. Halofuginone lactate (Halocur) has been approved for veterinary use in calves and lambs in some countries and has shown anti-*Cryptosporidium* activity, although it is not effective in completely eliminating oocyst production.

29.8.2 Recently discovered anti-*Cryptosporidium* leads and targets

Efforts over the past 20 years have resulted in several lead compounds with defined targets and anti-cryptosporidia potency *in vitro* at lower nanomolar levels. However, they are mostly in various preclinical and optimization stages. Even if one or more of these lead compounds (or analogues) are developed as therapeutic agents in the future, additional drug options are needed to diversify drug targets and overcome potential drug resistance.

29.9 Control and Management

In the absence of any innate resistance and marked effect of passive protection transmitted to the newborn kids through colostrum, the impact of the disease varies widely, depending on the susceptibility of the animals, the presence of carrier status and the stability of infection in the premises. The situation is further worsened by the fact that no satisfactory vaccine or specific cryptosporicidal drugs are available. Under these circumstances, effective control requires knowledge of the epidemiology of the disease coupled with the use of appropriate diagnostic tools, supportive treatment and segregation policy. Segregating affected animals should be followed by sound sanitary and management practices (Paul *et al.*, 2014).

Persistent diarrhoea severely affects nutritional status, growth and intellectual function. Addressing these challenges is extremely important, especially in developing countries. *Cryptosporidium* oocysts are highly infective, robust and resistant to disinfectants, highlighting the need for improved treatment options. To date, no safe and effective treatment for cryptosporidiosis has been identified, although efforts continue to direct resources toward this goal. *C. hominis* still appears to be prevalent in many settings, but zoonotic transmission should not be ignored. In line with the One Health initiative, general rules regarding sanitary barriers between humans and animals should be implemented in all settings. This reduces the risk of infection not only from *Cryptosporidium*, but also from other zoonotic pathogens. Since children and women are often responsible for caring for backyard livestock and usually also prepare feed and fetch water, focusing on this group for hygiene training and dissemination of the welfare of them and goats can be improved. Research that specifically focuses on the potential for *Cryptosporidium* infections between goats and their keepers is an important resource for lifting families and communities out of poverty (Utaaker *et al.*, 2021). It can provide more specific information about where to intervene without losing the value of goat keeping as a farm.

Cryptosporidium oocysts are widespread in the environment; they are the only life cycle stage involved in disease transmission under normal circumstances, and their minimization or elimination is an important intervention in infection control. Good husbandry and hygiene are central to on-farm cryptosporidiosis control, and fertilizer and slurry management are viable intervention points for farmers. Water and feeding troughs should be moved regularly to avoid faecal accumulation. The troughs should be raised or covered to avoid faecal contamination. Bedding should be adequate and thorough cleaning and disinfection should be done between different animal groups. If cryptosporidiosis remains a problem, mass prophylaxis with halofuginone lactate can be used to reduce the shedding of oocysts. There is no commercially available vaccine.

House decontamination is difficult due to the resistance of the oocysts and the ineffectiveness of bleach-based disinfectants. We recommend cleaning surfaces and utensils with detergent, rinsing and drying thoroughly. After cleaning, if specific cryptosporidian disinfection is desired, ammonia-based disinfectants, steam cleaning, or hydrogen peroxide with peracetic acid or silver nitrate can be used. Ammonium hydroxide can produce strong and pungent fumes and should only be used in open stables. In addition, this compound is ineffective against most bacteria and should be used as a general disinfectant. However, these methods may not be practical for routine implementation.

Advice for farmers to prevent zoonotic disease transmission is available from the Health and Safety Administration, which also provides guidance on preventing zoonotic disease transmission on open farms or farms open to the public. After touching animals, it is important that farm visitors should wash their hands, preferably with warm running water and liquid soap, and dry them with disposable towels, but alcohol gel is not suitable. Generic guidelines for investigating zoonotic diseases in the event of an outbreak have been published. In the UK, pets do not appear to pose a general public health risk from cryptosporidiosis, but they may pose individual risks, and immunocompromised patients should avoid contact with animal faeces and young pets.

The optimal management of *Cryptosporidium* to protect drinking water supplies is governed by the EU Water Framework Directive (2000/60/EU) (WFD). Elimination of direct animal access is achieved through farm management and fencing. To meet WFD requirements, England's Defra initiated a catchment-sensitive farming programme to control diffuse pollution, and revised codes of good farming practices to protect water, soil and air, integrating advice for farmers, growers and land managers. Other decentralized administrations in the UK have their own codes. The Food Standards Authority issued guidance to give UK farmers practical advice on how to reduce the risk of contamination of ready-to-eat crops when using fertilizers.

The risk of contamination and connectivity between agricultural waste and water sources upstream of collection points cannot always be mitigated and effective water treatment is required. The detection of multiple *Cryptosporidium* species and genotypes in individual watersheds indicates multiple sources of contamination and both sampling and analysis methods must be properly differentiated. In England, since the Water Supply (Water Quality) Regulations were amended in 2000, improved risk assessments, river basin protection and water treatment have been introduced and the reported incidence of cryptosporidiosis has declined, especially in the spring.

For other animals, especially in animal husbandry, primary prevention should be emphasized. This includes the isolation of causative risk factors from adult animals by limiting the number of farm or susceptible host animals at high risk of infection and keeping them at risk of infection. Possible *Cryptosporidium* species can be decreased. It spreads in herds of animals. In human habitation areas, livestock and their drinking water, the destruction of *Cryptosporidium* oocysts is caused by heat from agents such as hydrogen peroxide, steam, ethylene oxide, chlorine dioxide, ozone (O_3) and ultraviolet (UV) light sterilization processes, or can be managed by chemical disinfection. Sterilization of drinking water is used, but some disinfectants are generally not a viable method. However, all chemical disinfectants can be used to prevent and control cryptosporidiosis outbreaks and reduce mortality and morbidity in both humans and animals.

29.10 Conclusion

Cryptosporidiosis is recognized as an important zoonotic disease caused by a global protozoan parasite called *Cryptosporidium*. Cryptosporidiosis is becoming a major public health and veterinary concern because it affects humans and a wide variety of animal species within its host range. Fundamentally, the importance of infectious diseases has increased due to the high incidence of young children, immunocompromised people or patients with immunodeficiency syndromes, especially HIV/AIDS, and of patients infected with *Cryptosporidium* spp. It is also one of the leading causes of death. All domestic animals, farm animals, wildlife and humans are potential reservoir hosts for *Cryptosporidium* parasites. They infect food, surface water and other hosts via the faecal–oral route. The *Cryptosporidium* oocyst stage remains infective, resistant to a variety of environmental influences, and is also resistant to many common disinfectants, including chlorine disinfection commonly used in water treatment. The development of molecules and cell culture methods may explain the differences in infectivity and virulence between *C. parvum* isolated from different hosts. The management of cryptosporidiosis in small ruminants still requires the implementation of global knowledge on epidemiology, but also further research on disease prevention and treatment.

C. parvum is the most clinically important zoonotic cause of cryptosporidiosis, with extensive and abundant animal reservoirs, mainly in young livestock. Other *Cryptosporidium* species and/or genotypes may occur as human pathogens. This highlights the need to identify infectious isolates in human and animal reservoirs and ensure appropriate controls to prevent infection.

References

Editorial (2021) Bug of the month: *Cryptosporidium* Infection. *Journal of Hygiene Sciences* XIIV, 7–8. Available at: https://www.tulipgroup.com/JHS_magazine/2021/JHS_80.pdf (accessed 20 October 2024).

Giles, M., Chalmers, R., Pritchard, G., Elwin, K., Mueller-Doblies, D. *et al*. (2009) *Cryptosporidium hominis* in a goat and a sheep in the UK. *The Veterinary Record* 164(1), 24.

Paraud, C., Pors, I. and Chartier, C. (2010) Evaluation of oral tilmicosin efficacy against severe cryptosporidiosis in neonatal kids under field conditions. *Veterinary Parasitology* 170, 149–152.

Paul, S., Sharma, D.K., Boral, R., Mishra, A.K., Shivsharanappa, N. *et al*. (2014) Cryptosporidiosis in goats; a review. *Advances in Animal and Veterinary Sciences* 2(3S), 49–54. DOI: 10.14737/journal.aavs/2014/2.3s.49.54.

Pumipuntu, N. and Piratae, S. (2018) Cryptosporidiosis: A zoonotic disease concern. *Veterinary World* 11(5), 681.

Robertson, L.J., Johansen, Ø.H., Kifleyohannes, T., Efunshile, A.M. and Terefe, G. (2020) Cryptosporidium infections in Africa - how important is zoonotic transmission? A review of the evidence. *Frontiers in Veterinary Science* 7, 575881. DOI: 10.3389/fvets.2020.575881.

Utaaker, K.S., Chaudhary, S., Kifleyohannes, T. and Robertson, L.J. (2021) Global goat! is the expanding goat population an important reservoir of Cryptosporidium? *Frontiers in Veterinary Science* 8, 648500.

Xiao, L., Fayer, R., Ryan, U. and Upton, S.J. (2004) Cryptosporidium taxonomy: Recent advances and implications for public health. *Clinical Microbiology Reviews* 17(1), 72–97.

Zhu, G., Yin, J. and Cuny, G.D. (2021) Current status and challenges in drug discovery against the globally important zoonotic cryptosporidiosis. *Animal Diseases* 1(1), 1–10.

30 Sarcocystosis

Manaswini Dehuri*
Department of Veterinary Parasitology, College of Veterinary Sciences & Animal Husbandry, Odisha University of Agriculture and Technology, Bhubaneswar, India

Abstract
Sarcocystosis is a cyst-forming coccidial infection with heteroxenous life cycle of *Sarcocystis* spp. with a public health concern due to eating undercooked or raw meat. The most prevalent species are *Sarcocystis capracanis* and *Sarcocystis hircicanis*. In definitive or final hosts, the parasite shows no pathogenic effect, but severe symptoms are observed for intermediate hosts, leading to death of the fetus and abortion. The highest concentration of *Sarcocystis* in goats is in the oesophagus and tail muscles, followed by diaphragm muscle and cardiac muscle. The identification and diagnosis may be macroscopic and microscopic, serology and molecular.

Keywords: prey-predator, striated muscle, sarcocyst

30.1 Introduction

Sarcocystis is a genus of apicomplexan protozoan parasites of the class Sporozoasida, belonging to the family Sarcocystidae, having a broad host range and prevalent worldwide. It was regarded as a non-pathogenic agent but has been found associated with disease conditions in humans and animals, acting as an emerging disease of livestock in recent times. *Sarcocystis* is a Greek name, with *sarka* meaning flesh and *kystis* meaning bladder (encysted stage). Friedrich Miescher was the person who first documented this parasite in 1843, as white thread-like structures in skeletal muscle, which therefore became known as Miescher's tubules. Thereafter, *Sarcocystis* species were described mainly from striated muscles, less frequently from non-striated muscles and organs like the brain of mammals, reptiles and birds (Dubey *et al.*, 2016). *Sarcocystis* species are cyst-forming coccidian parasites that have heteroxenous life cycles, with an intermediate and a definitive host obligatory for the completion of the life cycle. The obligatory two-host life cycle was discovered in 1972 and was described as coccidians transmitted through faecal–oral routes, involving herbivores as intermediate hosts and carnivores as the definitive hosts (Dubey *et al.*, 1981).

Sarcocystosis infects mammals, birds and reptiles. Several *Sarcocystis* species are pathogenic, resulting in a severe disease that can lead to abortion and carcass condemnation. Some species are zoonotic in nature (Dubey, 2009). They can be found frequently in animal carcasses at slaughter, undermining the carcass value, and they have also been found associated with clinical disease. There is a potential public health concern owing to people eating undercooked or raw meat. Definitive hosts are infected through the ingestion of *Sarcocystis* parasites in muscle tissues and include carnivorous predators and scavengers, as well as humans. Intermediate

*Corresponding author: id-nishi.md@gmail.com

DOI: 10.1079/ 9781800622852.0030

hosts are infected by consuming sporocysts in feed or water contaminated by the final host faeces (Gjerde, 2013). The mature sarcocysts form due to multiplication of the protozoa inside striated muscles and final hosts are infected by consuming infected muscle tissues (Gjerde *et al.*, 2020). In definitive or final hosts, the parasite shows no pathogenic effect, but severe symptoms are observed for intermediate hosts. They are responsible for fetal deaths and abortion. Economic loss due to rejection of meat is also a major concern (Ren *et al.*, 2019).

In goats, the most prevalent species are *Sarcocystis capracanis* and *Sarcocystis hircicanis*. Although *S. gigantea* and *S. tenella* are prevalent in sheep, there have been only scarce reports in goats (Table 30.1).

The prevalence of *Sarcocystis* spp. in goats in different parts of the world is variable, ranging from 34% to 91.6% (Table 30.2) depending on the method of diagnosis.

Sarcocysts are usually cylindrical or spindle-shaped structures and their shape varies considerably. Macrocysts are visible to the naked eye and can reach up to 5 cm in diameter (Swar, 2021). Two forms of macroscopic sarcocysts are usually observed: fat and thin. Fat cysts are thick, round in shape and seem to grow in length and width (Chhabra and Samantaray, 2012). They are exclusively found in the oesophagus. Thin cysts are slim and slender and appear to grow mainly in length. Macrosarcocysts that are white, pale to creamy in colour, grain-sized and with multifocal nodules have been documented on the outer surface of the oesophagus (Meena *et al.*, 2022). Microcysts measure a few microns and are only visible with the aid of a microscope.

The highest concentration of sarcocysts in goats is in the oesophagus and tail muscles (suitable for detection in live animals), followed in frequency by diaphragm muscle and cardiac muscle (Saha and Ghosh, 1992; Shankar and Bhatia, 1993; Wadajkar *et al.*, 1995). *S. hircicanis* cysts have a thin wall with hairy processes, while *S. capracanis* cysts have a thick, radially striated wall and also a longer prepatent period (*S. capracanis* has a prepatent period of 9 days while *S. hircicanis* has 12–15 days). Larger sporocysts are observed in *S. hircicanis* (Sharma and Shah, 1992). The cyst wall of *S. capracanis* appears thick and radially striated with finger-like projections, while S. *hircicanis* possesses a thin sarcocyst wall with hair-like projections on its outer surface (Morsy *et al.*, 2011).

30.2 Life Cycle

The life cycle of *Sarcocystis* spp. was identified in 1972 during *in vitro* investigation of the gametogenic and oocyst phase of *S. falcatula* in poultry (Rommel *et al.*, 1972) (Fig. 30.1). Definitive and intermediate (predator and prey) hosts are required for completion of the life cycle (Odening, 1998).

Asexual stages are found especially in the intermediate host (prey animal). The intermediate host ingests food/water contaminated with the faeces of a definitive host containing oocysts or sporocysts. Inside the host, due to the action of gastric juices, sporozoites are liberated, which enter the gut and then lodge primarily in the arteries of endothelial cells (Valizadeh, 2021). Sporozoites divide to form motile merozoites, crescent in shape. They encyst in the muscles, forming metrocytes, which then transform to bradyzoites. They encyst in the skeletal, cardiac and smooth muscles of herbivores like goats (Fayer *et al.*, 2015; Khater *et al.*, 2020). Two types of

Table 30.1. Species of *Sarcocystis* affecting goats.

Sarcocystis sp.	Cyst	Transmission	Reference
S. capracanis	Microsarcocyst	Canids	Dubey *et al.*, 2016
S. hircicanis	Microsarcocyst	Canids	Lindsay and Dubey, 2020
S.moulei (S. caprafelis)	Macrosarcocyst	Felids	Lindsay and Dubey, 2020
S. gigantea (S. ovifelis)	Macrosarcocyst	Felids	Ghaffar *et al.*, 1989
S. tenella	Microsarcocyst	Canids	Hong *et al.*, 2016

Table 30.2. Prevalence of *Sarcocystis* spp. in goats in different regions of the world.

Area	Prevalence	Important findings	Reference
Rajasthan, India	68.28%	*Sarcocystis capracanis*, microcyst highest in oesophagus and lowest in heart. Cyst spindle shaped, septate with thick striated wall.	Singh, 1991
Bangalore, India	72.4%	The organ prevalence was found to be of 69.45%, 36.10%, 62.50% and 12.5% in oesophagus, heart, diaphragm and tongue, respectively.	Dafedar *et al.*, 2008
Malaysia	52.38% (light microscopy), 43.8% (histology), 90.48% (PCR)	The cysts were elongated to a spindle shape with a mean size of 393.30 × 81.6 µm and contained banana-shaped bradyzoites of size 12.32 × 2.08 µm.	Kutty *et al.*, 2015
Northen Iraq	34%	Highest infection in oesophagus (99%) and the lowest in the diaphragm (3%). Two forms of macroscopic sarcocysts: fat and thin. Fat cysts found in the oesophagus, thin cysts seen in the oesophagus, diaphragm and skeletal muscles.	Barham *et al.*, 2005
North-west Iraq	79.4%	Microcysts were highly observed in diaphragm muscles and the lowest in the heart muscle.	Valizadeh *et al.*, 2021
Sharkia province, Egypt	40%	The infection rate was higher in adult animals.	Nasr *et al.*, 2003
Cairo, Egypt	79.4%	Highest infection rate in skeletal muscles (77%) followed by diaphragm (74%), oesophagus (54.4%), tongue (43.5%) and the lower rate was recorded in heart muscles (38%).	Morsy *et al.*, 2011
Bahia, Brazil	91.6%	Microscopic cysts of *Sarcocystis capracanis* were detected	Bittencourt *et al.*, 2016
Kunming, China	77.3%	*Sarcocystis capracanis* and *Sarcocystis hircicanis* were identified	Hu *et al.*, 2016.
North-west Tunisia	50.4%	*Sarcocystis capracanis*	Amairia *et al.*, 2021

sarcocysts are present in goats: microsarocyst and macrosarcocyst.

The definitive host acquires the infection by ingestion of mature sarcocysts within the muscles of infected animals. The sarcocysts are digested, releasing bradyzoites, which are transferred to male (microgametes) and female (macrogametes), undergoing fusion to form zygotes, which then forms oocysts. The oocyst contains two sporocysts enclosing four sporozoites. On rupturing, sporocysts are released into the intestinal lumen and excreted through faeces (Fig. 30.2).

30.3 Pathogenesis

S. capracanis is the most pathogenic species in goats, causing fever, weight loss and abortion, and may even lead to death in a heavy infection (Dubey *et al.*, 1989). There is resultant weight

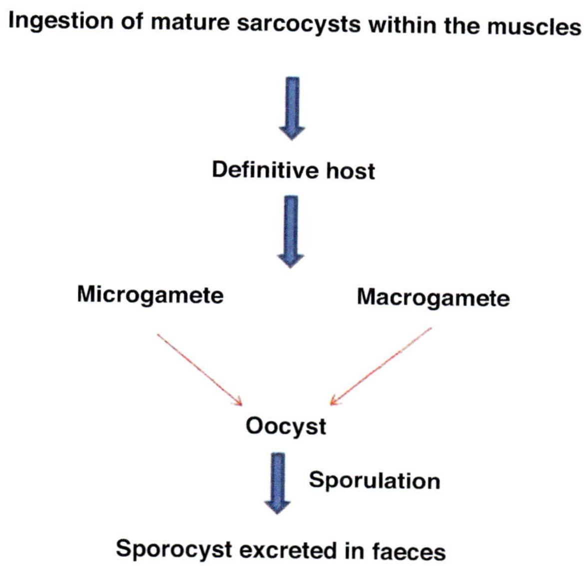

Fig. 30.1. Life cycle of *Sarcocystis* in a definitive host. (Author's own image.)

loss, anaemia, anorexia and reduced production parameters like milk production.

In an experimental study, *S. capracanis* was reported with a reduced packed cell volume and haemoglobin content, while there was an increase in alanine aminotransferase, lactic dehydrogenase, blood urea nitrogen and bilirubin values. The histological findings depicted vasculitis, cholangitis, hepatitis, generalized myositis, encephalomyelitis and thymic atrophy (Dubey *et al.*, 1981). Several forms of microscopic cyst, such as spindle, circular, elliptical, cylindrical and twisted, form in oesophagus. They appear as blue-coloured sarcocysts containing bradyzoites in the tunica muscularis (thin-walled and thick-walled). Single microcysts are surrounded by single layers of muscle fibres, while degeneration and necrosis of muscle bundles have been observed (Meena *et al.*, 2022). In animals infected with *Sarcocystis* spp., reduction in protein may be due to a decrease in gamma globulin (Gill *et al.*, 1988). There may be elevation in liver enzymes leading to degenerative changes, rupture of muscle fibres and sometimes myositis muscular cysts (Nevole *et al.*, 1986).

30.4 Diagnosis

In living animals, it is difficult to identify sarcocystosis and diagnosis may be macroscopic and microscopic, serological and molecular.

The most common methods of identification of *Sarcocystis* spp. depend on the morphology and size of the cyst.

30.4.1 Macroscopic examination

Fresh muscle samples, especially from oesophagus, heart and diaphragm tissue, are examined macroscopically for the presence of macroscopic *Sarcocystis* cysts and the shape, size, colour and consistency are noted.

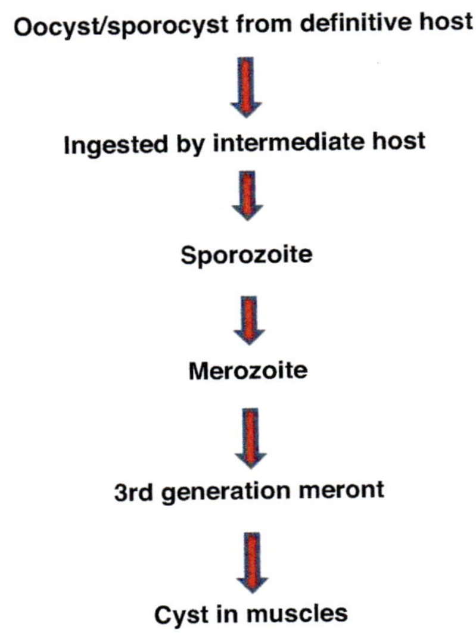

Fig. 30.2. Life cycle in an intermediate host. (Author's own image.)

30.4.2 Microscopic examination

Small pieces of fresh muscle (0.5 mm size) are compressed between two slides and examined microscopically under stereo microscope (Mowafy, 1993).

- For the digestion method, to 100 ml of digestion medium (2.5 g pepsin and 10 ml HCL in 1 litre of phosphate-buffered saline) 50 g (homogenized) muscle is added and placed in a shaking water bath at 37°C for 30 min. The suspension is then centrifuged for 10 min at 1500 rpm and the precipitate smear, fixed with absolute methanol, is stained with Giemsa and examined by light microscopy at 100× (Dubey *et al.*, 1989).
- Trypan blue staining can be used to visualize the dead and live bradyzoites in a bradyzoite suspension (10 µl) mixed with 0.4% Trypan blue stain (90 µl), examined under microscope. Dead bradyzoites appear blue in colour whereas live bradyzoites do not take any stain.
- In Diff-Quik staining, the smear is dipped in the Diff-Quik fixative (absolute methanol) five times and then eosin (for 1 s) followed by dipping the slide in methylene blue stain five times (for 1 s).
- For an impression smear/cytology, the smears from tissues collected at necropsy are fixed using methanol and stained with Giemsa and observed for cytopathological alterations.
- For histopathological examination, affected muscle pieces (0.5 cm thick) are fixed in 10% neutral buffered formalin, with section cutting to a thickness of 4–5 microns, stained with haematoxylin and eosin.

30.4.3 Molecular diagnosis

Molecular diagnosis of *Sarcocystis* spp., uses DNA markers like 18S rRNA, 28S rRNA, 18S rDNA, mitochondrial cytochrome C oxidase subunit one gene (cox1), and ITS1 region gene. Also DNA barcoding using the cox1 gene can identify genotypes (Hu *et al.*, 2016; El-Morsey *et al.*, 2019).

30.4.4 Serological techniques

Techniques like indirect fluorescent antibody technique (IFAT), indirect haemagglutination test (IHA) and enzyme-linked immunosorbent assay (ELISA) can be utilized for diagnosis. Serological tests appear to be more specific but have low sensitivity in diagnosing acute sarcocystosis.

30.4.5 Faecal examination

In final hosts, diagnosis of intestinal *Sarcocystis* infection is by faecal examination. *Sarcocystis* sporocysts and oocysts are shed fully sporulated in faeces, whereas those of *Neospora caninum*, *Toxoplasma gondii* and *Cystoisospora* spp. are shed unsporulated.

30.5 Immunity to Sarcocystosis

Subclinical infection in goats can lead to acquired protective immunity (Dubey *et al.*, 1981). Subclinical dose of *S. capracanis* in early pregnancy could cause fetal death without clinical disease. Immunization prior to pregnancy could protect *Sarcocystis*-infected goats from abortion (Dubey, 2001).

30.6 Control

- Salinomycin at 5 mg/kg body weight was found to be effective in experimental sarcocystosis (*S. capracanis*) in goats (Kumar *et al.*, 1988).
- Anticoccidials like Amprolium can also be recommended for treatment.
- The infected definitive host can shed millions of infectious *Sarcocystis* sporocysts over a period of time, thereby contaminating the environment.
- The sporocysts and oocysts remain viable in the environment for months and are resistant to freezing. The shedding of oocysts and sporocysts in faeces of the definitive hosts should be prevented.
- Control relies on interruption of the life cycle by preventing the carnivore definitive hosts from eating raw meat or offal of slaughtered or dead animals and then contaminating the feed and water of livestock with faeces.
- It is advisable not to feed uncooked meat or offal to carnivores.
- Cooking at high temperatures (heating food at 55°C for 20 min kills sarcocysts) and freezing can eliminate infection.
- The infected animal should be buried or incinerated and dead animals should never be left for animals or birds to devour.

References

Amairia, S., Rouatbi, M., Rjeibi, M.R., Gomes, J., Rekik, M. *et al.* (2021) Molecular detection of *Toxoplasma gondii* and *Sarcocystis* spp. co-infection in Tunisian Merguez, a traditional processed sausage beef meat. *Food Control* 121, 107618.

Barham, M., Stützer, H., Karanis, P., Latif, B.M. and Neiss, W.F. (2005) Seasonal variation in *Sarcocystis* species infections in goats in Northern Iraq. *Parasitology* 130(2), 151–156.

Bittencourt, M.V., Meneses, I.D., Ribeiro-Andrade, M., de Jesus, R.F., de Araújo, F.R. *et al.* (2016) *Sarcocystis* spp. in sheep and goats: Frequency of infection and species identification by morphological, ultrastructural, and molecular tests in Bahia, Brazil. *Parasitology Research* 115(4), 1683–1689.

Chhabra, M.B. and Samantaray, S. (2012) *Sarcocystis* and sarcocystosis in India: Status and emerging perspectives. *Journal of Parasitic Diseases* 37(1), 1–10.

Dafedar, A.M., Souza, P.E., Ananda, K.J. and Puttalakshmamma, G.C. (2008) Prevalence of sarcocystosis in goats slaughtered at an abattoir in Bangalore, Karnataka state. *Veterinary World* 1(11), 335–337.

Dubey, J.P. (2001) Recent developments in the biology of *Sarcocystis ncurona* and equine protozoal myeloencephalitis (EPM). *Journal of Veterinary Parasitology* 15, 91–102.

Dubey, J.P. (2009) The evolution of knowledge of cat and dog coccidia. *Parasitology* 136(12), 1469–1475.

Dubey, J.P., Calero-Bernal, R., Rosenthal, B.M., Speer, C.A. and Fayer, R. (2016) *Sarcocystosis of Animals and Humans*, 2nd edn. CRC Press, Boca Raton, Florida.

Dubey, J.P., Speer, C.A. and Fayer, R. (1989) *Sarcocystosis of Animals and Man*. CRC Press, Boca Raton, Florida.

Dubey, J.P., Weisbrode, S.E., Speer, C.A. and Sharma, S.P. (1981) Sarcocystosis in goats: Clinical signs and pathologic and hematologic findings. *Journal of American Veterinary Medical Association* 178(7), 683–699.

El-Morsey, A., Abdo, W., Sultan, K., Elhawary, N.M. and Abou Zaid, A.A. (2019) Ultrastructural and molecular identification of the sarcocysts of *Sarcocystis tenella* and *Sarcocystis arieticanis* infecting domestic sheep (*Ovis aries*) from Egypt. *Acta Parasitologica* 64, 501–513.

Fayer, R., Esposito, D.H. and Dubey, J.P. (2015) Human infections with *Sarcocystis* species. *Clinical Microbiology Reviews* 28(2), 295–311.

Ghaffar, F.A., Heydorn, A.O. and Mehlhorn, H. (1989) The fine structure of cysts of *Sarcocystis moulei* from goats. *Parasitology Research* 75, 416–418.

Gill, H., Charleston, A. and Moriarty, M. (1988) Immunosuppression in *Sarcocystis muris*-infected mice: Evidence for suppression of antibody and cell-mediated responses to a heterologous antigen. *Immune Cell Biology* 66(3), 29.

Gjerde, B. (2013) Phylogenetic relationships among *Sarcocystis* species in cervids, cattle and sheep inferred from the mitochondrial cytochrome c oxidase subunit I gene. *International Journal for Parasitology* 43(7), 579–591.

Gjerde, B., de la Fuente, C., Alunda, J.M. and Luzon, M. (2020) Molecular characterisation of five *Sarcocystis* species in domestic sheep (*Ovis aries*) from Spain. *Parasitology Research* 119, 215–231.

Hong, E.I., Sim, C., Chae, J.S., Kim, H.C., Park, J. *et al*. (2016) Ultrastructural and molecular identification of *Sarcocystis tenella* (Protozoa, Apicomplexa) in naturally infected Korean native goats. *Veterinary Medicine* 61, 374–381.

Hu, J.J., Liu, T.T., Liu, Q., Esch, G.W., Chen, J.Q. *et al*. (2016) Prevalence, morphology, and molecular characteristics of *Sarcocystis* spp. in domestic goats (capra hircus) from Kunming, China. *Parasitology Research* 115(10), 3973–3981.

Khater, H.F., Ziam, H., Abbas, A., Abbas, R.Z., Raza, M.A. *et al*. (2020) Avian coccidiosis: Recent advances in alternative control strategies and vaccine development. *Agrobiological Records* 1, 11–25.

Kumar, A., Srivastava, P.S. and Sinha, S.R.P. (1988) Chemotherapy of experimental caprine sarcocystosis in goats and young dogs with salinomycin (Coxistac Pfizer). *Journal of Veterinary Parasitology* 2, 129–132.

Kutty, M.K., Latif, B., Muslim, A., Hussaini, J., Daher, A.M. *et al*. (2015) Detection of sarcocystosis in goats in Malaysia by light microscopy, histology, and PCR. *Tropical Animal Health Production* 47, 751–756.

Lindsay, D.S. and Dubey, J.P. (2020) Neosporosis, toxoplasmosis, and sarcocystosis in ruminants: an update. *Veterinary Clinics of North America Food Animal Practice* 36(1), 205–222.

Meena, S., Dadhich, R., Sharma, S., Meena, D.S., Sharma, S.K. *et al*. (2022) Cytopathological and histopathological studies on *Sarcocystis* in oesophagus of goat. *The Pharma Innovation Journal* 11(7), 2236–2240.

Morsy, K., Saleh, A., Al-Ghamdi, A., Abdel-Ghaffara, F., Al-Rasheid, K. *et al*. (2011) Prevalence pattern and biology of *Sarcocystis capracanis* infection in the Egyptian goats: A light and ultrastructural study. *Veterinary Parasitology* 181(2–4), 75–82.

Mowafy, N.M. (1993) Sarcosporidiosis in rodents. PhD Thesis in Medical Science, Faculty of Medicine, Minia University, Egypt.

Nasr, S.S.M., Hussen, E.M. and Mekawy, S. (2003) Prevalence of *Sarcocystis* spp. in sheep and goats and its effect on some blood constituents in Sharkia province. *Kafrelsheikh Veterinary Medical Journal* 1(1), 6–84.

Nevole, M., Malota, L. and Koudela, B. (1986) Catalytic activity of selected serum enzymes in sarcocystosis in calves. *Acta Veterinaria Brno* 55, 81–84.

Odening, K. (1998) The present state of species-systematics in *Sarcocystis* lankester, 1882 (Protista, Sporozoa, Coccidia). *Systematic Parasitology* 41, 209–233.

Ren, M., Wu, Y., Zou, Y., Tu, Y., Wang, D. *et al*. (2019) Molecular characterization of *Sarcocystis* species isolated from Chinese buffaloes in Guizhou province based on 18S rRNA and cox 1 sequence. *Mitochondrial DNA Part B* 4(1), 637–641.

Rommel, M., Heydorn, A.O. and Gruber, F. (1972) Beiträge zum lebenszyklus der Sarkosporidien. 1. Die Sporozyste von S. tenella in den Fäzes der Katze [Life cycle of Sarcosporidia. 1. The sporocyst of S. tenella in cat feces. *Berliner Und Munchener Tierarztliche Wochenschrift* 85(6), 101–105.

Saha, A.K. and Ghosh, D. (1992) Prevalence of sarcocysts in black Bengal goats in Tripura. *Indian Veterinary Journal* 69, 82–83.

Shankar, D. and Bhatia, B.B. (1993) *Sarcocystis* infection in goats in Uttar Pradesh. *Indian Journal of Animal Science* 63, 284–287.

Sharma, R.K. and Shah, H.L. (1992) Occurrence of *Sarcocystis hircicanis* in the goat. *Indian Journal of Animal Science* 62, 561–563.

Singh, L. (1991) Studies on *Sarcocystis capracanis*. MVSc Thesis submitted to Rajasthan University of Veterinary and Animal Sciences, Bikaner, India.

Swar, S.O. and Shnawa, B.H. (2021) Recent advances in molecular characterization of *Sarcocystis* species in some meat producing animals: An updated review. *Asian Journal of Agriculture Biology* 2021(1), 1.

Valizadeh, H. and Ebrahimi, A. (2021) A study on the abundance of infection with *Sarcocystis* in goats slaughtered in the Tabriz slaughterhouse. *Journal of Food Safety & Hygiene* 7(3), 164–170.

Wadajkar, S.V., Shastri, U.V. and Narladkar, B.W. (1995) Caprine sarcocystosis: Clinical signs, gross and microscopic pathology. *Indian Veterinary Journal* 72, 224–228.

31 Echinococcosis

Vivek Agrawal*, Mukesh Shakya, A.K. Jayraw, Nidhi S. Choudhary, Nirmala Jamra, G.P. Jatav and Binita Kumari Singh
College of Veterinary Science and Animal Health, Mhow, NDVSU, Jabalpur, Madhya Pradesh, India

Abstract
Hydratidosis, or echinococcosis, is a cyclozoonotic disease that affects humans and animals. Four of the six species of *Echinococcus* pose major health risks. *Echinococcus granulosus* causes cystic echinococcosis, *E. multilocularis* alveolar, and *E. vogeli* and *E. oligarthrus* polycystic. The few *E. granulosus* strains known have evolved to specific life-cycle patterns and host assemblages. Some strains clearly qualify as species, whereas others do not. DNA analysis was used to identify *E. granulosus* genotypes (G1–10). The internal transcribed spacer (ITS) of rDNA has been studied in many parasites, including *Echinococcus*. These findings show that the ITS region of rDNA can provide an overall picture of genetic diversity and be a useful taxonomy marker. Cystic echinococcosis reduces the production of animal meat, milk and wool. Echinococcosis can be prevented by breaking the definitive–intermediate host life cycle. Education, occupational worker knowledge, stray dog management and strict organ and carcass disposal standards can help eradicate this deadly disease

Keywords: hydratidosis, Echinococcus, metacestode, genotypes, internal transcribed spacer (ITS)

31.1 Introduction

Echinococcosis is a zoonotic disease. It is also called hydatid disease or hydatidosis. Metacestode taeniid cestodes of the genus *Echinococcus* are responsible for echinococcosis infection in humans. Four of the six identified species are considered to constitute serious threats to human health. Cystic echinococcosis is caused by *Echinococcus granulosus*, alveolar echinococcosis by *Echinococcus multilocularis* and polycystic echinococcosis by *Echinococcus vogeli* and *Echinococcus oligarthrus*. The *E. vogeli* species is the smallest of the four. Carnivores serve as definitive hosts, housing the adult egg-producing form in the intestinal tract, whereas intermediate hosts are animals that are infected orally and evolve into the infective metacestode stage. Because the adult egg-producing form lives in the intestine of carnivores, they serve as definitive hosts. Echinococcosis is a disease caused by metacestodes that can affect humans and other animals. The *E. granulosus* species is known for having a fair amount of genetic diversity within it, which has resulted in the emergence of several distinct 'strains'. However, several of the types that are now known to be separate strains were, in fact, identified as species or subspecies quite a few years ago. Following a recent re-evaluation of the taxonomy of *Echinococcus* in light of phylogenetic analyses of deoxyribonucleic acid (DNA) sequence data, it has been suggested that its formal taxonomic position should be reinstated. Hydatidosis, or echinococcosis, is a cyclozoonotic disease that can affect both humans and animals. Therefore,

*Corresponding author: dragrawalin76@gmail.com

DOI: 10.1079/ 9781800622852.0031

it has significant implications for economies and public health, especially in developing countries (Ali *et al.*, 2020). The disease is found all across the world, but the rate at which it spreads varies greatly from one place to the next, due to differences in temperature and agroecology, as well as levels of education and development conditions (Al-Kitani *et al.*, 2017). It is more likely for *E. granulosus* to be found in developing nations than in developed nations, particularly in rural areas where there is close interaction between the dog, which is the definitive host, and a variety of domestic animals, any of which may act as an intermediate host (Torgerson *et al.*, 2000).

Echinococcus is distinguished from the second major genus in the family, *Taenia*, by the presence of a number of distinctive qualities that are exclusive to it. Adult *Echinococcus* species are just a few millimetres in length and typically have no more than six segments, whereas species of *Taenia* can grow to be several metres in length and consist of several thousand segments. In order to finish their life cycles, *Echinococcus* species need to infect two different mammalian hosts. The definitive host, a carnivore, will pass in its faeces segments known as gravid proglottids that contain eggs, as well as eggs that have been released from the segment. Eggs are consumed by an intermediate host, which allows for the development of the metacestode stage in a variety of the host's internal organs. When such infected organs of an intermediate host are consumed by an appropriate carnivore definitive host, the cycle is said to have been completed (Fig. 31.1). Eggs can be infectious for many months, or even up to around a year, if they are kept in a humid atmosphere at temperatures in the lower ranges (+4°C to +15°C) for an extended period of time. Eggs are highly resistant to environmental variables. Eggs laid by *Echinococcus* are particularly susceptible to drying out. At a relative humidity of 0%, eggs of *E. granulosus* were destroyed in just 1 day, but it took 4 days at a humidity level of 25%. Eggs of *E. granulosus* could not survive temperatures between 60°C and 80°C for more than a minute and a half. On the other hand, eggs laid by *Echinococcus* can tolerate temperatures as low as −40°C (Colli and Williams, 1972).

Eggs are the vectors via which the infection is passed on to the intermediate hosts, which include a diverse collection of mammalian species (Fig. 31.2). The keratinized embryophore gives way, allowing the oncosphere to emerge

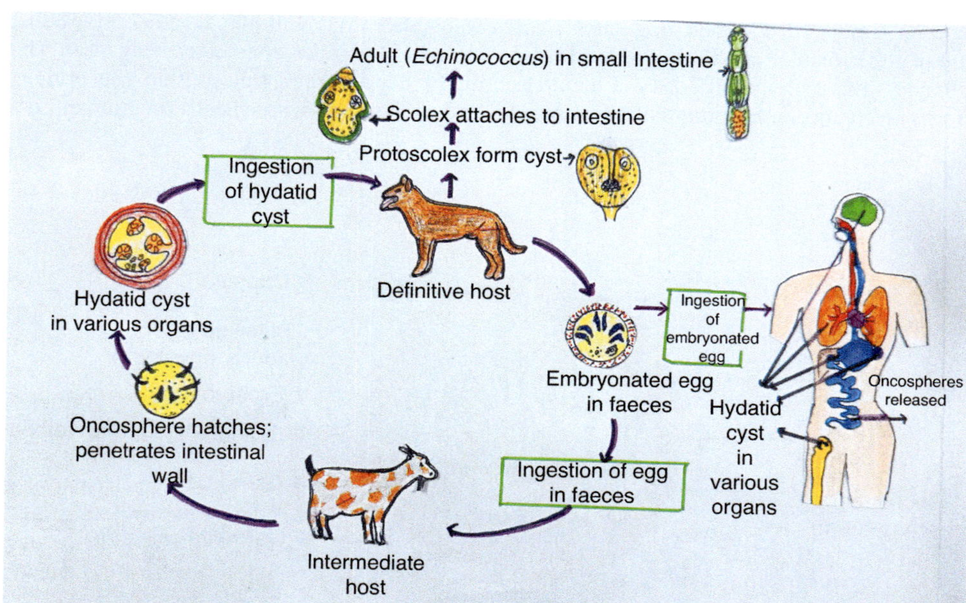

Fig. 31.1. Life cycle of *Echinococcus granulosus*. (Author's own image.)

from its confines. This process is catalysed by the action of enzymes in both the stomach and the small intestine. The secretion of bile is necessary for the activation of the oncosphere, which is responsible for penetrating the wall of the small intestine. After that, penetration is helped forward by the movements of the hook, and possibly also by the oncosphere's secretions. Once the oncosphere has gained entrance to a venule or a lacteal, it will be passively carried to the liver, where a portion of it will be maintained. Others make it to the lungs, and a small percentage of them may be carried on to the kidneys, spleen, muscles, brain, or other organs. It is possible to refer to any and all mammals, including humans, as 'intermediate hosts' in which metacestodes of *Echinococcus* species develop as a result of infection with eggs.

Echinococcus granulosus has low to intermediate host specificity. It has been found in domestic and wild ungulates belonging to eight different families, including bovids, in addition to primates and macropod marsupials. The most significant cycles for the perpetuation of *E. granulosus* involve domestic ungulates, of which it is stated that susceptible representatives can be found in every species. It is considered that the domestic form of *E. granulosus* arose from the form that is found in cervids, and that it became suited to domestic ungulates as a result of the spread of practices used in animal husbandry. There are several distinct life-cycle patterns involving domestic ungulates and dogs, and each one of them is maintained by the irresponsibility or ignorance of humans. There is no question that the cycle involving domestic dogs and sheep is the most significant one. Even while wild animals are involved in cycles in various parts of the world, the zoonotic significance of such cycles is very minor in comparison with the significance of domestic cycles.

The mature worm can vary in length from 2 mm to 7 mm (very rarely up to 11 mm), and it often has three or four segments (very rarely up to six) (Gill and Rao, 1967). It is usual for the genital pore to open posterior to the midpoint of the mature segment as well as the gravid segment. The penultimate segment has reached maturity. The uterus that is pregnant will have lateral sacculations that have matured to a significant degree (Fig. 31.3).

The metacestode stage consists of a bladder that is filled with fluid and is typically unilocular, though connecting chambers can also be present. The cyst is made up of an inner germinal or nucleated layer, which is supported externally by a stiff, elastic, acellular laminated layer of varying thickness. This layer is surrounded by an adventitial layer that is created by the host and is fibrous (Fig. 31.4).

In most cases, *E. granulosus* will create a cyst that is unilocular and has a single chamber. Sometimes cysts will join together to produce clusters of smaller cysts of varying sizes. This might happen randomly. Within the primary cyst of some hosts, specifically the human host,

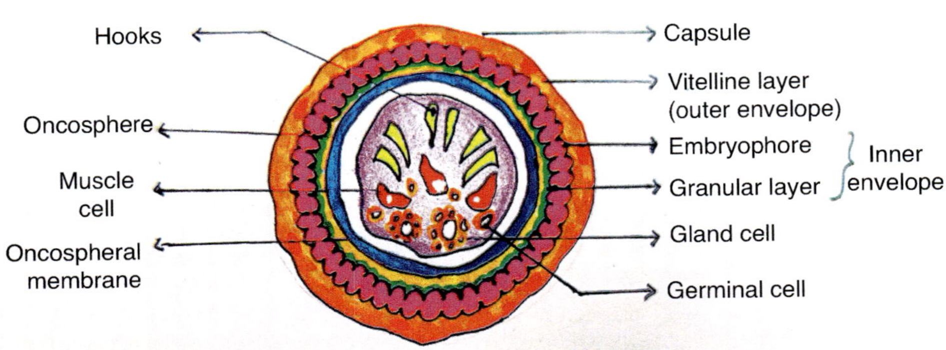

Fig. 31.2. Schematic diagram of *Echinococcus granulosus* egg. (Author's own image.)

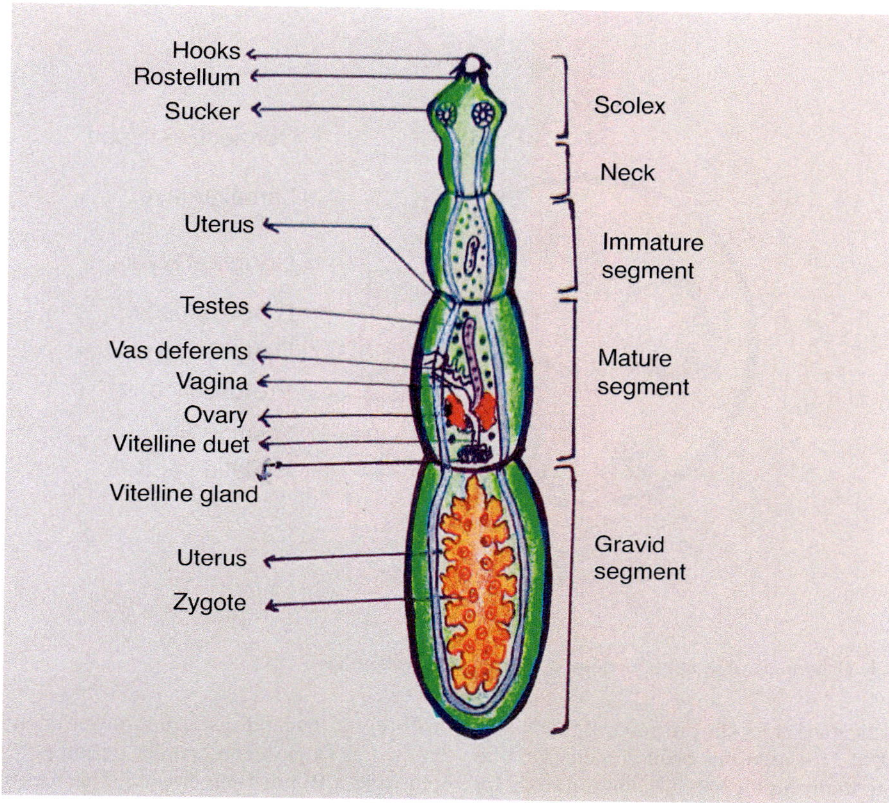

Fig. 31.3. Schematic diagram of adult *Echinococcus granulosus*. (Author's own image.)

it is possible for daughter cysts to emerge if the primary cyst grows to be an abnormally big size.

31.2 Epidemiological Significance of Various *Echinococcus Granulosus* Strains

There are a few distinct strains of *E. granulosus* that have been identified, and all of them appear to have evolved to certain life-cycle patterns and host assemblages. Some of these strains obviously merit the rank of species, while others do not. Biological characteristics have identified ten genotypes (G1–10) of *E. granulosus* variations based on DNA analysis (Thompson and McManus, 2002).

The concept of strain variety within the species *E. granulosus*, which was previously based on morphological and biological characteristics, has been mostly verified by recent genetic investigations. There are already a number of different molecular approaches available, any one of which might quite readily enable the identification of particular strains of *E. granulosus* by utilizing genetic markers. These kinds of investigations have the potential to help with the swift clarification of the epidemiological situation in a particular region, but they need to be carried out by a reference laboratory that has prior relevant experience.

The ITS region of rDNA, also known as the internal transcribed spacer, has been the subject of research on a variety of parasites, including *Echinococcus*. These studies have demonstrated that the ITS region of rDNA is able to not only provide an overall picture of the extent of genetic variation but also serve as an effective

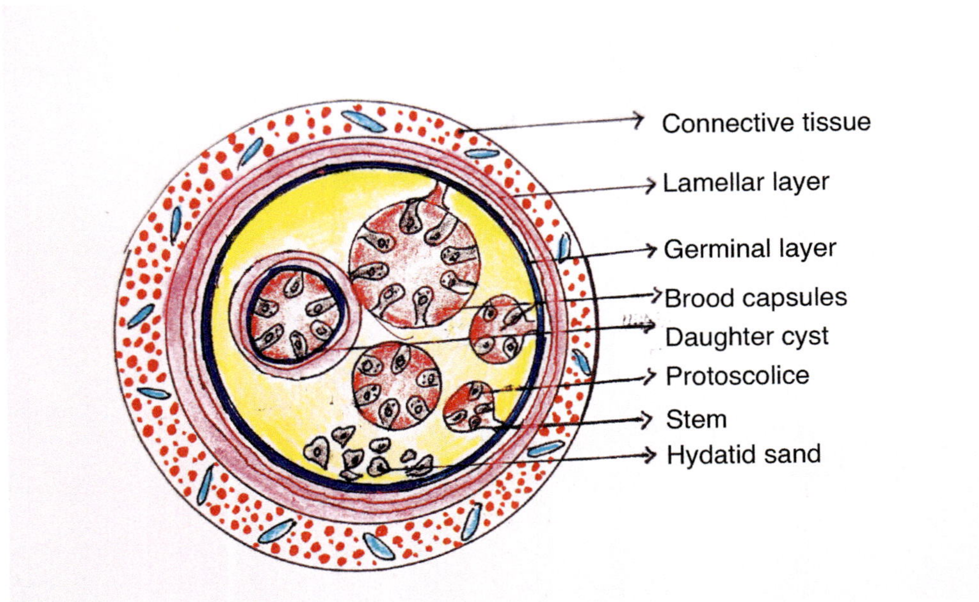

Fig. 31.4. Schematic diagram of hydatid cyst. (Author's own image.)

diagnostic marker for the purposes of taxonomy. The rDNA ITSI area has been demonstrated to be a potentially highly helpful genetic marker for identifying strains and species of *Echinococcus*, and small quantities of *Echinococcus* material can be classified using a technique known as polymerase chain reaction–restriction fragment length polymorphism (PCR–RFLP) fingerprinting. In addition, the rDNA ITSI region has been found to be a genetic marker that is potentially very useful for distinguishing strains and species of *Echinococcus*. This method, which may be altered in the future once additional restriction enzymes have been evaluated, provides a procedure that is the most reliable and technically reproducible for the routine laboratory identification of species and strains of *Echinococcus*. This is especially true when confirmation is obtained by sequencing mitochondrial DNA. In a recent study, the ITS1–PCR–RFLP fingerprinting technique and sequencing of the mitochondrial genes cytochrome C oxidase I (COI) and NADH dehydrogenase subunit I (NDI) were used to characterize 33 *E. granulosus* isolates collected from various regions and hosts in Argentina. The purpose of this study was to determine which genotypes occurred in humans with cystic hydatid disease. A novel technique known as single-strand conformation polymorphism (SSCP) has been created. This technique is technically quite straightforward, possesses a high-resolution capability when used in optimal conditions, and is an excellent choice for screening large sample sizes for nucleotide changes in short gene segments. The efficacy of SSCP was recently established for the classification of *Echinococcus* genotypes, and the method has been employed for the genetic analysis of a large number of isolates of *Echinococcus granulosus* collected from the People's Republic of China and from Argentina. For the purpose of molecular identification of *Echinococcus* species and strains, the PCR–RFLP fingerprinting approach and/or the determination of COI/NDI gene sequences by PCR/direct sequencing are probably the best methods that are now available.

Patients who have echinococcosis will have a different prognosis depending on the pathogenicity of the strains or species of *Echinococcus* they have contracted. Epidemiological evidence suggests that the sylvatic strain of *E. granulosus* in northern North America is infective to humans, causing a benign infection of low pathogenicity, with predominant localization of cysts in the lungs. This is due to the fact that the sylvatic strain lives in forest environments. Observations made in the field of epidemiology in the People's Republic of China have led researchers to hypothesize that *E. granulosus* strains found in particular parts of the country may not be as pathogenic. On the other hand, it has been hypothesized that there are locally virulent strains of *E. granulosus* present in certain regions of Kenya and Libya. There is also growing evidence from epidemiological studies that certain strains of *E. granulosus*, such as the kind that has adapted to horses, may not infect humans at all or may infect humans only very rarely. On the other hand, current isoenzyme and molecular research have validated what has been hypothesized for a long time based on epidemiological data, namely, that the sheep strain is infectious to human beings. In point of fact, until quite recently, the majority of *E. granulosus* material collected from human patients through surgical procedures belonged to the sheep strain. The exception to this was a single instance in the Netherlands, in which the bovine strain was typed through PCR-based molecular characterization processes. The findings of a study on the genetic variation and epidemiology of *E. granulosus* in Argentina reported for the first time the presence in humans of the Tasmanian sheep strain (G2 genotype) and the same genotypic strain (G6) previously identified in camels. These findings may have significant repercussions for the state of human health. On the basis of many pieces of circumstantial evidence, it was hypothesized that *E. granulosus* contracted from pigs would have a limited infectious potential for humans. In fact, recent research conducted at endemic foci in the Ukraine and Poland revealed that *E. granulosus* infections are quite common in dogs and pigs, but there was very little evidence of the disease in humans. Molecular genetic investigation of human cystic hydatid cases from Poland has, despite this, uncovered a hitherto unknown genotypic group (G9) of *E. granulosus*. According to the results of the molecular investigation, these patients did not have an infection with the strain that is often found in sheep. In its place, the hydatid parasite was shown to have a molecular affinity with the pig strain that had been previously defined, but it also had certain genetic changes. The findings of this study have raised a number of questions, the most important of which concerns the reservoir(s) of human hydatid disease in Poland. It is possible that pigs naturally host the newly detected genotype of *E. granulosus* that is present in humans there, but this has not yet been definitively established. The national numbers for cystic hydatidosis in slaughtered animals indicate that pigs have a prevalence that is five times higher than that of sheep.

Although camels in the Middle East and Africa are frequently found to be infected with *E. granulosus*, there has been some debate as to whether or not the disease may be transmitted to humans from camels. However, as mentioned previously, recent molecular genetic investigations of isolates obtained in Argentina have suggested for the first time that the camel strain genotype (G6) can infect people. This research was conducted in Argentina. Although it is difficult to get isolates of *E. granulosus* from these species, researchers are making an effort to do so. They are also attempting to study isolates from goats, given that the G6 genotype has also been discovered in goats in the past. In regions with a high concentration of intermediate host species, it is essential to determine whether or not each species harbours a unique strain of the pathogen and whether or not there is the potential for interactions between distinct cycles. For instance, *E. granulosus* is maintained in Great Britain through two separate cycles of transmission: sheep/dog and horse/dog. Interaction between the two cycles is highly unlikely because each cycle is associated with the maintenance of a different strain or species that exhibits different intermediate host specificity characteristics. The epidemiological facts are supported by the results of molecular characterization of parasite isolates from horses and sheep, which showed that the two host species are genetically distinct from one another. Developmental changes between species and strains of *Echinococcus*, in particular variation in the commencement of egg production, are likely to be a limiting issue in control programmes that require frequent, adult cestocidal treatment of definitive hosts in order to interrupt the cycle of transmission. This is because egg production begins at different times for different strains and species of *Echinococcus*. This has been shown to be the case in multiple strains of *E. granulosus*. For instance, the adult parasite of the cattle strain displays a precocious development in the definitive host with a short pre-patent phase of only 33–35 days. This is about a week earlier than the typical development of the parasite in sheep.

31.3 Economic Losses

Cystic echinococcosis can lower the yield and quality of meat, milk and wool from animals. It can also lower the birth rate, slow performance and growth and damage organs, especially the liver and lungs (Al-Shaibani *et al*., 2015) (Fig. 31.5). In addition, economic losses might occur as a result of the removal of infected viscera and deceased animals, as well as the prohibition on the export of animals and the products they produce if these are required to be free of cystic echinococcosis (CE). Echinococcosis in humans is a substantial threat to public health in a number of geographical areas across the globe. The necessity of surgical operations, hospital care and productivity losses in asymptomatic cases are the primary contributors to human casualties. The prevalence of hydatid cysts in significant food-producing animals was gathered from previously published abattoir-based epidemiological studies. These surveys indicated a prevalence of 5.39% in cattle, 4.36% in buffalo, 3.09% in pigs and 2.23% in sheep. In contrast, the prevalence of hydatid cysts was only 0.41% in goats. The most recent census of India's Department of Animal Husbandry, Dairying, and Fisheries served as a primary source for the collection of data pertaining to the animal population. A series of sensitivity analyses were carried out in order to determine the impact that various significant parameters had on the calculated economic losses. According to the findings of the study, the overall annual median loss amounts to Rs. 11.47 billion (about US$212.35 million). The cattle and buffalo industries were responsible for the majority of the losses, as they were responsible for 93.05% of the animal losses and 88.88% of the overall losses, respectively. The losses that were attributed to human hydatidosis were estimated to be Rs. 472.72 million (about US$8.75 million); however, it is likely that these numbers are an underestimate due to the fact that the disease is underreported in the country. When the proportion of human undiagnosed cases was increased

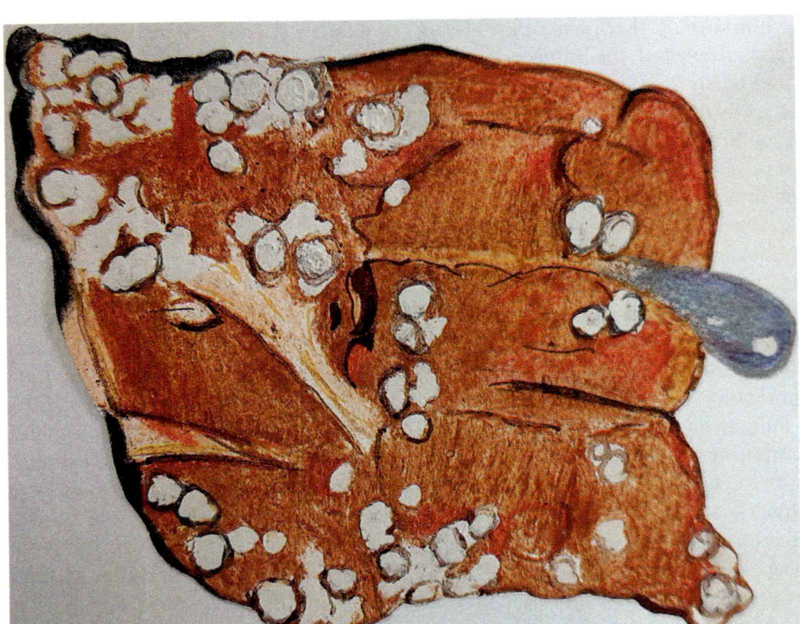

Fig. 31.5. Liver infected with hydatid cyst. (Author's own image.)

to 0.2%, the sensitivity analysis showed that the human losses more than quadrupled to Rs. 1953 million, which is equivalent to around US$36.17 million (Singh *et al.*, 2014). The findings underscore the critical necessity for the country to immediately implement a policy that is based on scientific research in order to control and manage the disease.

31.4 New Molecular Insights on Echinococcosis

31.4.1 Restriction fragment length polymorphism

The restriction fragment length polymorphism (RFLP) technique can be applied to various genomic areas in addition to ribosomal DNA (rDNA). In a Southern Blot procedure known as RFLP-SB, the DNA is first subjected to digestion by restriction enzymes, and then the fragments that are produced by this process are electrophoretically separated on an agarose gel, transferred to a nitrocellulose or nylon filter, and hybridized with a specific DNA probe that has been radioactively or otherwise tagged.

The rDNA RFLP technology has been coupled with the polymerase chain reaction (also known as PCR–RFLP or PCR-linked RFLP), which has resulted in a significantly simpler procedure. This was accomplished without a reduction in resolution or accuracy. A snippet of DNA that is defined by oligonucleotide primers at either end is amplified several million-fold using a thermostable form of Taq polymerase during the PCR process. The coding portions of ribosomal RNA genes are extremely well preserved; however, the non-coding spacer regions that separate them are only moderately well conserved. Ribosomal RNA genes are grouped into rDNA units. The sequence for PCR amplification was determined to be internal transcribed spacer 1 (ITS1), and primers were developed based on highly conserved areas at the 3' end of the 18S rRNA gene (forward primer BD1) and within the 5.8S rRNA gene (reverse primer 45). The PCR result, which includes the majority of the 5.85 gene and spans ITS1 of the rDNA repeat unit, has been amplified from a variety of *Echinococcus* isolates and digested with one of a number of restriction enzymes that cut 4-base bases. When agarose gel electrophoresis is used to assess samples from various species and strain groups, distinctive RFLP patterns are created. These patterns can be used to identify the samples (Bowles and McManus, 1993).

31.4.2 PCR-amplified deoxyribonucleic acid sequences

Using two conserved PCR primers, the nucleotide sequences (and inferred amino acid sequences) of segments of the mitochondrial cytochrome c oxidase subunit I (COI) gene and of the NADH dehydrogenase I (NDI) gene were determined. After PCR amplification of the variable segment that lies between the primers for a particular *Echinococcus* isolate, the variable segment is either manually or automatically sequenced in its entirety. Following this, the sequences acquired may be directly compared with sequences that have already been published for each of the four species of *Echinococcus* and each of the different genotypes of *E. granulosus*. The genotypic identification of a given isolate can then be identified as a result (Gasser *et al.*, 1999).

31.4.3 Random amplified polymorphic deoxyribonucleic acid–polymerase chain reaction

A technique known as random amplified polymorphic DNA–PCR, or RAPD–PCR, amplifies genomic DNA by the use of a single oligonucleotide primer with an arbitrary nucleotide sequence. This allows for the detection of polymorphisms in genomic DNA. This method is relatively straightforward; it requires only a tiny amount of DNA (about 25 ng), and it may be completed in a short amount of time. However, in order to produce results that can be relied upon, the conditions must first be very carefully managed, particularly in terms of the quantity and quality of the template DNA. As a result, it is recommended that RAPD–PCR be employed concurrently with either one of the other DNA techniques that are available (Taha, 2012).

31.4.4 Single-strand conformation polymorphism

A straightforward approach to mutation scanning, single-strand conformation polymorphism (also known as SSCP) has the potential to differentiate between two DNA sequences that only differ by a single nucleotide. The technique is predicated on the idea that the electrophoretic mobility of a single-stranded DNA molecule in a non-denaturing gel is directly proportional to the molecule's overall size and structure. The conformation of the molecule can be altered, and as a result, its electrophoretic mobility can be changed, if there is a mutation or a change in the base at a specific location in the main sequence. The direct visual display of sequence variation in PCR-amplified portions of the mitochondrial COI and NDI genes of *Echinococcus* species and *E. granulosus* genotypes has been accomplished by the application of SSCP. There is no need for DNA sequencing or restriction analysis when using this method, and a large number of samples can be evaluated in a very short amount of time. Despite the fact that the method requires very careful control, its advantages outweigh its drawbacks (Zhang *et al.*, 1999).

31.5 Diagnosis

Necropsy findings are the most important factor considered when making a diagnosis of cystic echinococcosis in intermediate hosts of *E. granulosus*. Clinical symptoms, particularly those with modest presentations, are commonly ignored because of this. However, ultrasound evaluation of cystic structures has also been performed in horses, thus it is not exclusive to the identification of conditions affecting smaller animals like sheep and goats. In Kenya, the detection of hydatid cysts was accomplished through ultrasound evaluation of the lungs and the liver.

It is necessary to do necropsies on intermediate hosts to look for cysts of *E. granulosus* in order to conduct baseline surveys and to monitor control efforts. Lungs and liver are the primary organs that are affected by this predisposition. When it comes to establishing the epidemiological status of *E. granulosus*, the age-dependent prevalence is the piece of evidence that is considered to be the most essential. It is imperative that the study be carried out with extreme caution so that organisms other than *E. granulosus* are not included in the results. When investigating the effects of age on the occurrence of a disease in young animals, it is absolutely necessary to take thin slices of both the liver and the lungs at a thickness of about 2 mm and to submit all lesions to staining and microscopy. For the purpose of histological analysis, material that has been preserved in formalin can be processed by the traditional staining processes. One distinguishing feature of metacestodes of *E. granulosus* is the presence of a PAS-positive acellular laminated layer, with or without an internal cellular nucleated germinal layer. It is possible to perform a differential diagnosis of larval cestodes utilizing techniques such as *in situ* hybridization antibody testing (IFAT) with monoclonal antibodies or PCR.

There is now no serological test available that is sensitive enough and specific enough to diagnose ovine hydatidosis, nor is there such a test available for any other species of animal. Nevertheless, the identification of exposure to *E. granulosus* at the flock or herd level by using mean values for serum antibody activity is conceivable when using hydatid cyst fluid antigens in ELISA. This method may be helpful in hydatid screening and surveillance programmes. It would be very helpful for monitoring hydatid prevention efforts if there was a way to identify exposure to *E. granulosus* in lambs using serology. Even an autopsy diagnosis can be difficult to make in this situation. In experimentally infected sheep, hydatid cyst fluid-reactive antibodies can be identified in the serum by 4 weeks after infection, particularly when large oral egg dosages were utilized. This is the case when the infection was carried out orally. However, reports of sensitivity of greater than 90% have been documented by groups utilizing antigen B-enriched hydatid fluid extracts in ELISA. This is despite the fact that the sensitivity of serological assays is very variable in spontaneous infections. Unless serum from monospecific helminth infections caused by organisms other than *Echinococcus* is tested, determining the specificity of an infection is challenging. Cross-reactivity has been documented to take place with infections caused by *T. hydatigena*, *T. ovis* and *F. hepatica* when this procedure is carried out. Unfortunately, very few investigations have been conducted to describe the difficulties associated with sensitivity and specificity in the immunodiagnosis of CE in animals. It is possible that recombinant antigens will increase specificity, but there will probably still be sensitivity issues

31.6 Treatment, Preventive Measures and Disease Management

Current means of treatment include surgery, which can be either conservative or laparoscopic, as well as percutaneous drainage, which consists of puncture, aspiration, injection and re-aspiration (PAIR) (Filice and Brunetti, 1997). These procedures are primarily helpful for liver cysts. Percutaneous drainage without re-aspiration is a procedure that can be used as an alternative to PAIR or surgery for the treatment of muscle, spleen, or kidney cysts.

In the therapy of patients with hydatid cysts in the liver and lungs, medical treatment with albendazole and mebendazole, which has proved successful, is useful. The use of combination chemotherapy with albendazole and praziquantel has been tried, and it has been discovered to be more effective than the use of either of these medicines alone. There were reports of flubendazole being effective either on its own or in conjunction with ivermectin. Infections caused by *E. granulosus* are treated with pre-surgical chemotherapy, which decreases the size and number of live protoscolices. Furthermore, it has been demonstrated that percutaneous treatment in combination with albendazole is more successful than surgical cystectomy (Elissondo *et al.*, 2009).

Echinococcosis can be controlled through preventive methods that break the life cycle between the definitive and intermediate hosts. These steps include completely preventing dogs from gaining access to infected raw offal by ensuring that any condemned offal that contains hydatid cysts is disposed of in an appropriate manner at abattoirs, local slaughterhouses, backyards and farms. Additional control methods include the introduction of appropriate meat inspection, the establishment of local slaughterhouses, the education of the people, the effective implementation of legislative measures, the burning or burial of condemned offal and the sterilization of offal, if it is going to be used as dog food. Specific control measures, such as the capture and euthanization of stray dogs, the registration of all privately owned dogs, the spaying and neutering of female dogs and the administration of praziquantel to all or the majority of dogs at regular intervals, such as once every 6–8 weeks, are recommended (Eckert and Deplazes, 2004). It is possible to avoid contracting the disease by adhering to stringent hygiene practices and routines, such as: washing one's hands after handling animals, in particular dogs; controlling the movement of food animals and dogs from diseased areas to clean areas; marking animals from infected flocks or herds and controlling their movement (Watson-Jones and Macpherson, 1988). *Echinococcus* vaccinations would ideally block oncosphere progression to hydatid cysts in sheep, and consequently stop the formation of adult gravid tapeworms in dogs (Pourseif *et al.*, 2018). Large controlled experiments with sheep have demonstrated that immunization with a recombinant oncospheral EG95 provides a significant degree of protection, lowering the cyst counts in vaccinated animals by roughly 90–100%. There is no vaccine for dogs, but research is under way. There has been some success in using community ultrasound surveys to educate people about potentially dangerous situations. Currently there are no effective human vaccinations against any kind of echinococcosis but there is research looking at potential vaccine candidates.

31.7 Conclusion

Proper education, raising awareness among occupational workers, managing stray dogs and implementing stringent rules surrounding the disposal of condemned organs and carcasses will assist to eradicate this disease. This will limit the risk of the disease being passed on to possible hosts in the area.

References

Ali, R., Khan, S., Khan, M., Adnan, M., Ali, I. *et al.* (2020) A systematic review of medicinal plants used against *Echinococcus granulosus*. *PLoS ONE* 15(10), e0240456.

Al-Kitani, F.A., Mansoor, M.K., Hussain, M.H., Al Rawahi, A.H., Saqib, M. *et al.* (2017) Sero-epidemiology of cystic echinococcosis (*Echinococcus granulosus*) in the livestock of Oman. *Veterinary Parasitology: Regional Studies and Reports* 8, 21–27.

Al-Shaibani, I., Saad, F.A. and Al-Mahdi, H. (2015) Cystic echinococcosis in humans and animals at Dhamar and Taiz governorates, Yemen. *International Journal of Current Microbiology and Applied Sciences* 4(2), 596–609.

Bowles, J. and McManus, D.P. (1993) Rapid discrimination of *Echinococcus* species and strains using a polymerase chain reaction-based RFLP method. *Molecular and Biochemical Parasitology* 57(2), 231–239.

Colli, C.W. and Williams, J.F. (1972) Influence of temperature on the infectivity of eggs of *Echinococcus granulosus* in laboratory rodents. *The Journal of Parasitology* 58(3), 422–426.

Eckert, J. and Deplazes, P. (2004) Biological, epidemiological, and clinical aspects of echinococcosis, a zoonosis of increasing concern. *Clinical Microbiology Reviews* 17(1), 107–135.

Elissondo, M.C., Ceballos, L., Alvarez, L., Sánchez Bruni, S., Lanusse, C. *et al.* (2009) Flubendazole and ivermectin *in vitro* combination therapy produces a marked effect on *Echinococcus granulosus* protoscoleces and metacestodes. *Parasitology Research* 105, 835–842.

Filice, C. and Brunetti, E. (1997) Use of PAIR in human cystic echinococcosis. *Acta Tropica* 64(1–2), 95–107.

Gasser, R.B., Zhu, X. and McManus, D.P. (1999) NADH dehydrogenase subunit I and cytochrome c oxidase subunit I sequences compared for members of the genus *Taenia* (Cestoda). *International Journal for Parasitology* 29(12), 1965–1970.

Gill, H.S. and Rao, B.V. (1967) On the biology and morphology of *Echinococcus granulosus* (Batsch, 1786) of buffalo–dog origin. *Parasitology* 57(4), 69.

Pourseif, M.M., Moghaddam, G., Saeedi, N., Barzegari, A., Dehghani, J. *et al.* (2018) Current status and future prospective of vaccine development against *Echinococcus granulosus*. *Biologicals* 51, 1–11.

Singh, B.B., Dhand, N.K., Ghatak, S. and Gill, J.P. (2014) Economic losses due to cystic echinococcosis in India: Need for urgent action to control the disease. *Preventive Veterinary Medicine* 113(1), 1–12.

Taha, H.A. (2012) Genetic variations among *Echinococcus granulosus* isolates in Egypt using RAPD-PCR. *Parasitology Research* 111, 1993–2000.

Thompson, R.A. and McManus, D.P. (2002) Towards a taxonomic revision of the genus *Echinococcus*. *Trends in Parasitology* 18(10), 452–457.

Torgerson, P.R., Carmona, C. and Bonifacino, R. (2000) Estimating the economic effects of cystic *Echinococcosis*: Uruguay, a developing country with upper-middle income. *Annals of Tropical Medicine & Parasitology* 94(7), 703–713.

Watson-Jones, D.L. and Macpherson, C.N.L. (1988) Hydatid disease in the Turkana district of Kenya: VI. man:dog contact and its role in the transmission and control of hydatidosis amongst the Turkana. *Annals of Tropical Medicine & Parasitology* 82(4), 343–356.

Zhang, L., Gasser, R.B., Zhu, X. and McManus, D.P. (1999) Screening for different genotypes of *Echinococcus granulosus* within China and Argentina by Single-Strand Conformation Polymorphism (SSCP) analysis. *Transactions of the Royal Society of Tropical Medicine and Hygiene* 93(3), 329–334.

32 Myiasis and Mange

Manaswini Dehuri*
Department of Veterinary Parasitology, College of Veterinary Science and Animal Husbandry, OUAT, Bhubaneswar

Abstract
The ectoparasitic infestation in goats leads to myiasis and mange in goats. The flies that cause myiasis mostly belong to family Calliphoridae. The different types of myiasis are wound, warble and nasal myiasis. The effectiveness of treatment depends on the application of insecticides and control of fly population. Mange infestations are caused by parasitic mites like *Sarcoptes*, *Psoroptes* and *Demodex* species. Mange causes allergic dermatitis, which occurs as discomfort and scratching-related skin conditions that lead to irritation, exudation, crusts and scabs forming on the skin, and has several clinical manifestations that can be treated by the use of acaricides.

Keywords: Calliphora fly, insecticides, scab, maggots

32.1 Myiasis in Goats

Myiasis is derived from Greek word *mya*, meaning fly, and was first proposed by the researcher F.W. Hope in 1840 to define diseases caused by dipterous larvae, instead of those caused by insect larvae in general (Hope, 1840). Myiasis has since been defined as the infestation of live vertebrates (humans and animals) with dipterous larvae. Myiasis-causing flies are one of the most devastating insects, responsible for significant economic losses that include reduced milk yield, body weight and fertility, as well as hide quality. In mammals, the dipteran larvae feed on the host's living or dead tissue, body fluids and ingested food. Depending on the location in the body and the relationship of the larvae with the host, a broad range of infestations is observed (Zumpt, 1965). Myiasis in goats is a major animal welfare problem that causes pain and suffering and, unless treated, will result in grave tissue injury, loss in production, reproduction losses and even death. Due to the importance of dairy husbandry, prevention and control of myiasis can be problematic, especially of lactating females in goat herds, due to the lengthy withdrawal periods for many of the insecticidal products (Sotiraki and Hall, 2012).

The families and genera that are usually incriminated in myiasis of goats are:

- Calliphoridae: Calliphora, Chrysomya, Lucilia, Protophormia;
- Sarcophagidae: Sarcophaga, Wohlfahrtia; and
- Oestridae: Oestrus, Przhevalskiana.

The main types of myiasis in goats are traumatic or wound myiasis, nasal myiasis and warble myiasis. The most common agents of these diseases in goats are *Wohlfahrtia magnifica*, *Oestrus ovis* and *Przhevalskiana silenus*, respectively.

*Corresponding author: nishi.md@gmail.com

 The Handbook of Zoonotic Diseases of Goats (ed. T. Rana)
DOI: 10.1079/ 9781800622852.0032

32.1.1 Traumatic or wound myiasis

Traumatic or wound myiasis is caused mainly by calliphorid and sarcophagid flies. Traumatic myiasis is defined as when larvae 'invade pre-existing wounds and enlarge them, or form wounds after having actively gained access to the tissue' (Zumpt, 1965). Most of the calliphorid species involved, such as *Lucilia sericata* and *Chrysomya albiceps*, are facultative dipteran flies that develop in live hosts as well as carrion (Figs. 32.1–32.3).

The obligate parasite causing traumatic myiasis of goats is the sarcophagid, *Wohlfahrtia magnifica* (wound myiasis fly), whose larvae move actively in the skin surface. *Lucilia* spp. can also be found at sites of wounds, where larvae tend to feed on necrotic tissues (Khalafallah, 2020). *W. magnifica* is an obligate parasite that requires a living host for development of its larvae: they cannot develop on carrion. A number of predisposing factors such as the level of worm burden (internal parasites), extent of soiling mostly by faeces, urine and ensuing bacterial contamination, temperature and humidity affect the level of infestation (Angulo-Valadez, 2009). All these factors affect the larval growth, multiplication and survival. The larvae may remain on the skin surface with little damage or they may bore inwards. Larger numbers of larvae create a larger wound. Death may result, usually from secondary effects, including toxaemia. The adult females lay larvae rather than eggs; the larvae moult from first to second instars within 6–8 hours and undergo a second moult to third instars. About 5–7 days after larvipositing, they drop from the wound to the ground, into which they burrow for pupation (Ruiz-Martinez *et al.*, 1989). When larvae leave the wound, it can become secondarily infested by facultative species. Traumatic myiasis gives rise to a severe penetrative infestation of dermal tissues by larvae. Sites infested include the mucous membranes, head and body orifices,

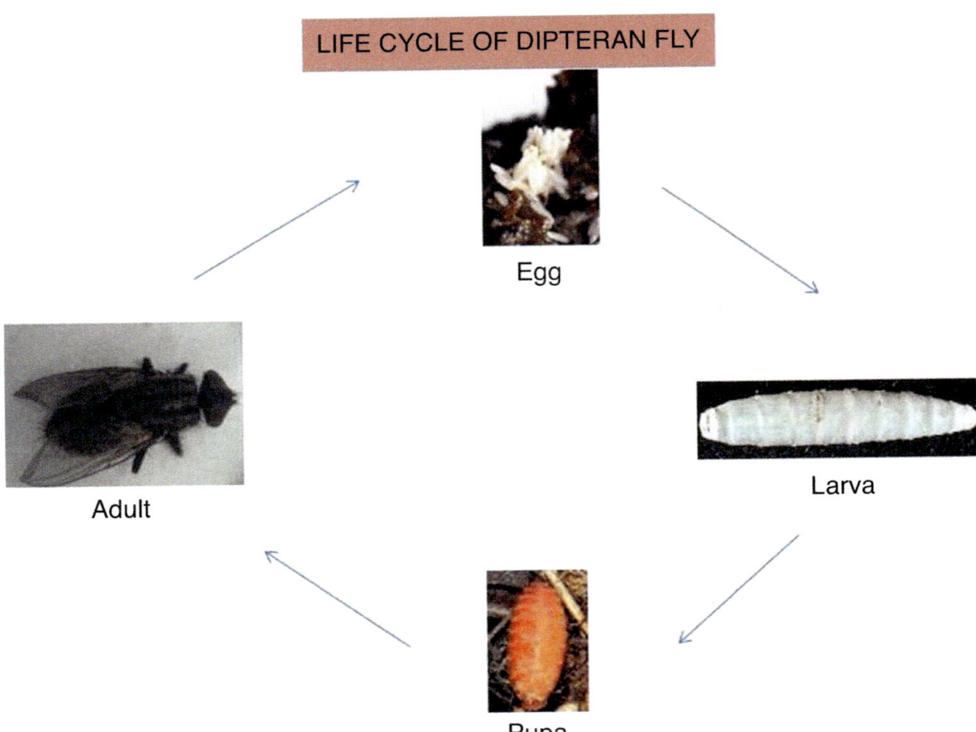

Fig. 32.1. Life cycle of dipteran fly. (Author's own image.)

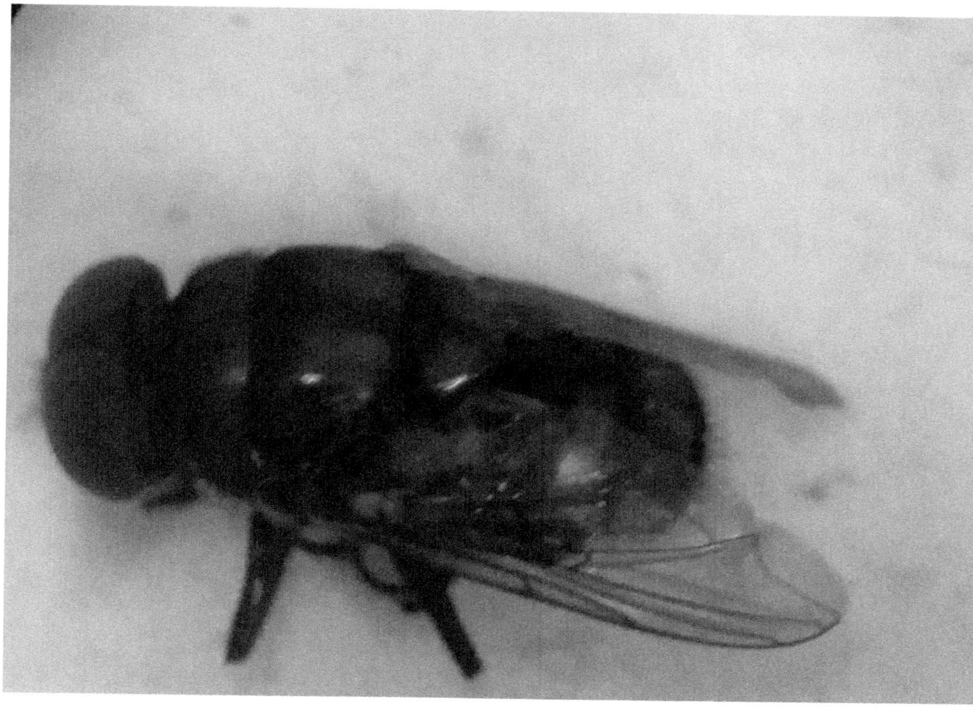

Fig. 32.2. *Chrysomya* fly. (Author's own image.)

especially the genitalia of both female and male hosts. The prevalence in males is frequently greater than in females and causes, in effect, a temporary castration (Farkas *et al.*, 2009).

32.1.2 Nasal myiasis

Nasal myiasis is caused by larvae of *Oestrus ovis* (Diptera: Oestridae). The adult nose-bot fly does not cause any harm to animals, but larvae live in the nostrils of goats. The larvae are obligatory parasites of nasal and sinus cavities (Zumpt, 1965). The development of larvae in the nasal–sinus cavities can cause severe clinical signs, including breathing difficulties and nasal discharge which, together with the annoyance caused by the adult flies, may lead to significantly reduced animal production and economic losses. Larvae mature in the head sinuses and nasal membranes become inflamed as a result of larvae migrating to and from the head sinuses. Infected animals develop symptoms that include grinding of teeth, loss of appetite, excessive head shaking and nasal discharge. The nasal discharge may contain blood. When mature bot flies are present, goats exhibit unusually excitable behaviour. Secondary infections can develop at the sites of migration. *O. ovis* flies are equipped with olfactory sensilla, which allow for the detection of various host-related odour volatiles (Poddighe *et al.*, 2010). Gadding, searching for shade during the day and sneezing are typical behaviours in the proximity of larvipositing flies. The main pathophysiological mechanisms involve mast cells and eosinophils, which destroy the larvae in sensitized animals (Lashari, 2016). The intense eosinophilic reaction can have side effects on the nasal mucosa and, more generally, as significant accumulation of eosinophils in tissues can have important consequences on other parasites living in these locations (e.g. gastrointestinal strongyles), which have been reported in goats. *O. ovis* infection elicits an IgM and IgG systemic antibody response. Ivermectin is very effective against *O. ovis* larvae in all

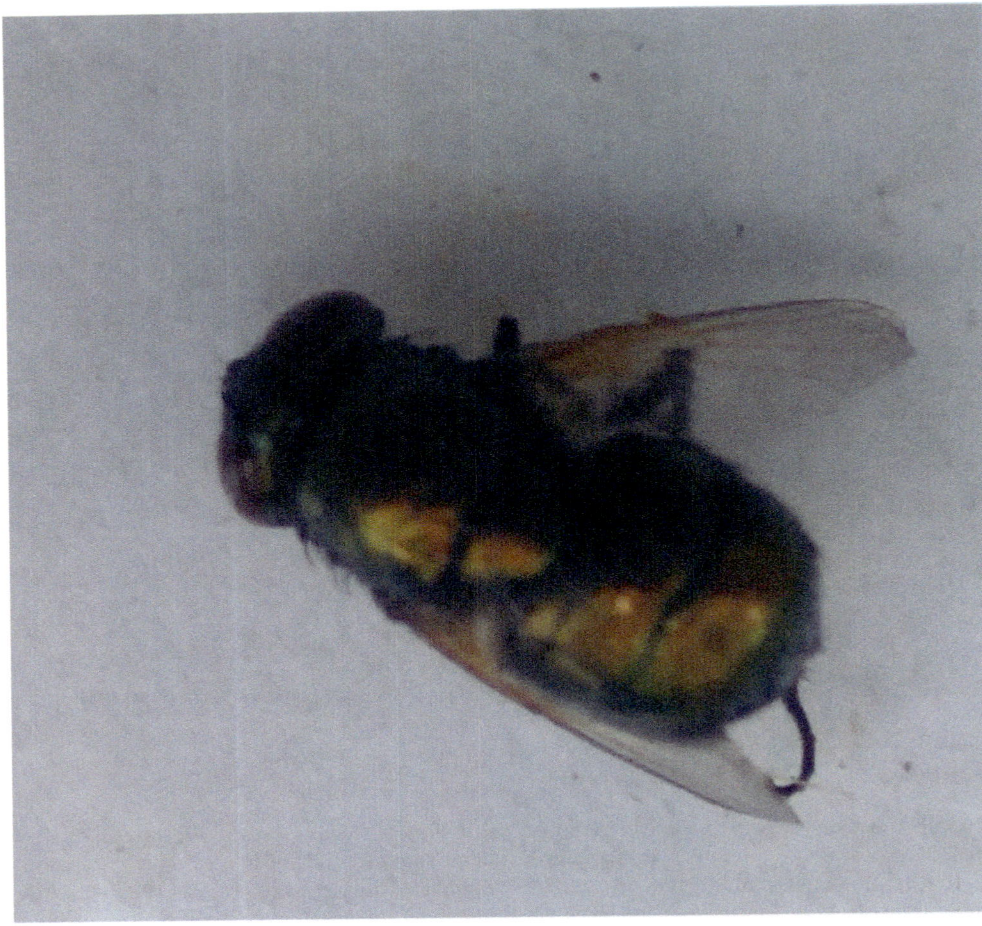

Fig. 32.3. *Lucilia* fly. (Author's own image.)

stages. Eprinomectin and doramectin are other medications that are effective.

32.1.3 Warble myiasis

Goat warble fly infestation is a myiasis caused by the larval stages of *Przhevalskiana* species, flies that belong to the family Oestridae, subfamily Hypodermatinae, whose larvae mature under the skin of goats, mainly in the back, flank and, rarely, in other subcutaneous regions (Zumpt, 1965). The three species that cause warble myiasis are *P. silenus*, *P. aegagri* and *P. crossii*, with prevalence in flocks ranging from 30% to 90% (Tassi *et al.*, 1989). After mating, female flies lay their eggs on goat hairs and first-instar larvae emerge in 5–6 days, penetrating the subcutaneous tissue by means of the collagenolitic enzymes of salivary and intestinal glands. The larvae are found in the subcutaneous tissue of the animal's back and flanks and develop into their second and third stages, thus causing warbles. *P. silenus* larvae do not migrate in their hosts, either subcutaneously or to any internal organs (Oryan *et al.*, 2009).

A study in Iran showed that *P. silenus* larva infested 5.3% of the goat population (Azizi *et al.*, 2007). The factors predisposing to wound myiasis in goats has been reported as open wound, shearing wound, caseous lymphadenitis, foot rot, faecal staining, ophthalmo- or facial eczema, horn fracture, rumen fistula and posterior paralysis. Also poor hygiene, presence of draining wounds, reduced level of farmers' consciousness and immobility affect occurrence of myiasis (Amin *et al.*, 1997). According to a study in Northen India, *P. silenus* infestations cause an overall loss of Rs. 73.26 million annually, in which reduced growth alone contributed 49% of the total losses (Yadav *et al.*, 2012).

32.1.4 Control of myiasis

Management practices can help to reduce myiasis by good grazing and insecticide use. The effectiveness of treatment is dependent on the timing of application and the seasonal effects of temperature and rainfall. Regular inspection and treatment of affected animals can help reduce myiasis prevalence. The fly populations can be controlled by the use of traps, and parasitoid wasps also offer some promise. In livestock, myiasis is controlled primarily through the prophylactic and therapeutic use of diazinon, the pyrethroids like deltamethrin and cypermethrin, the macrolide compound ivermectin and, in recent years, the insect growth regulators cyromazine, dicyclanil and diflubenzuron (Wall, 2012).

32.2 Mange in Goats

All around the globe, mange infestations caused by parasitic mites are a common problem of small ruminants and can occur during grazing, treatment and overcrowding that facilitate rapid development of mites. The goat mites feed on blood, lymph, skin waste, or sebaceous secretions. The mites devour by piercing the skin, scavenging from the skin surface, or sucking from skin lesions. The spread of infestation is facilitated by poor health care, starvation or lack of awareness about mange mites. Also, sex hormones may contribute to immunosuppression that acts as a predisposing factor. The impact of the mange in causing skin damage leads to reduced performance in the tanning industry, which affects the country's foreign exchange. Mange causes allergic dermatitis due to infestations of mites, occurs as discomfort and scratching-related skin conditions that lead to irritation, exudation, crusts and scabs forming on the skin, and has several clinical manifestations. Mites are obligate parasites that spend their entire life cycles, from egg to adult, on the host. In goats, there may be many species of burrowing mites (scabies mite (*Sarcoptesscabiei*), goat follicle mite (*Demodex caprae*)) and non-burrowing mites (psoroptic ear mite (*Psoroptes cuniculi*) and chorioptic scab mite (*Chorioptesbovis*).

Mange causes great financial loss to farmers due to livestock deaths and poor production and reproduction performance. It is also an important factor for downgrading or refusal of the skin of mange-infested animals in the tannery. Besides, the effect of the disease on skin damage severely limits the performance of tannery plants and thus also limits the country's foreign currency earnings.

Intense pruritus, manifested over the face, pinnae, neck, limbs, or over the body and associated with the presence of papules, crusts, excoriations and hypotrichosis-alopecia, on an erythematous or hyperpigmented, lichenified, thick and folded skin make up the typical clinical picture of sarcoptic mange as it appears in the goat. The affected animals usually die at the final stage of the disease, preceded by anorexia, emaciation or cachexia, and lethargy (Dorny *et al.*, 1994).

In cases of mange-infected goats, reduced values of haemoglobin, total erythrocyte count, total platelet count, pack cell volume, neutrophils and monocytes were observed, whereas total leukocyte count, lymphocytes and eosinophils increased significantly. The activity of alanine aminotransferase, total protein, zinc and copper were significantly decreased while aspartate aminotransferase activity increased in mange-infested goats (Shah *et al.*, 2022).

32.2.1 Sarcoptic mange (scabies)

Scabies is a highly contagious disease in goats, caused by the mite *Sarcoptes scabiei* var. *caprae*, and it is mainly transmitted by close contact (Fig. 32.4). *Sarcoptic* mange is caused by

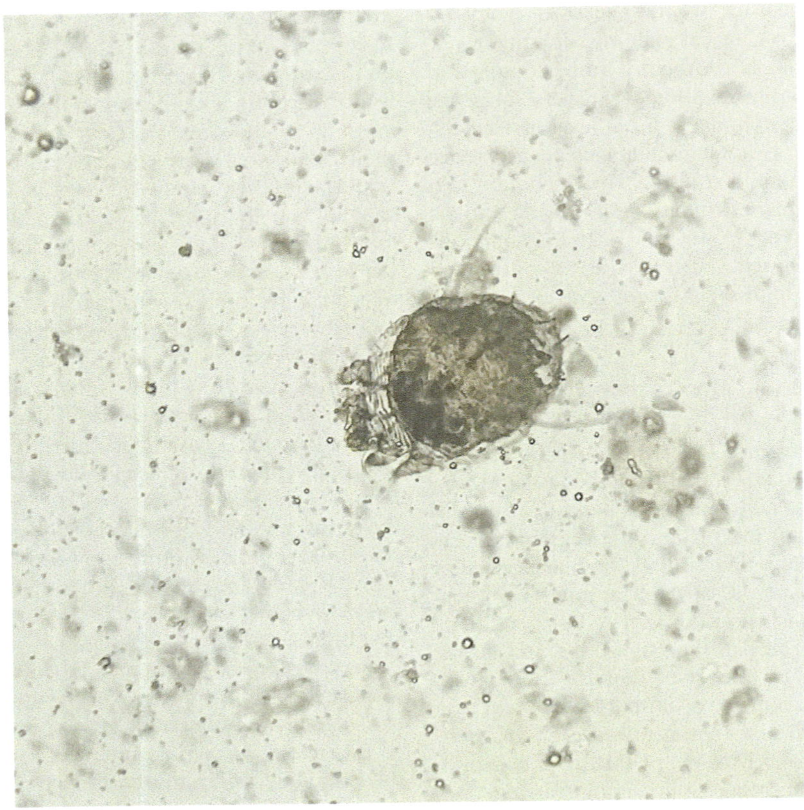

Fig. 32.4. *Sarcoptes* mite. (Author's own image.)

burrowing mites that are globular in shape and is characterized by extreme pruritus, scratching and rubbing against inanimate objects. In female mites, the first two pairs of legs end in unsegmented pedicels, while the third and fourth pairs end in hair/setae. In male mites, setae are present only in the third pair of legs. The dorsal surface of mites contains triangular spines and scales.

The female mite burrows under the skin to lay eggs; the eggs hatch and moult to larvae and the larvae produce new burrows. The larvae moult further to nymphs and adults and the life cycle is completed within 2–3 weeks. Due to constant scratching, there is restlessness, abrasion and degradation of the skin and firmly attached scabs are formed. The infection starts from the head and then spreads to the whole body. Lesions result directly from the mechanical damage due to the presence of the mites. This damage occurs as the mites feed and move about, and from irritating secretions from the mites. Additionally, an immune-mediated hypersensitivity to foreign antigens from the mites produces inflammation. As the host responds to inflammation by rubbing or other types of self-mutilation, the lesions increase in size and severity. Itching is a frequent symptom in cutaneous hypersensitivity reactions and also represents the first clinical feature for sarcoptic mange. The infection produces itchy, chronic, encrusted lesions and loss of hair. There is intense pruritus, observed over the face, pinnae, neck, limbs and all over the body, associated with the presence of papules, crusts, excoriations, hypotrichosis and alopecia. The skin is erythematous or hyperpigmented, and lichenified, thick and folded skin makes up the typical clinical picture of sarcoptic mange in the goat. The affected animals usually die at the final stage of the disease, preceded by anorexia, emaciation or cachexia, and lethargy (Scott, 1988) (Dorny *et al.*, 1994). *Sarcoptes scabei* not only causes direct economic loss to the farmer through animal mortality and poor growth and reproduction, but also the skin of mange-infested animals often must be downgraded or rejected at the tannery. This leads to economic losses to the tannery industry.

32.2.2 Psoroptic scabies

This is due to *Psoroptes cuniculi*, a non-burrowing mite that is highly contagious and transmitted readily from one animal to another by direct contact. They are ovoid mites, about 0.75 mm in length, with four pairs of brownish legs and sharp, pointed, brownish mouth parts. The eggs are large (250 μm) and oval. They feed superficially on lipid emulsion of skin cells, bacteria and lymph of host skin, produced as a result of a hypersensitivity reaction to the mite's faeces. At the site of puncture, the serum on the skin becomes mixed with debris, which soon dries, hardens and forms a crust or scab. As the lesion develops, the skin becomes thickened, hard and wrinkled. In the ears, they cause crusting leading to head shaking. The lesions grow, the centre becomes dry and covered in a yellow crust, whilst the border areas become moist. The host scratches its skin due to the intense itching. The disease is primarily seen during the winter season and goats become restless and exhausted, suffering from weight loss and poor growth rates. *P. cuniculi* is a cause of otitis in goats, with head shaking and scratching being the typical signs of irritation. Although the infestation is generally benign, with clinical signs limited to behavioural changes, animals with severe mite infestations shows symptoms of internal otitis, due to bacterial superinfection. *Psoroptes* mites also cause decline in reproductive performance in goats by causing lesions and consequently irritation of the scrotum (Littlejohn, 1968).

32.2.3 Chorioptic mange (foot scabies)

This mange is caused by a mite known as *Chorioptes caprae*, also known as *Chorioptes ovis*, *Chorioptes equi*, *Chorioptes bovis* and *Chorioptes cuniculi* as well as *Chorioptes texanus*. It is a non-borrowing mite that affects skin, particularly the legs and fore feet, but also the base of the tail and upper rear surface of the udder. Infected animals may stamp or scratch infected areas, causing skin damage. The mites are transmitted by direct contact and contaminated fomites. They have a lifespan of 60 days and complete their life cycle on the body of the host in 3 weeks. The clinical signs of animals with chorioptic mange include alopecia, pruritus, thickening and wrinkling of the skin with scabs, crust and fissures on the feet and tail (Reddy *et al.*, 2013). *Chorioptes* mites generally have a small round body and unsegmented pedicel with cup-shaped suckers. The mites reside in groups on the surface of the skin, usually on the lower parts of the legs and around the feet, and spread to the inner surfaces of the thighs and to the udder and abdomen in severe cases. The visible lesions usually occur initially around the feet and are more evident during winter when the flock is housed together. Lesions caused by *Chorioptes* are mostly observed on farms with poor management and nutrition. The lesions on the legs and in the interdigital space are usually benign, consisting only of hair loss and of dry crusts. These mites are also associated with a high incidence of interdigital myiasis. Severe infestation leads to decreased meat and milk production as well as poor hide quality, which may result in heavy economic loss in the leather industry.

32.2.4 Follicular mange (demodectic scabies)

Demodectic mange is quite common in goats and is caused by *Demodex caprae* (Fig. 32.5). The mites are host-specific and they infest the sebaceous or oil glands of the skin, which become filled with a thick, cheesy substance that contains lots of mites. The swollen glands look like nodules and are found at the base of the neck in front of the shoulders, back, hips, flanks, ears and jaws and may eventually spread all over the whole body. The elongated body of the mite is divided into the anterior part, which bears the head; the thorax, with legs attached (short and stout); and the abdomen. The mites have sucking mouth parts. *Demodectic* mange is found deep in

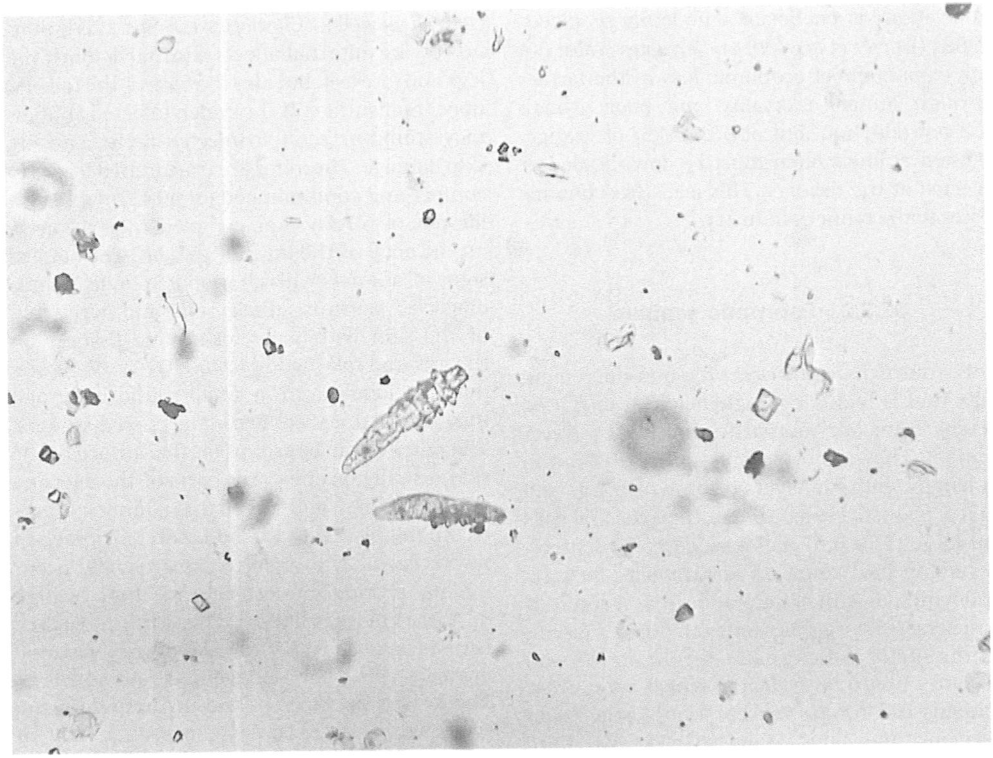

Fig. 32.5. *Demodex* mite. (Author's own image.)

the skin and causes pustules, redness, scaling, nodules and hair loss. It occurs most commonly in kids, pregnant does and dairy goats (Dalapati *et al.*, 1997). The nodules contain a thick, waxy, greyish material. Transmission requires prolonged contact, such as when suckling, hence most infections are acquired in the early weeks of life and seen on the muzzle, neck and withers.

32.3 Prevalence of Myiasis Flies and Mange Mites

Table 32.1 shows the prevalence of carriers for myiasis and mange in goats.

32.4 Diagnosis for Mange

The infected animal is clinically examined for the presences of skin lesions like scales, crust, alopecia and clinical signs of itching. Skin scraping is commonly used for diagnosis of dermatological conditions such as mange infestation. The blade is dipped in drops of mineral oil before scratching the skin. The skin is deeply scraped for burrowing mites until the capillary fluid oozes out. Skin scrapings from mange-like lesions from clinically suspected animals are collected in a clean container for detailed laboratory examination. Multiple skin scrapings from the edges of visible active mange-like lesions for mites are collected and preserved in 70% alcohol. The samples are processed in the laboratory by direct smear and sedimentation methods and examined under microscope using low power of magnification. Skin scrapings collected from the goats with mange-like skin lesions are dissolved in 10% potassium hydroxide solution for microscopic examination for the presence of mites. Also, concentration and flotation of multiple scrapings may increase chances of finding the mites and eggs. Skin biopsies are

Table 32.1. Prevalence of myiasis flies and mange mites in goats from different regions of the world.

Region	Prevalence %	Salient findings	Reference
Tamil Nadu, India	Myiasis in goats (9.85%). *Chrysomyabezziana* and *Musca domestica*	The prevalence was significantly ($P <$ 0.05) higher in females, in adults, in summer and in Boer goats. Lambing and kidding in adults and tagging in lambs/kids were the most important predisposing factors for myiasis. Lesions of cutaneous myiasis were located more frequently on the head and genitals.	Soundararajan *et al*., 2021
Egypt	(2.11%) infested with *Przhevalskiana silenus* fly	Nodule caused by *P. silenus* larvae were recovered from 32.65% slaughtered goats.	Morsy *et al*., 1998
Jammu, India	47.22% of warble fly (*Przhevalskianasilenus*)	Highest prevalence in > 3 years Adult fly is active in April to June.	Yadav *et al*., 2011
Chittagong, Bangladesh	69%	Infestation highest in goats aged above 6 months (75.5%), cross-breeds (34.2%) and females (64.5%) Foul odorous abscess with wound, umbilical infection, dirtiness, faecal and urine contamination and bed sores were the most habitual risk factors. Most exposed sites were vagina and perineal region, inter digital space, tail, brisket, navel, scrotum, inguinal region and gums.	Imtiaz *et al*., 2014.
Southern Ethiopia	*Demodex* (2.86%), *Psoroptes* (8.1%), *Sarcoptes* (23.7%)	Goats with poor body condition score (43.6%), adult goats (37.6%), males (60.2%) more than females (39.8%) were the most infected. Skin lesions most frequent on the head region followed by legs and thoracic region.	Fesseha *et al*., 2021
Malaysia	*Chorioptes texanus*-(20.7%), *Psoroptes cuniculi* (19.3%), *Sarcoptes scabiei* (18.6%) and *Demodex canis* var. *caprae* (0.4%)	Higher incidence of *Chorioptes* was detected in young goats.	Dorny *et al*., 1994
Anand, India	55.56%	Higher prevalence of sarcoptic mange in 1–2 years of age and in females.	Shah *et al*., 2022
Multan, Pakistan	35.50%	Prevalence was highest (46.15%) in age group of 28–50 months and in females.	Lashari *et al*., 2016.
Eastern Ethiopia	7.5 %	*Sarcoptes* and *Demodex* spp. higher prevalence in poor body condition.	Seid *et al*., 2016

also collected from different sites from goats with mange-like skin lesions and fixed in 10% neutral-buffered formalin. The skin biopsies are routinely processed, sectioned and stained with haematoxylin and eosin for histopathological studies. Serological tests like ELISA have been documented to be utilized in detection of sarcoptic mange.

Another way to detect mites, especially ear mites, is to scrape the outer edge of the lesion with a blunt blade, transfer the scrapings to a sheet of black paper, and examine the material under bright light. If the material is slightly warmed by sunlight or a lamp, the mites become active and are plainly visible with a hand lens.

32.5 Treatment for Mange Mites

Treatment for mange mites is complicated, as the severity of mange infestation often influences the number of treatments required to eliminate infestation and the overall success of acaricide treatment. In designing treatment protocols, it is important to treat all in-contact animals, including domestic animals, and ensure that human beings follow proper biosecurity protocols to avoid becoming a source of mite infestation (Madeleine *et al.*, 2019). In the case of *Psoroptes* mites, goats and cattle kept with sheep may be temporary carriers and may even develop lesions of short duration, so they should be included when the flock is treated.

For demodectic mange, ivermectin injected at 0.2 mg/kg body weight administered subcutaneously is effective, though it does not result in the immediate elimination of the mites. The affected animals should be isolated for at least 2 weeks following treatment for full recovery. Amitraz administration topically at a concentration of 0.025% is also recommended. While treating lactating goats, caution should be exercised. Treatment of *Sarcoptes*-infested goats with ivermectin at 200 μg/kg body weight along with topical application of amitraz (5%) twice a week for six applications, supported by vitamin A injection given twice a week, yielded complete recovery of skin 20 days post treatment (Kottadamane *et al.*, 2016). Treatment with injectable moxidectin solution at 0.2 mg/kg, applied subcutaneously every 15 days for four times, showed reduction in pruritus after the first treatment, although satisfactory healing of cutaneous lesions was not witnessed until 6 weeks (Nektarios *et al.*, 2011).

Some researchers have reported chemical dipping (0.05% diaznon, 0.1% lime sulfur and triclorfon) as an effective way of treating scabies in goats (Bates *et al.*, 2005). Chorioptic mange treatment initiated with ivermectin (0.2 mg/kg), administered subcutaneously for 3 weeks, did not remove the lesion, but treatment with amitraz (0.05%) for 3 weeks resolved the lesions (Jesse *et al.*, 2016). Topical application of permethrin or lime sulfur along with parenteral ivermectin and vitamin A supplementation are effective for the therapeutic management of chorioptic mange in goats (Chaithanya *et al.*, 2021).

In goats infested with both *Sarcoptes* and *Psoroptes* mites, ivermectin injection (0.2 mg/kg subcutaneously), dexamethasone injection at 1 mg/10 kg and multivitamin injection at 10 mg/kg intramuscular (repeated on alternate days) showed improvement 6 weeks after commencement of therapeutic medication and full recovery at 10 weeks (Marimuthu *et al.*, 2015; Hamel *et al.*, 2015). Intensive use of ivermectin, however, can lead to resistance, so it needs a synergistic product for rapid treatment of infested animals. Permethrin 5% can be used as a synergistic acaricide (Currie and McCarthy, 2010) for treatment of mange for faster recovery.

There has been scarce experiment regarding use of traditional herbals against mange infection. The oil of *Jatropa curcas* was found more efficacious in controlling sarcoptic mange in sheep and can be used as an adjunct for rapid recovery with lesser applications of main therapy (Dimri and Sharma, 2004). Similarly, oil of *Cedrus deodara* was effective in hastening recovery from sarcoptic mange with good haematological parameters (Sharma *et al.*, 1997).

References

Amin, A.R., Shoukry, A., Morsy, T.A. and Mazyad, S.A. (1997) Studies of wound myiasis among sheep and goats in North Sinai Governorate, Egypt. *Journal of Egypt Society of Parasitology* 27(3), 719–737.

Angulo-Valadez, C.E., Cepeda-Palacios, R., Ascencio, F., Jacquiet, P., Dorchies, P. *et al.* (2009) Relationships of systemic IgG antibody response and lesions caused by *Oestrusovis* L. larvae (Diptera: Oestridae) in infected goats. *Revista Electronica de Veterinaria* 10, 1–13.

Azizi, H., Pourjafar, M., Darabi, S., Assadian, F. and Kahkesh, F.A. (2007) Survey of seasonal infestation with Przhevalskiana larvae in slaughtered goats and sheep in South-Western Iran. *Pakistan Journal of Biological Sciences* 10, 3940–3943.

Bates, P., Rankin, M., Clifford, D. and Stubbings, L. (2005) Shower dipping in diazinon or cypermethrin dip wash to control ovine Psoroptic mange (sheep scab). *Veterinary Record* 156(20), 655.

Chaithanya, C., Biju, P.H., Sindhu, O.K., Janus, A., Ravindran, R. *et al.* (2021) *Chorioptes texanus* causing mange in goats: Comparison of two therapeutic protocols. *Journal of Veterinary and Animal Sciences* 52(4), 357–361.

Currie, B.J. and McCarthy, J.S. (2010) Permethrin and ivermectin for scabies. *New England Journal of Medicine* 362(8), 717–725.

Dalapati, M.R., Bhowmik, M.K., Sarkar, S. and Sasmal, N.K. (1997) Demodicosis of goats: Haematological and biochemical changes. *Tropical Animal Health and Production* 29(4), 240–242.

Dimri, U. and Sharma, M.C. (2004) Effects of sarcoptic mange and its control with oil of *Cedrus deodara*, *Pongamia glabra*, *Jatropha curcas* and benzyl benzoate, both with and without ascorbic acid on growing sheep: Epidemiology; assessment of clinical, haematological, cell-mediated humoral immune responses and pathology. *Journal of Veterinary Medicine. A, Physiology, Pathology, Clinical Medicine* 51(2), 71–78.

Dorny, P., Van Wyngaarden, T., Vercruysse, J., Symoens, C. and Jalila, A. (1994) Survey on the importance of mange in the aetiology of skin lesions in goats in Peninsular Malaysia. *Tropical Animal Health and Production* 26(2), 81–86.

Farkas, R., Hall, M.J., Bouzagou, A.K., Lhor, Y. and Khallaayoune, K. (2009) Traumatic myiasis in dogs caused by *Wohlfahrtia magnifica* and its importance in the epidemiology of wohlfahrtiosis of livestock. *Medical and Veterinary Entomology* 23(1), 80–85.

Fesseha, H., Etana, E. and Mathewos, M. (2021) Mange mites of goats in Malle District of South Omo Zone, Southern Ethiopia. *Veterinary Medicine* 12, 159–168.

Hamel, D., Joachim, A., Löwenstein, M., Pfister, K., Silaghi, C. *et al.* (2015) Treatment and control of bovine sarcoptic and psoroptic mange infestation with ivermectin long-acting injectable (Ivomec(®) Gold). *Parasitology Research* 114(2), 535–542.

Hope, F.W. (1840) On insects and their larvae occasionally found in the human body. *Transactions of Royal Entomology Society London* 2, 256–271.

Imtiaz, M.A., Rahman, M.A., Islam, K., Barua, M., Alim, M.A, *et al.* (2014) Prevalence and associated risk factors of myiasis in different areas of Chittagong, Bangladesh. *Research Journal of Veterinary Practice* 2(2), 22–27.

Jesse, F.F.A., Hambali, I.U., Abba, Y., Sadiq, M.A., Bitrus, A.A. *et al.* (2016) Therapeutic options in management of a clinical case of chorioptic mange in a goat. *Resident Journal of Veterinary Practice* 4(2), 39–41.

Khalafallah, S.S., Metawea, Y.F. and El Sayad, E.E.M. (2020) Epidemiology and control of mange in sheep and goat in Menofia Governorate, Benha. *Veterinary Medical Journal* 39, 111–116.

Kottadamane, M.R., Satheesha, S.P., Chandrashekhar, G. and Nagaraj, L. (2016) Clinical management of sarcoptic mange in goat case report. *International Journal of Science, Environment and Technology* 5(3), 1879–1881.

Lashari, M.H. and Tasawar, Z. (2016) Prevalence of *Sarcoptes scabiei* var. *caprae* infestation in goats of Multan, Pakistan. *Journal of Applied Animal Science* 9(2), 49–56.

Littlejohn, A.I. (1968) Psoroptic mange in the goat. *Veterinary Record* 82, 6.

Madeleine, L., Pam, L. and Scott, C. (2019) The treatment of sarcoptic mange in wildlife: A systematic review. *Parasites & Vectors* 12, 99.

Marimuthu, M., Abdullah, F.F.J., Mohammed, K., Adamu, L., Tijjani, A. *et al.* (2015) Comparative treatment approach for Sarcoptes and Psoroptes mite infestation in a Boer cross. *Journal of Advanced Veterinary and Animal Research* 2(1), 84–88.

Morsy, T.A., Shoukry, A., Mazyad, S.A. and Abou Gamra, M.M. (1998) The goat warble fly, *Przhevalskiana silenus* (Brauer) in North Sinai. *Egypt. Journal of Egypt Society of Parasitology* 28(2), 373–378.

Nektarios, D., Giadinis, R.F., Papaioannou, N., Papadopoulos, E., Karatzias, H, *et al.* (2011) Moxidectin efficacy in a goat herd with chronic and generalized sarcoptic mange. *Veterinary Medicine International* 2011, 476348.

Oryan, A., Razavi, S.M. and Bahrami, S. (2009) Occurrence and biology of goat warble fly infestation by *Przhevalskiana silenus* (Diptera, Oestridae) in Iran. *Veterinary Parasitology* 166, 178–181.

Poddighe, S., Dekker, T., Scala, A. and Angioy, A.M. (2010) Olfaction in the female sheep bot fly. *Die Naturwissens Chaften* 97(9), 827–835.

Reddy, B.S., Sivajothi, S. and Raju, K.G. (2013) Chorioptic mange and its therapeutic management in caprines. *Intas Polivet* 14, 329–330.

Ruiz-Martinez, I., Soler-Cruz, M.D., Benitez-Rodriguez, R., Perez-Jimenez, J.M. and Diaz-Lopez, M. (1989) Postembryonic development of *Wohlfahrtia magnifica* (Schiner, 1862) (Diptera: Sarcophagidae). *Journal of Parasitology* 75, 531–539.

Scott, D.W. (1988) *Large Animal Dermatology*. WB Saunders, Philadelphia, Pennsylvania.

Seid, K., Amare, S. and Tolossa, Y.H. (2016) Mange mites of sheep and goats in selected sites of Eastern Amhara region, Ethiopia. *Journal of Parasitic Disease* 40(1), 132–137.

Shah, K.S., Mandali, G.C., Rao, N., Patel, A.C. and Panchal, R.P. (2022) Epidemiology and hemato-biochemical changes in mange infested goats. *Indian Journal of Veterinary Science and Biotechnology* 18(2), 123–125.

Sharma, D.K., Saxena, V.K., Sanil, N.K. and Singh, N. (1997) Evaluation of oil of *Cedrus deodura* and benzyl benzoate in sarcoptic mange in sheep. *Small Ruminant Research* 26, 81–85.

Sotiraki, S. and Hall, M.J.R. (2012) A review of comparative aspects of myiasis in goats and sheep in Europe. *Small Ruminant Research* 103(1), 75–83.

Soundararajan, C., Sivakumar, T. and Pandian, A.S.S. (2021) Epidemiology and factors associated with cutaneous myiasis in sheep and goats under coastal region of Tamil Nadu. *Indian Journal of Small Ruminants* 27(1), 12.

Tassi, P., Puccini, V. and Giangaspero, A. (1989) Infection by the warble fly *Przhevalskiana silenus* Brauer, 1858, in the Italian goats. An update up to 1988. *Parasitologia* 31(2–3), 239–250.

Wall, R. (2012) Ovine cutaneous myiasis: Effects on production and control. *Veterinary Parasitology* 189, 44–51.

Yadav, A., Katoch, R., Khajuria, J.K., Katoch, M. and Agrawal, R. (2011) Prevalence and biology of goat warble fly infestation by *Przhevalskiana silenus* in Jammu province, India. *Tropical Animal Health Production* 43(8), 1487–1492.

Yadav, A., Katoch, R., Khajuria, J.K., Katoch, M. and Rastogi, A. (2012) Economic impact of *Przhevalskiana silenus* infestation in native goats of Northern India. *Tropical Animal Health Production* 44(3), 581–587.

Zumpt, F. (1965) *Myiasis in Man and Animals in the Old World*. Butterworths, London.

33 Toxoplasmosis

J. Jyothi* and M. Bhavya Sree
P.V. Narasimharao Telangana Veterinary University, Hyderabad

Abstract

Toxoplasma gondii is the parasitic zoonotic agent that causes toxoplasmosis. It is spread globally, as a goat disease, and its prevalence varies by region from 11% to 96%. Because asexual stages develop in mammals and birds, they are regarded as intermediate hosts. Because sexual phases can be found in cats, they are regarded as the definitive host. Consuming raw or improperly cooked goat's meat or milk, as well as undercooked food that has encountered infected meat or milk, can result in *T. gondii* infection in humans.

Keywords: toxoplasmosis, Toxoplasma gondii, goats, tachyzoite, bradyzoite, abortions

33.1 Introduction

Toxoplasmosis, a widespread zoonotic disease, is caused by *Toxoplasma gondii* (Tenter *et al.*, 2000). All warm-blooded animals, including sheep and goats, are susceptible to *T. gondii* infection. Fever, anorexia, dyspnoea, embryonic resorption and mummification, abortion and neurological symptoms are the primary clinical manifestations.

Geographically, toxoplasmosis has a global distribution. *T. gondii* has been recognized as one of the most significant causes of reproductive illnesses in sheep and goats in several countries, including South Africa, Argentina, China and the USA. In Brazil, there are a few reports of miscarriages with lesions and diagnostic confirmation of goat reproductive losses caused by toxoplasmosis.

In goat herds, *T. gondii* infection has been linked to abortions and reproductive losses. Congenital transplacental transmission may also contribute to the maintenance and dissemination of the protozoan infection in flocks (Dubey, 2010).

33.2 Prevalence and Incidence

Goats are frequently infected with *T. gondii*, especially in regions where breeding is intensive. Anti-toxoplasmal antibodies have been reported as being present in goat herds with an average prevalence of 31% worldwide, with a regional range of 11% to 96%. In 14% of herds, toxoplasma infection caused clinical illness (Robert-Gangneux and Dardé, 2012). All the findings were based on herds that experienced pre-natal mortality and provided samples to diagnostic laboratories. Therefore, it is likely that the data overestimate the true prevalence.

33.3 Source of Toxoplasmosis Infection

Meat from domestic animals harbouring *T. gondii* is considered an important infection source for humans (Robert-Gangneux and Dardé, 2012).

*Corresponding author: jyothirvm1027@gmail.com

 The Handbook of Zoonotic Diseases of Goats (ed. T. Rana)
DOI: 10.1079/ 9781800622852.0033

Multiplication occurs in many body organs, particularly the brain and muscles and the placenta of pregnant animals, when a susceptible animal consumes oocysts on pasture or feed. After 1–2 weeks, the immune system of the host limits the organism's growth, which causes tissue cysts. The cysts might live a lifetime in the tissues of the hosts. When a susceptible cat consumes either tissue cysts or oocysts, *T. gondii*'s life cycle is finished.

33.4 Pathological Importance

T. gondii has been identified as a substantial contributor to small-ruminant abortions. When susceptible goats are infected while pregnant, abortions, stillbirths and neonatal death are the most frequently reported symptoms of toxoplasmosis. Early-stage *T. gondii* infection in goats can result in the fetus's death and reabsorption, which manifests as infertility or barrenness.

In sheep, infection with *T. gondii* is typically undetectable. Infection in mid-gestation is more likely to result in abortion and the birth of feeble lambs, while infection in late gestation results in the birth of live, infected and immune lambs.

Because the disease cannot spread laterally, afflicted goats are safeguarded for life and do not pose a threat to other animals.

33.5 Epidemiological Importance

Humans may become infected with *T. gondii* when they consume raw or improperly cooked infected meat, particularly from poultry, goats, mutton and wild game, as well as uncooked foods that have been in contact with infected meat. Cat oocysts can accidentally be eaten by humans if they ingest them in dirt or from a litter box.

An acutely infected pregnant woman can transmit toxoplasmosis transplacentally to the developing fetus, which can result in serious illness in the fetus.

33.6 Diagnostic Methods

There are several methods for the diagnosis of toxoplasmosis, including serological detection of antibodies in the blood serum of goats. High serum levels of the antibody immunoglobulin G (IgG) usually occur after the infection and persist for several months. Serodiagnostic testing of fetuses may be crucial, since maternal antibodies do not cross the placenta. Necropsy and pathological alterations provide reliable indicators of toxoplasmosis. Focal inflammation and fetal cotyledon necrosis at the placenta may be the most significant macro-pathological alterations. Intestinal myocarditis, lung necrosis and localized granulomatosis in the liver may be noticed. In the fetus, alterations in the brain include central calcification, non-purulent encephalitis and localized persistent inflammation.

Goat meat may ultimately be tested for cysts and *T. gondii* vegetative form using a digestive technique.

Molecular techniques based on nucleic acid amplification can be used in addition to serology or in situations where employing serological methods is not possible, such as the diagnosis of young animals that have taken colostrum, or the detection of intrauterine *T. gondii* infection at early stages of gestation when the fetus is not immunocompetent (Hurtado *et al.*, 2001).

33.7 Prevention and Therapy

Goats typically contract an illness from oocyst-contaminated feed or pasture. Illness rates can be decreased by keeping feed covered to minimize its contamination by cat faeces, keeping cats out of livestock barns and limiting stray cat populations on farms. The danger of infection is also decreased by giving goats anti-coccidial medications such monensin and decoquinate constantly during their pregnancies

To identify the reason for an abortion outbreak in their flocks or herds, farmers may need the help of a veterinary diagnostic laboratory. Control strategies for toxoplasma abortion in goats include chemotherapy preventive treatment of pregnant goats with anticoccidial medications and inoculation with a live vaccine or by exposing susceptible animals to infection prior to conception. Because there is a considerable period between infection and abortion, treating goats with toxoplasma-effective medications during an abortion outbreak is not helpful in preventing abortions, but it can greatly reduce subsequent *T. gondii* infections

Ewes treated with monensin and administered toxoplasma oocysts orally gave birth to more live lambs. Since overdosing on monensin has been known to result in fatalities, the drug is not approved for use in goats and can only be administered by a veterinarian. The anticoccidial medication decoquinate is approved for use in sheep and may also be used in goats. Although it is safer and more pleasant than monensin, it still requires a veterinarian's prescription if used to help prevent toxoplasmosis in pregnant ewes. It has been shown that medications like the combination of sulfamezathine and pyrimethamine can lower the severity of a toxoplasma-related abortion outbreak, but it is likely to be too late to use therapy by the time acute toxoplasmosis is discovered in a flock or herd.

In the 1980s, a vaccine employing the live attenuated strain (S48) of *T. gondii* was created in New Zealand and used to immunize sheep. The vaccine is the most efficient method of control for toxoplasmosis in sheep now available. It creates a mild, short-lived infection in the inoculated sheep but protects it from clinical sickness and chronic infection. However, we lack the necessary data and expertise to apply it to stop toxoplasmosis in goats.

33.8 Discussion

Cats are the definitive hosts of *T. gondii* and are considered as the main risk factor for toxoplasmosis in goats.

Transplacental transmission is an important route of infection. Exogenous transplacental transmission in goats indicates that oocyst ingestion plays an important role in the maintenance of endemicity of *T. gondii* in goats. Placentas can show signs of active protozoan infection in the cotyledonary tissue by having mononuclear infiltration, necrotic and calcified regions, and *T. gondii* DNA. The fetus's gestational oxygen supply may be reduced because of toxoplasma infection.

Indirect immunofluorescent antibody tests (IFATs) are more effective than ELISA for detecting *T. gondii* antibodies in serum samples from aborted ovine fetuses.

33.9 Conclusion

The toxoplasmosis review in this chapter has examined the epidemiology, transmission and seroprevalence of the disease in various populations. Livestock, cats, wild animals that roam free and birds are the principal vectors for the transmission of toxoplasma infection. Consuming raw or partially cooked foods contaminated with *T. gondii* may spread the illness. One of the determining elements for illness epidemiology is socioeconomic status.

Toxoplasmosis is one of the neglected infections that need to be brought to the public's attention and to that of academics, policy makers, healthcare workers and veterinary professionals. Increased efforts should be made to inform people about toxoplasmosis caused by *T. gondii*.

In addition, some reports in the literature suggest that the meat of animals intended for consumption should be properly tested and marked as 'toxoplasma-free meat' (Kijlstra and Jongert, 2008, 2009).

References

Dubey, J.P. (2010) *Toxoplasmosis of Animals and Humans*, 2nd edn. CRC Press, Boca Raton, Florida.

Hurtado, A., Aduriz, G., Moreno, B., Barandika, J. and García-Pérez, A.L. (2001) Single tube nested PCR for the detection of *Toxoplasma gondii* in fetal tissues from naturally aborted ewes. *Veterinary Parasitology* 102, 17–27.

Kijlstra, A. and Jongert, E. (2008) Control of the risk of human toxoplasmosis transmitted by meat. *International Journal for Parasitology* 38, 1359–1370.

Kijlstra, A. and Jongert, E. (2009) Toxoplasma-safe meat: Close to reality? *Trends in Parasitology* 25, 18–22.

Robert-Gangneux, F. and Dardé, M.L. (2012) Epidemiology of and diagnostic strategies for toxoplasmosis. *Clinical Microbiology Reviews* 25, 264–296.

Tenter, A.M., Heckeroth, A.R. and Weiss, L.M. (2000) *Toxoplasma gondii*: From animals to humans. *International Journal for Parasitology* 30, 1217–1258. DOI: 10.1016/S0020-7519(00)00124.

34 Giardiasis

M. Reza Najafi[1]* and Negin Esfandiari[2]
[1]Department of Pathobiology, Faculty of Veterinary Medicine, Urmia University, Urmia, Iran; [2]Department of Food Hygiene and Quality Control, Division of Epidemiology, Faculty of Veterinary Medicine, University of Tehran, Tehran, Iran

Abstract
Giardiasis is an infection of the intestine caused by the protozoan flagellate parasite, *Giardia* spp. The majority of veterinary health-related infections are caused by *G. duodenalis*, a species complex of several genotypes that exhibit host specificity. Production animals, companion animals and wildlife can all be affected. Humans also encounter the disease frequently. *Giardia* infection frequently happens in some species without overt or apparent clinical indications.

Most infections begin after consuming water or food that has been contaminated with cysts. Humans and animals can contract the sickness brought on by the parasite. The parasite has a direct life cycle; when the infective cyst is released through the host's faeces, it encysts and becomes immediately contagious. Giardiasis, although asymptomatic in most humans and goats, leads to economic losses mostly in developing countries. This chapter reviews giardiasis in goats in all its aspects.

Keywords: Giardiasis, Goats, Zoonoses, Protozoan

34.1 Introduction

In looking for microorganisms in his own stool samples and being able to precisely define this parasite's characteristics, Anton van Leeuwenhoek, a pioneer of microscopy, is credited with discovering *Giardia* for the first time in 1681 (Fink *et al.*, 2020). Giardiasis is an infection of the intestine caused by the protozoan flagellate parasite, *Giardia* spp. The majority of veterinary health-related infections are caused by *Giardia duodenalis* (also known as *G. intestinalis* and *G. lamblia*), a species complex of several genotypes that exhibit host specificity. Production animals, companion animals and wildlife can all be affected (Fig. 34.1). Humans also encounter the disease frequently. *Giardia* infection frequently happens in some species, especially ruminants and also wild mammals, without overt or apparent clinical indications (Robertson, 2021). In contrast to other intestinal flagellates, *Giardia* trophozoites are present in the small intestine rather than the caecum and colon (Bowman, 2020).

Most infections begin after consuming water or food that has been contaminated with cysts (Fink *et al.*, 2020). Humans and animals, including dogs, cats, cows, goats and lambs, could contract the sickness brought on by the parasites. Contaminated surface waters are one of the parasite's main environmental reservoirs. *Giardia* cysts can survive in the environment for long periods of time, and water chlorination by itself will not render

*Corresponding author: m.rezanajafiparasitol@gmail.com

DOI: 10.1079/ 9781800622852.0034

them inactive (ECDC, 2022). Cysts are ingested by the faecal–oral route, which can result from direct human-to-human, animal-to-human, or animal-to-animal contact, or indirectly from the intake of contaminated food or drink (Sing, 2015).

Giardia muris in mice, *Giardia agilis* in amphibians and *Giardia psittaci* in birds are a few examples of *Giardia* species that are recognized as distinct, but that is about where conventional nomenclature ends (Bowman, 2020). The genotypic distribution of *G. duodenalis* members is changing. Another name for genetic variances (genotypes) is assemblages (Constable *et al.*, 2017). There are eight assemblages, each having their main host associations: Assemblages A and B are mostly linked with humans, whereas Assemblages C and D are with dogs, Assemblage E is with hoofed stock (such as cattle, sheep, goats, pigs, horses and so on), Assemblage F is with cats, Assemblage G is with rats and Assemblage H is with seals (Bowman, 2020). It is essential to keep in mind that there is additional genetic diversity inside assemblages (called intra-assemblage variability), and that several sub-assemblages have been identified and given the names AI, AII, BIII and BIV. Sub-assemblage isolates are genetically similar but not identical (Sing, 2015). While Assemblage F has been discovered in AIDS patients and other immunocompromised individuals, canine Assemblages C and D have never been detected in a human body in the United States. The majority of zoonoses research has been on Assemblage A, which is present in humans and several other species. The Assemblage A subtype AII infection most frequently affects humans, whereas the subtype AI infection more frequently affects animals when they contract Assemblage A (Bowman, 2020). Studies have consistently found that Assemblage E predominates in sheep and goat populations, while Assemblage A is only occasionally found. Rarely has Assemblage B been discovered in sheep (Jafari *et al.*, 2014). This shows a possibility of zoonotic potential of goats. With the exception of a little increase in intraepithelial lymphocytes, the acute pathophysiology of giardiasis does not involve trophozoite invasion of the small intestine tissues or overt inflammatory cell infiltration. Several factors, including the host immune system's condition, the host's age and nutritional health, the strain's genotype, the infectious dose and perhaps co-infections, have been suggested to explain the disease's diversity (Halliez and Buret, 2013) (Fig. 34.2).

34.2 Morphology

The trophozoite, which is the replicative stage, and the cyst, which is the infective stage, are the two phases that make up *Giardia*'s direct life cycle

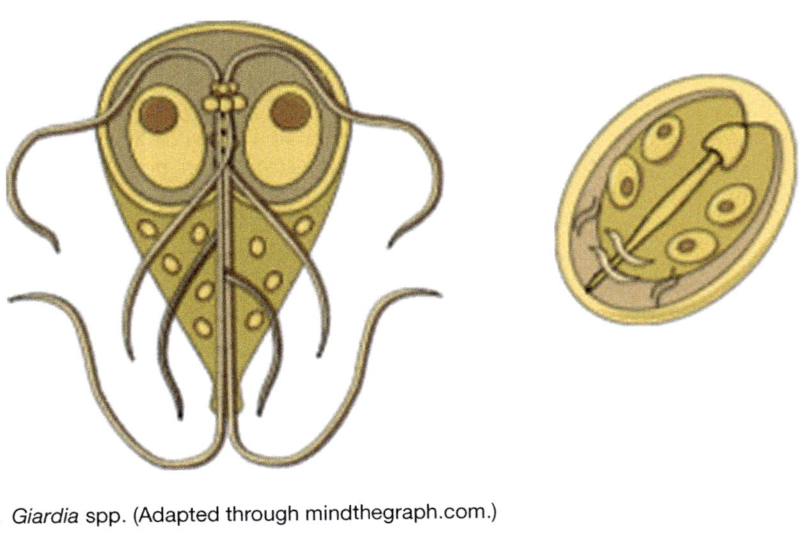

Fig. 34.1. *Giardia* spp. (Adapted through mindthegraph.com.)

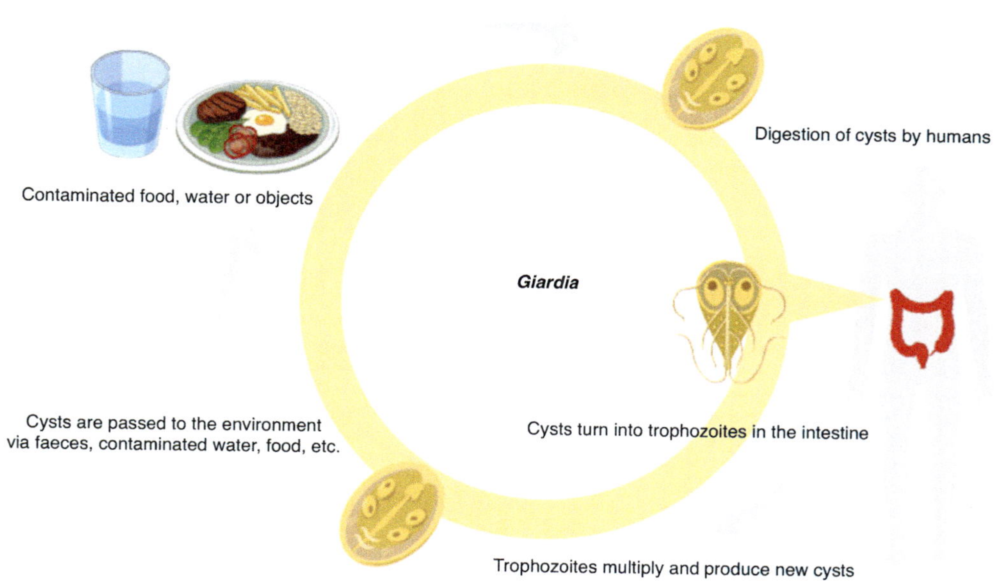

Fig. 34.2. Cycle in *Giardia* spp. infection. (Adapted through mindthegraph.com.)

(Sing, 2015). The trophozoites are pear-shaped or drop-shaped; on their flattened ventral side, they have an extensive adhesive system (known as a discus) and the typical eight symmetrically distributed flagella (Mehlhorn, 2016). Two anterior nuclei, two thin axostyles, eight flagella in four pairs, two darkly stained median bodies and two slender flagella are present (Taylor *et al.*, 2015). The trophozoites grow to a maximum length of 20 μm and a maximum width of 7–10 μm. The trophozoites travel via the faeces to the colon after separating from the host's duodenal wall, where they retract their flagella and expel a thin cyst wall. The nuclei of this cyst, which is ovoid-shaped and measures 10–14 μm in length, are doubled inside it. As a result, each cyst seems to have four nuclei (Mehlhorn, 2016).

34.3 Life Cycle

Giardia has a direct life cycle: when the infective cyst is released through the host's faeces, it encysts and becomes immediately contagious. In cool, moist places, the cysts can spread infection for several months and quickly build up in the environment (Fig. 34.3). Additionally, the cysts are more resistant to chlorine treatment than the majority of microorganisms, which is why contaminated swimming pools and drinking water have been connected to numerous *Giardia* epidemics (Bedi *et al.*, 2022). *Giardia* is one of the few protozoans that can be made to go through its entire life cycle in a laboratory setting (Fink *et al.*, 2020). *Giardia* cysts are comparatively resistant to environmental factors; they can endure 4°C in water for 11 weeks, in soil for 7 weeks and in cattle faeces for 1 week, but they cannot endure freezing. They are resistant to chlorination, and even thorough environmental sanitation cannot stop re-infection (Constable *et al.*, 2017). Cysts can also survive for 3 months in humid food (Mehlhorn, 2016).

The cysts can contaminate surfaces, food and water, and when consumed during this infective stage of their life cycle, they can result in giardiasis. Cysts from contaminated food, drink, hands, surfaces, or objects that are swallowed can cause infection. They move from the mouth, oesophagus and stomach into the small intestine where, through a process known as excystation, each cyst produces two trophozoites. The trophozoites then consume

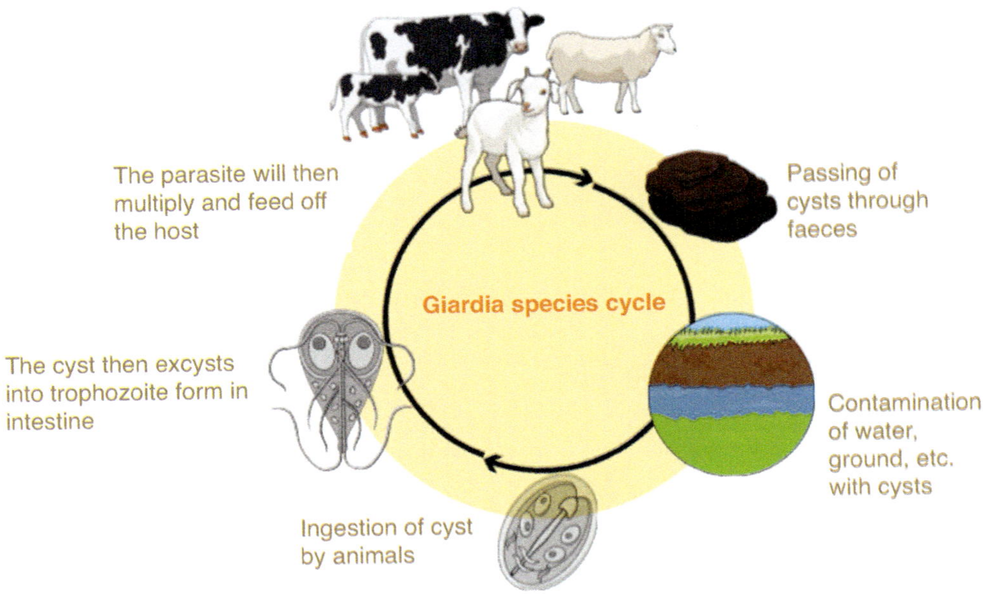

Fig. 34.3. Life cycle of *Giardia* spp. (Adapted through mindthegraph.com.)

the infected person's or animal's nutrients and feed on them. The trophozoites remain in the small intestine, where they can be free or attached to the inner lining of the small intestine and reproduce by splitting in two, through a process known as longitudinal binary fission. The trophozoites then advance towards the colon and undergo encystation, reverting to cyst form. The stage most frequently discovered in stools is the *Giardia* cyst. The cysts can spread quickly after passing in the faeces or immediately (CDC, 2022).

34.4 Signs and Symptoms in Goats

Typically, non-pathogenic *Giardia* spp. live in the intestines of horses, cattle, sheep and goats. However, in certain situations, such as in animals that are immunocompromised, underweight, or extremely young, they may induce infections (Mehlhorn, 2016) (Fig. 34.4).

Severe infections are uncommon. Rarely the signs of a catarrhal enteritis coupled with diarrhoea appear. Single cysts are already excreted 4–5 days after an infection, which is the prepatent period, and the patency goes on for months (Mehlhorn, 2016). The incubation period varies greatly, depending on the immune status or fitness of the animal (Mehlhorn, 2016).

Ruminants with *G. duodenalis* infections are often asymptomatic, but subclinical signs like slow growth, decreased feed conversion efficiency and persistent diarrhoea are occasionally seen (Jafari *et al.*, 2014).

G. duodenalis parasites are often found in the faeces of healthy animals and, when present, in the faeces of animals with diarrhoea, *G. duodenalis* is usually detected alongside other putative aetiological agents, making it difficult to attribute pathogenicity. Dehydration, acidosis and electrolyte depletion are all pathophysiological effects of diarrhoea, which is also linked to hypoglycaemia in newborns. If left untreated, these physiological abnormalities frequently result in death (Smith and Sherman, 2022).

Regardless of the cause, diarrhoea may be accompanied by some degree of gastrointestinal discomfort, potential abdominal distension and most likely a loss of appetite. Kids and lambs have been known to develop a chronic type of giardiasis that lasts for several weeks and is accompanied by gassy, watery brown stools. Dehydration results from persistent or severe

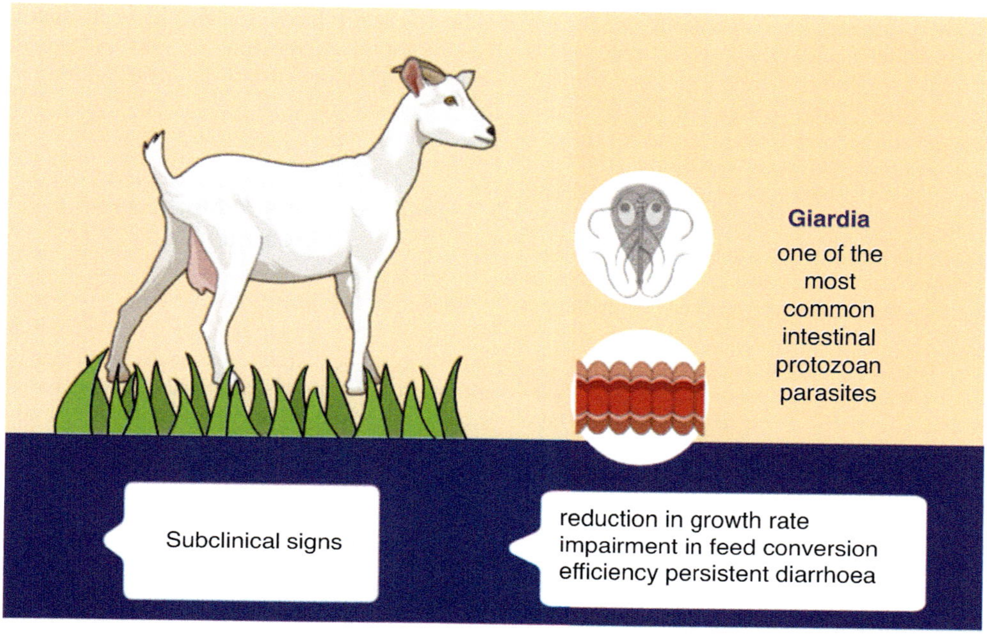

Fig. 34.4. Subclinical signs of giardiosis. (Adapted through mindthegraph.com.)

diarrhoea. Animals who are severely dehydrated have depression, dry mouth and a progressive loss of the sucking reflex. Animals that are affected become increasingly helpless until they are unable to stand. Hypovolaemia and impaired peripheral circulation result from fluid loss. The body temperature may drop below normal, the eyes may become sunken, the pinch reaction of the skin slows down and the extremities may feel cold (Smith and Sherman, 2022).

Diarrhoea-related electrolyte and acid–base imbalances can cause hyperaesthesia, opisthotonos and terminal convulsions, among other neurological abnormalities. Kids who are dehydrated and have diarrhoea have a severe metabolic acidosis that is potentially fatal due to the loss of bicarbonate in the stool and the development of l-lactate brought on by inadequate peripheral perfusion (Smith and Sherman, 2022).

Neonatal giardiasis resulted in prolonged periods for lambs to attain slaughter weight and lower carcass weight in experimentally infected lambs, according to an analysis of production parameters in bottle-reared and infected animals (Bowman, 2020).

Giardia has a prepatent period of 7–8 days and a patency of 60–112 days without signs of giardiasis, according to investigations on calves. *Giardia* trophozoites caused episodes of diarrhoea and soft stools in 6-week-old specific pathogen-free (SPF) lambs, and these symptoms occurred concurrently with the discovery of *Giardia* cysts in the faeces. Infected lambs gained weight less quickly without eating less than controls did, and they took longer to reach market weight (Constable *et al.*, 2017).

34.5 Pathology

Giardia lamblia (another name for *G. duodenalis*) lives in the duodenum and upper small intestine, where it is closely applied or attached to the epithelium by means of a suction disc. A small intestinal biopsy's ultrastructural analysis frequently reveals that the epithelial microvilli at the flagellates' attachment sites have been damaged. Giardiasis has been associated with epithelial damage, increased epithelial cell turnover, villus shortening and disaccharidase deficiency, among other symptoms (Mehlhorn, 2016). Villus atrophy, crypt hypertrophy and a rise in intraepithelial lymphocytes are possible. Trophozoites, which are linked to the brush border of epithelial cells by their concave surface, can be seen between villi (Taylor *et al.*, 2015).

Additionally, *Giardia* infections have been linked to increased permeability, apoptosis, diffuse shortening of microvilli, decreased disaccharidase activity and loss of epithelial barrier function. Recent research revealed that *Giardia* infection can result in chloride ion hypersecretion. The host immune system, specifically CD8 +cells, and parasite products, potentially a toxin, are likely to be responsible for these modifications (Thompson *et al.*, 2008).

Injury may result from the parasite's removal. However, it is unclear whether the symptoms of maldigestion and malabsorption, as well as the villus atrophy and crypt hyperplasia seen in response to *Giardia* infection, are direct consequences of the parasite load or produced by the host's immune response (Mehlhorn, 2016).

34.6 Clinical Pathology and Necropsy

Measuring PCV, total plasma protein, serum sodium, potassium, bicarbonate, blood glucose and blood gases might help assess the severity of electrolyte deficits, acidosis and hypoglycaemia in neonatal diarrhoea cases. A loop of gut can be tied off and removed during a necropsy, then it can be sent unopened and refrigerated to the laboratory. Additionally, formalinized tissues from diverse gastrointestinal tract segments and important organs should be submitted for histopathological analysis. In some of these situations, histological analysis can be beneficial, and immunohistochemistry is now available for identifying some intestinal pathogens, such as *Giardia* and *Cryptosporidium* (Smith and Sherman, 2022).

Necroscopic findings are in the upper small intestine. Even though there are frequently no macroscopic changes, the jejunum may have more intraepithelial lymphocytes, moderate to severe widespread inflammation, villus atrophy, distorted crypts and a decrease in the villus-to-crypt ratio. Histologically, trophozoites can be found on the mucosa and in stained mucosal scrapings from the small intestine (Constable *et al.*, 2017).

34.7 Diagnostic Methods and Treatment

Giardia-induced diarrhoea is most common in 2- to 4-week-old lambs, kids and fawns, but not always. The diarrhoea is usually temporary, although sick animals can shed cysts for many weeks after they appear clinically normal. Finding the pathogen in faeces does not necessarily imply that it is the cause of the diarrhoea, especially in older animals. *Giardia* can be detected in herds with no history of neonatal diarrhoea, so detecting *Giardia* in herds where newborn animals have diarrhoea is doubtful. These animals, however, may be a source of illness for others, including people. The classic method of diagnosing giardiasis is to identify the organism on iodine-stained wet mounts of faeces or tissue (Pugh *et al.*, 2020).

Giardiasis must be diagnosed correctly in order to be treated and prevented from spreading to other individuals. Although immunologically based tests and molecular approaches are also available and are utilized for diagnostic or research purposes in developed countries, the laboratory diagnosis of *Giardia* spp. is mostly reliant on discovering and demonstrating a microscopic cyst in stool samples (Hooshyar *et al.*, 2019).

ELISA tests for the identification of giardiasis became widely accessible starting around 2006. It was also known that trophozoites could be seen in direct smears of diarrhoeal faeces, but stationary flotations and centrifugal flotations in sodium nitrate or saturated sugar solution would not be of significant value in identifying cysts in stool samples, because they collapse and can be challenging to identify when they do float. Currently, a number of in-house antigen detection kits are available, and veterinarians frequently employ the IDEXX SNAP Giardia test in-house (Bowman, 2020).

An immunofluorescent antibody staining (IFAT) of the cyst walls may be a quick and easy technique to detect them in laboratories equipped with a fluorescent microscope. There are several commercial IFAT kits available, with antibodies typically linked to fluorescein isothiocyanate (Robertson, 2021).

Numerous nucleic acid amplification techniques (NAATs) are capable of detecting *Giardia intestinalis* (*G. duodenalis*) DNA and could one day replace current diagnostic methods for *Giardia* infections. Methods involving fluorescent microspheres (Luminex) or DNA isothermal amplification (loop-mediated isothermal amplification (LAMP)) are two of the most promising of these techniques (Heyworth, 2014).

The main objective of therapy is to keep the animals physiologically stable while the diarrhoea runs its course, because many cases of diarrhoea are self-limiting. This plan's implementation includes relocating the goat kid to a warm, dry location to maintain a healthy body temperature as well as administering the right fluid treatment to combat dehydration, electrolyte depletion, hypoglycaemia and acidosis. Depending on how severe the condition is, either parenteral or oral therapy may be employed. Goat kids with a dehydration level of up to 7% can use oral fluids; however, if the level is higher than 8%, they should have intravenous fluids with bicarbonate supplementation (Smith and Sherman, 2022).

Instead of eradicating cyst shedding, drug therapy approaches should probably attempt to stop clinical symptoms. In both large and small ruminants, it has been demonstrated that fenbendazole and albendazole (5–20 mg/kg per day, for 3 days) decrease cyst shedding while also having some therapeutic benefits such as reduced diarrhoea and increased weight gain (Robertson, 2021).

Using metronidazole (20 mg/kg, 0.5 ml/10 kg orally or subcutaneous daily) has also been suggested, but metronidazole is banned from use in food-producing animals in the European Union (Matthews, 2009).

During the acute period of diarrhoea, it is best to proceed slowly when introducing milk or milk-substitute products to goat kids. Lactose in milk-based feeds may remain undigested in the gut and encourage a hyperosmotic diarrhoea on top of the already-existing enteritis, because there will likely be some disturbance of digestive function (Smith and Sherman, 2022).

34.8 Epidemiology of Disease

Giardia lamblia (*G. duodenalis*) is the most common protozoal intestinal parasite found around the world. Giardiasis is particularly prevalent in places with low sanitation and inadequate water treatment facilities (Leung *et al.*, 2019).

Giardiasis is transmitted through the faeces of people and mammals, and the pathogen is transferred by the faecal–oral pathway. Human giardiasis outbreaks are most commonly waterborne and triggered by contaminated drinking water, while other pathways have been documented (Zhang *et al.*, 2012). As mentioned in the Introduction, human-to-human, animal-to-human and animal-to-animal contacts, as well as intake of contaminated food and water, are some of the many probable transmission pathways (Sing, 2015).

Giardia prevalence in small ruminants has been reported to range from 4% to 44% worldwide (Geurden *et al.*, 2008). The prevalence of *Giardia* in goats varies from 10% to >40%, depending on the age, location and diagnostic method. Young goats have a high infection rate, which supports the idea that they significantly contribute to the *Giardia* cyst contamination of the environment, according to a Spanish study. According to a study conducted in Nigeria, the frequency of giardia was high (46.9%) in goats, with pre-weaned (3-month-old) goats having a substantially greater prevalence (58.1%) than those that were older than 3 months (38.2%) (Siwila, 2017). Goat farm prevalence ranges from 66% to 95% (Sing, 2015).

Goats in Belgium and Côte d'Ivoire were found to have zoonotic genotype A infections, according to other investigations. According to another study, goats in Malaysia have genotypes A and B. These results imply that goats might be a potential zoonotic infection source (Siwila, 2017).

In the study in Belgium (Geurden *et al.*, 2008), with 35.8% prevalence in goat kids, six goat kids tested positive for the zoonotic Assemblage A, indicating that they may be a source of zoonotic diseases.

The Assemblages have a stronger potential to be spread in underdeveloped countries with poor sanitation, where people live near domestic animals and share the same untreated water.

Due to diagnostic bias, tests for *Giardia* are more frequently requested if there is a travel history, therefore the source country is typically thought to be the one visited most recently. Many human diagnoses are made after travel in the developed world (Bowman, 2020).

34.9 Prevention and Control

Giardia cysts are immediately infective when passed in the faeces and thrive in damp and cold environments, where they can remain infective for months. For animals, particularly those living in crowded settings, cysts are a source of infection and reinfection. Therefore, faeces should be removed as soon as possible (at least daily) and potentially infectious waste should be disposed of (Robertson, 2021).

Giardia cysts are so small that they might also be carried from faeces to food or water by the wind or by flies. Cooking food and boiling water can help prevent the spread of infection to humans (Mehlhorn, 2016).

Through increased hygiene and sanitation, direct faecal–oral transmission of giardiasis can be largely reduced. Giardiasis in livestock and companion animals can be controlled by employing good husbandry and farm management methods (Dixon, 2021). Faeces should be promptly and frequently removed, and subsequent disinfection helps to reduce environmental pollution. Most quaternary ammonium compounds, steam and boiling water can inactivate cysts. After cleaning, areas should be given ample time to completely dry off, because cysts are prone to desiccation (Robertson, 2021).

Goat kids who have been exposed should, whenever possible, be transferred to a clean pen or, at the very least, temporarily removed from pens that have been contaminated by diarrhoea. Dry and clean bedding is ideal. Regardless of the feeding method, all tools and equipment need to be cleaned and sanitized between feedings. In order to prevent feedstuff contamination from faeces, kid pens should, whenever possible, be set up such that food may be fed in trays or buckets outside the pen (Smith and Sherman, 2022).

To reduce the risk of waterborne transmission, it is advised to use numerous barriers, such as restricting access for people and animals to watersheds and reservoirs, and treating the water using flocculation, filtration and disinfection. Foodborne transmission is frequently linked to eating fresh produce, and there are several preventive steps that should be done before, during and after harvest, as well as by food handlers and consumers, to reduce the risk of contamination or to get rid of or inactivate parasites (Dixon, 2021).

34.10 Public Health Aspect

Giardiasis in small ruminants is of unclear public health significance. While some studies contend that these animals are probably not a significant zoonotic reservoir, others contend that they are, arguing that sheep and goats should be viewed as significant epidemiological reservoirs. Some outbreaks have also been linked to diseases in small ruminants. This parasite has been linked to widespread outbreaks in communities where the transmission method has been shown to be contaminated drinking water (Robertson, 2009).

Goats have a number of traits that make them ideal livestock to raise in their backyards for those with little means. These traits include their grazing habits, which allow them to consume vegetation that other domestic animals avoid; their small size requires less space than larger animals and they are less expensive to purchase and maintain; and they have the ability to adapt to adverse climatic circumstances. These settings are prone to poor hygiene and sanitation standards, which lowers the barrier between human and livestock and increases the risk of zoonotic and anthroponotic diseases (Utaaker *et al.*, 2017).

Given that an adult goat excretes 1–3 kg of faeces each day, it is obvious that there is a high risk of faecal parasites contaminating the environment, particularly water. Before taking preventive actions, appropriate studies should be launched if water contamination from a certain population of sheep or goats is suspected. These investigations should look into prevalence as well as species and genotype (Robertson, 2009).

The epidemiological traits of *G. duodenalis* are well-suited for creating infectious foci in areas with high population densities and extensive animal husbandry, as they include a low infectious dose, cysts that become infectious immediately after excretion, and robustness that allows them to survive for months in the environment (Utaaker *et al.*, 2017).

Considering all this, whether goats are a reservoir of *Giardia* or not, we will be discussing the disease in humans in the spirit of One Health. Giardiasis in humans is regrettably not a top health concern in most nations, but numerous authors have underlined the impact of the parasite on patient well-being and quality of life, as well as its effect on human health (Siwila, 2017). Giardiasis has been a part of the World Health Organization's 'neglected diseases initiative' since 2004. According to reports, the infection rate among asymptomatic children ranges from 8 to 30% in underdeveloped nations and 1–8% in industrialized areas (Hooshyar *et al.*, 2019).

Giardia is a parasite that has a broad host range, although its pathogenic potential and negative effects are best understood in humans. It is thought to be the cause of 280 million human cases annually. Around 200 million individuals in Asia, Africa and Latin America have symptomatic giardiasis, with 500,000 deaths a year being recorded (Siwila, 2017).

Giardiasis is more common in developing nations with inadequate water sanitation systems, where it affects 20% or more of the population. In contrast, the United States has an estimated yearly prevalence of 1% and adequate water sanitation. *Giardia* was discovered to be the second most prevalent pathogen among children between 1 and 2 years old and the fourth most prevalent pathogen in the stools of infants younger than 1 year old in locations where giardiasis is endemic (Fink *et al.*, 2020).

Most *Giardia* infections in humans are asymptomatic, but they can occasionally cause acute diarrhoea that can progress to chronic diarrhoea (Bowman, 2020). *Giardia* infections typically result in clinical disease that is self-limited (Bedi *et al.*, 2022). Symptoms start to show 1–2 weeks after consuming cysts and they typically last for 3–4 days (Sing, 2015).

Sometimes giardiasis symptoms can become very severe. In these cases, nausea, vomiting, abdominal swellings, abdominal pain with cramping spells, and significant sporadic watery slimy diarrhoeas are frequently observed. These diarrhoeas can cause a potentially fatal loss of water in children and AIDS patients. Giardiasis impairs the parasitized host cells' ability to absorb nutrients, particularly vitamins from meals (Mehlhorn, 2016).

Giardiasis may cause long-term effects and sequelae in an uninformed community. Investigations following a significant waterborne outbreak in Norway revealed that at least 5% of infected people acquired persistent post-infectious fatigue syndrome and that 10% of infected people had persistent symptoms with a mean disease duration of 7 months. In addition, clinical studies and epidemiological research have linked giardiasis to the emergence of allergic reactions, reactive arthritis and irritable bowel syndrome (IBS) (Sing, 2015).

Children in daycare facilities, child care providers, institutionalized individuals, visitors to locations where the disease is endemic, consumption of tainted or polluted water, immunodeficiency, cystic fibrosis and oral–anal sex are among the risk factors for infection (Leung *et al.*, 2019).

It is clear that zoonotic diseases have a catastrophic effect on the human population, from the effect on human life to the financial losses experienced by people who lose animals or have reduced production of animal products to the significant losses to a country's economy. *Giardia*, although asymptomatic in most human and goat cases, is no exception, from inducing more severe disease in goat kids leading to economic losses (mostly in developing countries), to its zoonotic potential for humans, and being able to cause long-term consequences ranging from allergies to IBS in them.

Considering all this, research concentrating on the One Health approach needs to be prioritized because of the close ties between animals, humans and the environment, so that effective control measures can be adopted.

Acknowledgement

All figures were made using the website mindthegraph.com

References

Bedi, J.S., Vijay, D. and Dhaka, P. (2022) *Textbook of Zoonoses*. John Wiley & Sons, Chichester, UK. DOI: 10.1002/9781119809548.

Bowman, D.D. (2020) *Georgis' Parasitology for Veterinarians*, 11th edn. Saunders. DOI: 10.1016/B978-0-323-54396-5.00001-5.

CDC (2022) *Giardia*. US Centers for Disease Control and Prevention. Available at: https://www.cdc.gov/parasites/giardia/pathogen.html (accessed 5 December 2022).

Constable, P.D., Hinchcliff, K.W., Done, S.H., Grunberg, W. and Radostits, O.M. (2017) *Veterinary Medicine: A Textbook of the Diseases of Cattle, Horses, Sheep, Pigs, and Goats*. Elsevier, St Louis, Missouri. Available at: http://sutlib2.sut.ac.th/sut_contents/H111504.pdf (accessed 2 December 2022).

Dixon, B.R. (2021) *Giardia duodenalis* in humans and animals – transmission and disease. *Research in Veterinary Science* 135, 283–289. DOI: 10.1016/J.RVSC.2020.09.034.

ECDC (2022) Giardiasis (lambliasis). In: *Annual Epidemiological Report for 2019*. European Centre for Disease Prevention and Control, Stockholm. Available at: https://www.ecdc.europa.eu/en/publications-data/giardiasis-lambliasis-annual-epidemiological-report-2019 (accessed 2 December 2022).

Fink, M.Y., Shapiro, D. and Singer, S.M. (2020) *Giardia lamblia*: Laboratory maintenance, lifecycle induction, and infection of murine models. *Current Protocols in Microbiology* 57(1), e102. DOI: 10.1002/CPMC.102.

Geurden, T., Thomas, P., Casaert, S., Vercruysse, J. and Claerebout, E. (2008) Prevalence and molecular characterization of *Cryptosporidium* and *Giardia* in lambs and goat kids in Belgium. *Veterinary Parasitology* 155(1–2), 142–145. DOI: 10.1016/j.vetpar.2008.05.002.

Halliez, M.C.M. and Buret, A.G. (2013) Extra-intestinal and long term consequences of *Giardia duodenalis* infections. *World Journal of Gastroenterology* 19(47), 8974. DOI: 10.3748/WJG.V19.I47.8974.

Heyworth, M.F. (2014) Diagnostic testing for Giardia infections. *Transactions of the Royal Society of Tropical Medicine and Hygiene* 108(3), 123–125. DOI: 10.1093/TRSTMH/TRU005.

Hooshyar, H., Rostamkhani, P., Arbabi, M. and Delavari, M. (2019) *Giardia lamblia* infection: Review of current diagnostic strategies. *Gastroenterology and Hepatology from Bed to Bench* 12(1), 3.

Jafari, H., Jalali, M.H.R., Shapouri, M.S.A. and Hajikolaii, M.R.H. (2014) Determination of *Giardia duodenalis* genotypes in sheep and goat from Iran. *Journal of Parasitic Diseases* 38(1), 81–84. DOI: 10.1007/S12639-012-0199-8.

Leung, A.K., Leung, A.A.M., Wong, A.H.C., Sergi, C.M. and Kam, J.K.M. (2019) Giardiasis: An overview. *Recent Patents on Inflammation & Allergy Drug Discovery* 13(2), 34–39. DOI: 10.2174/1872213X13666190618124901.

Matthews, J.G. (2009) *Diseases of the Goat*, 4th edn. Wiley-Blackwell, Hoboken, New Jersey.

Mehlhorn, H. (2016) *Animal Parasites: Diagnosis, Treatment, Prevention*. Springer, Cham, Switzerland. DOI: 10.1007/978-3-319-46403-9/COVER.

Pugh, D.G., Baird, N., Edmondson, M.A. and Passler, T. (2020) *Sheep, Goat, and Cervid Medicine*, 3rd edn. Elsevier Health, Philadelphia, St Louis and New York. Available at: http://www.sciencedirect.com:5070/book/9780323624633/sheep-goat-and-cervid-medicine (accessed 5 December 2022).

Robertson, L.J. (2009) *Giardia* and *Cryptosporidium* infections in sheep and goats: A review of the potential for transmission to humans via environmental contamination. *Epidemiology and Infection* 137(7), 913–921. DOI: 10.1017/S0950268809002295.

Robertson, L.J. (2021) Giardiasis in animals (Lambliasis). In: *MSD Veterinary Manual*. Available at: https://www.msdvetmanual.com/digestive-system/giardiasis-giardia/giardiasis-in-animals (accessed 2 December 2022).

Sing, A. (2015) *Zoonoses – Infections Affecting Humans and Animals: Focus on Public Health Aspects*. Springer, Dordrecht, Netherlands. DOI: 10.1007/978-94-017-9457-2/COVER.

Siwila, J. (2017) Giardiasis: Livestock and companion animals. In: Rodriguez-Morales, A.J. (ed.) *Current Topics in Giardiasis*. IntechOpen, London. DOI: 10.5772/INTECHOPEN.70874.

Smith, M.C. and Sherman, D.M. (2022) *Goat Medicine*, 3rd edn. Wiley Blackwell.
Taylor, M.A., Coop, R.L. and Wall, R.L. (2015) *Veterinary Parasitology*, 4th edn. Wiley Blackwell. DOI: 10.1002/9781119073680.
Thompson, R.C.A., Palmer, C.S. and O'Handley, R. (2008) The public health and clinical significance of *Giardia* and *Cryptosporidium* in domestic animals. *The Veterinary Journal* 177(1), 18–25. DOI: 10.1016/J.TVJL.2007.09.022.
Utaaker, K.S., Myhr, N., Bajwa, R.S., Joshi, H., Kumar, A. *et al*. (2017) Goats in the city: Prevalence of *Giardia duodenalis* and *Cryptosporidium* spp. in extensively reared goats in Northern India. *Acta Veterinaria Scandinavica* 59(1), 86. DOI: 10.1186/s13028-017-0354-4.
Zhang, W., Zhang, X., Wang, R., Liu, A., Shen, Y. *et al*. (2012) Genetic characterizations of *Giardia duodenalis* in sheep and goats in Heilongjiang province, China and possibility of zoonotic transmission. *PLoS Neglected Tropical Diseases* 6(9), e1826. DOI: 10.1371/journal.pntd.0001826.

35 Dermatophytosis (Ringworm)

Kabita Roy[1], Saindla Rakesh[1] and Tanmoy Rana[2*]
[1]Department of Veterinary Medicine, College of Veterinary Science & Animal Health, NDVSU, Jabalpur, Madhya Pradesh, India; [2]Department of Veterinary Clinical complex, West Bengal University of Animal & Fishery Sciences, Kolkata, India

Abstract

The domestication of goats dates back to about 9000–7000 BC. Goats are one of the most economically important livestock in the world. A goat is often described as a poor man's cow (or mini-cow) because of its immense contribution to the poor man's economy. Goat rearing is the backbone of the economy of small and landless farmers in India. India occupies the world's second position in terms of goat population and first in milk production. In addition to milk and meat, good-quality skin and valuable fibre such as Pashmina contribute 8% of livestock gross domestic product (Soodan *et al.*, 2020).

Despite being immune to many illnesses, goats frequently suffer from dermatological conditions. Skin conditions lead to worse leather quality and a drop in tannery profits. Huge financial losses are incurred by farmers as a result of the deterioration in the skin and hide quality, the decline in meat and milk production, culling and mortality losses.

Mycotic infections have been viewed as a serious public health issue in many parts of the world (Torres-Rodriguez *et al.*, 1986). They are more common in developing and economically underdeveloped nations. Ectoparasitic infestations, dermatophytosis/ringworm, as well as bacterial, viral, nutritional, environmental and miscellaneous conditions, are the most frequent dermatological conditions encountered in goats.

Keywords: mycotic infections, dermatophytosis, skin disease, zoonosis

35.1 Introduction

Dermatophytosis, a fungal skin disease of both animals and humans, is highly contagious in goats and is of zoonotic significance (Torres-Rodríguez, 1986). Dermatophytosis is a superficial fungal infection of the hair and keratinized layers of the epidermis brought on by keratinophilic and keratinolytic genera such as *Microsporum*, *Trichophyton* and *Epidermophyton* (Rudramurthy and Shaw, 2017). The classical lesions are circular and are known as ringworm. Clinically, the disease is characterized by alopecia patches ranging from being annular to uneven to diffuse, with scaling, erythema and yellowish crusts that typically appear on the face, neck and limbs. Classically, multiple animals are often affected. In otherwise healthy goats, dermatophytosis typically resolves spontaneously after 3–4 months (Scott, 2018). The disease is also economically significant, because it has an impact on the quantity and quality of fibre, hides and leather.

35.2 Aetiology

Fungi belonging to the genera *Microsporum*, *Trichophyton* and *Epidermophyton* cause

*Corresponding author: tanmoyrana123@gmail.com

DOI: 10.1079/ 9781800622852.0035

dermatophytosis in goats. These septate fungi, or dermatophytes, are a family of closely-related organisms that depend on keratin for growth.

Dermatophytes are further divided into geophilic species, zoophilic species and anthropophilic species based on their principal habitat. While zoophilic species primarily feed on animals, geophilic species survive as saprophytes in the soil (Soodan, 2020). Anthropophilic species are those that normally affect humans. Dermatophytes reproduce asexually and are referred to as fungi imperfecti (Dubos and Hirsch, 1966).

Ringworm in goats is rare. Chandran (2021) reported that dermatophytosis in goats is caused by *Trichophyton mentagrophyte*. The most common dermatophyte in goats is *Trichophyton verrucosum*, which is followed by *T. mentagrophytes*, *Trichophyton equinum* and *Microsporum canis* (Nweze, 2011). Biswas *et al.* (2015) reported that the most prevalent dermatophyte species found in goats was *Microsporum gypseum*, followed by *T. verucossum*, *T. mentagrophytes* and *Trichophyton rubrum*.

Isolation of different species of pathogenic dermatophytes from the goat population by various authors is shown in Table 35.1.

35.3 Epidemiology

While the disease is spread globally, the occurrence may vary from country to country. Dermatophyte prevalence varies with climate and natural reservoir (Pier *et al.*, 1994). The overall incidences of dermatophytosis in goats reported by various authors in different states of India and abroad are shown in Table 35.2. The great variation in incidence reports may be caused by a number of variables, including management styles, population size, geoclimatic conditions, hygiene practices, animal breed, virulence and isolated species of fungi.

Table 35.1. Species isolated.

Species isolated	Reference
Trichophyton mentagrophyte	Chandran (2021)
Microsporum gypseum	Biswas *et al.* (2015)
Trichophyton verucossum	
Trichophyton mentagrophytes	
Trichophyton rubrum	
Trichophyton mentagrophyte	Mitra (1998)
Microsporum gypseum	
Trichophyton verrucosum	Nweze (2011)
Trichophyton mentagrophytes	
Trichophyton equinum	
Microsporum canis	

Table 35.2. Overall incidences of dermatophytosis in goats.

State or country	Incidence (%)	Reference
Kerala	38.23	Chandran (2021)
West Bengal	6.10	Biswas *et al.* (2015)
Uttar Pradesh	0.12	Mitra (1998)
Egypt	18.60	Abd-Elmegeed *et al.* (2020)
Iran	12.55	Rahbari (1986)
Nigeria	8.90	Nweze (2011)

35.4 Transmission

A number of variables, such as host preference, susceptibility, native habitat of the fungus, virulence of the infecting pathogens, site of infection, nutritional status of the host and local environmental factors, might affect the transmission and progression of dermatophyte infection (Gentles and Graham-Jones, 1968).

The most typical way for ringworm to spread is through direct contact with infected animals or people, but indirect contact with inanimate items is also possible. Up to 20% of healthy animals in an infected population will act as 'carrier animals' and spores can dwell on the skin without creating sores. The spores of ringworm fungi survive for many months, and in some cases years, in the farm environment and may spread to susceptible hosts by asymptomatic carriers or by fomites like brushes, gates and feed carts (Abdalla, 2019).

35.5 Risk Factors

Risk factors include age, breed, sex, season/ climate and management.

35.5.1 Age

Regarding age-based studies on the prevalence of dermatophytosis in goats, very few reports are readily available. Mitra (1998) reported that young animals (below 6 months of age) are more susceptible to dermatophytosis than adults (above 6 months of age). Young animals are usually confined and are thereby exposed to constant infection from the crowded infected animals of the herd with which they come into close contact. The thick skin of adult animals with high levels of unsaturated fatty acids also contributes to the disease's reduced prevalence in the adult population (Dey *et al.*, 2006). However, Biswas *et al.* (2015), Abd-Elmegeed *et al.* (2020) and Chandran (2021) reported that goats older than 6 months were more susceptible to dermatophytosis than goats younger than 6 months. They opined that lesser prevalence in young kids might be due to their lesser exposure to infected surroundings.

35.5.2 Breed

The disease has a greater impact on goats of exotic and mixed breeds than on non-descript goats. This may be due to the disease-resistant nature of the non-descript breeds of goats.

35.5.3 Sex

Ringworm infection is more likely to affect male animals than females. This may be attributed to male goats being housed in close contact for long periods for fattening purpose and the contagious aspect of the disease (Abd-Elmegeed *et al.*, 2020). Biswas *et al.* (2015) opined that the increased incidence of dermatophytosis in males could be attributed to interactions between male goats and other goats as a result of flock breeding tendencies. Sex was not, however, recognized as a risk factor for dermatophytosis in various studies.

35.5.4 Season and climate

A high incidence of clinical cases in the winter and of spontaneous recovery in the spring is common, but outbreaks also occur during the summer months. It is possible that, because of the close confinement of animals during winter, there is an opportunity for the easy spread of infection (Dey *et al.*, 2006; Abd-Elmegeed *et al.*, 2020; Chandran, 2021).

35.5.5 Management

Poor nutrition, overcrowding, immunosuppression and stress may predispose goats to dermatophytosis. Dermatophytosis is more likely to affect animals housed in close proximity to sick animals, animals kept in warm, moist and poorly ventilated locations, or animals that are bathed too frequently. Lanolin, a natural barrier to pathogenic organisms, is broken down by frequent washing and trimming of sheep and goats, making the skin more vulnerable to diseases (Abdalla, 2019).

35.6 Pathogenesis

The spores of zoophilic dermatophytes from the environment infect susceptible goats through abrasions on the skin. Keratin provides nourishment to the dermatophytes, and hence skin is the predilection site for them. The spores germinate into hyphae and invade the stratum corneum and walls of the hair follicles (Roberson *et al.*, 2012). The superficial dead and desquamating layers of the skin and appendages are colonized by these fungi. The deeper living tissues are exposed to fungal metabolic products that are irritating and cause localized inflammation.

As a result, inflammation raises the temperature of the tissue beneath the diseased area, creating a hotspot in the lesion's centre. Low temperatures between 0°C and 30°C are perfect for dermatophytes to thrive. The higher temperatures of the hotspot cause the fungus to move towards the periphery of the lesion, where the temperature is comparatively low, thus producing concentric ring-shaped lesions; the name 'ringworm disease' is derived from such lesions. While the periphery of the ring may contain actively growing fungi, the centre of the ring is made up of dead, desquamated cells that matt by oozing secretions. Secondary bacterial infection may produce micro-abscesses in the superficial epidermis together with suppurative folliculitis. The severity of the infection is determined by the virulence of the infecting strain or species, the anatomical location of the infected site and local environmental factors (Soltys, 1963).

35.7 Clinical Findings

Areas of alopecia that ranged from being annular to uneven to diffuse, skin erythema and inflammation, scaling and crusting were the most common clinical symptoms observed in dermatophytic infections (Saravanan *et al.*, 2012; Kalaiselvi *et al.*, 2014; Chandran, 2021). The affected goats rarely showed signs of pruritus. Though the lesions can appear anywhere, they are most frequently found on the face, head, ear pinnae, neck and legs. Chandran (2021) reported alopecia of the ear pinnae of the affected goat, followed by the lesions at the lips, trunk, legs, feet, mucocutaneous junctions, periorbital areas and neck. Saravanan *et al.* (2012) reported alopecia on the ear pinnae, periocular and around the nasal and axillary region of the affected kid.

35.8 Clinico-Pathological Findings

In goats with dermatophytosis, a complete blood count (CBC) study may show neutrophilia and lymphocytopenia (Chandran, 2021). Neutrophilia and lymphocytopenia may be a result of stress factors or may be related to secondary bacterial infections.

35.9 Diagnosis

Dermatophytosis is diagnosed based on the clinical signs, but direct microscopic inspection of skin scrapings from the periphery of the lesions and culture should be recommended to confirm the diagnosis.

35.9.1 Collection of samples

The material that is most frequently used to isolate fungus is hair. Alcohol should be used to disinfect the affected skin and the advancing lesion border should be scraped using a sterile disposable scalpel's blunt edge. Sterile tweezers can be used to remove hairs and scales. Skin scrapings or hair plucks for direct microscopical examination and culture should be collected from the periphery of the lesions, since the strictly aerobic fungi will die under the crust in the centre of the lesions, forming anaerobic conditions (Roberson *et al.*, 2012).

35.9.2 Direct microscopic examination

Skin scrapings collected from the active peripheral lesions are treated with 10% potassium hydroxide and examined under the microscope. This is a quick and accurate way to identify spores and hyphae, among other fungal components. Fungal spores invading hairs may indicate ectothrix or endothrix invasion of hairs. Skin scrapings subjected to direct microscopic analysis may contain hair fragments with thick, rough and uneven surfaces as well as arthrospores (Chandran, 2021).

35.9.3 Fungal culture

The gold standard test for the diagnosis of dermatophytosis is the isolation and identification of the organism (Moriello *et al.*, 2017). The selective and differentiating medium used for dermatophyte detection and identification is called dermatophyte test medium (DTM). The morphology and alkaline metabolite production, which is indicated by the phenol red indicator turning the yellow-coloured medium to pink-red, can be used to identify the growth on the DTM (Rudramurthy and Shaw, 2017).

The pigmentation, rate of growth, colonial morphology and microscopic analysis of the fungal colony are used to confirm the organism. Wet preparations can be stained with lactophenol cotton blue (LPCB) dye to examine fungus structures, which are generally spindle or boat-shaped with rough, thick walls. The macroconidia of *Trichophyton* species are far less numerous in culture and have an elongated, cigar or pencil shape (Quinn *et al.*, 2013).

35.9.4 Wood's lamp examination

This technique is insensitive and nonspecific for the identification of *Microsporum canis* and is positive in approximately 50% of the cases. When positive, it helps select areas for culture. However, a negative result does not rule out dermatophyte infection.

A Wood's lamp (wavelength 340–450 nm) is used to examine the animal. The animal is examined in a dark room with the light 10–30 cm from the skin.

Yellow-green or apple-green fluorescence of the hair is a positive result. False-positive assessments are common, as topical products, drugs, soaps and bacteria (*Pseudomonas* sp.) or occasional individual scales can fluoresce as well, but they should not be associated with the hair shafts. A lack of fluorescent areas does not rule out dermatophytosis. In the case of negative results, fungal culture is performed using the McKenzie toothbrush technique.

35.9.5 Skin biopsy

Haematoxylin and eosin or other specialized stains, such as Periodic Acid Schiff (PAS) and Grocott Methenamine Silver (GMS), are used to stain samples of diseased skin for histopathological examination. A skin biopsy may reveal a mixture of orthokeratotic and parakeratotic hyperkeratosis (Krametter-Froetscher *et al.*, 2005).

35.9.6 Molecular identification

Conventional methods of diagnosis take time, because it could take up to 4 weeks or more to give the final results. For clinical and epidemiological reasons, PCR–RFLP methods are an effective assay to quickly identify and distinguish between dermatophyte species, even closely-related strains (Mohammadi *et al.*, 2015).

35.9.7 Differential diagnosis

1. Dermatophilosis
2. Staphylococcal folliculitis
3. Contagious viral pustular dermatitis ('orf')
4. Zinc-responsive dermatitis
5. Pemphigus foliaceus (Scott, 2018)

35.10 Treatment

Dermatophytosis in healthy goats usually resolves spontaneously within 3 months and thus recovery may not be directly related to the therapy used. Other animals within the herd may also be infected at a clinical or subclinical level. These animals should be examined and treated if the infection is detected. Therapy usually involves a combination of both topical and systemic treatment. The duration of treatment should be at least 1 month and can be as long as 2 months to get a complete recovery (Saevik *et al.*, 2001).

35.10.1 Topical treatment

Although topical therapy is unlikely to be successful in curing an infection on its own, it may assist in lessening environmental pollution and the spread of infection to owners and other animals. In the majority of instances, a combination of topical and systemic medication is best. If the lesions are generalized or extensive, the entire coat should be clipped. In cases of focal lesions, the coat should be clipped around focal lesions for a distance of approximately 5 cm. Commonly used topical agents in the treatment of dermatophytosis include:

- Tincture iodine, 2% (Smith and Sherman, 2009; Pal, 2015);
- Tincture iodine:glycerine (1:1) (Chandran, 2021); and
- Miconazole nitrate, 2% (Pal, 2001).

35.10.2 Systemic treatment

- Gresiofluvin @ 25 mg/kg body weight orally (Saravanan *et al.*, 2012)
- Ketoconazole @ 10 mg/kg body weight orally (Saevik *et al.*, 2001)
- Ivermectin @ 200 μg/kg body weight by subcutaneous injection (Jameel *et al.*, 2014)

35.10.3 Additional treatment

Environmental decontamination should be tried, due to the widespread dissemination of infected hairs from affected animals and the protracted survival of arthrospores. It is advisable to clean everything thoroughly and use disinfectants whenever possible.

Antibiotic therapy should be utilized in conjunction if there is a concomitant bacterial overgrowth or superficial pyoderma (Koutinas *et al.*, 2007).

35.11 Vaccination

A live attenuated vaccine of *T. verrucosum* has been used to manage sheep and goat dermatophytosis (Lund and DeBoer, 2008).

35.12 Zoonotic Importance

Farm and companion animals can significantly cause dermatophyte infection in humans. *Trichophyton tonsurans*, *Microsporum canis* and *Microsporum audouinii* are typically the agents responsible for human infections (Gupta and Summerbell, 2000). Isolation of *T. rubrum* from a kid increases the zoonotic potential of the disease and indicates goats as a source of infection for humans (Debnath, 2012).

35.13 Conclusion

Dermatophytosis, or ringworm, is a serious zoonotic skin condition that affects both humans and animals. It is caused by fungi of genera such as *Microsporum*, *Trichophyton* and *Epidermophyton*. The most typical way that ringworm spreads is through direct contact with infected humans or animals. Clinically, it is distinguished by alopecia patches ranging from being annular to uneven to diffuse, scaling, erythema and yellowish crusts that typically appear on the face, neck and limbs. The gold standard test for the diagnosis of dermatophytosis is frequently regarded as isolation in DTM and identification of the organism. For effective control and prevention of dermatophytosis/ringworm infection, a precise early diagnosis, treatment of affected goats with a suitable therapeutic regimen coupled with environmental decontamination are strongly advised. Since it has zoonotic significance, controlling dermatophytosis/ringworm is crucial from both an animal and a public health standpoint.

References

Abdalla, W.G. (2019) An over view of ovine and caprine dermatophytosis. *South Asian Journal of Research in Microbiology* 5(2), 1–10.

Abd-Elmegeed, M., El-Mekkawi, M.F., El-Diasty, E.M. and Fawzi, E.M. (2020) Dermatophytosis among ruminants in Egypt: The infection rate, identification and comparison between microscopic, cultural and molecular methods. *Zagazig Veterinary Journal* 48(2), 116–127.

Biswas, M.K., Debnath, C., Mitra, T., Baidya, S. and Pradhan, S. (2015) Studies on dermatophytoses in sheep and goat in West Bengal, India. *Indian Journal of Animal Health* 54(2), 109–114.

Chandran, C. (2021) Dermatological disorders in goats with special reference to mange and dermatophytosis. MVSc thesis (Veterinary Clinical Medicine, Ethics and Jurisprudence), Kerala Veterinary and Animal Sciences University, Pookode, Wayanad.

Debnath, C. (2012) Studies on some important epidemiological aspects of dermatophytoses in animals and man in and around Kolkata. MVSc thesis (Veterinary Public Health), West Bengal University of Animal and Fishery Sciences, Belgachia, Kolkata.

Dey, A., Bhowmik, M.K. and Biswas, P. (2006) Dermatophytosis in sheep due to *Trichophyton mentagrophytes*; occurrence, haemato-biochemical and pathomorphological changes. *Indian Journal of Veterinary Pathology* 30(2), 22–24.

Dubos, R.J. and Hirsch, J.G. (1966) *Bacterial and Mycotic Infections of Man*, 4th edn. Pitman Medical Publishing Co, London; J.B. Lippincott, Philadelphia.

Gentles, J.C. and Graham-Jones, O. (1968) *Some Diseases of Animals Communicable to Man in Britain*. Pergamon Press, Oxford, UK.

Gupta, A.K. and Summerbell, R.C. (2000) Tinea capitis. *Medical Mycology* 8(4), 255–287.

Jameel, G.H., Minnat, T.R., Humadi, A.A. and Al-Ezzy, A.I.A. (2014) Hematological and histopathological effects of ivermectin in treatment of ovine dermatophytosis in Diyala province, Iraq. *International Journal of Science and Research* 3(11), 1389–1394.

Kalaiselvi, G., Daniel, N.J.C. and Vidhya, M. (2014) Ringworm infection in a goat. A clinical case report. *Indian Journal of Veterinary and Animal Sciences Research* 43(5), 386–387.

Koutinas, A.F., Saridomichelakis, M.N., Argyroudis, S., Koutinas, C.K., Karatzanos, P. *et al*. (2007) Clinical, histopathological and therapeutic considerations in a flock of sheep with facial staphylococcal-associated dermatitis. *Veterinary Dermatology* 18(4), 211–216.

Krametter-Froetscher, R., Hauser, S. and Baumgartner, W. (2005) Zinc-responsive dermatosis in goats suggestive of hereditary malabsorption: Two field cases. *Veterinary Dermatology* 16(4), 269–275.

Lund, A. and DeBoer, D.J. (2008) Immunoprophylaxis of dermatophytosis in animals. *Mycopathologia* 166, 407–424.

Mitra, S.K. (1998) Dermatophytes isolated from selected ruminants in India. *Mycopathologia* 142(1), 13.

Mohammadi, R., Abastabar, M., Mirhendi, H., Badali, H., Shadzi, S. *et al*. (2015) Use of restriction fragment length polymorphism to rapidly identify dermatophyte species related to dermatophytosis. *Jundishapur Journal of Microbiology* 8(6), e17296.

Moriello, K.A., Coyner, K., Paterson, S. and Mignon, B. (2017) Diagnosis and treatment of dermatophytosis in dogs and cats. Clinical consensus guidelines of the World Association for Veterinary Dermatology. *Veterinary Dermatology* 28(3), 266–268.

Nweze, E.I. (2011) Dermatophytoses in domesticated animals. *Revista do Instituto de Medicina Tropical de Sao Paulo* 53, 94–99.

Pal, M. (2001) Dermatophytosis in goat and its handler due to *M. canis*. *Indian Journal of Animal Science* 71, 138–140.

Pal, M. (2015) Diagnosis and management of *Trichophyton verrucosum* in ruminants a report of 4 animals. *Intas Polivet* 16(2), 464–466.

Pier, A.C., Smith, J.M.B., Alexiou, H., Ellis, D.H., Lund, A. *et al*. (1994) Animal ringworm – its aetiology, public health significance and control. *Journal of Medical and Veterinary Mycology* 32(sup.1), 133–150.

Quinn, P., Markey, B., Carter, M. and Carter, G.R. (2013) *Clinical Veterinary Microbiology*, 2nd edn. Mosby, St Louis, Missouri.

Rahbari, S. (1986) Ringworms in ruminants of Iran. *Journal of Veterinary Faculty of Tehran* 41(1), 89–98.

Roberson, J.R., Baird, A.N. and Pugh, D.G. (2012) Diseases of the integumentary system. In: Pugh, D.G. and Baird, D.N. (eds) *Sheep and Goat Medicine*, 2nd edn. Saunders. Elsevier, Maryland Heights, Missouri, pp. 256–290.

Rudramurthy, S.M. and Shaw, D. (2017) Overview and update on the laboratory diagnosis of dermatophytosis. *Clinical Dermatology Review* 1(3), 3.

Saevik, B.K., Bergvall, K., Holm, B.R., Saijonmaa-Koulumies, L.E., Hedhammar, A. *et al*. (2001) *Muller and Kirk's Small Animal Dermatology*, 6th edn. W.B. Saunders, Philadelphia.

Saravanan, M., Sasikala, V., Ranjithkumar, M., Sarma, K. and Mondal, D.B. (2012) Clinical articles: Dermatophytosis due to *Trichophyton mentagrophytes* in a kid. *Indian Veterinary Journal* 89(2), 63.

Scott, D.W. (2018) *Color Atlas of Farm Animal Dermatology*, 2nd edn. Wiley and Sons, Hoboken, New Jersey, pp. 132–133.

Smith, M.C. and Sherman, D.M. (2009) *Goat Medicine*. Wiley-Blackwell, Hoboken, New Jersey.

Soltys, M.A. (1963) *Bacteria and Fungi Pathogenic to Man and Animals*. Baillière Tindall and Cox, London.

Soodan, J.S., Kumar, S. and Singh, A. (2020) Effect of goat rearing on farmers' income. *International Journal of Livestock Research* 10(8), 89–97.

Torres-Rodríguez, J.M., Balaguer-Meler, J., Ventin-Hernandez, M. and Martin-Casabona, N. (1986) Multicenter study of dermatophyte distribution in the metropolitan area of Barcelona (Catalonia, Spain). *Mycopathologia* 93(2), 95–97.

Index

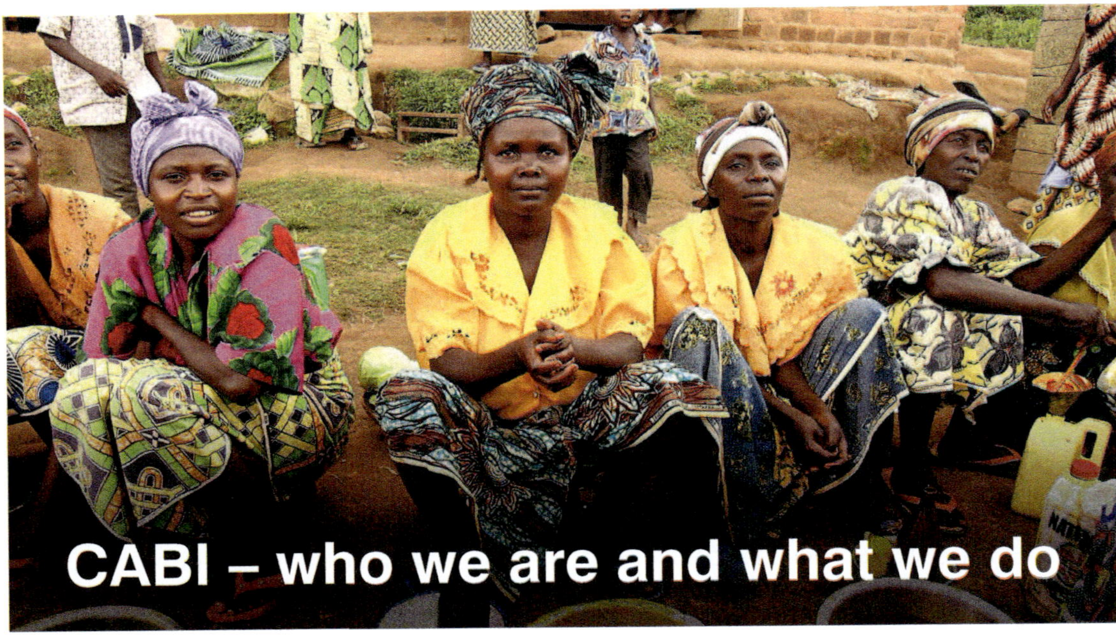

This book is published by **CABI**, an international not-for-profit organisation that improves people's lives worldwide by providing information and applying scientific expertise to solve problems in agriculture and the environment.

CABI is also a global publisher producing key scientific publications, including world renowned databases, as well as compendia, books, ebooks and full text electronic resources. We publish content in a wide range of subject areas including: agriculture and crop science / animal and veterinary sciences / ecology and conservation / environmental science / horticulture and plant sciences / human health, food science and nutrition / international development / leisure and tourism.

The profits from CABI's publishing activities enable us to work with farming communities around the world, supporting them as they battle with poor soil, invasive species and pests and diseases, to improve their livelihoods and help provide food for an ever growing population.

CABI is an international intergovernmental organisation, and we gratefully acknowledge the core financial support from our member countries (and lead agencies) including:

UKaid from the British people | Ministry of Agriculture People's Republic of China | Australian Government Australian Centre for International Agricultural Research | Agriculture and Agri-Food Canada | Ministry of Foreign Affairs of the Netherlands | Schweizerische Eidgenossenschaft Confédération suisse Confederazione Svizzera Confederaziun svizra Swiss Agency for Development and Cooperation SDC

Discover more

To read more about CABI's work, please visit: **www.cabi.org**

Browse our books or explore our online products at:
https://www.cabidigitallibrary.org

Interested in writing for CABI? Find our author guidelines here:
https://www.cabidigitallibrary.org/books/authors